Handbook of
Kidney
Transplantation

Fourth Edition

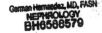

Handbook of Kidney Transplantation

Fourth Edition

Edited by

GABRIEL M. DANOVITCH, MD
Medical Director, Kidney Transplant Program,
UCLA Medical Center;
Professor, Department of Medicine,
David Geffen School of Medicine at UCLA,
Los Angeles, California

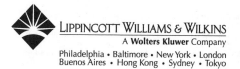

LIPPINCOTT WILLIAMS & WILKINS
A **Wolters Kluwer** Company

Philadelphia • Baltimore • New York • London
Buenos Aires • Hong Kong • Sydney • Tokyo

Acquisitions Editor: Lisa McAllister
Developmental Editor: Joanne Bersin
Production Superviser: Melanie Bennitt
Production Editor: Joanne Bowser
Manufacturing Manager: Ben Rivera
Cover Illustration: Patricia Gast
Compositor: TechBooks
Printer: R.R. Donnelley—Crawfordsville

Library of Congress Cataloging-in-Publication Data

Handbook of kidney transplantation / edited by Gabriel M. Danovitch.—
4th ed.
    p. ; cm.
    Includes bibliographical references and index.
    ISBN 0-7817-5322-8 (pbk.)
    1. Kidney—Transplantation—Handbooks, manuals, etc.
2. Transplantation of organs, tissues, etc.—Handbooks, manuals, etc.
I. Danovtich, Gabriel M.
    [DNLM: 1. Kidney Transplantation.   WJ 368 H236 2005]
RD575.H236   2005
617.4′610592—dc22

                                                2004010377

Care has been taken to confirm the accuracy of the information presented and to describe generally accepted practices. However, the authors, editor, and publisher are not responsible for errors or omissions or for any consequences from application of the information in this book and make no warranty, expressed or implied, with respect to the currency, completeness, or accuracy of the contents of the publication. Application of this information in a particular situation remains the professional responsibility of the practitioner.

The authors, editor, and publisher have exerted every effort to ensure that drug selection and dosage set forth in this text are in accordance with current recommendations and practice at the time of publication. However, in view of ongoing research, changes in government regulations, and the constant flow of information relating to drug therapy and drug reactions, the reader is urged to check the package insert for each drug for any change in indications and dosage and for added warnings and precautions. This is particularly important when the recommended agent is a new or infrequently employed drug.

Some drugs and medical devices presented in this publication have Food and Drug Administration (FDA) clearance for limited use in restricted research settings. It is the responsibility of the health care provider to ascertain the FDA status of each drug or device planned for use in their clinical practice.

                                      10 9 8 7 6 5 4 3 2 1

Cover: Schematic diagram of the structure of a representative class I MHC molecule (HLA-A2). The α_1 and α_2 domains form a peptide-binding site with the binding groove, which faces the T-cell receptor at the top (see Chaps. 2 and 3). (This remarkable structure is described in detail by PJ Bjorkman, MA saper, B Samraoni, et al. Structure of the human class I histocompatibility antigen, HLA-A2, *Nature* 1987;329:506. Reprinted with permission.)

In honor of my mother, Gertrude Danovitch, who remains, in her later years, a source of inspiration to three generations of loving progeny.

Contents

Contributing Authors

Samhar I. Al-Akash, M.D.   *Consultant Physician, Division of Pediatric Nephrology, King Faisal Specialist Hospital, Riyadh, Saudi Arabia*

William J. C. Amend, Jr., M.D.   *Attending Physician, Department of Medicine, University of California—Moffitt/Long; Professor of Clinical Medicine, Department of Medicine, Kidney Transplant Service, University of California at San Francisco, San Francisco, California*

Suphamai Bunnapradist, M.D.   *Director, Nephrology Fellowship Training Program; Medical Director, Kidney-Pancreas Transplant Program, Cedars-Sinai Medical Center; Assistant Professor, Department of Medicine, David Geffen School of Medicine at UCLA, Los Angeles, California*

J. Michael Cecka, Ph.D.   *Director of Clinical Research, UCLA Immunogenetics Center, UCLA Medical Center; Professor, Department of Pathology, David Geffen School of Medicine at UCLA, Los Angeles, California*

Arthur H. Cohen, M.D.   *Director, Anatomic Pathology, Department of Pathology, Cedars-Sinai Medical Center; Professor, Department of Pathology and Medicine, David Geffen School of Medicine at UCLA, Los Angeles, California*

Gabriel M. Danovitch, M.D.   *Medical Director, Kidney Transplant Program, UCLA Medical Center; Professor of Medicine, Department of Medicine, David Geffen School of Medicine at UCLA, Los Angeles, California*

Robert B. Ettenger, M.D.   *Professor, Department of Pediatrics, Head, Department of Pediatric Nephrology, and Vice Chairman, Clinical Affairs, David Geffen School of Medicine at UCLA, Los Angeles, California*

Fabrizio Fabrizi, M.D.   *Staff Nephrologist, Division of Nephrology and Dialysis, Maggiore Hospital, IRCCS, Milano, Italy*

Robert S. Gaston, M.D.   *Medical Director of Kidney and Pancreas Transplantation, University Hospital; Professor of Medicine and Surgery, School of Medicine, Division of Nephrology, University of Alabama at Birmingham, Birmingham, Alabama*

Marci H. Gitlin, M.S.W., L.C.S.W.   *Clinical Social Worker, UCLA Medical Center; Adjunct Professor, Department of Social Welfare, UCLA, Los Angeles, California*

William G. Goodman, M.D. *Associate Director, General Clinical Research Center, UCLA Medical Center; Professor, Department of Medicine, David Geffen School of Medicine at UCLA, Los Angeles, California*

H. Albin Gritsch, M.D. *Surgical Director, Department of Urology, Renal Transplant Program, UCLA Medical Center; Associate Professor, David Geffen School of Medicine at UCLA, Los Angeles, California*

Susan Weil Guichard, R.D., C.S.R. *Renal Dietitian, UCLA Kidney and Pancreas Transplant Program, UCLA DaVita Dialysis Center, UCLA Medical Center, Los Angeles, California*

Sundaram Hariharan, M.D. *Chief, Division of Nephrology, Department of Medicine, Froedtert Memorial Lutheran Hospital; Professor of Medicine, Division of Nephrology, Medical College of Wisconsin, Milwaukee, Wisconsin*

Andy Hwang, PHARM.D. *Research Associate, Department of Medicine, David Geffen School of Medicine at UCLA, Los Angeles, California*

Bertram L. Kasiske, M.D. *Director, Division of Nephrology, Hennepin County Medical Center; Professor, Department of Medicine, University of Minnesota, Minneapolis, Minnesota*

Elizabeth A. Kendrick, M.D. *Assistant Clinical Professor of Medicine, Division of Nephrology, David Geffen School of Medicine at UCLA, Los Angeles, California*

Bernard M. Kubak, M.D., Ph.D. *Associate Professor of Infectious Disease/Medicine, Division of Infectious Disease, David Geffen School of Medicine at UCLA, Los Angeles, California*

Didier A. Mandelbrot, M.D. *Staff Nephrologist, Department of Medicine, UMass Memorial Hospital; Associate Professor, Department of Medicine, University of Massachusetts, Worcester, Massachusetts*

Cynthia L. Maree, M.D. *Senior Clinical Fellow, Division of Infectious Diseases, David Geffen School of Medicine at UCLA, Los Angeles, California*

Paul Martin, M.D. *Clinical and Medical Director, Center for Liver and Kidney Disease and Transplantation, Cedars-Sinai Medical Center; Professor of Medicine, David Geffen School of Medicine at UCLA, Los Angeles, California*

Kirk J. Murphy, M.D. *Attending Psychiatrist, Department of Psychiatry, UCLA Medical Center; Assistant Clinical Professor, Department of Psychiatry, Neuropsychiatric Institute, David Geffen School of Medicine at UCLA, Los Angeles, California*

Cynthia C. Nast, M.D. *Attending Pathologist, Department of Pathology, Cedars-Sinai Medical Center; Professor of Pathology, Department of Pathology, David Geffen School of Medicine at UCLA, Los Angeles, California*

David A. Pegues, M.D. *Epidemiologist, Department of Infectious Diseases, UCLA Medical Center; Professor of Clinical Medicine, Division of Infectious Diseases, David Geffen School of Medicine at UCLA, Los Angeles, California*

John D. Pirsch, M.D. *Director of Medical Transplant Service, Department of Medicine and Surgery, University of Wisconsin Hospital and Clinic; Professor, Department of Medicine and Surgery, University of Wisconsin Medical School, Madison, Wisconsin*

Nagesh Ragavendra, M.D. *Chief, Ultrasound Section, UCLA Medical Center; Clinical Professor of Radiology, Department of Radiology, David Geffen School of Medicine at UCLA, Los Angeles, California*

Elaine F. Reed, Ph.D. *Director, UCLA Immunogenetics Center; Professor, Department of Pathology and Laboratory Medicine, David Geffen School of Medicine at UCLA, Los Angeles, California*

J. Thomas Rosenthal, M.D. *Professor, Department of Urology, David Geffen School of Medicine at UCLA, Los Angeles, California*

Meena Sahadevan, M.D. *Staff Nephrologist, Division of Nephrology, Hennepin County Medical Center; Assistant Professor, Department of Medicine, University of Minnesota, Minneapolis, Minnesota*

Mohamed H. Sayegh, M.D. *Research Director, Department of Immunogenetics and Transplantation, Brigham & Women's Hospital; Associate Professor, Department of Medicine, Harvard Medical School, Boston, Massachusetts*

Christiaan Schiepers, M.D. Ph.D. *Department of Nuclear Medicine, UCLA Medical Center; Professor, Department of Molecular and Medical Pharmacology, David Geffen School of Medicine at UCLA, Los Angeles, California*

Robyn S. Shapiro, J.D. *Partner and Chair, Health Law Group, Michael Best & Freidrich, L.L.P; Ursula von Der Ruhr Professor and Director, Center for the Study of Bioethics, Medical College of Wisconsin, Milwaukee, Wisconsin*

Nauman Siddqi, M.D. *Faculty Physician, Department of Medicine, Froedtert Memorial Lutheran Hospital; Assistant Professor of Medicine, Division of Nephrology, Medical College of Wisconsin, Milwaukee, Wisconsin*

Jennifer Singer, M.D.   *Assistant Professor, Department of Urology, David Geffen School of Medicine at UCLA, Los Angeles, California*

Craig Smith, M.D.   *Associate Professor, Department of Diabetes, Endocrinology, and Metabolism, City of Hope National Medical Center, Duarte, California; Associate Professor, Department of Surgery and Urology, David Geffen School of Medicine at UCLA, Los Angeles, California*

Hans W. Sollinger, M.D., Ph.D.   *Chairman, Division of Organ Transplantation, Department of Surgery, University of Wisconsin Hospital; Folkert O. Belzer Professor of Surgery, Chairman, Division of Organ Transplantation, Department of Surgery, University of Wisconsin Medical School, Madison, Wisconsin*

Stephen J. Tomlanovich, M.D.   *Medical Director, Kidney Transplant Service, Department of Medicine and Surgery, University of California at San Francisco Medical Center; Clinical Professor, Department of Medicine and Surgery, University of California at San Francisco, San Francisco, California*

Flavio Vincenti, M.D.   *Clinical Professor, Department of Medicine, University of California at San Francisco, San Francisco, California*

Peter Zimmerman, M.D.   *Associate Professor, Department of Radiology, David Geffen School of Medicine at UCLA, Los Angeles, California*

Preface

The publication of the fourth edition of the *Handbook of Kidney Transplantation* coincides with the fiftieth anniversary of two critical milestones in the history of modern medicine. The modern era of transplant immunology can be said to have begun with the description of actively acquired immunologic tolerance in rats by Peter Medawar and his colleagues at University College, London in 1953, while the modern era of clinical transplantation began on December 23, 1954, when Joseph Murray and his colleagues at Harvard performed the first kidney transplantation between identical twin brothers. Both these pioneers were rewarded with the Nobel Prize for their contributions.

In many ways, the promise of these momentous events has been fulfilled in the half century that has followed. The mere fact that organ transplantation is the subject of a handbook such as this reflects the extent to which it has become normative medical practice. Hundreds of thousands of lives have been saved and quality years have replaced years of suffering. Our understanding of the complex immunobiology of the immune response has advanced and has brought widespread benefits well beyond the field of organ transplantation. A broad armamentarium of immunosuppressive medications is now available, and innovative surgical techniques serve to expand the donor pool and minimize morbidity. National and international organ-sharing organizations are an accepted part of the medical landscape.

Modern organ transplantation can be visualized as a complex edifice that rests on a triangular base. In one corner is the basic research that is the life-blood of improvement and innovation. Nowhere in medicine is the term "translational medicine" more relevant or does research reach the bedside with greater speed. In another corner is clinical transplant medicine, a new medical subspecialty that requires compulsive, detail-oriented clinical care, and both organ-specific and broad expertise. In the third corner are the ethical underpinnings of the whole transplant endeavor, an endeavor that is utterly dependent on human altruism and love, and an absolute trust among medical staff, patients, and families that is the bedrock of societal acceptance of organ donation, from both the living and the deceased.

The edifice is strong, but its strength cannot be taken for granted. The immune system still has many secrets it has yet to reveal. As this text describes, the ultimate goal of donor-specific tolerance, either complete or near complete, appears closer than ever. Clinical xenotransplantation, however, a procedure that could provide the ultimate answer to the organ donor shortage, remains remote. The availability of new immunosuppressive agents has permitted the introduction of innovative immunosuppressive regimens designed to minimize toxicity. Yet the success of clinical transplantation—with low mortality, high graft survival, and a low incidence of rejection episodes—has, paradoxically, made it more difficult to prove the benefit of new approaches. Because the demand for organs greatly outstretches supply, patients with advanced kidney disease who do not have a living donor may be faced with an interminable, and often morbid, wait for an organ from a deceased donor. The need for living donors has, on the one hand, provided a stimulus to develop ingenious new techniques and approaches to facilitate donation, and on the other hand, has spawned an illegal global market in purchased organs.

The 4-year intervals between the publication of each of the editions of the *Handbook of Kidney Transplantation* are a reflection of the rate of change in the world of organ transplantation. This fourth edition has been thoroughly updated and revised to reflect the most current knowledge and practice in the field. Like its predecessors, its mission is to make the clinical practice of kidney transplantation fully accessible to all those who are entrusted with the care of our long-suffering patients.

Gabriel M. Danovitch

Handbook of Kidney Transplantation

Fourth Edition

Options for Patients with Kidney Failure

William G. Goodman and Gabriel M. Danovitch

Before 1970, therapeutic options for patients with kidney failure were quite limited. Only a small number of patients received regular dialysis because few dialysis facilities had been established. Patients underwent extensive medical screening to determine their eligibility for ongoing therapy, and treatment was offered only to patients who had renal failure as the predominant clinical management issue. Patients with other systemic illnesses apart from kidney failure were not considered for chronic dialysis therapy. Kidney transplantation was in the early stages of development as a viable therapeutic option. Transplant immunology and immunosuppressive therapy were in their infancy, and for most patients, a diagnosis of chronic renal failure was a death sentence.

In the decade that followed, the availability of care for patients with kidney failure grew rapidly throughout the medically developed world. In the United States, the passage of Medicare entitlement legislation, in 1972, to pay for maintenance dialysis and renal transplantation, provided the major stimulus for this expansion. This trend continues unabated, at least for hemodialysis.

Despite numerous medical and technical advances, patients with kidney failure who are treated with dialysis often remain unwell. Constitutional symptoms of fatigue and malaise persist despite better management of anemia with erythropoietin. Progressive cardiovascular disease (CVD), peripheral and autonomic neuropathy, bone disease, and sexual dysfunction are common, even in patients who are judged, using established, objective criteria, to be treated adequately with dialysis. Patients may become dependent on family members or others for physical, emotional, and financial assistance. Rehabilitation, particularly vocational rehabilitation, remains poor. Such findings are not unexpected, however, because the most efficient hemodialysis regimens currently provide only 10% to 12% of the small-solute removal of two normally functioning kidneys. Removal of higher-molecular-weight solutes is even less efficient.

For most patients with kidney failure, kidney transplantation has the greatest potential for restoring a healthy, productive life. Renal transplantation does not, however, occur in a clinical vacuum. Virtually all transplant recipients have been exposed, at least to some extent, to the adverse consequences of chronic kidney disease (CKD). Practitioners of kidney transplantation must consider the clinical impact of CKD on the overall health of renal transplantation candidates when this therapeutic option is first considered. They must also remain cognizant of the potential long-term consequences of previous and current CKD (see Chapter 6) during what may be decades of clinical follow-up after successful renal transplantation (see Chapter 9).

STAGES OF CHRONIC KIDNEY DISEASE

Table 1.1 summarizes the stages of CKD as defined by the National Kidney Foundation Disease Outcome Quality Initiative (K/DOQI). The purpose of this classification is to permit more accurate assessments of the frequency and severity of CKD in the general population, enabling more effective targeting of treatment recommendations. Note that the classification is based on estimated values for glomerular filtration rate (GFR) and that the terms kidney failure or end-stage renal disease (ESRD) are used for patients with values less than 15 mL per minute. It has been estimated that close to 20 million adults in the United States have CKD that can be categorized as stage 1, 2, 3, or 4, whereas approximately 300,000 have overt kidney failure, or stage 5 CKD. The known population of patients with ESRD thus represents only the "tip of the iceberg" of progressive CKD. It is also evident from Table 1.1 that most, if not all, kidney transplant recipients can be regarded as having some degree of CKD because their kidney function is rarely normal.

A discussion of the management of CKD in the general population is beyond the scope of this text. Strict blood pressure control and the use of angiotensin-converting enzyme inhibitors, both in diabetic patients and in those with proteinuria from other glomerular diseases, are standard practice. There is less certainty, however, about the benefits of these agents in patients without significant proteinuria. Low-protein diets may delay the onset of kidney failure or death in patients with established CKD, but there is insufficient evidence to recommend restricting dietary protein intake to less than 0.8 g/kg per day on a routine basis. Lipid-lowering agents and lifestyle changes, particularly smoking cessation, may slow disease progression. Many of the concerns and treatment recommendations that pertain to the long-term management of kidney transplant recipients, which are discussed in Chapter 9, also apply to patients with CKD.

Estimation of Glomerular Filtration Rate

Measurements of GFR provide an overall assessment of kidney function both in the transplant and nontransplant settings. The GFR is measured best by the clearance of an ideal filtration

Table 1.1. **Stages of chronic kidney disease (CKD)**

Stage	Description	GFR (mL/min/1.73m^2)
1	Kidney damage with normal or increased GFR	>90
2	Kidney damage with mild decrease in GFR	60–90
3	Moderate decrease in GFR	30–59
4	Severe decrease in GFR	15–29
5	Kidney failure	<15 or dialysis

GFR, glomerular filtration rate.

marker such as inulin or with radiolabelled filtration markers (see Chapter 12). In clinical practice, GFR is usually estimated from measurements of creatinine clearance or serum creatinine levels to circumvent the need for timed urine specimen collections. Several equations have been developed to estimate GFR after accounting for variations in age, sex, body weight, and race. The most popular and easiest to use among these is the Cockcroft-Gault formula

Creatinine clearance (mL/min)

$$= \frac{(140 - \text{age in years}) \times \text{weight in kg}}{72 \times \text{serum creatinine (mg/dL)}} \times 0.85 \text{ for females}$$

The MDRD (Modification of Diet in Renal Disease) equation uses a formula based on serum creatinine, age, gender, and race. It should be noted that neither equation has been formally validated in renal transplant recipients.

DEMOGRAPHICS OF THE END-STAGE RENAL DISEASE POPULATION

United States

Each year, the United States Renal Data System (USRDS) provides updated demographic information about patients with kidney disease who are treated either with dialysis or renal transplantation in the United States. The 2002 report is based on data updated through March 2002 that are complete only through December 2000. At that time, 275,000 patients were receiving maintenance dialysis in the United States (Table 1.2). This number continues to increase at an annual rate of approximately 5%. By the year 2010, it is expected to reach 520,000. The average age of the dialysis population also continues to increase each year. Nearly half of patients undergoing regular dialysis are older than 65 years of age, and the mean age of those beginning treatment is greater than 60 years. This phenomenon has been described as the "gerontologizing" of nephrology, and it accounts for the increasing age of patients being evaluated for, awaiting, and undergoing renal transplantation (see Chapters 3 and 6).

In the ESRD population, men slightly outnumber women, and 37% of patients are black. The prevalence of blacks in the ESRD population thus exceeds by threefold their percentage in the general population of the United States. Despite improvements in the clinical management of both diabetes mellitus and hypertension, these two diagnostic categories remain by far the most common causes of ESRD. In Hispanic and Native American patients, the burden of diabetes is particularly heavy, and for those who have survived for 1 year on dialysis, the incidence of diabetes is 74% and 82%, respectively.

Older patients and those with diabetes are more likely to be accepted for dialysis in the United States than in other countries. Moreover, patients now beginning dialysis in the United States have more comorbid medical conditions than those accepted for treatment in the 1980s. Congestive heart failure is present in 35% of the incident dialysis population, whereas coronary artery disease can be found in up to 40% of the incident dialysis population in some published reports.

Table 1.2. **Demographics of the dialysis population in the United States (point prevalence as of 2002)**

Demographic	Percentage
Age (yr)	
<20	<1
20–44	17
45–64	39
65–74	24
>75	20
Sex	
Male	53
Female	47
Race	
Black	37
White	55
Asian	4
Native American	2
Primary ESRD diagnosis	
Diabetic nephropathy	40
Hypertension	28
Glomerulonephritis	12
Cystic kidney disease	3
Other[a]	18

[a] Nearly 10% of patients with end-stage renal disease have a failed transplant.
From: United States Renal Data System. Excerpts from the 2002 Annual Data Report. *Am J Kidney Dis* 2003;41(Suppl 2), with permission.

In contrast to the steady rise in the number of patients receiving regular dialysis, the number of deceased donor kidney transplants performed each year has remained steady at approximately 9,000. The annual number of living donor transplants has increased, however, and it is now greater than the number of deceased donor transplants, largely due to an increase in the number of transplants from living donors who are not biologically related to the recipient (see Chapter 5). The number of patients receiving dialysis who are awaiting deceased donor renal transplantation is progressively rising, reaching more than 60,000 by early 2004. Fig. 1.1 graphically illustrates the gap between the supply of and the demand for deceased donor kidneys. Consequently, the average waiting time for a cadaveric renal transplant has increased substantially, and it is now measured in years (see Chapter 3).

Worldwide

The worldwide dialysis population is estimated to be greater than 1.1 million persons and is likely to reach 2,000,000 by 2010. Compared to Japan, Taiwan, and the United States, most countries have a lower incidence of treated ESRD (Fig. 1.2). This difference reflects, in part, the high incidence of ESRD in blacks in the United States. Other factors, such as limitations on the

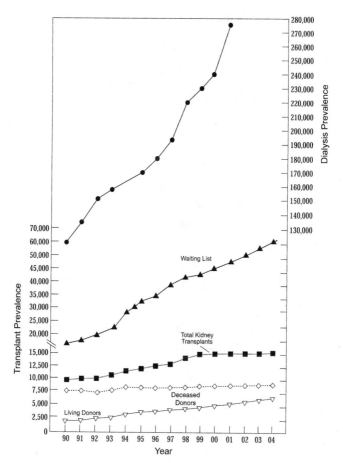

Fig. 1.1. Comparative numbers of patients receiving dialysis and awaiting and receiving transplants in the United States between 1990 and 2004. (From US Renal Data System 2003 and United Network for Organ Sharing, www.unos.org, accessed April 2004, with permission.)

availability of dialysis for elderly patients in some countries, also play a role. There is no age restriction for providing dialysis in the United States, and this largely explains the steady rise in the average age of the U.S. dialysis population.

Modalities for the management of ESRD vary among countries. For example, in the United Kingdom, Australia, and Canada, home dialysis is used extensively, whereas this therapeutic approach is uncommon in Japan. Age is an important factor for patient selection in many countries. Renal transplant rates from

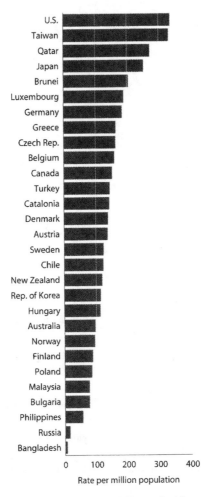

· **Incidence of ESRD**

Fig. 1.2.   Incidence of end-stage renal disease incidence rates per
1 million population for selected countries and for the United States
for 2000. [From US Renal Data System 2003 annual data report: Atlas
of end-stage renal disease in the United States. *Am J Kidney Dis*
2003;42(Suppl 5):176:Fig. 12.2, with permission.]

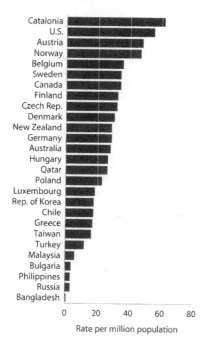

· Transplant rates

Fig. 1.3.   Renal transplants rates per 1 million total population
for selected countries as of 2000. [From US Renal Data System 2003
annual data report: Atlas of end-stage renal disease in the
United States. *Am J Kidney Dis* 2003;42(Suppl 5):179:Fig 12.10.]

both deceased and living donors vary considerably among industrialized countries (Fig. 1.3). Certain legal constraints and cultural barriers to the acceptance of brain-death criteria or living
donation (see Chapters 5 and 16) are important determinants of
national transplantation rates.

TREATMENT OPTIONS FOR END-STAGE RENAL DISEASE: DIALYSIS

Hemodialysis

Hemodialysis is the predominant technique for treating ESRD
throughout the world. In the United States, 87% of patients start
their ESRD care with hemodialysis. The procedure can be done
either in medical facilities specifically designed for this purpose or
in the patient's home. When performed in a dialysis facility, hemodialysis treatments typically range in length from 2.5 to 5 hours,
and they are usually done three times a week. For highly motivated patients with a suitable living environment and a willing

assistant, usually a spouse, hemodialysis can be done at home, freeing the patient from the need to visit a dialysis center and to adhere to a rigid treatment schedule.

During dialysis, solutes are removed by diffusion across a semipermeable membrane within a dialyzer, or artificial kidney, from blood circulated through an extracorporeal circuit. Fluid retained during the interval between treatments is removed by regulating the hydrostatic pressure across the membrane of the dialyzer. Most hemodialysis machines now control fluid removal, or ultrafiltration, using volumetric systems controlled by electronic microcircuits to ensure accurate and predictable results. Hemodialysis is generally well tolerated, although ultrafiltration can cause hypotension, nausea, and muscle cramps. Older patients and those with established CVD may tolerate the procedure less well. Vascular access failure from repeated cannulation procedures and the need for intermittent heparinization to prevent clotting in the extracorporeal blood circuit are additional concerns, particularly in diabetic patients. Over only a few hours, the intermittent nature of hemodialysis, which results in rapid changes in extracellular fluid volume, blood solute concentrations, and plasma osmolality, may contribute to fatigue and malaise after treatment.

Most dialysis membranes are cellulosic, and they provide reasonably efficient removal of low-molecular-weight solutes. Urea clearances of 180 to 240 mL per minute are readily achieved during hemodialysis. The efficiency of solute removal declines markedly, however, as molecular weight increases. Thus, the clearance of vitamin B_{12}, which has a molecular weight of about 1,350 daltons, rarely exceeds 40 to 60 mL per minute, a value far less than that provided by two normal kidneys.

Although the minute-by-minute removal of low-molecular-weight solutes during hemodialysis may exceed that provided by normal endogenous renal function, the intermittent nature of hemodialysis as employed in clinical practice substantially undermines the overall efficiency of this form of renal replacement therapy. Even for patients receiving 12 to 15 hours of hemodialysis per week, adequate solute clearance is provided for less than 10% of a 168-hour week. During the remaining 153 to 156 hours of each week, no additional solute removal is achieved unless there is some residual endogenous renal function. This residual function needs to be considered when recommending native kidney nephrectomy before transplantation (see Chapter 6).

Concerns regarding dialysis efficiency and adequacy have received considerable attention in the nephrology literature in recent years, particularly with respect to their impact on patient morbidity and mortality. Annual mortality rates in the United States are higher than in Europe, where the average weekly duration of hemodialysis is considerably longer. In addition, favorable outcomes in several small studies using alternative dialysis regimens, such as nightly, nocturnal hemodialysis or short-duration hemodialysis six times per week, serve to underscore the potential benefits of greater treatment duration and cumulative weekly solute removal on various clinical outcomes. The decline in annual mortality in the U.S. ESRD population in recent years corresponds temporally with educational efforts to raise clinician awareness about the need for more efficient weekly dialysis prescriptions and with the more widespread use of objective measures of dialysis efficiency to monitor ongoing therapy. The K/DOQI guidelines published and updated by the National Kidney Foundation are an invaluable resource for the management of patients with CKD.

The hemodialysis procedure requires access to the patient's circulation to provide continuous blood flow to the extracorporeal dialysis circuit. For ongoing hemodialysis therapy, an autologous arteriovenous (A-V) fistula is the most reliable type of vascular access and the one whose use is associated with the best prognosis. Long-term patency is greatest with A-V fistulas, and the incidence rates of thrombosis and infection are low. A-V grafts that use synthetic materials are often placed in elderly patients and in diabetic patients whose native blood vessels may be inadequate for the creation of a functional A-V fistula. Complication rates are considerably higher, however, with grafts than with fistulas. Thrombosis is a recurrent problem, and it frequently occurs because of stenosis at the venous end of the graft, where it forms an anastomosis with the native vein. Infections and the formation of pseudoaneurysms are more common with grafts than with fistulas.

Temporary venous dialysis catheters are used to establish vascular access when hemodialysis must be started urgently. Other venous catheters, designed to be used over longer intervals, have been increasingly used as a method for providing vascular access in patients undergoing regular hemodialysis, particularly when treatment is first begun or when permanent access sites require surgical revision. Reliance on these approaches should be limited, however, and permanent access should be established using A-V fistulas or A-V grafts as soon as ESRD is deemed to be inevitable. Stenotic lesions in large proximal veins in the thorax are an increasingly recognized complication of indwelling venous dialysis access catheters. These may involve the subclavian and innominate veins and the superior vena cava. Their presence can interfere with successful placement of permanent vascular access by producing venous hypertension that interferes with venous blood return from A-V fistulas or grafts. The sustained use of venous dialysis access catheters should be avoided. Early referral of patients with CKD to nephrologic care and elective placement of dialysis access, preferably in the form of an arterial autologous fistula, reduces morbidity. This become particularly important for patients who do not have a living kidney donor and who thus are likely to experience a prolonged wait on the deceased donor transplant waiting list (see Chapter 6).

Peritoneal Dialysis

Peritoneal dialysis is an alternative to hemodialysis that exploits the fluid and solute transport characteristics of the peritoneum as an endogenous dialysis membrane. In the United States, 11% of patients start dialysis with this technique, but the percentage is falling. In Australia and New Zealand, peritoneal dialysis is more popular and accounts for more than 40% of prevalent dialysis patients. Peritoneal dialysis can be done either as *continuous ambulatory peritoneal dialysis* (CAPD) or as *continuous cycling peritoneal dialysis* (CCPD). Access to the peritoneal cavity is achieved by surgically placing a Silastic catheter (often called a Tenckhoff catheter) of varying design through the abdominal wall. Surgery is done several weeks before starting treatment, and patients are trained subsequently to perform their own dialysis procedures.

Peritoneal dialysis is accomplished by instilling a specified volume of peritoneal dialysis fluid, typically between 1,500 and 3,000 mL, into the abdominal cavity by gravity-induced flow, allowing the fluid to remain in the abdomen for a defined period, and then draining and discarding it. During each dwell period, both solute removal and ultrafiltration are achieved. Solute removal occurs by diffusion down a concentration gradient from the extracellular fluid into peritoneal dialysate, with the peritoneal membrane acting as a functional semipermeable dialysis membrane. The efficiency of removal of small solutes is relatively low compared with hemodialysis, whereas the clearance of higher-molecular-weight solutes is somewhat better. Ultrafiltration is accomplished by osmotic water movement from the extracellular fluid compartment into hypertonic peritoneal dialysate that contains a high concentration of dextrose, ranging from 1.50 to 4.25 gram percent. The lower rates of solute removal that characterize peritoneal dialysis are offset by prolonged treatment times.

For CCPD, an automated cycling device is used to regulate and monitor the dialysate flow into and out of the abdominal cavity. Four to ten dialysis exchanges, ranging from 1 to 3 L each, are done nightly over 8 to 10 hours. A variable amount of dialysate is left in the abdomen during the day to provide additional solute and fluid removal. For CAPD, dialysis is done 24 hours a day, 7 days a week, using manual exchanges of peritoneal dialysate four or five times per day.

Peritoneal dialysis has certain advantages over hemodialysis, including the maintenance of relatively constant blood or serum levels of urea nitrogen, creatinine, sodium, and potassium. Hematocrit levels are often higher than for patients receiving hemodialysis, and gradual and continuous ultrafiltration may provide better blood pressure control. Because it is a form of self-care, peritoneal dialysis promotes patient independence.

The major complication of peritoneal dialysis is bacterial peritonitis. Its frequency varies considerably among patients and among treatment facilities, but it occurs with an average frequency of one episode per patient per year. When bacterial peritonitis is diagnosed promptly and treatment is begun immediately, infections are generally not severe and resolve within a few days with appropriate antibiotic therapy. Episodes of peritonitis are an ongoing threat, however, to the long-term success of peritoneal dialysis, and they can lead to scarring of the peritoneal cavity and to the loss of the peritoneum as an effective dialysis membrane. In the past, gram-positive organisms, such as *Staphylococcus epidermidis* or *S. aureus,* accounted for most cases of peritonitis, but almost half of episodes are now caused by gram-negative bacteria. Fungal peritonitis typically causes extensive intraabdominal scarring and fibrosis, and it often leads to the failure of peritoneal dialysis as an effective mode of treatment.

Table 1.3.   Comparison of hemodialysis and peritoneal dialysis

Advantages	Disadvantages
Hemodialysis	
Short treatment time	Need for heparin
Highly efficient for small solute removal	Need for vascular access
	Hypotension with fluid removal
Socialization occurs in the dialysis center	Poor blood pressure control
	Need to follow diet and treatment schedule
Peritoneal dialysis	
Steady-state chemistries	Peritonitis
Higher hematocrit	Obesity
Better blood pressure control	Hypertriglyceridemia
Dialysate source of nutrition	Malnutrition
Intraperitoneal insulin administration	Hernia formation
Self-care form of therapy	Back pain
Highly efficient for large solute removal	
Liberalization of diet	

With few exceptions, hemodialysis has no medical advantage over peritoneal dialysis. Both effectively manage the consequence of uremia (Table 1.3). Matters of individual lifestyle and other psychosocial issues should be considered when selecting a particular mode of dialysis. Home hemodialysis provides an opportunity for independence and rehabilitation, but it can be a cause of substantial emotional stress for the dialysis assistant and other family members. In some home settings, neither hemodialysis nor peritoneal dialysis is advisable. In-center hemodialysis can provide ongoing social interaction for older, single patients who have few friends or family members available to provide support.

Technical Advances in Dialysis

Numerous technical and procedural advances have significantly improved the quality of life for patients who require renal replacement therapy by dialysis.

Hemodialysis

The development of synthetic dialysis membranes with higher hydraulic conductance and increased permeability for higher-molecular-weight solutes has made it possible to increase the overall efficiency of hemodialysis. Many of the newer hemodialysis membranes are considered to be biologically more compatible than previously used materials. Cytokine release and complement activation during dialysis are less, and these differences may have long-term benefits. The use of advanced microcircuits and automated controls in modern dialysis equipment permits precise control of the rate of fluid removal, and the capacity to vary dialysate sodium concentrations can improve tolerance of the dialysis procedure in some patients. With better mass transport characteristics, some dialyzers can achieve equivalent amounts of solute removal with shorter treatment times than older, less-efficient models.

The use of high-efficiency hemodialysis has grown in popularity, particularly among patients for whom the shortened treatment time is appealing. The long-term consequences of this approach are not known, however, and there are concerns that manifestations of uremia or inadequate dialysis may develop after months or years. Indeed, guidelines for implementing and monitoring dialysis prescriptions in the United States have increasingly recognized the critical role of cumulative weekly procedure length as a key element for maintaining hemodialysis adequacy. The amount of dialysis achieved can be measured objectively by the term Kt/V, where K represents the rate of urea clearance by the dialyzer; t represents the duration, in minutes, of the treatment session; and V represents the volume of distribution for urea. The current K/DOQI guideline recommends a Kt/V of at least 1.2.

As noted previously, longer dialysis sessions and more frequent treatments have been reported to provide better blood pressure, extracellular volume, and metabolic control in patients with kidney failure. *Such findings suggest that more dialysis is better than less dialysis.* More dialysis reduces the substantial disparity between the amount of solute removal provided by the standard thrice-weekly hemodialysis schedule and that achieved by normal endogenous renal function. The impact of alternative dialysis regimens on long-term clinical outcomes, on morbidity, and on mortality are not yet known.

Peritoneal Dialysis

Efforts continue to lower the risk for bacterial contamination and peritonitis in patients undergoing peritoneal dialysis. The devices that establish the connections among peritoneal dialysis catheters, fluid transfer sets, and plastic bags containing peritoneal dialysate are continually being refined for both CAPD and CCPD.

Long-Term Complications of Dialysis

As survival for patients on regular dialysis improves, a number of debilitating complications of either long-term renal failure or protracted dialysis may develop, even in well-rehabilitated and medically adherent patients. As the waiting time for deceased donor renal transplants inexorably increases (see Chapter 3 and Fig. 1.1), these complications are more likely to manifest clinically. Their presence may affect the medical indications for transplantation, and they may influence the choice of renal transplantation as a therapeutic option (see Chapter 6). The longer patients receive dialysis, the greater the risk for posttransplant morbidity, mortality, and graft loss (see Chapter 6 and Fig 1.4). The following discussion concentrates on those long-term complications that are most relevant to the posttransplant course.

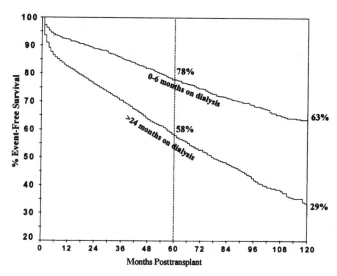

Fig. 1.4. Unadjusted graft survival in 2,405 recipients of paired kidneys with short compared to long ESRD time. (From Meier-Kriesche HU, Kaplan B. Waiting time on dialysis as the strongest modifiable risk factor for renal transplant outcomes: a paired donor kidney analysis. *Transplantation* 2002;74:1377, with permission.)

Cardiovascular Disease

The incidence of CVD in the CKD population has been described as reaching epidemic proportions. Even in the early stages of CKD, factors that contribute to the excess risk for CVD can be identified. Nearly all patients at some time during their clinical course develop hypertension, and many require multiple antihypertensive medications. The incidence of hypertension and diabetes as primary causes of CKD is increasing more rapidly than that of other diagnoses. Proteinuria and the associated hyperlipidemia, increases in extracellular fluid volume, anemia, high plasma levels of thrombogenic factors, and homocysteine all represent additional cardiovascular risk factors. Uremia per se may contribute to atherogenesis and to the development of cardiomyopathy, although there is some disagreement on this issue.

Patients with kidney disease have a greater risk for developing left ventricular hypertrophy (LVH) than those in the general population, even in the early stages of CKD. The prevalence of LVH varies directly with the degree of renal dysfunction. At the time that regular dialysis is begun, 50% to 80% of patients have LVH, and the prevalence of coronary artery disease may reach 40%.

Patients receiving regular dialysis have an adjusted death rate from all causes that is estimated to be 3.5 times higher than that in the general population, and the overall first-year mortality rate of hemodialysis patients in the United States is 21.7%. CVD accounts for 50% of this mortality, occurring at a rate of 9% per year, which is 10 to 20 times greater than in the general population. Hypertensive patients have worse outcomes after dialysis, and patients with LVH have a two- to threefold higher death rate from cardiac causes. Progressive calcification of the coronary arteries occurs over the years spent on dialysis and can be recognized even in young adult dialysis patients. Soft-tissue calcification may also affect heart valves and the pelvic and peripheral vasculature.

Vascular calcification is recognized increasingly as a complication of long-term dialysis, and it may be caused by, at least in part, the replacement of aluminum-based medications with calcium salts as phosphate-binding agents. Mortality rates after myocardial infarction in dialysis patients are substantially higher than in the general population, a finding that probably reflects the severity of underlying CVD. The passage of time in patients receiving regular dialysis reflects ongoing exposure to multiple cardiovascular risk factors, and worsening myocardial function has been described, particularly during the first year of treatment. These observations may explain the consistent finding that posttransplant prognosis worsens the longer patients are treated with dialysis before a renal transplant (Fig. 1.4).

Anemia

The routine administration of recombinant erythropoietin (epoetin alfa) to treat the anemia of CKD and ESRD has had an enormously beneficial impact on morbidity. Fatigue, depression, cognitive impairment, sexual dysfunction, and LVH all improve with adequate treatment of anemia. The degree to which anemia is corrected is, to a large extent, determined in the United States by Medicare reimbursement policies that govern the target level of hemoglobin. The K/DOQI target is currently 11 to 12 g/dL. Successful treatment of anemia in dialysis patients is closely linked to replenishment of iron stores. Darbepoetin alfa (Aranesp) is a protein that stimulates erythropoiesis and is closely related to erythropoietin. Because its terminal half-life is approximately threefold longer than that of epoetin alfa, darbepoetin alfa can be administered less frequently.

Renal Osteodystrophy

Secondary hyperparathyroidism and high-turnover bone disease often develop in patients with ESRD. Several factors contribute to excess parathyroid hormone (PTH) secretion in patients with renal failure. These factors include hypocalcemia, diminished renal calcitriol production, skeletal resistance to the calcemic actions of PTH, alterations in the regulation of pre-pro-PTH gene transcription, reduced expression of receptors for vitamin D and calcium in the parathyroid glands, and hyperphosphatemia caused by diminished renal phosphorus excretion. Progressive parathyroid gland hyperplasia occurs often. Severely affected patients experience bone pain, skeletal fracture, and substantial disability. Hypercalcemia and soft-tissue and vascular calcifications may develop. Treatment with one of several vitamin D sterols may lower plasma PTH levels and restore bone formation and bone-remodeling rates toward normal. Episodes of hypercalcemia and hyperphosphatemia occur frequently, however, during vitamin D therapy. Newer therapeutic agents, such as calcimimetic compounds, may offer an alternative for controlling excess PTH secretion in patients undergoing dialysis without aggravating disturbances in calcium and phosphorus metabolism.

Low-turnover lesions of renal osteodystrophy include osteomalacia and adynamic bone. In the past, osteomalacia was found in patients with tissue aluminum accumulation, but aluminum-related bone disease is now uncommon. Most ESRD patients with osteomalacia have evidence of vitamin D deficiency, mineral deficiency, or both.

The adynamic lesion of renal osteodystrophy occurs in patients with normal or only modestly elevated serum PTH levels. It can also be a manifestation of aluminum toxicity, and affected patients have severe bone pain, muscle weakness, and fractures. When aluminum is not the cause, patients with adynamic lesions have few symptoms, but episodes of hypercalcemia occur more often than in patients with high-turnover skeletal lesions. Adults with adynamic bone may be at increased risk for vertebral fracture. Adynamic renal osteodystrophy is more common in patients undergoing peritoneal dialysis than in those treated with hemodialysis, and it can develop after the treatment of secondary hyperparathyroidism with large intermittent doses of calcitriol, or 1,25-dihydroxyvitamin D. The impact of transplantation on uremic bone disease is discussed in Chapter 9.

Uremic Neuropathy

Peripheral neuropathy is a feature of chronic renal failure, and encephalopathy will develop if appropriate renal replacement therapy is not begun. A mild stable sensory neuropathy is common even in nondiabetic dialysis patients; it is usually largely sensory and detected clinically by impaired vibration and position sense. It may be a source of pain and "restless legs." Occasionally, a devastating polyneuropathy develops is be reminiscent of Guillain-Barré syndrome. Neuropathy can recover dramatically after successful transplantation. It may also improve substantially after intensification of dialysis treatment.

Severe encephalopathy is rare in patients who receive effective amounts of dialysis. Impairments in the ability to concentrate and minor memory loss represent more subtle manifestations of cognitive impairment in dialysis patients, and improvement after transplantation is gratifying. Autonomic neuropathy in nondiabetic patients receiving dialysis can be recognized by impaired heart rate variability, and it may account for wise variations in blood pressure during dialysis procedures. Autonomic dysfunction is also reversible after renal transplantation.

Neuropathy contributes to sexual dysfunction in many dialysis patients. About half of men suffer from erectile dysfunction; menstrual disturbances and infertility are common in women. Improvement after transplantation is variable and is discussed in Chapter 9.

Amyloidosis

Patients undergoing long-term dialysis may develop a unique form of amyloidosis in which the amyloid deposits are composed of β_2-microglobulin, a protein that is present normally on the surface of all cells. β_2-Microglobulin is released into the circulation, freely filtered at the glomerulus, and subsequently degraded by cells of the proximal tubule. In renal failure, β_2-microglobulin accumulates in the plasma, and it eventually forms amyloid deposits in various tissues.

Tendons and articular cartilage are the most common sites of β_2-microglobulin deposition, and the amyloid deposits at the wrist may cause carpal tunnel syndrome. Cystic lesions at the proximal ends of long bones are frequently seen. Patients have typically been treated with dialysis for at least 5 years, and amyloid deposits can be documented in most patients after 8 years. Severe disease with joint deformity can lead to marked disability, and the clinical course is progressive. Renal transplantation may result in symptomatic improvement, but there is little evidence that amyloid deposits disappear after successful transplantation.

Interactions between blood constituents and hemodialysis membranes, particularly cellulosic membranes, are thought to promote the development of dialysis-related amyloidosis by stimulating β_2-microglobulin production. Amyloid deposition can occur, however, in patients receiving peritoneal dialysis. Blood–membrane contact may thus not be essential for its development. Disease prevalence has been reported to be lower with improved water purification methods during dialysate production, with certain high-permeability dialysis membranes, and with bicarbonate-containing dialysate. Only symptomatic relief is available for patients with dialysis-related amyloidosis.

Acquired Cystic Disease and Cancer of the Kidney and Urinary Tract

Patients on all forms of maintenance dialysis are at increased risk for cancer, especially of the kidney and urinary tract. The risk increases with time. Kidney cancer rates are elevated nearly fourfold. The pattern of risk is consistent with causation through acquired cystic disease. Urothelial cancer risk is increased by approximately 50%, presumably as a result of the carcinogenic effects of certain primary renal diseases.

Patients with CKD of any cause can develop acquired cystic disease involving the kidneys after several years of treatment by dialysis. The condition is characterized by multiple, usually bilateral, renal cysts in small, contracted kidneys and is, therefore, easily distinguishable from adult polycystic kidney disease. Cysts may become infected, bleed, or cause localized pain, and they can undergo malignant transformation. "Suspicious" cysts should be imaged at regular intervals, and concern about malignant transformation may be an indication for pretransplant nephrectomy. The capacity for malignant transformation should not be forgotten in the posttransplant period.

Dialysis Access Failure

Early referral before the initiation of regular hemodialysis is required is essential for establishing optimal long-term vascular access. For patients managed with hemodialysis, reliable vascular access is a life-sustaining aspect of medical care. Vascular access failure not only threatens the near-term well-being of patients, but has long-term implications with regard to the success of ongoing renal replacement therapy. Access-related morbidity accounts for almost 25% of all hospital stays for ESRD patients and for close to 20% of the cost of ESRD care.

As discussed previously, A-V fistulas are the gold standard for long-term vascular access for hemodialysis. A-V grafts almost invariably undergo thrombosis; their 3-year cumulative patency rate has been estimated to be approximately 50%. Because the number of sites that can be used for permanent vascular access placement is limited, the choice of A-V grafts for long-term vascular access conveys the risk of ultimately losing all remaining vascular access sites, rendering further hemodialysis technically impossible.

TREATMENT OPTIONS FOR ESRD: TRANSPLANTATION

The relative prevalence of the major ESRD treatment options between 1987 and 2004 in the United States is shown in Fig. 1.1. Deceased donor transplantation accounts for half of all kidney transplants in the United States, the remainder being from living donors. A critical shortage of donor organs is the major limitation to expanding the use of this therapeutic modality. The rate of renal transplantation varies considerably among patient groups. Transplantation rates are lower in older patients, who represent a relatively high-risk group (see Chapter 6). Transplantation rates tend to be lower in black ESRD patients, partly for reasons that constrain access to deceased donor organs (see Chapter 3). A tendency to restrict access to transplantation based on race, gender, insurance status, and type of dialysis center has also been described.

Patient and graft survival rates in the United States are shown graphically in Chapter 3 (see Figs. 3.4 and 3.5). Mean 1-year graft survival for all types of living donor transplants is approximately 95%. In many centers, it is 90% or greater for all match grades of deceased donor transplants.

Patient Survival

Difficulties with Data Analysis

To help select the most appropriate therapeutic option for patients with advanced CKD, clinicians and patients are understandably interested in comparative survival rates among various treatment modalities. Such comparisons are difficult, however, because data in the literature often do not reflect the fact that patients change treatment modalities frequently and that the characteristics of patients selected for each modality may differ substantially when therapy is begun. For dialysis patients, a number of comorbid factors can adversely affect survival; these include increased age, diabetes, coronary artery disease, chronic obstructive pulmonary disease, and cancer. Overall, blacks have a better survival rate on dialysis than do nonblacks, whereas certain renal diagnoses, such as amyloidosis, multiple myeloma, and renal cell cancer, are associated with poorer prognoses. Nutritional status, as measured by serum albumin and prealbumin levels, has been increasingly recognized as an important predictor of survival during long-term dialysis (see Chapter 18). If these factors are not considered, accurate comparisons among therapeutic modalities cannot be made.

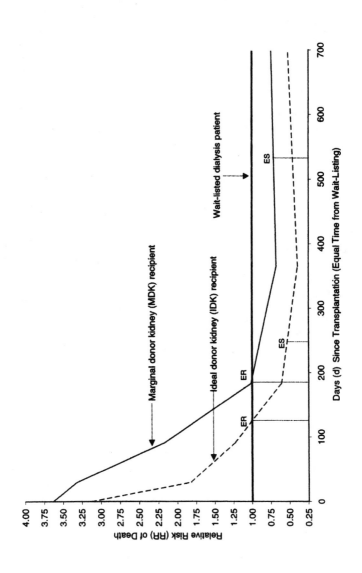

Comparison of Treatment Modalities

Most of the data comparing survival rates for patients treated with hemodialysis, CAPD, and deceased donor kidney transplantation suggest that an individual's state of health before treatment, rather than the treatment modality itself, is the most important factor in determining survival. Healthier dialysis patients are more likely to be placed on the waiting list for transplantation. The annual mortality rate for dialysis patients awaiting a transplant is approximately 6%, a value that is several-fold lower than the overall mortality rate among all patients treated with dialysis. Wait-listed dialysis patients enjoy a further reduction in the relative risk for death if they subsequently receive a transplant rather than continue to receive dialysis. This phenomenon is illustrated graphically in Fig. 1.5, which records the relative risk for death for dialysis patients who were placed on a deceased donor transplant waiting list. The long-term survival rates were better for transplant recipients who received either an "ideal" or "marginal" donor kidney (see Chapter 5). This survival benefit was detected within the first posttransplant year despite the higher mortality rates associated with the surgical procedure and with immunosuppressive therapy. The magnitude of the survival benefit varies according to the quality of the transplanted kidney and the patient characteristics at the time of placement on the waiting list (Fig. 1.6). It is most marked for young diabetic patients.

Cost of Therapy

The annual cost of medical care for patients undergoing chronic hemodialysis in the United States is about $50,000. Medical costs during the first year after renal transplantation are considerably higher and are estimated to be nearly $100,000. The cost of care is less, however, after the first posttransplant year when compared with the cost of dialysis, despite the approximately $10,000 annual cost of immunosuppressive therapy (see Chapter 19). The mean cumulative costs of dialysis and transplantation are about the same for the first 4 years of therapy. Thereafter, overall costs are lower after successful renal transplantation.

Survival by Diagnosis

When the most common causes of kidney disease are assessed by the Cox proportional hazards model, only diabetes mellitus has an adverse effect on patient survival. Other common causes of

Fig. 1.5. Survival benefit of transplantation versus remaining on the waiting list for recipients of "ideal" (*interrupted line*) and "marginal" (*solid line*) kidneys (see Chapter 5). Note that in the early period after a transplant the risk of death is higher for transplant recipients than for wait-listed patients. Within a short period, somewhat longer for recipients of marginal kidneys, the risk of death (*ER*) and chances of survival (*ES*) equalize. Thereafter, transplantation has a persistent survival benefit. (From Ojo AO, Hanson JA, Meier-Kriesche H, et al. Survival in recipients of marginal cadaveric donor kidneys compared with other recipients and wait-listed transplant candidates. *J Am Soc Nephrol* 2001;12:589, with permission.)

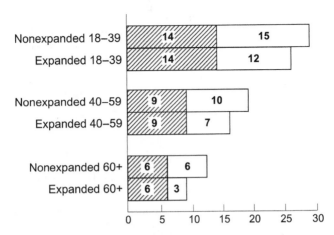

Fig. 1.6.   Projected Lifetime on wait-list (hatched bars) and extra lifetime after deceased donor kidney transplant (open bars) by age and quality of kidney, 1995–2001. The term "expanded" is discussed in Chapter 5. (From Scientific Registry of Transplant Recipients, 2002)

renal failure do not significantly affect survival. The survival rate of patients with ESRD caused by other less-common renal diseases, such as collagen vascular disease and vasculitis, is generally similar to that of nondiabetic patients with common causes of ESRD. Not surprisingly, systemic and renal malignancies confer a poorer prognosis.

Quality of Life

Most studies demonstrate that the quality of life of patients receiving peritoneal dialysis exceeds that of patients receiving hemodialysis in a dialysis center. Home hemodialysis patients reportedly have a high quality of life, although selection factors, such as the level of patient motivation and the patient's overall health status at the beginning of treatment, make it difficult to attribute this higher quality of life to the modality alone.

Most dialysis patients select renal transplantation with the hope of improving their quality of life, and recipients of successful transplants consistently report a better quality of life than do patients undergoing either peritoneal dialysis or home hemodialysis. Life satisfaction, physical and emotional well-being, and the ability to return to work are all significantly better in transplant recipients than in dialysis patients. Transplantation often corrects or improves some complications of uremia that are typically not reversed fully by dialysis; these include anemia, peripheral neuropathy, autonomic neuropathy, and sexual dysfunction (see Chapter 9). The quality of life for recipients of living donor transplants compares favorably to that seen in the general population.

INITIATION OF END-STAGE RENAL DISEASE THERAPY

An in-depth discussion of the indications for starting renal replacement therapy is beyond the scope of this text. Most patients with progressive renal failure develop symptoms of kidney failure and will require treatment for ESRD when the GFR falls to below 15 mL per minute or the serum creatinine level increases to more than 10 mg/dL. Many patients, particularly those with diabetes, develop symptoms at lower serum creatinine levels and at higher GFR values. Hemodialysis or peritoneal dialysis access should be arranged sufficiently far in advance so that treatment can be started when needed, rather than on an urgent or emergency basis. Patients can then be spared the suffering and risk that are inevitably associated with advanced CKD. Because permanent vascular access for hemodialysis requires 4 to 8 weeks to mature, placement should be undertaken early so that the use of temporary venous catheters for dialysis access can be avoided. For peritoneal dialysis, peritoneal catheter placement can be delayed until dialysis is more imminent because only 2 to 4 weeks is required before the access can be used.

K/DOQI guidelines recommend that dialysis be initiated when the weekly Kt/V falls below 2.0 which corresponds to a GFR of less than 10.5 mL per minute per 1.73 m^2. The decision to start dialysis is a clinical one, however, and it should be based on the plasma levels of creatinine, urea nitrogen, and selected electrolytes, as well as on a careful assessment of uremic symptoms. Outcomes after dialysis are better for patients who start early rather than late and who start electively rather than emergently.

Predialysis or preemptive transplantation is discussed in Chapter 6. It is the preferred therapeutic modality for ESRD in terms of morbidity, mortality, and long-term graft survival, but only 2% of ESRD patients receive preemptive transplantation. The current allocation algorithm (see Chapter 3) allows patients who have not yet started dialysis to accrue waiting-time points when their GFR is 20 mL per minute or less. The very long waiting time for deceased donor organs makes it unlikely, however, that a predialysis patient without a living donor will be allocated a kidney. Predialysis patients who are placed on the deceased donor transplant waiting list and those prepared for living donor transplantation should be warned explicitly not to delay establishing access for dialysis should it become necessary before a donor organ is available. Such an approach avoids the need for an unduly hurried pretransplantation preparation that can be dangerous and emotionally stressful both for patients and caregivers.

SELECTED READINGS

Bolton WK. Renal Physician Association clinical practice guideline: appropriate patient preparation for renal replacement therapy: guideline number 3. *J Am Soc Nephrol* 2003;14:1406–1410.

Davis MR, Hruska KA. Pathophysiological mechanisms of vascular calcification in end-stage renal disease. *Kidney Int* 2001;60:472–479.

Dhingra RK, Young EW, Hulbert-Shearon TE, et al. Type of vascular access and mortality in US hemodialysis patients. *Kidney Int* 2002;61:1443–1451.

Ganesh SK, Hulbert-Shearon, Port FK, et al. Mortality differences by dialysis modality among incident ESRD patients with and without coronary artery disease. *J Am Soc Nephrol* 2003;14:415–424.

Goodman WG, Goldin J, Kuizon BD, et al. Coronary-artery calcifications in young adults with end-stage renal disease who are undergoing dialysis. *N Engl J Med* 2000;342:1478–1483.

Hariharan S, Johnson CP, Bresnahan BA. Improved graft survival after renal transplantation in the United States, 1988 to 1996. *N Engl J Med* 2000;342:605–612.

Himmelfarb J. Success and challenge in dialysis therapy. *N Engl J Med* 2002;347:2068–2070.

Levey AS. Clinical practice. Nondiabetic kidney disease. *N Engl J Med* 2002;347:1505–1511.

Luke RG, Beck LH. Gerontologizing nephrology. *J Am Soc Nephrol* 1999;10:1824–1827.

Lysaght M. Maintenance dialysis population dynamics: current trends and long-term implications. *J Am Soc Nephrol* 2002;13:S37–S40.

Parfrey PS, Foley RN. The clinical epidemiology of cardiac disease in chronic renal failure. *J Am Soc Nephrol* 1999;10:1606–1615.

Pereira BJ. Optimization of pre-ESRD care: the key to improved dialysis outcomes. *Kidney Int* 2000;57:351–365.

Schwab SJ. Vascular access for hemodialysis. *Kidney Int* 1999;55:2078–2083.

Stewart JH, Buccianti G, Agadoa L, et al. Cancers of the kidney and urinary tract in patients on dialysis for end-stage renal disease: analysis of data from the United States, Europe, and Australia and New Zealand. *J Am Soc Nephrol* 2003;14:197–207.

US Renal Data System. Excerpts from the USRDS 2003 annual data report: atlas of end-stage renal disease in the United States. *Am J Kidney Dis* 2003;42[Suppl 5]:4–224.

Xue JL, Ma JZ, Louis TA, et al. Forecast of the number of patients with end-stage renal disease in the United States to the year 2010. *J Am Soc Nephrol* 2001;12:2753–2758.

Transplantation Immunobiology

Didier A. Mandelbrot and Mohamed H. Sayegh

The immune response to a transplanted graft can be divided into three phases: recognition of foreign antigens, activation of antigen-specific lymphocytes, and the effector phase of graft rejection. If the transplant is between genetically different individuals of the same species, it is referred to as an *allogeneic* graft, or allograft. This allograft stimulates an immune response (alloresponse), which is mediated by alloreactive lymphocytes. This chapter focuses on the immune response to allografts. However, grafts can also be *autologous* (from an individual back into that same individual), *syngeneic* (between genetically identical individuals), or *xenogeneic* (between individuals of different species).

The principal function of the immune system is to defend against infections. Fundamental to this function is the capacity of the immune system to discriminate between self and non-self antigens. The system is highly evolved in its ability to defend against various microbial infections, and normally does not react against self—the tissues of the host. The immune response to allografts is one example of a response to non-self antigens. Because transplantation is an unlikely event in the life of any organism, it has long been surprising that the immune system retains such a powerful ability to recognize and reject transplanted allografts. The explanation can now be provided in considerable detail.

THE RECOGNITION OF ALLOGRAFTS

Genetics of Allograft Rejection

Studies of the acceptance and rejection of tissue grafts exchanged between inbred mice established the following four basic principles that govern graft rejection:

1. Grafts exchanged between members of one inbred strain (syngeneic grafts) will survive.
2. Grafts between animals of different inbred strains (allografts) will be rejected.
3. Grafts from a parent to an F1 offspring of two different strains will survive (because the F1 offspring recognizes the graft from the homozygous parent as "self").
4. Grafts from an F1 offspring to a parent will be rejected (because the parent recognizes the graft from the heterozygous F1 as "non-self").

These results led to the realization that graft rejection was controlled by genes whose inheritance followed simple mendelian rules. The genes that determine the rejection or acceptance of tissue grafts are present in a locus on chromosome number 6 that was named the major histocompatibility complex (MHC) (Fig. 2.1A). the gene products are MHC antigens or molecules. In humans, syngeneic grafts are those between identical twins— they survive because donor and recipient have identical MHC

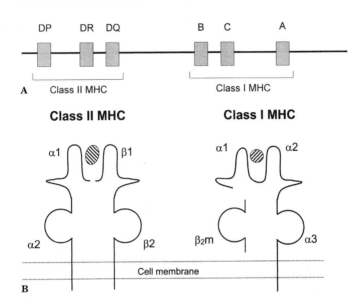

Fig. 2.1.   A: Schematic map of the human MHC genes found on chromosome 6. B: Structure of MHC. The MHC class I molecule is composed of a polymorphic α chain noncovalently attached to a nonpolymorphic β_2-microglobulin chain ($\beta_2 m$). The α chain has three domains ($\alpha 1$, $\alpha 2$, and $\alpha 3$). The MHC class II molecule has a similar overall structure to class I, except that both α and β chains are polymorphic, and each has two domains ($\alpha 1$, $\alpha 2$ and $\beta 1$, $\beta 2$, respectively). Both class I and class II bind a peptide (cross-hatched) in their polymorphic region.

molecules. When donors and recipients of grafts differ in their histocompatibility antigens, the allogeneic grafts are rejected. Genes other than MHC play smaller roles in graft rejection, and are called minor histocompatibility genes. MHC incompatibilities lead to more vigorous rejection than to minor incompatibilities, and, in general, the greater the differences in the MHC, the more rapid the rejection.

Major Histocompatibility Complex Molecules

The central event in the initiation of an alloresponse is the recognition of MHC/peptide complexes by a T-cell receptor. The MHC encodes a group of highly diverse cell surface proteins. Although these gene products were discovered in the 1940s to be the principal determinants of graft rejection, and thus named histocompatibility genes, their broader importance in controlling all immune responses to foreign antigens was only established in the 1960s. Many details of the structure and function of MHC molecules have since been established, and these are relevant to all responses to self and non-self antigens. Unlike antibody molecules, which can bind to essentially any class of molecule, including carbohydrates, lipids, and proteins, the antigen receptors of T cells primarily recognize peptides that are bound to MHC molecules. Consequently, T-cell activation is critically dependent on the MHC.

There are two types of MHC molecules: class I and class II molecules. In humans, the MHC genes are called human leukocyte antigen (HLA) genes, and include the class I genes HLA-A, HLA-B, and HLA-C, and the class II genes HLA-DP, HLA-DQ, and HLA-DR. There are two critical features of MHC molecules that determine their importance as histocompatibility antigens. First, they are highly *polymorphic:* unlike most proteins, which are the same in all humans, such as structural proteins or enzymes, each MHC locus can express any one of hundreds of different molecules. For example, HLA-A1, HLA-A2, HLA-A3, and so on are different enough from each other to determine self and non-self, and different molecules are expressed in each individual. Each of the MHC loci is polymorphic, and the set of different MHC molecules, or *alleles,* expressed on one chromosome is called a *haplotype.* A *genotype* is the sum of two haplotypes. The second critical feature of the MHC is that its genes are *codominantly expressed*—an individual expresses alleles from both chromosomes at each locus. Therefore, the MHC genotype of an individual consists of 12 different MHC molecules (two alleles from each of six loci). This explains why grafts from an F1 offspring are rejected by each parent: the F1 will express MHC molecules derived from both parental alleles, and the parent will recognize the other parent's alleles as foreign.

The evolutionary benefit of the extensive polymorphism of MHC molecules is that a wide variety of microbial peptides can be bound and presented to T cells, thus successfully initiating responses to infections. However, this same polymorphism creates a practical barrier to successful organ transplantation, because the chances of matching the MHC of an unrelated organ donor to that of a recipient is low. The degree of MHC matching between an allograft donor and recipient plays a role in determining the chances of a successful graft survival. In clinical transplantation, the most important MHC genes are HLA-A, -B, and -DR. The antigenic determinants of their six alleles are the focus of attempts at HLA matching to improve graft survival (see Chapter 3 and Fig 3.3).

The molecular structure of MHC molecules has been meticulously defined. A class I molecule is composed of a polymorphic α or heavy chain (44 kDa) and a noncovalently associated invariable (nonpolymorphic) light chain, β_2-microglobulin (12 kDa) (Fig. 2.1B). A class II molecule is composed of polymorphic α and β chains of similar molecular weight (32 kDa), covalently bound to each other (Fig 2.1B). A critical feature of both classes of MHC is the presence of a peptide-binding groove (see front cover). The specific amino acids that line this groove determine which specific peptides can bind for presentation to T cells. Class I molecules bind peptides that are 9 to 11 amino acids long, while class II molecules bind peptides that are 13 to 30 amino acids long.

Class I and class II MHC molecules have different expression patterns. Class I molecules are expressed on essentially all nucleated cells, while class II molecules are expressed only on professional antigen-presenting cells (APCs), including dendritic cells,

B lymphocytes, and macrophages. Cytokines play an important role in modifying the expression of MHC molecules. For example, interferons (IFNs), particularly IFN-γ, upregulate levels of MHC class I. IFN-γ also increases MHC class II levels on macrophages, and can induce class II expression on cells not traditionally considered APCs, including endothelial and epithelial cells. Thus, during an immune response to an allograft, essentially all cells in the graft can express both MHC class I and class II molecules.

Both class I and class II molecules are stably expressed at the cell surface only if peptides are present in their binding grooves. Class I molecules bind peptides derived from proteins in the cytoplasm of cells, which are often proteins that are synthesized intracellularly, such as viral proteins (the cytosolic, or endogenous, pathway). In contrast, class II molecules bind extracellular proteins that have been brought into a cell's vesicles by endocytosis (the vesicular, or exogenous, pathway). In both cases, the complex of MHC molecule and peptide is recognized by a T-cell receptor (TCR) to initiate T-cell activation. In the absence of a microbial infection or foreign graft, the peptides presented by MHC molecules are derived from self proteins, and some of these peptides have been shown to be derived from self MHC molecules. The significance of the self MHC peptides present on MHC molecules is unclear, but their possible immunologic role has led to efforts to design MHC peptide molecules as therapies to block the rejection of allografts.

Pathways of Alloantigen Presentation

Although the immune system evolved primarily to respond to foreign microbial peptides presented by self MHC molecules, the strong response to allografts is highly conserved in evolution. In humans, between 1% and 10% of T cells respond to a given allogeneic MHC molecule. During their maturation in the thymus, T cells that respond to self antigens are deleted (*negative selection*), while those that are specific for foreign peptides displayed by self MHC molecules are allowed to develop (*positive selection*). These same positively selected T cells also recognize foreign MHC molecules in grafts and induce graft rejection. The nature of the MHC molecules recognized by alloreactive T cells varies according to the pathway of alloantigen presentation.

Direct Antigen Presentation

The response of recipient T cells to intact MHC/peptide complexes on APCs from a graft is called *direct allorecognition*. That is, the APCs in the graft directly present alloantigens (the foreign MHC molecules) for recognition by alloreactive T cells. The high alloreactivity of the T cell repertoire is a result of cross-reactivity: T cells that normally recognize self MHC/microbial peptide complexes (Fig. 2.2A) are capable of recognizing foreign MHC/peptide complexes because the complexes are structurally similar. The T cells responding to direct antigen presentation recognize determinants on the allogeneic MHC molecule itself (Fig. 2.2B), as well as structures determined by both MHC and peptide (Fig. 2.2C). The peptides presented by foreign MHC molecules may be derived from polymorphic proteins (i.e., MHC antigens) or nonpolymorphic proteins (e.g., an enzyme from a metabolic pathway).

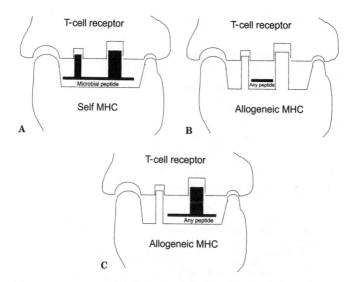

Fig. 2.2.   A: During development, T cells are selected for their ability to recognize microbial peptides (found in the central peptide groove) in the context of self MHC (identified by residues surrounding the peptide groove). These T cells cross-react with a three-dimensional structure that can be formed entirely by an allogeneic MHC molecule (B), or a combination of structures from the allogeneic MHC molecule and any peptide that happens to be in the peptide groove (C).

Indirect Antigen Presentation

A recipient's T cells can also respond to donor MHC peptides presented on the recipient's own APCs. This pathway is called *indirect allorecognition*, to distinguish it from the direct response to intact MHC on donor APCs (Fig. 2.3). In indirect antigen presentation, donor MHC molecules are shed from their cell surface, taken up by recipient APCs, processed, and presented as peptides on recipient MHC molecules. The indirect alloresponse is analogous to the immune response to invading microbes, which are also presented to T cells as peptides displayed by self MHC molecules. Several types of experiments have demonstrated the importance of indirect allorecognition in graft rejection. For example, skin grafts from MHC class II-deficient mice are rejected in a CD4 T-cell–dependent manner. In this experiment, CD4 T cells (which are class II MHC-restricted) cannot be stimulated by the direct pathway, because no MHC class II is present on donor cells. Therefore, they must be responding to recipient APCs presenting allopeptides on recipient class II molecules.

It is generally assumed that indirect antigen presentation is most important for activating CD4 T cells, because class II molecules present peptides derived from exogenous sources, unlike class I molecules, which usually present peptides derived from endogenous sources. However, cross-priming of CD8 cells

Direct antigen presentation

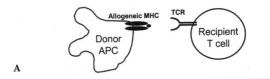

A

Indirect antigen presentation

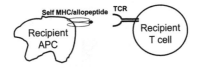

B

Fig. 2.3.   A: In direct antigen presentation, recipient T cells recognize intact allogeneic MHC molecules on the surface of donor APCs. B: In indirect antigen presentation, recipient T cells recognize allopeptides in the context of self (recipient) MHC. The allopeptides are derived from donor MHC molecules that have been processed, then brought to the cell surface by recipient MHC.

has been demonstrated, whereby MHC class I molecules can be loaded with peptides from exogenous sources. This suggests the possibility that CD8 cells also may be able to respond to indirect antigen presentation.

Acute rejection of an allograft is primarily dependent on direct allorecognition, with the ratio of T cells reactive by the direct pathway:indirect pathway estimated at 100:1. However, experimental evidence suggests that in chronic rejection, the indirect pathway may be more important. Because chronic rejection is a major cause of graft loss (see Chapter 9), there is great interest in understanding the indirect pathway with the goal of developing therapeutic approaches to block this pathway.

Minor Histocompatibility Antigens

Although the MHC is the major barrier to allotransplantation, studies in humans and mice have demonstrated that non-MHC molecules, referred to as minor histocompatibility antigens, can also mediate rejection. In fact, some mouse models of skin and cardiac transplantation have demonstrated that minor incompatibilities can lead to rejection that is as rapid as that seen in grafts with MHC mismatches. The clinical importance of minor antigens is demonstrated by the fact that MHC-matched, unrelated individuals, unlike identical twins, require immunosuppression to prevent graft rejection. By definition, this alloresponse is targeting minor antigens. The mechanism of the alloresponse to minor antigens is similar to the response to microbial antigens, in that host MHC molecules present foreign peptides to host T cells.

Sites of T-cell–Antigen-Presenting Cell Interactions

After transplantation, the first foreign antigens encountered by recipient T cells are on the vascular endothelium of the graft. Resting endothelium expresses MHC class I, and activated endothelium also expresses MHC class II molecules. Not surprisingly, inflammation of the endothelium, referred to as endothelitis or vasculitis, is one of the hallmarks of acute graft rejection (see Chapter 13).

In addition, when an organ is transplanted, donor leukocytes are carried to the recipient as passenger leukocytes with the graft. These leukocytes are found in lymphoid tissue and in most other organs of the body, scattered within the parenchyma. The most important of these cells are dendritic cells, which are potent APCs because of their ability to express high levels of MHC molecules, as well as critical accessory molecules that facilitate T-cell activation. Passenger leukocytes play an important role in allograft rejection, and in several models, the removal of these cells before transplantation prolongs graft survival. For example, both the culture of thyroid cells before transplantation and the use of antibodies to deplete dendritic cells from islet allografts prolong graft survival.

Passenger leukocytes may stimulate direct alloresponses of graft-infiltrating T cells, and may also shed MHC molecules that are be taken up and presented by infiltrating monocytes, thereby stimulating an indirect alloresponse of infiltrating T cells. In addition, passenger dendritic cells are able to migrate out of a graft and traffic to recipient lymphoid tissue, where they can again elicit either a direct or indirect alloresponse. Thus, the recipient's lymphoid organs are also an important site of T cell–APC interactions.

Role of Graft Injury and Ischemia in the Alloresponse

The surgical procedure required to transplant a graft produces an inflammatory response to the injury, as well as to the ischemia that develops in the organ before its vessels are reconnected. This process, also referred to as ischemia–reperfusion, is chronologically the first event after transplantation, and its importance has been clearly demonstrated using syngeneic grafts. In particular, the process of cutting and reattaching vessels, restoring blood flow to an ischemic organ, leads to the production of inflammatory cytokines, and the recruitment of cells, such as macrophages, into the graft. Thus, the immune response is primed, so that antigen-reactive cells are recruited to the site of injury. If no alloantigens are encountered, as in a syngeneic graft, the inflammatory response subsides with a time course similar to that of any repair from injury. But if alloantigens are present, the antigen-specific immune response leads to graft rejection. The clinical importance of graft ischemia is highlighted by studies showing that acute rejection episodes are more frequent with grafts having prolonged ischemia time before transplantation. In addition, living unrelated kidney transplants (which are completely MHC mismatched but have short ischemia time) are more successful than well-matched deceased donor transplants, which have more prolonged ischemia time (see Chapter 3).

ROLLING   ADHESION   TRANSMIGRATION

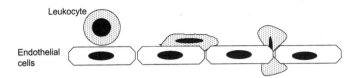

Fig. 2.4. **Leukocyte recruitment. Expression of selectins slows the flow of leukocytes in blood vessels, and causes them to roll along the endothelium. Release of chemokines activates the leukocytes, and expression of high-affinity integrins causes firm adhesion to endothelial cells. Firmly adherent cells then transmigrate through the endothelial cell layer into the interstitial site of injury.**

Leukocyte Recruitment

For a leukocyte to exit from a blood vessel and home in on a site of tissue injury, such as an allograft, a complex series of interactions between *adhesion* molecules must take place. Leukocyte homing can be divided into three steps (Fig. 2.4). In the first, endothelial cells are activated, leading to the expression of *selectins*. The binding of selectins to their ligands on leukocytes slows their flow, and the leukocytes start rolling along the endothelium. This step allows circulating cells to sample various environments. The second step involves the secretion of *chemokines*, which attract more leukocytes to the site of inflammation, and leads to the firm attachment of leukocyte to endothelium. This firm adhesion is mediated by *integrins* on leukocytes binding to their ligands, either on the endothelial cell surface or in the extracellular matrix. The third step is the extravasation of leukocytes into surrounding tissue. One of the most extensively studied adhesive interaction is between the integrin leukocyte factor antigen (LFA)-1 (CD11a/CD18) and intercellular adhesion molecule (ICAM)-1 (CD54). These molecules are particularly important as an antigen-independent component of the immune response because, in addition to their role in leukocyte extravasation, they are critical to adhesive interactions between T cells and APCs.

Many of the steps involved in leukocyte recruitment have been studied specifically in the context of transplantation. Ischemic injury causes increased production of several cytokines, including interleukin (IL)-1, which upregulates expression of selectins. Cytokines produced following the trauma of transplantation also induce expression of several other adhesion molecules, including E-selectin, ICAM-1, and vascular cell adhesion molecule (VCAM)-1. Chemokines are also upregulated in the context of graft infiltration. Several adhesion molecules have been studied as potential targets to block graft rejection. For example, antibodies to LFA-1 or ICAM-1 prolong graft survival in animals, and preliminary studies in humans show promise in mitigating rejection.

LYMPHOCYTE ACTIVATION

T Lymphocytes

The critical importance of T cells in the rejection of allogeneic grafts has long been recognized from diverse models in which T cells are genetically absent or impaired. T-cell recognition of alloantigen is the primary event leading to activation, proliferation, and differentiation of alloreactive T cells, and T-cell-dependent rejection.

The T-Cell Receptor for Antigen

The T-cell receptor (TCR) is a heterodimer composed of an α and a β polypeptide chain, both of which have variable (V) and constant (C) domains. Additional diversity in the peptide-binding region, which includes the V domain, is provided by joining (J) segments, and on the β chain only, a diversity (D) segment. A second TCR heterodimer, comprising γ and δ chains, has been described, but has not been shown to play a role in the alloresponse. TCRs are associated on the T-cell surface with the CD3 complex, made up of several polypeptide chains that are important for the cell surface expression of the TCR, and for transmitting signals into the T cell. The critical importance of CD3+ cells is demonstrated by the fact that one of the most potent immunosuppressive agents used in clinical transplantation is muronomab OKT3, which binds to and inactivates T cells (see Chapter 4 Part II).

Intracellular Signaling

To transduce molecular events at the surface of T cells into the nucleus, and modify the expression of genes that regulate cell function, a complex machinery is required. A number of signaling pathways have been identified in T cells, and many steps in these pathways have been targets for blocking the alloresponse. Engagement of the TCR induces phosphorylation of TCR-associated proteins such as the ζ (zeta) chain, as well as a variety of adapter proteins. These phosphorylation events lead to the activation of several biochemical pathways, including the calcineurin pathway, the protein kinase C pathway, and the Ras– and Rac– mitogen-activated protein (MAP) kinase pathways.

Of these pathways, the calcineurin pathway (Fig. 2.5) is the best characterized, since it is the site of action of the potent immunosuppressive agents cyclosporine and tacrolimus. Within minutes of TCR engagement, phosphorylation of ZAP-70 (ζ-associated protein of 70 kDa) leads to the phosphorylation of PLCγ1 (phospholipase C γ1), which hydrolyzes a membrane phospholipid phosphatidylinositol 4,5-bisphosphate (PIP$_2$) into inositol 1,4,5-trisphosphate (IP$_3$) and diacylglycerol (DAG). IP$_3$ leads to an increase in cytosolic calcium, which binds calmodulin, forming a complex that activates several enzymes, including the phosphatase calcineurin. Calcineurin dephosphorylates NFAT (nuclear factor of activated T cells), allowing NFAT to translocate from the cytoplasm to the nucleus. Once in the nucleus, NFAT binds to regulatory sequences and increases the transcription of genes for several cytokines, including the T-cell growth factor, IL-2. Cyclosporine exerts its immunosuppressant

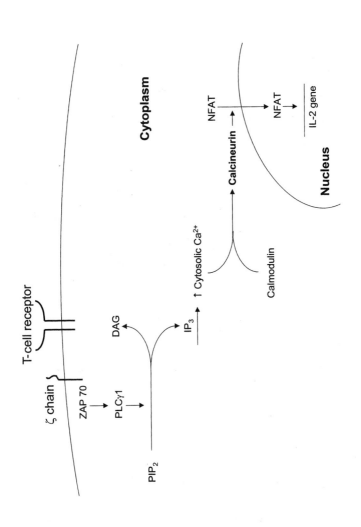

effect by binding to an intracellular protein, cyclophilin, and the cyclosporine–cyclophilin complex inhibits the activity of calcineurin. Tacrolimus (originally known as "FK") binds to FK-binding protein (FKBP) and the tacrolimus/FKBP complex similarly inhibits the activity of calcineurin (see Plate 1). Hence the drugs are both referred to as calcineurin inhibitors (see Chapter 4, Part I).

CD4 and CD8 Subsets of T Cells

Most mature T cells carry either the CD4 or CD8 protein on their cell surface. CD4 molecules define the "helper" subset of T cells, and directly bind MHC class II molecules. CD8 molecules define the "cytolytic" subset of T cells, and directly bind MHC class I molecules. However, exceptions to this functional division of T cells exist. For example, CD4 cells restricted to MHC class II, in certain systems, have cytolytic function, and CD8 cells produce many, although not all, of the regulatory cytokines made by CD4 cells. Generally, CD4 T cells are thought to mediate the initial recognition of an allograft, and to help amplify and coordinate the subsequent immune response, including providing help to CD4 and CD8 effector T cells. For example, in a model of mouse heart transplantation, CD4-deficient mice are unable to reject grafts, while CD8-deficient mice do reject grafts. This is one of several models where a CD4 T-cell-mediated delayed-type hypersensitivity (DTH) response is sufficient to cause rejection, without requiring the cytolytic function of CD8 cells. However, in other experimental models, antibody blockade of CD8 cells prevents rejection, suggesting the need for CD8 cells to destroy a graft. Taken together, these data are a testament to the overlapping functions, or redundancy, of various components of the alloresponse, and the ability of the immune system to compensate for specific impairments and still cause the destruction of a transplanted organ.

Type 1 and Type 2 T-Cell Responses

Upon activation, T cells produce a variety of cytokines to regulate the immune response. With persistent antigenic stimulation, T cells can often be shown to differentiate into one of two different types with distinct cytokine profiles. Type 1 helper T cells (called Th1 cells) secrete cytokines that include IL-2, IFN-γ, IL-12, and tumor necrosis factor (TNF). These cytokines stimulate DTH reactions, cytolytic activity and production of opsonizing and complement-fixing IgG antibodies. Type 2 helper cells (Th2 cells)

$\leftarrow$

Fig. 2.5. Intracellular signaling in T cells. One of the many signal cascades by which cell surface events are transduced into cellular changes. The activation of calcineurin is inhibited by cyclosporine and tacrolimus, decreasing T-cell production of IL-2 and other cytokines, and thus impairing T-cell proliferation. DAG = diacylglycerol; IL-2 = interleukin-2; IP$_3$ = inositol 1,4,5-trisphosphate; NFAT = nuclear factor of activated T cells; PIP$_2$ = phosphatidylinositol 4,5-bisphosphate; PLCγ1 = phospholipase C γ1; and ZAP-70 = ζ-associated protein of 70 kDa.

secrete cytokines that include IL-4, IL-5, IL-10, and IL-13, which activate eosinophils and stimulate production of immunoglobulin (Ig) E antibody. The regulation of these two types of responses has been most extensively studied in CD4 helper cells, but the polarization of responses also appears to apply to CD8 cytolytic cells. IFN-γ and IL-12 promotes deviation to type 1 responses, while IL-4 promotes type 2 responses. In addition, IFN-γ inhibits type 2 responses, while IL-4 inhibits type 1 responses, so that responses become increasingly polarized once they are initiated.

In recent years, there has been great interest in the role of cytokine deviation in transplant rejection because of the hypothesis that type 1 responses lead to rejection, while type 2 responses might mediate tolerance of grafts. This hypothesis developed in part from the findings that type 1 cytokines promote effector functions such as DTH and cytolytic activity, while type 2 cytokines antagonize these activities. Several experimental studies have shown that acute rejection is associated with an expansion of type 1 cytokines, while prolonged survival is associated with reduced levels of these cytokines. However, other studies have shown that rejection is associated with the production of both type 1 and type 2 cytokines, while tolerance is associated with a decrease in both types of cytokines. Furthermore, attempts to effect graft rejection by manipulating cytokines have been largely unsuccessful, suggesting that the type 1/type 2 hypothesis is limited in its therapeutic applicability to alloresponses. For example, IL-4 does not induce tolerance in mice, and mice deficient in IL-2 or IFN-γ still are able to reject grafts. Thus, it appears that type 2 responses are not purely immunosuppressive, and their associated effector functions may also contribute to graft rejection.

T-Cell Costimulation

The specificity of the immune response is determined by the interaction between the TCR of a T cell and the MHC/peptide complex on an APC. However, several other molecular interactions between T cells and APCs are essential for T-cell activation (Table 2.1). The idea that two distinct signals are required for lymphocyte activation was proposed more than 30 years ago. Since then, it has been demonstrated that T-cell activation requires one signal through the TCR, and a second, or costimulatory, signal through accessory molecules. These accessory molecules play

Table 2.1. Some critical T-cell accessory molecules and their ligands

T Cell	APC
TCR	MHC/peptide
CD28	B7-1/B7-2
LFA-1	ICAM-1
CD2	LFA-3
CD4	MHC class II
CD8	MHC class I

two important roles. The first role is to provide adhesive strength to keep the T cells and APCs in contact with each other, thus providing time for the TCR to sample antigens on the APC. Integrins, particularly LFA-1 on T cells binding to ICAMs on APCs, are perhaps the most important adhesion molecules for T-cell activation. The second role of accessory molecules is to cooperate with TCR-initiated signals in the process of T-cell activation. The most potent second signals regulating T-cell clonal expansion and differentiation are provided by the B7/CD28 family of molecules.

CD28 is expressed on most T lymphocytes, and engagement of CD28 increases T-cell proliferation by a variety of mechanisms, including the production of IL-2 and other cytokines. APCs express two ligands for CD28: B7-1 (CD80) and B7-2 (CD86). Expression of both B7 molecules is upregulated on APCs that have been activated by a variety of inflammatory stimuli, including microbial infection and cytokines. B7-1 and B7-2 can both provide T-cell costimulation through CD28, and in many experimental models, they play overlapping roles. However, B7-1 and B7-2 have distinct patterns of expression and binding kinetics for CD28, suggesting significant differences in the roles of the two molecules. B7-1 and B7-2 also regulate T cells by binding cytotoxic T-lymphocyte antigen (CTLA)-4, which inhibits T-cell proliferation.

The immunosuppressive drugs in current use are extremely potent in blocking transplant rejection, but none of these drugs is antigen specific, so they also strongly suppress immune responses to infections. Therefore, the goal of transplantation immunology is to specifically block responses to transplantation antigens, without producing global immunosuppression. One approach to this goal is to induce T-cell anergy, or antigen-specific unresponsiveness. *In vitro* models demonstrate that one way to induce anergy is to provide a T-cell with an antigen-specific signal through its TCR in the absence of CD28 engagement (Fig 2.6). In these models, subsequent exposure of the cell to both TCR and CD28 signals no longer can activate the T cell. Targeting the B7/CD28 pathway holds great promise for achieving antigen-specific unresponsiveness because the timing of transplantation can be controlled so as to coincide with the administration of agents that block CD28 engagement. If blockade of CD28 were only required at the time of initial antigen exposure, a graft recipient would not be exposed to the infectious risks of long-term immunosuppression. In addition, T-cell responses to transplant antigens could be prevented, without the need to identify the specific antigen.

In a wide variety of experimental models in animals, and in preliminary human trials, blockade of B7 molecules has been shown to significantly prolong graft survival. However, in most *in vivo* models of B7 blockade, anergy limited to specific antigens has been difficult to demonstrate. One reason for this difficulty may be the complexity of costimulation. For example, there is increasing evidence that engagement of CTLA-4 is important in inducing tolerance (Fig. 2.6). Because B7 blockade affects signaling through both CD28 and CTLA-4, and these molecules have opposing effects, the net result is highly dependent on the experimental system. Manipulation of this pathway may also be complicated by the existence of additional molecules, homologous to B7 or to

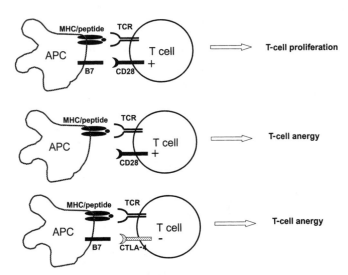

Fig. 2.6.   T cells require costimulation for activation. If both TCR and CD28 are engaged, T cells proliferate and differentiate. If the TCR is engaged in the absence of B7 costimulation, T cells fail to proliferate and become anergic. Binding of B7 to CTLA-4 is also important in inducing anergy.

CD28, that have been recently discovered. These molecules of the CD28 superfamily transduce both stimulatory and inhibitory signals to T cells (Fig. 2.7, left side). For example, B7h on APCs stimulates T cells by binding ICOS (inducible costimulator), and PD-L1 and PD-L2 inhibit T cells by binding PD-1. The interaction between these pathways is still being defined, but understanding their regulation is likely to improve therapies targeting costimulation.

Another molecular interaction that is critical in immune responses is that between the CD40 molecule on APCs and CD40 ligand (CD154, CD40L) on T cells. CD40 engagement plays a critical role in activating B cells, dendritic cells, and monocytes, and also upregulates expression of the B7 molecules. B7 interactions with CD28 and CTLA-4, in turn, are critical in T-cell regulation. There is also some evidence that engagement of CD154 directly stimulates T cells. The CD40/CD154 pathway has been the subject of great interest because of its importance in the activation of both APCs and T cells, and blockade of this pathway in experimental models of transplantation has proved to be extremely effective. In addition, a number of other pathways in the same family as CD40/CD154, the TNF/TNFR (tumor necrosis factor receptor) family, are also important in T-cell–APC interactions (Fig. 2.7, right side). In experimental models, blockade of TNF and CD28 superfamily pathways appears to be synergistic, and this approach has already shown potential clinical applicability in studies of nonhuman primates.

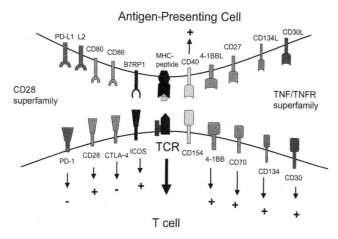

Fig. 2.7. Schematic of major costimulatory molecules belonging to the CD28 and TNF/TNFR (tumor necrosis factor receptor) superfamilies. Signals transduced into cells can either be stimulatory (+) or inhibitory (–). ICOS = inducible costimulator.

B Lymphocytes

The importance of B cells and antibodies in the rejection of an allograft is most dramatically illustrated by hyperacute rejection. This process occurs within 24 hours of transplantation in patients who were previously sensitized to allogeneic MHC molecules through previous transplants, blood transfusions, or pregnancy (see Chapter 3). Currently, hyperacute rejection is rare, because a cross-match test to detect these antibodies is performed prior to proceeding with transplantation. The role of B cells and antibody in cell-mediated acute allograft rejection is less clear, because B-cell recognition of a graft, in the absence of T cells, is insufficient to mediate rejection in mouse models, and the complete absence of immunoglobulin in mice does not slow cardiac allograft rejection.

Some acute rejection episodes have a humoral component, and this component is best identified by the presence of the complement protein C4d in biopsy specimens. Although the histologic findings in these cases are variable, the presence of C4d seems to correlate with the presence of donor-specific antibodies (see Chapter 13). Thus, B cells are less important than T cells in initiating an alloresponse, but antibody formation can play a role in the effector phase of graft destruction. Antibodies may be important in chronic rejection.

EFFECTOR MECHANISMS OF GRAFT DESTRUCTION

Once CD4 T cells recognize foreign class II MHC molecules, they play a critical role in regulating various arms of the effector response. The initial inflammatory response to the injury associated with transplantation, sometimes referred to as *innate immunity*, is antigen independent. This response is mediated by neutrophils and cells of the monocyte lineage, including macrophages and dendritic cells. The antigen-specific activation of CD4 T cells leads to expression of cell surface molecules and production of cytokines, which, in turn, further stimulates monocytes. This cooperation between CD4 T cells and monocytes, or DTH response, plays an important role in the destruction of a graft.

The activation of CD4 T cells and production of cytokines also stimulates the activation and proliferation of cytolytic CD8 T cells and natural killer (NK) cells. Upon recognition of class I MHC molecules on graft cells, the CD8 T cells cause cell death by two main mechanisms. The first mechanism is the release of soluble cytotoxic factors such as granzymes and perforin. The second mechanism is the upregulation of Fas ligand on T cells, which binds Fas (CD95) on target cells. When Fas is engaged on cells of a graft, these cells undergo apoptosis, or programmed cell death.

The production of cytokines by CD4 T cells also stimulates B cells. Upon binding of specific antigen by the B cell receptor, or cell surface immunoglobulin, B cells proliferate and differentiate into plasma cells. Plasma cells release soluble immunoglobulins, or antibodies, which can bind allogeneic cells. Antibodies can cause cell damage by fixing complement or by mediating antibody-dependent cellular cytotoxicity (ADCC).

TOLERANCE

Tolerance broadly refers to the absence of immune responses to specific antigens. During development, one of the critical functions of immune system is to prevent responses directed toward self antigens, thus preventing autoimmune disease. This is achieved both by *central tolerance* in the thymus, and by *peripheral tolerance* in extrathymic lymphoid tissue. During T-cell development, the vast majority of T cells found in the thymus have undesirable reactivities, so are deleted or made unresponsive by negative selection. T cells that recognize foreign antigen in the context of self MHC are positively selected and allowed to circulate in the blood. The process of negative selection is imperfect, so autoreactive T cells can be found in the periphery. Autoimmunity is usually prevented by the process of peripheral tolerance.

Peripheral tolerance is maintained by a number of mechanisms, including clonal deletion, anergy, and suppression. In contrast to clonal deletion of T cells, anergic T cells are still present but unable to respond, for example, because of the absence of costimulatory signals. The phenomenon of suppressor cells has long been demonstrated by adoptive transfer experiments, in which transfer of cells from tolerant animals can induce tolerance in naive animals. However, the molecular phenotype of suppressor cells, including their cell surface molecules and soluble factors produced, is just starting to be characterized. For example, a subset of T cells expressing CD25, the IL-2 receptor α chain, appears to be important in suppressing a variety of immune responses.

In the context of transplantation, tolerance can be defined as the absence of a destructive immune response to a graft, in a host with otherwise intact immunity. A variety of experimental approaches have tried to take advantage of basic mechanisms of tolerance in an attempt to induce transplantation tolerance. Early animal studies demonstrated that intrathymic injection of soluble antigen can induce central tolerance. More recently, tolerance has been induced by ablation or immunosuppression of a recipient's immune system, and reconstitution with both donor and recipient bone marrow, thus generating a chimeric immune system that does not reject donor organs.

A variety of approaches have been taken to inducing peripheral tolerance. For example, T cell deletion has been induced by programmed cell death, or apoptosis. The blockade of T-cell costimulatory signals has induced anergy, and the manipulation of the cytokine environment has suppressed T-cell activation. Novel strategies have used the immunomodulatory effects of peptides derived from amino acid sequences found in MHC molecules.

Despite the success of many potent immunosuppressive regimens in prolonging graft survival, the acquisition of antigen-specific tolerance remains a goal, rather than the clinical reality of transplantation. However, approaches to tolerance induction in animal models are increasingly successful in achieving this goal, and many of these approaches are approaching human trials. The term "prope tolerance," or "near tolerance," has been used to describe the situation that is achieved when a graft continues to function well in the face of minimal immunosuppression or after discontinuation of immunosuppression. Early clinical trials suggest that in the short-term this may be a more realistic goal than the much sought after full tolerance.

IMMUNOLOGIC MONITORING

The clinical diagnosis of renal allograft rejection currently relies on the histologic evaluation of a biopsy specimen. Because biopsies are usually performed only after a rise in creatinine is observed, several days and often weeks elapse between the start of graft rejection and the initiation of treatment. This delay allows tissue to be damaged, and shortens the survival of the graft. Biopsies are also not ideal as a technique to diagnose rejection because they are invasive, so cannot be repeated as frequently as desired to closely monitor a graft. As a result, several approaches have been attempted to monitor the immune response to a graft noninvasively. Ideally, an immune assay would detect rejection in its earliest stages. In addition, it would allow the accurate monitoring of the alloresponse so that immunosuppression could be adjusted to minimize exposure of the patient to side effects while maximally preserving the graft.

One of the oldest assays of alloreactivity is the mixed lymphocyte response (MLR). In this assay, cells from the donor are inactivated, and then mixed with lymphocytes from the recipient or responder. The degree of proliferation of responder cells, which are mostly CD4 T cells, reflects alloreactivity. A related assay is the cell-mediated lympholysis (CML), which measures the killing of donor cells by CD8 T cells. These assays are essentially *in vitro* versions of *in vivo* transplantation, and are commonly used in animal models. However, their clinical utility in renal transplantation is limited because of the many examples where the MLR and CML do not correlate with clinical rejection.

Immune reactivity has also been assayed by mixing a transplant recipient's T cells with peptides that correspond to donor MHC molecules. These peptides can be designed to reflect indirect antigen recognition, and reactivity to these peptides may prove to be particularly useful in predicting chronic rejection.

Another approach has been to measure the frequency of alloreactive T cells per volume of blood. In particular, an enzyme-linked immunospot (ELISPOT) assay for IFN-γ-producing cells is able to accurately quantitate small numbers of alloreactive T cells responding either to cells or peptides. However, the correlation between IFN-γ-producing cells and clinical transplant rejection remains to be proved.

Assays of B-cell function can also be performed, in that alloreactive antibodies in blood can be detected pretransplant, as in a standard cross-match, and specific antibodies can also be quantitated. These assays do not reliably correlate with alloreactivity posttransplant, but may prove to be useful in assessing chronic rejection.

One of the most promising recent developments in immune monitoring is the measurement of gene expression of the molecules important in causing graft damage. For example, renal biopsy levels of messenger ribonucleic acid (mRNA) for perforin, granzyme B, and Fas-L correlate well with the histologic diagnosis of rejection. The correlation with rejection is particularly strong if more than one of these three cytotoxic mediators is elevated. The utility of these measurements for the noninvasive diagnosis of rejection has been demonstrated for samples obtained from blood and from urine.

Although noninvasive assays of rejection have yet to be clinically used, it is likely that in the future such an assay, or possibly a panel of available assays, will greatly improve the management of immunosuppression in renal transplant recipients. In addition, such assays should be critical in evaluating novel immunosuppressive drugs and regimens.

XENOTRANSPLANTATION

Xenotransplantation involves the transplantation of tissues between different species. Initial interest was based partly on ethical concerns about using organs from humans. Currently, organs transplanted from animals to humans are viewed as a potential solution to the severe shortage of organs. Several major hurdles remain to the clinical application of xenotransplantation. From a public health point of view, the greatest concern is that novel infectious agents might be introduced from animals into human populations. In addition, immune responses to xenografts have several unique features not present in responses to allografts. For example, primates reject pig kidneys in a hyperacute fashion as a consequence of preformed antibodies to cell surface sugars such as Gal-alpha(1–3)-Gal. These xenoreactive natural antibodies are similar to the isohemagglutinins that recognize blood groups A and B, and the hyperacute rejection they produce is dependent on activation of complement. Porcine xenografts are particularly susceptible to complement-mediated injury because they lack the complement regulatory proteins (such as decay accelerating factor) that are present on human tissues.

A number of approaches have been used to prevent hyperacute rejection of xenografts. These include depleting xenoreactive antibodies from the recipient's circulation and administering reagents that inhibit complement. Genetic modification of porcine grafts also shows promise, because kidneys from transgenic pigs expressing human complement regulatory proteins minimize hyperacute rejection, and knockout pigs that lack Gal-alpha-(1–3)-Gal have now been generated.

If hyperacute rejection of xenografts could be entirely prevented, they would still be susceptible to acute vascular and cellular rejection. Antigens targeted by vascular rejection include MHC molecules and other xenoantigens found on endothelium. The effectiveness of currently available immunosuppressant strategies in blocking acute rejection of xenografts is currently being explored.

CONCLUSIONS

The last 20 years has seen an explosion of knowledge about the molecular interactions responsible for immune responses to allografts. MHC molecules are known to play a role in immune responses to all microbes, but were originally described as transplantation antigens, and continue to play a critical role as such. The recognition by the TCR of MHC/peptide complexes is the central antigen-specific event in the response to grafts, but the fact that each graft expresses a unique set of antigens has made the development of broadly applicable therapies targeting the MHC extremely difficult. Lymphocyte activation is a complex process with many molecular interactions having been described. New interactions continue to be reported, and further work is required in understanding the interactions between various pathways, as well as areas of redundancy. Many of these molecules have been considered as targets for therapy of transplant rejection, and the years to come are likely to yield continued progress in developing increasingly specific treatments, with concomitant decreases in toxicities.

SELECTED READINGS

Briscoe DM, Sayegh MH. A rendezvous before rejection: where do T cells meet transplant antigens? *Nat Med* 2002;8:220–221.

Calne RY. Probe tolerance: the future of organ transplantation—from the laboratory to the clinic. *Transplantation* 2004;77:930–932.

Cantrell D. T cell antigen receptor signal transduction pathways. *Annu Rev Immunol* 1996;14:259–274.

Delves PJ, Roitt IM. The immune system. *Part I. N Engl J Med* 2000; 343:37–49.

Delves PJ, Roitt IM. The immune system. *Part II. N Engl J Med* 2000: 343:108–117.

Hancock WW. Chemokines and transplant immunobiology. *J Am Soc Nephrol* 2002;13:821–824.

Lakkis FG. Role of cytokines in transplantation tolerance: lessons learned from gene-knockout mice. *J Am Soc Nephrol* 1998;9:2361–2367.

Mandelbrot DA, Sayegh MH. Novel costimulation pathways. *Curr Opin Organ Transplant* 2003;8:25–33.

Marrack P, Kappler J. The antigen-specific, major histocompatibility complex-restricted receptor on T cells. *Adv Immunol* 1986;38:1–30.

Mauiyyedi S, Colvin RB. Humoral rejection in kidney transplantation: new concepts in diagnosis and treatment. *Curr Opin Nephrol Hypertens* 2002;11:609–618.

Sayegh MH. Why do we reject a graft? Role of indirect allorecognition in graft rejection. *Kidney Int* 1999;56:1967–1979.

Sayegh MH, Turka LA. The role of T-cell costimulatory activation pathways in transplant rejection. *N Engl J Med* 1998;338:1813–1821.

Schwartz RS. Diversity of the immune repertoire and immunoregulation. *N Engl J Med* 2003;348:1017–1026.

Springer TA. Traffic signals for lymphocyte recirculation and leukocyte emigration: the multistep paradigm. *Cell* 1994;76:301–314.

Strom TB, Suthanthiran M. Prospects and applicability of molecular diagnosis of allograft rejection. *Semin Nephrol* 2000;20:103–107.

Tilney NL, Guttmann RD. Effects of initial ischemia/reperfusion injury on the transplanted kidney. *Transplantation* 1997;64:945–947.

Wu Z, Bensinger SJ, Zhang J, et al. Homeostatic proliferation is a barrier to transplantation tolerance. *Nature Medicine* 2004;10: 87–91.

Histocompatibility Testing, Cross-Matching, and Allocation of Kidney Transplants

J. Michael Cecka and Elaine F. Reed

The human major histocompatibility complex, a cluster of genes on chromosome 6, encodes human leukocyte antigens (HLAs) and other products that play integral roles in controlling the immune response (see Chapter 2, Fig. 2.1). The HLA antigens are also major barriers to transplantation of organs and tissues between individuals. Antibodies directed against donor HLA antigens that might arise as a result of pregnancies, blood transfusions, or transplantation cause hyperacute or accelerated acute graft rejection when they are present before transplantation. Additionally, recent evidence implicates their appearance after transplantation with accelerated acute rejection and with chronic graft dysfunction and loss. The allogeneic donor HLA antigens themselves are the main immunologic targets of rejection on the graft. The degree of histocompatibility (the similarity between the constellation of HLA antigens of the donor and recipient) affects long-term graft survival and for that reason, HLA matching has been incorporated into kidney allocation in the United States and in many other countries. This chapter describes the HLA antigens and their genetics, methods to identify them, anti-HLA antibodies and the means to detect and characterize them, and the important roles each plays in kidney transplantation and allocation.

THE HUMAN MAJOR HISTOCOMPATIBILITY COMPLEX

Nomenclature

One of the most notable features of the major histocompatibility complex is the remarkable degree of polymorphism exhibited by its gene products. Even when we limit the discussion to the products of the HLA-A, -B, and -DR loci, which are most commonly encountered in clinical kidney transplantation, there are 88 recognized antigens encoded by more than 1,000 distinct alleles (Table 3.1) and the number of new alleles is still increasing. Obviously, keeping track of this diversity requires a specialized nomenclature. The HLA antigens were identified and characterized over a 40-year period beginning with the discovery of the MAC (now HLA-A2) antigen by Dausset in Paris in 1958. A series of international workshops beginning in 1964 and held approximately every 4 years until 1987 established a nomenclature for the HLA antigens, naming unique antigens in the sequence they were officially recognized: A1, A2, A3, Bw4, B5, Bw6, B7, B8, and so on. The antigens were identified using antisera obtained primarily from multiparous women. As the field evolved, new antisera were discovered that could "split" some HLA antigens into narrower specificities. HLA-A9 was split into HLA-A23 and -A24 and HLA-A10 was split into HLA-A25, -A26, -A34, and -A66, for example. Table 3.1 lists the broad parent antigens for splits in parentheses.

The already complicated HLA nomenclature became more complex when deoxyribonucleic acid (DNA) technologies for HLA testing were developed in the mid-1980s. To accommodate the growing numbers of alleles that could be identified by their unique nucleotide sequences within the antigen designations, the established serologic nomenclature was modified to associate alleles with antigens whenever possible, and four-digit designations were developed in which the antigen designation makes up the first two digits and the sequential allele designation makes up the third and fourth digits. The first allele for HLA-A1 is HLA-A*0101, which includes the locus (A), an asterisk (*) to indicate the typing was performed by DNA methods, the serologic antigen (01), and the allele number (01). As the number of alleles grows, it may be necessary to modify this convention to accommodate three-digit allele numbers. The naming of HLA class II antigens is similar even though two distinct polypeptides encoded by separate genes combine to form the antigen. The DR antigens are distinguished by their DR β_1 subunit; therefore, the first allele of DR1 is DRB1*0101. There are some exceptions that may be confusing. The HLA-B14, -B15, -B40, and HLA-DRB1*03 allele series include distinct antigens that are both immunogenic and antigenic. The HLA-B62 antigen, for example, is encoded by HLA-B*1501, 1504, 1505, 1506, 1507, and many other B15 alleles, while HLA-B75 is encoded by HLA-B*1502, 1508, 1511, and so on. HLA-DRB1*0301 is HLA-DR17, while HLA-DRB1*0302 is HLA-DR18. The correlation between alleles and antigens is updated periodically in the *HLA Dictionary* and in the series "Nomenclature for factors of the HLA system" (see Selected Readings).

Although the number of HLA antigens, alleles, and combinations is very large, the frequencies of individual antigens, alleles and combinations vary considerably. The most common HLA antigen is A2, which is found in roughly 50% of individuals from populations around the world. Approximately 96% of whites with European ancestry who express HLA-A2 have the HLA-A*0201 allele. Northern Chinese and many Hispanics who express HLA-A2 have the HLA-A*0206 allele. HLA-B8 is found in 30% of Scots and the frequency declines as populations in Europe and more distant areas are analyzed, except in those areas that were colonized by the British—South Africa, India, Australia—where the frequency is higher. Thus, certain antigens and alleles are common, while others are very rare, and, in fact, no frequencies have been established yet for the majority of alleles because they have not been encountered or detected among donors and recipients. Some HLA antigens are racially limited. Thus, HLA-B54 is found almost exclusively in persons from Japan and nearby Asian countries. HLA-A36 is relatively common among blacks, but is very rare in other populations.

The additional HLA polymorphism that has been revealed through the application of DNA technologies has provided interesting insights into the role of HLA in many autoimmune diseases, but its significance in clinical kidney transplantation remains to be seen. Allele differences between the donor and

Table 3.1. Recognized human leukocyte antigen (HLA) specificities

No. of Alleles	Antigen	No. of Alleles	Antigen
HLA-A		3	B53
4	A1	1	B54(22)
32	A2	7	B55(22)
6	A3	5	B56(22)
5	A11	5	B57(17)
1	A23(9)	2	B58(17)
21	A24(9)	1	B59
2	A25(10)	3	B60(40)
12	A26(10)	4	B61(40)
4	A29(19)	15	B62(15)
7	A30(19)	2	B63(15)
4	A31(19)	1	B64(14)
3	A32(19)	1	B65(14)
3	A33(19)	2	B67
2	A34(10)	1	B70
1	A36	2	B71(70)
1	A43	2	B72(70)
3	A66(10)	1	B73
10	A68(28)	5	B75(15)
1	A69(28)	3	B76(15)
3	A74(19)	1	B77(15)
1	A80	4	B78
		1	B81
HLA-B		1	B82
14	B7		
6	B8	**HLA-DR**	
4	B13	6	DR1
17	B15	3	DR2
7	B18	10	DR3
16	B27	35	DR4
28	B35	2	DR6
2	B37	3	DR7
4	B38(16)	26	DR8
19	B39(16)	1	DR9
13	B40	1	DR10
3	B41	39	DR11(5)
2	B42	8	DR12(5)
11	B44(12)	36	DR13(6)
3	B45(12)	33	DR14(6)
1	B46	10	DR15(2)
3	B47	8	DR16(2)
5	B48	3	DR17(3)
1	B49(21)	2	DR18(3)
1	B50(21)	14	DR51
17	B51(5)	19	DR52
3	B52(5)	10	DR53

Note: The numbers in parentheses represent prior designations.
Data modified from Bodmer JG, Marsh SGE, Albert ED, et al. Nomenclature for factors of the HLA system, 1999. *Hum Immunol* 1999;60:361–395, with permission.

recipient of bone marrow transplants lead to graft-versus-host disease. However, extensive analysis of HLA allele-level mismatches among HLA antigen-matched kidney transplant recipients has revealed no substantial effect of allele-level HLA mismatches on graft survival rates.

Structure and Function of Human Leukocyte Antigen Molecules

The HLA antigens are grouped into two classes based on their general structural similarities and tissue distribution. The class I HLA-A, -B, and -C locus antigens consist of an α heavy chain of 45 kDa with three globular external domains, a transmembrane region, and an intracellular domain. The structure is stabilized by β_2-microglobulin (which is not encoded in the major histocompatibility complex) associated with the $\alpha 3$ domain. The class I antigens are expressed on all nucleated cells and interact primarily with CD8+ T cells. The class II HLA (HLA-DR, -DQ, -DP) antigens consist of two noncovalently linked chains: an α chain of 35 kDa and a β chain of 31 kDa. Both chains are transmembranes with two globular extracellular domains. The constitutive expression of class II antigens is limited to antigen-presenting cells (dendritic, macrophage, and monocyte cells) and B lymphocytes, but these antigens can be induced on activated T cells and endothelial cells, including the glomerular endothelium, renal tubular cells, and capillaries.

The three-dimensional structures of several HLA molecules have been solved crystallographically. These reveal a remarkably similar organization of the outermost domains of both class I and class II molecules (see front cover). The $\alpha 1$ and $\alpha 2$ domains of class I and the $\alpha 1$ and $\beta 1$ domains of class II form a platform of beta-pleated sheet with 2 looping α helices forming a groove facing away from the cell. During synthesis and assembly of the HLA antigens, peptides are added to the groove (intracellularly derived peptides in the endoplasmic reticulum for class I, and extracellularly derived peptides in endocytotic vesicles for class II). The class I and class II molecules differ with regard to the ends of the groove that are closed in class I and open in class II molecules, permitting longer peptides to be accommodated on class II molecules. The HLA antigens with their associated peptides are exposed to T cells, which may recognize foreign peptides in the context of the HLA molecules. The HLA molecules normally play a key signaling role in the immune response, and for this reason they are important transplant antigens. Allogeneic HLA antigens differ from the recipient's own HLA antigens in the general area where peptides are displayed and they display foreign peptides, including those derived from allogeneic HLA molecules directly to the recipient's immune system or indirectly after processing by recipient antigen-presenting cells.

Alloantigenic sites are clustered in the $\alpha 1$ and $\alpha 2$ domains of the class I molecule and in the external domain of the DR β chain. Some antigenic determinants are shared by many HLA antigens. These are called public specificities. Unique determinants are known as private specificities. Both private and public specificities are often associated with distinct amino acid sequences. The Bw4 and Bw6 public specificities are good examples

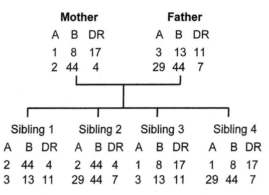

Fig. 3.1. Inheritance of haplotypes and HLA profile in four theoretical siblings. Sibling 1 is a one-haplotype match to siblings 2 and 3 and a zero-haplotype match to sibling 4.

of public antigens. All HLA-B antigens express either Bw4 or Bw6. The antigenic determinant that defines these specificities is affected by amino acids in positions 80 and 83 of the class I molecule sequences located in the exposed part of the α_1 helix. Class I molecules with arginine at position 83 and threonine or isoleucine at position 80 are recognized by anti-Bw4 antisera and include the HLA-B13, -B17, -B27, -B37, -B38, -B44, -B47, -B49, -B51, -B52, -B53, -B57, -B58, -B59, -B63, and -B77 antigens. The HLA-A23, -A24, -A25, and -A32 antigens also have the characteristic arginine at position 83 and react with anti-Bw4 antibodies. All other B-locus antigens have glycine at position 83 and asparagine at position 80, and react with anti-Bw6 antibodies. Antigenic determinants recognized by antibodies with private specificities are located on other parts of the HLA molecules.

Inheritance

Each parental chromosome 6 provides a haplotype or linked set of major histocompatibility complex (MHC) genes to the offspring (Fig. 3.1). Haplotypes are usually inherited intact from each parent, although crossover between the A and B locus occurs in approximately 2% of offspring, resulting in a recombination (and a new haplotype). The child carries one representative antigen from each of the class I and class II loci of each parent. A child is, by definition, a one-haplotype match to each parent unless recombination has occurred.

HLA haplotypes are inherited in a mendelian fashion. Statistically, there is a 25% chance that siblings will share the same parental haplotypes (two-haplotype match), a 50% chance they will share one haplotype (one-haplotype match), and a 25% chance that neither haplotype will be the same (zero-haplotype match). In the latter case, 25% to 100% of other parental chromosomes may still be shared, and these other chromosomes include other "minor" histocompatibility antigens, which can also initiate rejection reactions.

Haplotypes, Genotypes, and Phenotypes

Consider an individual with the following HLA profile or phenotype: A1, A24, B8, B44, DR4, DR15. From this phenotypic information alone it is not possible to identify haplotypes because it is not known which antigens are linked on each chromosome.

Consider another individual with the following HLA phenotype: A1, A3, B7, B8, DR4, DR12. If this second individual is the biologic parent, offspring, or sibling of the first individual, it becomes possible to identify a shared haplotype of the family as A1, B8, DR4. The first individual also has an unshared haplotype A24, B44, DR15, and the second individual an unshared haplotype A3, B7, DR12. These haplotypes should appear in the parents and other siblings. A kidney transplanted between these two individuals would be a one-haplotype matched graft, and the A1, B8, and DR4 antigens would be genotypically identical in the donor and recipient because they are encoded by the same inherited genes.

If these two individuals are not related, it is not possible to identify the haplotypes. Thus, in transplants from living-unrelated or deceased donors, the haplotypes are unknown, and only the phenotypic identity of individual HLA antigens can be determined. The two individuals whose HLA phenotypes are listed would be called a three-antigen match or a three-antigen mismatch (see "Human Leukocyte Antigen Matches and Mismatches," below). Sharing of minor histocompatibility antigens is serendipitous.

Linkage Disequilibrium

Although it is not possible to identify an individual's haplotypes from the phenotypic HLA typing information alone, within racial or ethnic populations, certain HLA determinants are inherited together more often than would be expected by chance (e.g., HLA-A1, -B8, -DR17, and HLA-A2, -B44, -DR7 among whites). If the HLA antigens A1, B8, and DR17 were distributed randomly, the probability of finding them together would be much less than 1%; however, the HLA-A1,-B8, -DR17 combination is found in approximately 5% to 6% of whites, significantly above the predicted incidence. This phenomenon is known as linkage disequilibrium and represents the inheritance of haplotypes within racial groups.

Human Leukocyte Antigen Matches and Mismatches

It is not always possible to identify two HLA specificities at each HLA locus. Consider the HLA phenotypes for the following two unrelated individuals:

1. A2,—; B27, B13; DR17, DR4
2. A2, A3; B8, B14; DR17,—

The absence of the second A-locus antigen in individual 1 and the second DR-locus antigen in individual 2 could result from a failure to identify the second antigen. More often, it reflects the inheritance of the same antigen (A2 and DR17 in these cases) from both parents (the individuals are homozygous at these loci). Among whites, the latter is usually the case. A kidney transplanted between these two individuals would be described as a one A and one DR match, but this terminology does not take into account homozygosity in the A and DR loci of individuals 1 and 2, respectively. If individual 1 were a donor for individual 2, it would be more informative to describe the combination as a zero A, two B, and one DR mismatch. If individual 2 were a donor for individual 1, the combination would be a one A, two B, and zero DR mismatch. Antigenic differences in the donor kidney are potential targets of rejection; therefore, the convention of counting the number of donor HLA antigens that are *not* shared by the recipient provides an estimate of the antigen dose.

Identical and Fraternal Twins

The differentiation between identical twins and two-haplotype–matched fraternal twins is important because the recipient of a transplant from an identical twin requires no immunosuppression. The procedure is immunologically equivalent to an auto-transplantation. Two-haplotype–matched siblings, whether they are fraternal twins or not, differ in their minor histocompatibility antigens, and immunosuppression is required. Monozygotic, or identical, twins share a single placenta and amniotic sac at birth. However, such information may be unavailable or unreliable when the patient and donor are evaluated as adults. A variety of methods have been used to identify monozygotic twins, including skin grafting from the potential twin donor to the recipient (the graft would be rejected if the twins were fraternal). Today, several genetic polymorphisms can be exploited to determine identity at many genetic loci providing a high degree of confidence that twins are identical. Extended blood groups include markers that are determined by many genes on different chromosomes. Analysis of short tandem repeats (STRs), which, as the name implies, are short nucleotide sequences that are repeated a variable number of times, provide a high probability of identifying differences between individuals. STRs are often used in monitoring engraftment of HLA-identical bone marrow transplants, so they are exquisite markers of individuality.

TISSUE-TYPING TECHNIQUES

The Microcytotoxicity Test

The microcytotoxicity test developed by Terasaki and McClelland in 1964 was the international standard test for HLA typing for more than 30 years. This serologic test is performed in small plastic trays with a grid of small flat-bottomed wells, each of which contains 1 μL of a selected antiserum suspended in 5 μL of mineral oil to prevent drying. One microliter of a lymphocyte suspension (at a concentration of 2×10^5/mL) from the individual to be typed is added to each well, mixed, and incubated. Complement is added and after another incubation, a vital dye is added to indicate the proportion of dead cells in each well when examined under the microscope. Using the products of an immune response (antibodies) to measure the targets of an immune response (HLA antigens) has a certain inherent logic. If an antigen had provoked an antibody response, its immunologic importance was demonstrated. However, the HLA-typing antisera are seldom monospecific (i.e., they do not recognize a single private specificity), so in most cases it is necessary to examine the patterns of reactivity with several antibodies to determine the HLA type.

DNA Typing Methods

It is now more common to type individuals by DNA-based rather than serologic methods. Using the extensive DNA sequence data available, oligonucleotide primers and probes that specifically hybridize to sites that are unique to an HLA locus, allele, or group of alleles have been developed and are commercially available for HLA typing. Three basic methods used in conjunction with polymerase chain reaction (PCR) employ sequence-specific oligonucleotide probes (SSOPs), sequence-specific primers (SSPs), and sequencing-based typing (SBT). SSOP is based on first amplifying genomic DNA using locus- or group-specific primers and then detecting the hybridization of specific oligonucleotide probes tagged with enzymatic or fluorescent markers to the amplified product. In commercial kits, the process is often reversed, with the probes attached to mylar strips or to microparticles that can be hybridized with the labeled PCR product to produce a series of colored bands or fluorescent beads when hybridization occurs. The developed strips can be read manually or scanned, and the microparticles read on a flow cytometer. SSP depends on DNA amplification using group- or allele-specific primers and detecting an amplified product of the correct size by gel electrophoresis. The size is determined by running an agarose gel that separates the PCR products according to their size. SBT uses group-specific primers to sequence polymorphic regions of the gene, and alleles can be assigned based on the nucleotides identified at key positions in the sequence. Even with these molecular approaches to HLA typing, it is difficult to produce reagents that uniquely recognize each individual HLA antigen. As with serology, it is often necessary to identify patterns of primer and probe reactivity in order to determine the HLA type. Computer programs assist in the analysis of primer and probe patterns, which are more difficult to analyze unaided because of the added complexity of the HLA genes.

It is difficult to identify HLA alleles without performing sequence-based typing, because the differences between alleles may be determined by single nucleotide differences. However, SSP and SSOP can easily provide low or intermediate levels of typing, identifying the recognized HLA antigens and major allele groups, respectively. This level of typing is sufficient for renal transplantation in most cases.

DNA-based typing offers several advantages over serology, including greater accuracy and reproducibility of the reagents. Viable lymphocytes are not required. Typing can be performed on any tissue containing nucleated cells. Buccal swabs can provide sufficient DNA for tissue typing, and may be preferable to drawing blood from infants or from those who are squeamish about needles. Samples can be dried on filter paper and stored without refrigeration for extended periods. The oligonucleotide reagents are more easily standardized and controlled, and they can be synthesized when needed.

The accuracy of DNA typing is better than has been achieved using serology. The more difficult HLA specificities, those for which highly specific alloantiserum is rare or not widely available, can be accurately identified using DNA testing. For example, HLA-DR6 and its splits, -DR13 and -DR14, have been troublesome for many years because antisera could not be obtained. It is now known that HLA-DR6 is composed of at least 69 alleles of HLA-DR13 and HLA-DR14. Laboratories around the world generally have been successful in typing the DR13 and DR14 splits of DR6 by using DNA typing. For the most part, the concordance of DNA and serologic typing for HLA has been high for the broad specificities, but DNA is clearly the superior method.

ANTI-HUMAN LEUKOCYTE ANTIGEN ANTIBODIES

Patients who have circulating anti-HLA antibodies are at high risk of hyperacute rejection (the immediate and usually irreversible destruction of the transplanted kidney) or of accelerated acute rejection (an early and rapid antibody-mediated rejection that is not easily controlled with immunosuppression). The presence of preformed anti-HLA antibodies restricts the number of compatible donors for the sensitized patient to those who do not express the HLA antigens to which the patient is sensitized. Sensitized patients often must wait substantially longer for a crossmatch–compatible kidney. Evaluation of HLA antibodies in the serum of a transplant candidate is the transplant equivalent of ABO blood group typing for a blood transfusion. The consequence of proceeding with transplantation or transfusion with the presence of reactive antibody is similar. The former produces red blood cell lysis and a transfusion reaction, and the latter results in hyperacute rejection. Assiduous attention to pretransplant lymphocyte cross-matching has virtually eliminated hyperacute rejection as a clinical threat.

Origins of Alloantibodies

During pregnancy, the semi-allogeneic fetus develops and is tolerated within the mother for 9 months. At birth and during the pregnancy, the mother is exposed to paternal HLA antigens of the fetus and may become immunized and produce anti-HLA antibodies to the mismatched HLA antigens derived from the father. Sera from multiparous women were collected and screened against large panels of lymphocytes to identify HLA-typing reagents for the microcytotoxicity test. Among patients awaiting a kidney transplant, sensitization occurs in up to 25% of women with a history of pregnancy and is usually highest in those with multiple pregnancies. Exposure to allogeneic HLA antigens also occurs following blood or platelet transfusion and loss of an organ transplant, and anti-HLA antibodies can develop as a result of viral or bacterial infections.

The specificity of anti-HLA antibodies an individual produces upon exposure to allogeneic HLA molecules is influenced by the individual's immunologic history and by the individual's own HLA type. Antibodies are generally not produced against self HLA antigens. Anti-HLA antibodies can be directed against private specificities such as HLA-A1, or against public specificities such as Bw6. Antibodies to private specificities recognize an epitope that is unique to a particular HLA molecule or a limited group or family of closely related alleles, whereas antibodies

Table 3.2.   HLA antigen cross-reactive groups

A1C	A1 3 11 29 30 31 32 36 74 80
A2C1	A2 B17 57 58
A10C	A10 19 25 26 29 30 31 32 33 34 66 74
A9C	A2 9 23 24 28 68 69
A28C	A2 28 68 69
B5C	B5 18 35 37 51 52 53 58 78
B7C	B7 8 13 40 41 42 48 60 61 81
B8C	B8 14 16 18 38 39 64 65
B12C	B12 13 21 37 40 44 45 47 49 50 60 61
B21C	B5 15 17 21 49 50 51 52 53 57 58 62 63 70 71 72 73 75 76 77 78
B22C	B7 22 27 42 46 54 55 56 73 81 82
B27C	B7 13 27 40 41 42 47 60 61
Bw4	A9 23 24 25 32 B5 13 16 17 27 37 38 44 47 49 51 52 53 57 58 59 63 77
Bw6	B7 8 14 18 22 35 39 40 41 42 45 46 47 48 50 54 55 56 60 61 62 64 65 67 70 71 72 73 75 76 78 81

to public specificities recognize an epitope that is shared by more than one HLA molecule. Public epitopes are responsible for cross-reactivity observed in HLA alloantiserum. HLA antigens that share epitopes can be grouped into the major cross-reactive groups (CREGs) listed in Table 3.2.

Measurement of Anti-Human Leukocyte Antigen Antibodies

The first cross-match results were reported by Patel and Terasaki in 1968, and showed that among 30 patients transplanted with a positive cytotoxicity cross-match, 24 suffered hyperacute rejection and 3 others lost their grafts within the first 3 months. As a result of these convincing results, all patients now undergo a cross-match test prior to transplantation. In the same article, the authors reported that patients could be screened beforehand against a panel of normal individuals representative of the local donor pool. Patients who had no positive tests against the panel had a very low incidence of hyperacute rejection. Thus, patients could be screened in advance of a final cross-match to determine whether they had antibodies against a panel of donors and the result would provide an estimate of how often the patient would have a positive cross-match against donors who became available.

The screening process must ensure a true negative cross-match with the intended donor by accounting for all relevant antibodies and avoiding a false-positive cross-match with clinically irrelevant antibodies. Information from anti-HLA antibody testing is used to (a) predict the likelihood of finding a cross-match-compatible donor; (b) avoid transplantation with a donor carrying HLA antigens to which the patient is sensitized; (c) select the optimal cross-match method to ensure maximum sensitivity for antibody detection; and (d) avoid a false-positive cross-match with a donor by excluding clinically irrelevant antibodies.

Isolation of Lymphocytes

Lymphocytes are the best target for detecting antidonor HLA antibodies and donor lymphocytes are required for final cross-matches. Panels of local donor lymphocytes are also used for screening patients' sera, although alternative methods are available. Immunomagnetic beads coated with monoclonal antibodies provide the simplest method for the selective separation of lymphocytes from whole blood or a suspension of mononuclear cells. Anti–T-cell or anti–B-cell monoclonal antibodies are used to coat the immunomagnetic beads. When mixed with a blood sample, the target cells adhere to the beads, and after placing the tube against a magnet to hold the beads in place, the remaining cells in the supernatant may be removed to another tube or discarded. The target cells may be used on the beads.

Another simple method for cell isolation uses a monoclonal antibody-complement cocktail. The reagent contains complement, a density gradient medium, and monoclonal antibodies against the cells that are to be eliminated from the suspension. When buffy coat cells are added to the mixture and incubated, red blood cells, granulocytes, and platelets are lysed. After centrifugation, purified lymphocytes are deposited on the bottom of the tube, and the fragments of the other cells remain in the supernatant. The main advantage of this technique is that the isolation of lymphocytes takes place in one tube, eliminating the possibility of switching samples.

Cytotoxicity

The complement-dependent lymphocytotoxicity (CDC) assay is the most common method for anti-HLA antibody screening. The patient's serum is incubated separately with B cells and T cells from a panel of donors selected to represent the HLA antigens commonly found in the local population. Complement is added and cell lysis detected, as noted previously. Prolonging the complement incubation time increases the sensitivity of the test and enhances the detection of low-titer antibodies. The results are usually expressed as the percentage of panel cells that are killed by the serum. The anti-HLA antibodies that are detected are called panel-reactive antibody (PRA). Thus, on a 50-cell panel, a positive reaction against 30 donors represents a PRA of 60%. Simplistically, the finding of 60% PRA on the T-cell panel suggests that 60% of donors will be unacceptable for the patient because there are circulating antibodies that react with one or more of the donors' HLA antigens.

Immunoglobulin (Ig) G antibodies reactive to HLA class I antigens (found on both T and B cells) are the most important. These antibodies react with T cells at $37°C$ ($98.6°F$) (and are sometimes called T warm antibodies). The importance of anti-DR and DQ antibodies (reactive to B cells) remained unclear for a long time. However, there is a large body of evidence showing that both antibodies directed against HLA class I and class II antigens pose significant risks to transplant outcome. There are several reports of hyperacute and accelerated rejection caused by anti-DR or anti-DQ antibodies.

IgM antibody is characterized by reactivity at $4°C$ $(39.2°F)$ and its activity can be removed by heating the serum to $55°C$ $(131°F)$ or by treatment with a reducing agent, such as dithiothreitol (DTT). IgM antibody is often autoantibody and is commonly detected in the sera of patients with autoimmune disorders such as systemic lupus erythematosus. IgM antibodies can usually be ignored.

More Sensitive Tests for Measuring Human Leukocyte Antigen Antibodies

The CDC assay typically detects high-affinity antibodies that efficiently activate complement. Many of the public antibodies that are typically present in the sera of highly sensitized patients cannot be detected by the standard CDC assay. Antibodies to CREGs often exhibit a cytotoxicity-negative, adsorption-positive reactivity as they bind to lymphocytes, but do not always fix complement and hence are not cytotoxic. Many anti-CREG antibodies appear to react with a private HLA specificity when tested in a standard cytotoxicity assay. However, when tested with a more sensitive technique such as antiglobulin, enzyme-linked immunoabsorbent assay (ELISA), or flow cytometry, reactivity toward the associated CREG specificity becomes apparent. These augmented screening tests are summarized below.

Antihuman Globulin

The cytotoxicity test can be enhanced by adding antihuman globulin (AHG) to the microcytotoxicity plate after adding the patient's serum and before addition of complement. AHG promotes complement fixation by cross-linking bound HLA antibody. The AHG test is more sensitive than the standard CDC test and detects lower titer and noncytotoxic antibodies. The AHG reagent must be standardized using sera known to have noncytotoxic anti-HLA antibodies because its titer and specificity may vary.

Enzyme-Linked Immunosorbent Assay

ELISA uses solubilized or purified class I and class II HLA antigens (pooled from a panel of many donors) that have been chemically attached to a test plate. Patient serum is added, followed by an enzyme-labeled second antibody reactive to human IgG. The reaction is measured in an ELISA reader. Interpretation of the test results is based on comparisons of optical-density measurements of test wells to those of positive and negative antigen wells. Neither viable lymphocytes nor complement fixation is required, and the assay is not confounded by interference from cytotoxic drugs such as antithymocyte globulin or muronomab OKT3. The presence or absence of anti-HLA antibodies can be readily detected using pooled soluble antigens, which is a low cost, rapid assay for the detection of antibody. Targeted HLA specificities can further be determined using a panel of HLA antigens from individual donors plated in separate wells on the test plate. Innovations of this technique that use purified HLA antigens have improved identification of class I and class II specificities.

Flow Cytometry

Flow cytometry is the most sensitive antibody assay. To determine PRA, a mixture of target cells composed of lymphocytes from five to ten donors is used. Target cell mixtures are selected to represent CREGs and DR antigens. The patient's serum is mixed with target cells; the cells are washed and then incubated with monoclonal mouse anti-CD3 (a pan T-cell marker) antibody conjugated with phycoerythrin and an antihuman IgG antibody conjugated with fluorescein. The T cells that stain red can be gated using a flow cytometer, making the amount of green fluorescence proportional to the concentration of anti-T-cell antibodies present in the serum. Alternatively, microparticles coated with purified HLA class I or class II antigens can be used as antibody targets. These microparticle tests offer the advantage of purified target antigens and may be prepared from individual donors to allow antibody specificities to be determined. Recently, recombinant HLA class I molecules representing single HLA antigens have been produced and coupled to microspheres for antibody detection. The use of recombinant HLA molecules provides a powerful tool to assess the presence or absence of specific antidonor HLA antibodies in the patient's serum and assist in the analysis of anti-HLA antibodies in the highly sensitized patient.

Determination of the Specificity of Antihuman Leukocyte Antigen Antibodies

It is often possible to determine the HLA target specificities (a list of HLA antigens that react with the patient's serum) by analyzing reaction patterns against the HLA types of the panel donors. Determination of antibody specificity is based on a statistically significant correlation between the pattern of serum reactivity and the pattern of a particular HLA antigen in the panel. Precise definition of antibody specificity may be affected by the presence of multiple antibodies or the panel size and composition of the panel phenotypes. When multiple antibodies are present in a serum, antibodies to more frequent HLA antigens may mask the recognition of antibodies to less-frequent antigens. This problem is reduced by using large panels of target cells or by using recombinant HLA antigens. Testing sera at multiple dilutions can also aid in determining antibody specificities because it is common for the different antibodies to have distinct titers. The specific HLA antigens to which a patient has made antibodies is important information. If a patient has a clearly defined antibody to HLA-A1, potential donors expressing HLA-A1 would not be acceptable without intervention (see "Desensitizing the Sensitized Patient," below).

Pretransplant Cross-Match

The cross-match test is the final pretransplant immunologic screening step. Using the previously described HLA antibody screening assays, the potential donor's lymphocytes serve as the target cells for the patient's serum. The presence of cytotoxic IgG antidonor HLA antibodies is a strong contraindication to transplantation. Most transplant centers use the more sensitive AHG augmentation or flow cytometry, in addition to the cytotoxicity test, to detect even low levels of historical antibody. ELISA tests using isolating donor antigens have yet to gain widespread acceptance.

Patients with high PRA have accumulated on waiting lists because of the difficulty in finding suitable cross-match-negative donors. To expedite the cross-match procedure, screening tray sets with recent serum samples from sensitized patients are prepared either quarterly or monthly. Separate tray sets are made for patients with blood groups A or AB, B, and O and a "preliminary" cross-match is performed by testing donor cells on the appropriate tray set at the time of donor HLA typing. Sensitized patients with a positive cross-match are excluded, but those with a negative preliminary cross-match and 80% or more PRA receive special consideration in the ranking of candidates (see "Allocation of Deceased Donor Kidneys in the United States"). When the preliminary cross-match is negative, a final cross-match using either AHG or flow cytometry is performed with recent or fresh sera. When sera from waiting patients are collected monthly and are available in the laboratory, a final cross-match can usually be performed without obtaining a fresh sample from the patient. This allows the laboratory to perform final cross-matches for a deceased donor kidney before organ procurement in most cases, avoiding delays in transplantation. Some centers allow older sera to be used if the patient is not sensitized and has not received a recent blood transfusion.

IgM autoantibodies can cause false-positive lymphocytotoxic cross-match test results. The most straightforward approach to detecting autoantibodies is the autocross-match. Adsorption of the antibody on autologous cells can remove the antibody and render the serum negative. Alternatively, DTT is used to eliminate IgM autoantibodies. If the serum contains a mixture of auto- and alloantibodies of the IgG isotypes, autoadsorption would be required to remove the autoantibody and leave behind the alloantibody. When the autoantibody is of the IgM isotype, the IgG alloantibody would remain even after DTT treatment. A serum that reacts with lymphocytes, but not with purified HLA class I and/or class II antigens (as detected by flow cytometry or ELISA) is also suggestive of autoantibodies. Sera from patients with demonstrated IgM autoantibodies should be heated or treated with DTT to eliminate IgM before the final cross-match to avoid a false-positive result. Not all IgM antibodies are benign. IgM antibodies with anti-HLA specificity are associated with hyperacute or accelerated rejections in isolated cases. Thus, the patient's antibody profile should be thoroughly evaluated before transplantation. When testing is performed by flow cytometry, the specificity of the second antibody can be used to determine the antibody class. Typically, these tests employ antihuman IgG antibody; therefore, IgM reactions are not detected.

Flow Cytometry Cross-Match

The flow cytometry cross-match test (FCXM) is a very sensitive cross-match test. Although a positive lymphocytotoxic cross-match is a contraindication to kidney transplantation, the place of the flow cytometry cross-match is still somewhat controversial. The test can detect very low levels of circulating antibodies. Positive flow cytometry cross-matches are associated with a higher rate of early acute rejection episodes and a lower 1-year graft survival rate. Hyperacute rejection has not been reported, however, and some transplants across a positive FCXM have no early problems (if the cytotoxic cross-match is negative). The T-cell FCXM is particularly useful for sensitized and retransplant candidates whose antibody levels may have fallen but who can mount a rapid memory response upon challenge. Low levels of circulating antibody have a more profound effect when the cadaver donor is older or the kidney quality is uncertain. The potential for false-positive reactions is responsible for much of the uncertainty about the role of the flow cytometry cross-match. Positive, particularly weakly positive, flow cross-match results should be supported by the patient's sensitization history or be consistent with a determination that the patient has anti-HLA antibodies. When the flow cross-match detects antidonor HLA antibodies, there is a substantial risk for adverse outcomes after transplantation.

Desensitizing the Sensitized Patient

More than 25% of renal transplant candidates are highly sensitized. Two approaches based on the use of intravenous immune globulin (IVIG) are currently used to reduce HLA allosensitization and facilitate transplantation of highly sensitized patients. The first therapy is based on infusion of high-dose IVIG (2 g/kg), which has been demonstrated to be a potent inhibitor of anti-HLA antibodies and to permit transplantation with minimal risk of rejection. IVIG can also be used as therapy in the treatment of patients experiencing humoral rejection (see Chapter 4, Part IV). There are several proposed mechanisms of action of high dose IVIG in highly sensitized patients, including inhibition of anti-HLA antibody in an idiotypic manner, elimination of HLA-reactive T and B cells, inhibition of cytokines involved in immunoglobulin synthesis, and blockade of T-cell activation (see Table 4.6).

A second approach uses a combined regimen of cytomegalovirus (CMV)-IVIG therapy and plasmapheresis. Plasmapheresis rapidly depletes donor-specific antibody and administration of CMV-IVIG blocks resynthesis of anti-HLA antibodies. Treatment is continued until donor-specific anti-HLA antibodies are no longer detected in the patient's serum. CMV-IVIG and plasmapheresis is also effective in reducing HLA allosensitization in highly sensitized patients and is a successful therapy for the treatment of humoral rejection. Combined plasmapheresis and IVIG is also reportedly effective in removing anti-A or anti-B isoagglutinins before successful transplantation across ABO blood group barriers. The precise immunomodulatory mechanisms of the combined therapy are unknown, but appear to function in a long-term, donor-specific manner.

IMMUNE MONITORING

Current methods used to diagnose renal allograft rejection depend on changes in blood chemistry markers, such as creatinine levels or blood urea nitrogen (BUN). However, these markers are, at best, surrogate markers for rejection, and clearly rejection must precede the deterioration in graft function. Although diagnosis of rejection by histopathologic examination of renal biopsies remains the gold standard (see Chapter 13), there is a need for a less-invasive approach for the early detection of immunologic events leading to rejection. A promising area in the study of renal allograft rejection is the identification of biomarkers of immune alloreactivity to the graft. Monitoring the immune response to the allograft will permit the early identification of patients at risk of rejection and graft loss, optimization of drug regimens, monitoring responses to therapy following intervention, and to guide the development of new immunosuppressive therapies. Immune monitoring might aid in differentiating rejection from other forms of graft dysfunction such as primary nonfunction and drug toxicity. The potential of this approach to reduce the cost associated with graft rejection while maximizing patient and graft survival is tremendous. The following outlines some of the common and newly developed cellular and humoral assays to assess the immune status of the transplant recipient.

Monitoring Anti-Human Leukocyte Antigen Antibodies After Transplantation

Acute humoral rejection occurs during the early posttransplant period and can lead to rapid deterioration of graft function (see Chapter 8). The primary histopathologic feature is the deposition of complement in the graft as measured by C4d immunostaining (see Chapter 13). Humoral rejection may also play a role in chronic rejection. Studies show that patients developing anti-HLA antibodies after transplantation are at high risk of both acute and chronic rejection and graft loss. The development of donor-specific anti-HLA antibodies to class I and/or class II antigens following renal transplantation strongly correlates with C4d deposition in the graft and appears to be a specific marker of antibody-dependent vascular injury. Anti-HLA antibody production may also predict chronic allograft rejection. Immune monitoring of anti-HLA antibodies can be used to guide immunotherapy and permit early intervention.

The methods and approaches for the detection of anti-HLA antibodies are identical to those used in pretransplant evaluation. Detection of anti-HLA antibodies by complement-dependent lymphocytotoxicity has the benefit of being a functional test and antibodies that fix complement are clearly detrimental to the graft. However, the more recently developed solid-phase flow cytometry and ELISA tests using purified HLA antigen are more useful for posttransplant monitoring because they are more sensitive and can identify the isotype and specificity of the anti-HLA antibody. Alternatively, the production of anti-HLA antibodies can be monitored by directly cross-matching recipient sera with donor lymphocytes using complement-dependent lymphocytotoxicity and flow cytometry methods.

Cellular Tests

The mechanisms underlying allograft rejection are not completely understood, although it has become increasingly clear that recipient T cells become activated upon direct recognition of HLA/peptide complexes present on the membrane of passenger dendritic cells of donor origin. This vigorous response, which appears to violate the rule of self–MHC restriction, is driven primarily by antigenic mimicry. T cells activated via the direct recognition pathway are thought to be important for initiation of early acute rejection. However, these directly activated T cells seem to play a less-important role following the departure of donor dendritic cells from the graft, because upon recognition of donor HLA molecules on "nonprofessional" antigen-presenting cells (APCs) that lack costimulatory elements, they may become anergized. Several recent studies indicate that the indirect recognition pathway, which is stimulated by allopeptides presented by professional APCs of host origin, is a major contributor to rejection, especially chronic rejection. T-helper cells engaged in the direct and indirect pathway provide lymphokines required for the proliferation and maturation of cytotoxic T cells and of anti-HLA antibody-producing B cells. The T-helper cells may also produce cytokines, invoking a delayed-type hypersensitivity response. The direct recognition pathway is thought to be the primary mediator of acute allograft rejection and can be measured *in vitro* by the strength of the antidonor mixed lymphocyte culture (MLC) assay and cell-mediated lympholysis (CML) reactivity exhibited by recipient T cells.

Cell-Mediated Lympholysis and Mixed Lymphocyte Culture Assays

The CML assay measures the cytotoxic T-cell reactivity to mismatched HLA class I antigens of the donor. The MLC assay measures the capacity of recipient leukocytes to respond to HLA class II differences expressed by donor leukocytes. The degree of T-cell proliferation when leukocytes from the recipient are cocultured with irradiated leukocytes from the donor represents a functional measure of the degree of histocompatibility differences between individuals. T-cell proliferation or cell division is measured by incorporation of radioactive thymidine into proliferating cells. Alternatively, cell division can be followed using a novel flow cytometric assay that uses the intracellular fluorescent label carboxyfluorescein diacetate succinimidyl ester (CSFE) to tag proliferating cells. The intensity of the CSFE tag is reduced at each cell division, thereby permitting the extrapolation of the number of cells responding to an antigen. Another approach for determining cell activation and proliferation involves the measurement of the nucleotide adenosine triphosphate (ATP). The cell produces ATP during activation with a mitogen or specific antigen and the quantity is directly related to the strength of the immune response. ATP is measured by addition of firefly luciferase and luciferin in the presence of magnesium ions.

Traditionally, the CML and MLC tests were used in the pretransplant evaluation of donor–recipient pairs. More recently, these tests have been used in the posttransplant setting to identify patients who are hyporesponsive and who display decreased alloresponses to the donor. Donor antigen-specific hyporesponsiveness, defined as a significantly lower MLC or CML between the recipient and donor after transplantation, has been observed in recipients of kidney, heart, lung, and liver transplants. Several studies report that the hyporesponsive state is associated with a lower incidence of chronic rejection and improved graft outcome. However, not all investigations confirm this finding and variation may be explained by differences in the techniques used and interpretation of test results. For instance, the CML assay primarily measures class I alloreactivity via the direct pathway, whereas the MLC test recognizes class II differences between the recipient and donor by both the direct and indirect recognition pathways.

Precursor Frequency Analysis

The indirect recognition allorecognition pathway is thought to play an important role in mediating chronic allograft rejection. Patients who are at risk of chronic rejection of heart, renal, lung, and liver allografts can be identified by an increased capacity for indirect recognition of donor HLA allopeptides. Persistent allopeptide reactivity and epitope spreading are both characteristic of chronic allograft rejection. The precursor frequency of alloreactive T cells recognizing mismatched donor MHC, measured by limiting dilution analysis, provides a means of assessing the indirect pathway. T-cell precursor frequency can also be measured by an enzyme-linked immunosorbent spot assay (ELISPOT), which has the advantage of detecting cytokine-secreting antigen-specific cells. In the ELISPOT assay, tissue culture plates are coated with antibodies specific for the cytokine of interest and cells, together with antigen, are added to the plates. Cytokines produced by the antigen-specific cells are detected using a secondary reporter antibody. Cytokine-secreting cells are enumerated using an automated computer-assisted image analyzer. Alternatively, cytokine-secreting antigen-specific T cells can be detected using flow cytometry. Following activation, the secreted cytokines are captured onto the surface of the cell and enumerated using an anticytokine antibody conjugated with a fluorescent dye. Both the ELISPOT and flow assays are up to 400-fold more sensitive than the detection of cytokines in supernatants and can detect antigen-specific cells at the single-cell level.

Tetramers

Antigen-specific T cells can also be detected using HLA class I and class II tetramers. The HLA tetramer is created by generating recombinant HLA class I or class II molecules that are folded together with antigenic peptides to form monomers conjugated with biotin. The monomers are assembled into tetramers by adding avidin conjugated with a fluorochrome. Antigen-specific T cells can be detected at a frequency of 10^{-4} to 10^{-5} and tetramers have been used to monitor immunity to infectious agents, vaccines, autoantigens, and tumors by flow cytometry. Their potential use in monitoring alloimmune responses is currently unknown and may be hindered by the numerous peptides typically presented by MHC molecules.

Cellular assays have been used to detect alloantigen-specific T cells both in the peripheral blood and in the allograft. Characterization of graft-infiltrating cells identifies populations of cells that are likely participating in pathological processes such as transplant rejection. The ability to detect interleukin (IL)-2+ T cells in graft infiltrates correlates with both acute and chronic rejection. The disadvantage of this approach is that it involves obtaining a biopsy sample, which is an invasive procedure and clearly not suitable for routine monitoring.

In addition to identifying patients at risk of rejection, the cellular assays described above may be useful for monitoring the effectiveness of immunosuppressive agents and for identifying patients who can successfully undergo withdrawal of immunosuppressive drugs. Currently, immunosuppressive drugs are administered based on body weight and drug dose is monitored using biochemical assays. Unfortunately, these biochemical assays do not provide an indication of the effectiveness of the drug regimen on immune function. Because the major immunosuppressive agents used inhibit calcineurin, a key enzyme involved in T-cell activation, assays quantitating mitogen or antigen-specific T-cell activation in the peripheral blood of transplant recipients have the potential to evaluate the effectiveness of an immunosuppressive regimen. Monitoring studies will also permit real-time analysis of the immune response to changes in therapy, ultimately offering individualized therapy.

Gene Expression Assays

Technological advances in the field of molecular genetics allow measurement of the expression of immune activation and effector molecules involved in transplant rejection. Perforin and granzyme B, the cytotoxic T-lymphocyte effector molecules, are upregulated in the blood, urine, and graft of patients undergoing acute renal allograft rejection and serve as useful diagnostic markers. Increased expression of chemokines, cytokines, and/or HLA class II genes can also serve as sensitive and differential markers of rejection. Rapid measurement of gene expression by real-time PCR provides an accurate assessment of ribonucleic acid (RNA) levels in recipient blood or the donor allograft that can be used to diagnose rejection in the clinical setting. The main limitation of monitoring expression of immune activation genes for diagnosis of rejection is that these same markers can also be elevated during viral and bacterial infections.

DNA microarrays have also been used to provide global insights into the mechanisms of allograft dysfunction and rejection. Although the cost of this technology precludes it from being used as a monitoring tool, genome-wide analysis by microarrays has the potential to identify novel surrogate markers of graft rejection that can be validated in a larger number of clinical samples using real-time PCR.

The immune response to the transplant is dynamic and it is unlikely that one single assay will accurately assess the immune status of the patient. It is likely that a panel of assays will be used to monitor different components of the immune response (humoral and cellular) to provide an accurate profile of the patient.

IMMUNOLOGIC EVALUATION OF TRANSPLANTATION CANDIDATES

Candidates for renal transplantation today fall into one of two categories: those with a potential living donor and those without. Figure 3.2 outlines the initial immunologic evaluation of these candidates. Once a patient is identified as a suitable candidate for transplantation, HLA typing and antibody-screening tests are performed using the tests outlined above. The HLA type permits assessment of donor and potential recipient pairs

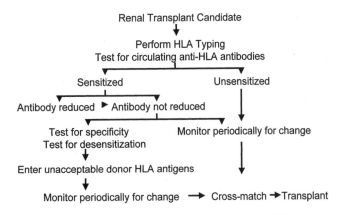

Fig. 3.2. Strategy for immune monitoring of patients waiting for transplantation.

for degree of histocompatibility, as well as evaluation of sensitization and cross-match results. In the case of sibling donors, the HLA-identical sibling kidney provides superior long-term graft survival and less immunosuppression is needed. The HLA-A, -B, and -DR types are required to list a patient as a candidate for a deceased donor kidney with the national Organ Procurement and Transplantation Network (OPTN), which is currently maintained by the United Network for Organ Sharing (UNOS). The sensitization status of the patient is also determined prior to transplantation to identify those patients who are at risk for hyperacute or accelerated acute rejection. The patient's PRA level is another important element in listing a renal candidate with UNOS, because patients with a PRA greater than 20% receive special ranking in organ allocation. A panel screening by cytotoxicity should be followed by a more sensitive test to identify unsensitized patients. Autoantibodies and other antibodies that do not pose a significant risk of hyperacute or accelerated rejection should be identified before transplantation, and for those without a living donor, these antibodies should be characterized before a deceased donor kidney is offered. Thus, patients with IgM antibodies should be identified and retested after reduction. When the PRA is less than 75%, there is a reasonable chance that specific antibodies can be identified either through analysis of the panel types or by using a microparticle test with coupled HLA antigens. For patients who will wait for a deceased donor kidney or when the living donor transplant will be delayed, it is necessary to monitor changes in patterns of sensitization and reevaluate patients periodically to keep abreast of their current sensitization status.

Patients with a suitable living donor can proceed to a preliminary cross-match against their donor(s) and, if negative, can be transplanted. When there are multiple potential donors, the evaluation of each donor can be tailored to determine whether antibodies are directed against the specific mismatched donor HLA antigens, and whether desensitization procedures could permit successful transplantation with one or more potential donors. For patients without a living donor, it is important to investigate and characterize sensitization early in the process, before a deceased donor kidney is offered.

The Role of ABO Blood Groups in Transplantation

The ABO blood group antigens behave as strong transplantation antigens, and transplantation across ABO barriers usually leads to irreversible hyperacute rejection. In principle, the same criteria determine kidney distribution according to ABO as do blood transfusions with group O (the universal donor) and group AB (the universal recipient). The disproportionate percentage of waiting patients who are type O or type B generally mandates that blood group identity rather than blood group compatibility determines the distribution of deceased donor kidneys. Exceptions are made for blood group AB patients who may be offered A or AB kidneys, and for zero-HLA antigen mismatched kidneys, which can be offered to an ABO-compatible recipient if an ABO-identical recipient is not available. For living-related donor transplantation, ABO compatibility is adequate.

Attempts have been made to overcome blood group barriers when there is a willing ABO-incompatible living donor by removing blood group isoagglutinins with plasmapheresis or immunoabsorption, often in conjunction with splenectomy. ABO-incompatible transplantations have now been performed successfully at many centers, with the largest experience in Japan and Korea, where deceased donor transplantation is not well established (see Chapter 5). Exchange programs are also being testing at several transplant programs, allowing paired exchanges between unrelated individuals who are both incompatible with their intended recipients but reciprocally compatible with the patient from the other pair.

In white populations, approximately 20% of blood group A individuals can be defined as A_2; these patients have reduced levels of A antigen on graft endothelium. They may permit an exception to the ABO-incompatibility barrier because A_2 kidneys can be safely transplanted into O or B recipients with low preoperative titers of isoagglutinin. Transplantation of A_2 kidneys into O or B recipients is routine in some centers.

Table 3.3 lists the distribution of the major ABO groups among deceased donors and different ethnic groups of potential kidney transplant recipients. If all ethnic groups contributed equally to the donor pool and all ethnic groups suffered end-stage renal disease in direct proportion to their representation in the general population, waiting times for the different ethnic groups and blood group categories would be the same. In fact, whites contribute disproportionately to the donor pool and blacks contribute disproportionately to the recipient pool because kidney disease is more common in blacks. As a result, patients with blood group O or B wait longer for a blood group-identical donor.

Role of Human Leukocyte Antigen Matching in Transplantation

The HLA antigens are strong transplant antigens that may engage large numbers of T cells (estimates of up to 100 times as many T cells as nominal protein antigens have been reported).

Table 3.3.   Percent distribution of ABO blood groups among kidney donors and according to ethnicity on the transplant waiting list

Blood Group	Donors	White	Black	Asian	Waiting List[a]
O	47	50	53	44	53
A	38	34	22	23	28
B	11	13	22	27	17
AB	4	3	3	5	3
n	5,630	21,916	19,586	3,365	54,919

[a] Waiting list including all ethnicities was compiled by the United Network for Organ Sharing research department as of June 13, 2003.

Secondary responses to HLA antigens may occur as a consequence of prior exposures to allogeneic HLA through pregnancy, blood transfusion, or previous transplantation. Despite remarkable improvements in immunosuppression during the past 20 years, the difference in 10-year graft survival rates between recipients of deceased donor kidneys with no HLA-A, -B, or -DR antigens mismatched and recipients of completely mismatched grafts is approximately 18%. The effect of HLA matching is illustrated in Fig. 3.3, which shows data from the University of California at Los Angeles (UCLA) Transplant Registry for U.S. transplants performed between 1978 and 1984 (before the introduction of cyclosporine) and data from the UNOS Scientific Renal Transplant Registry for U.S. transplants performed between 1995 and 2000.

Among recipients of living donor transplants, however, the effect of HLA matching on long-term graft survival differs from the effect on deceased donor transplants as shown in Fig. 3.4. Although transplants between HLA-identical siblings provide the best long-term success rates (79% of these grafts will still survive at 10 years), the number of HLA antigen mismatches has little effect on the survival of mismatched grafts. Surprisingly, kidneys from genetically unrelated donors have had nearly the same long-term graft survival rates as grafts between one haplotype-matched siblings or parents and their offspring (approximately 64% at 10 years). This observation has fueled a rapid increase in the number of unconventional living donor transplants during the past decade, so that now there are more living than deceased kidney donors in the United States. The results of living donor transplants are superior to those of deceased donor transplants, even for recipients of HLA-matched kidneys (Fig. 3.4).

Reduction of the number of potential targets for rejection reactions should lead to fewer rejection episodes, regardless of the immunosuppression. This expectation is supported by the data shown in Fig. 3.5. Whether the donor is a relative or an unrelated individual, the incidence of early rejection episodes increases with each additional HLA antigen mismatched between the donor and recipient. However, it is difficult to find HLA-matched kidney donors outside the patient's immediate family. Recognition of the special immunologic status of HLA-matched transplants has led to the development of a national organ distribution for the sharing

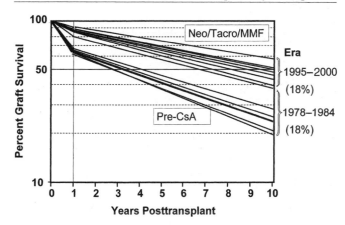

Fig. 3.3. Impact of HLA matching on long-term graft survival among recipients of deceased donor transplants reported to the UCLA Transplant Registry between 1978 and 1984 and to the OPTN/UNOS Registry between 1995 and 2000. The survival curves show an orderly decrease in graft survival rates from zero to six HLA-A, -B, and -DR mismatches between the donor and recipient during the precyclosporine (*Pre-CsA*) era and during the era of more modern immunosuppression with Neoral (*Neo*), tacrolimus (*Tacro*), and CellCept (*MMF*). Ten years after transplantation, the graft survival rates comparing recipients with HLA-matched grafts to patients with completely HLA-mismatched grafts differed by 18% in each era. (The 10-year graft survival rates for the more recent era were projected assuming a constant rate of graft loss after the first year.)

of donor kidneys for HLA-matched recipients. Initially, mandatory sharing was limited to patients who matched the donor at all six HLA-A, -B, and -DR antigens. Only approximately 3% of patients received a six-antigen-matched graft under these stringent criteria. The rules were relaxed in 1990 to allow sharing for homozygous donors and recipients. The proportion of HLA-matched transplants increased to approximately 8% with the relaxed criteria. In 1995, an HLA-matched kidney was defined as one with no HLA antigens that were not in common with the recipient (no mismatch). This new definition meant that homozygous donors would be allocated to heterozygous recipients and the proportion of matched grafts increased to approximately 17% of deceased donor transplants. To achieve this level of matching, each donor's HLA type is compared with those of all waiting patients in the United States (approximately 60,000 at the beginning of the year 2004).

Antigens are considered as "matches" using definitions that take into account the capability of HLA laboratories to distinguish one antigen from another. For example, a donor's HLA-B14 antigen would match a recipient typed as B14 or B64 or B65 (splits of B14). A donor with HLA-DR16 would match a recipient with DR2, DR15, or DR16. These equivalences are based on laboratories reaching greater than 90% consensus in their ability to type the "split" antigens. So far, there is no evidence

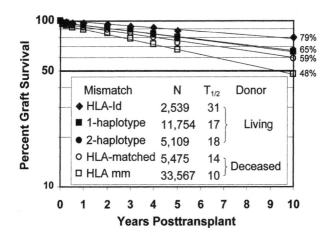

Fig. 3.4. Projected 10-year graft survival rates for recipients of living donor kidney transplants according to the HLA-haplotype match. HLA-identical sibling kidneys have the highest 10-year graft survival rate (79%) and half-life (31 years) followed by living donor kidneys mismatched for one or two HLA haplotypes. Even poorly matched kidneys from living donors have better 10-year graft survival rates than HLA-matched or HLA-mismatched deceased donor kidneys. The graft half-life is the number of years before half of the grafts that survive at 1 year will fail or the patient will die with a functioning graft. The half-life was used to estimate 10-year graft survival rates. mm, Mismatched; N, number; $T_{1/2}$, half-life. (Data are from the OPTN/UNOS Registry for living donor transplants performed between 1996 and 2001.)

that marked improvements in graft survival could be achieved by matching kidneys at the allele level. In fact, many recipients with HLA-mismatched kidney grafts continue to have good function many years after transplantation, suggesting that some HLA mismatches may be more deleterious than others. If those combinations could be identified, it would reduce the number of HLA specificities that should be matched for organ sharing. A recent trial of matching for CREGs suggests that donors and patients matched for these antigen groups may benefit from better graft survival and have fewer positive cross-matches.

ALLOCATION OF DECEASED DONOR KIDNEYS IN THE UNITED STATES

The establishment of the OPTN through the National Organ Transplant Act of 1984 (see Chapter 17) required the development of uniform national policies to describe how organs from deceased donors would be distributed to recipients. This was to insure that patients awaiting a transplant anywhere in the United States would be transplanted in an established order. To operate this system, the country is divided into organ procurement regions and areas (Fig. 3.6), with regional organ procurement

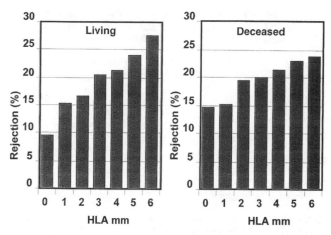

Fig. 3.5. The relationship between HLA-A, -B, and -DR mismatches between the kidney donor and recipient on early treated rejection episodes (within the first 6 months after transplantation). Recipients of living donor grafts are shown at the left and recipients of deceased donor grafts on the right. mm = Mismatched. (Data are from the OPTN/UNOS Registry for first transplants performed between 1996 and 2002.)

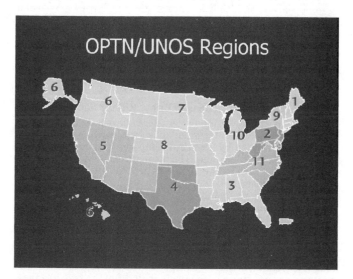

Fig. 3.6. United Network for Organ Sharing (UNOS) regions of the United States.

Table 3.4.   United Network for Organ Sharing (UNOS) point system for allocation of deceased donor kidneys as of June 2003

Factor	Points	Condition
Time waiting[a]	1	each year of waiting time
Quality of HLA match		0-A, B, DR mismatch[b]
	2	0 DR mismatch
	1	1 DR mismatch
Panel-reactive antibody	4	>80% PRA and negative crossmatch
Pediatric recipient	4	age <11 yr
	3	ages 11–17 yr
Organ donor[c]	4	
Expanded criteria donor		longest waiting patient[d]

[a]Defined from the time a patient is activated on the UNOS computer. In the event of a total point tie the longest waiting patient is allocated the kidney.
[b]All 0-A, B, DR mismatched organs are involved in the national mandatory sharing program.
[c]Previous living donor in need of a kidney transplant.
[d]See text.

organizations (OPOs) operating according to agreed upon distribution and sharing criteria. To be placed on the transplant waiting list, a patient must fulfill certain listing criteria (see Chapter 6). Renal transplant recipients must either be receiving chronic dialysis or, if they are not on dialysis, have a glomerular filtration rate estimated at 20 mL per minute or less. No priority is given for specific disease states, although many diabetics are now listed for a kidney and pancreas and receive transplants more quickly (see Chapter 14). The distribution of kidneys by the OPOs to patients on the waiting list is discussed next.

The Point System for Deceased Donor Kidney Allocation

The order in which waiting patients are offered each kidney that becomes available is determined by a set algorithm and waiting patients are ranked by a central computer that currently is located in Richmond, Virginia. The ultimate decision as to whether or not to accept an offer for a given patient falls to the responsible physician or surgeon; however, whenever an offer is declined, a reason must be provided to UNOS. Table 3.4 shows the point system used to rank waiting patients. The patient's rank within each blood group is determined by the time the patient has been waiting and the quality of HLA match with the donor, with additional points awarded to sensitized patients who have a negative crossmatch, children, and anyone who has previously donated an organ and now requires a kidney transplant. The point system has been adjusted several times based upon analyses of the transplant results reported to UNOS. A key change to the allocation scheme was made early in 1990, when it was noted that pediatric donor kidneys had very poor survival rates when transplanted to pediatric recipients. The initial expectation was that pediatric kidneys should be preferentially offered to pediatric recipients and the original algorithm did that. The revised allocation provides additional points for very young and for older pediatric patients so they will be transplanted more quickly with the first suitable kidney.

The HLA component of the local allocation algorithm has been the most frequently modified part of the scheme. The importance of matching in determining graft outcome is well established. The extent to which matching should determine local kidney distribution remains controversial. Points for HLA-A matches were dropped in 1990 after analyses showed no survival benefit for this category of matched patients. With growing concerns about racial equity in transplantation, the B-locus matching points were eliminated in 2003, and were replaced with 2 points for zero HLA-DR mismatches and 1 point for one DR mismatch. These changes may produce small increases in the rate of graft loss.

The allocation system was originally designed to balance fairness (the waiting time component) with medical utility (HLA matching to improve survival). But much has changed over the years. The waiting list for a kidney transplant has grown from 13,000 in 1988 to 60,000 in 2004, but the number of deceased donor kidneys procured annually only increased from 7,000 to about 9,000 in the past 10 years (see Fig 1.1) The widening gap between the supply and demand for kidneys means that the wait for a kidney transplant can vary from several months to several years. The organ shortage has resulted in a marked expansion of the limits of acceptability for deceased donors. In fact, nearly all of the increase in deceased donor kidneys over the past decade has resulted from accepting older so-called expanded criteria donors (ECDs) (see Chapter 5). More than one-third of ECDs are older than age 50 years and many have comorbid diseases that would have excluded them from consideration as donors a few years ago. In 1988, 95% of the kidneys that were procured for transplantation were transplanted, meaning that only 5% of kidneys procured were discarded. In 2002, the percentage discarded had increased to 16%. At the same time, transplant candidates are aging. More than half were older than age 50 years as of June 2003. The longer waiting times combined with an aging candidate list has resulted in a growing number of patients who die before receiving a transplant. The higher graft survival rates of recent transplants also affect the relative influence of medical utility. It may be more important to avoid delays that could result in organs being discarded than to provide an advantage for a local patient with a slightly better HLA match. Thus, the concepts of fairness and utility are dynamic and the system for allocating kidneys needs to revisited and studied periodically to insure that it still serves the patients.

Allocation of Expanded Criteria Donor Kidneys

Expanded criteria donors have been defined as donors older than age 60 years or age 50 to 59 years with two additional risk factors, including a history of hypertension, death as a result of cerebrovascular accident, or an elevated terminal serum creatinine. ECD kidneys, which account for approximately 15% of deceased donor kidneys, have at least a 70% increased risk of failing within 2 years, when compared with standard criteria kidneys. (On the positive side this means that if a standard kidney has a 2-year graft survival of 88%, an ECD kidney has an estimated survival at 2 years of approximately 80%.) In 2003, the allocation of ECD kidneys was changed in an effort to speed their placement in an appropriate recipient in the hopes of achieving a reduction in cold ischemia time and a reduction in the percentage discarded because of increased cold ischemia time. ECD kidneys are offered only to those patients who have agreed to accept them, who have been informed of the risk, and who understand that these kidneys are more likely to fail. ECD kidneys are offered nationally for HLA-matched recipients, but the decision to accept them must be made within 2 hours; otherwise, ECD kidneys are allocated to local patients according to their waiting time alone. Appropriate candidates for ECD kidneys are discussed in Chapter 6.

Whether or not these recent changes to the point system for local kidney allocation will have their intended effects, is not known. However, with more than 1,000 deceased donor kidney transplants performed each month in the United States, data should accrue quickly. It is important to remember that the allocation system merely ranks the waiting patients for each donor kidney that becomes available. Often the patients who are ranked at the top of the list are also those who are most broadly sensitized against potential donor antigens and who will have a positive cross-match against most donors. Their chances of transplantation will be increased with more histocompatible donors or if they can be desensitized.

SELECTED READINGS

Bunce M, Young NT, Welsh KI. Molecular HLA typing—the brave new world. *Transplantation* 1997;64:1505–1513.

Carpenter CB. Improving the success of organ transplantation. *N Engl J Med* 2000;342:647–648.

Cecka JM. The UNOS Renal Transplant Registry. In: Cecka JM, Terasaki PI, eds. *Clinical transplants 2002*. Los Angeles: UCLA Immunogenetics Center, 2003:1–20.

Chua MS, Sarwal M. Microarrays: new tools for transplantation research. *Pediatr Nephrol* 2003;18:319–327.

Danovitch GM, Cecka JM. Allocation of deceased donor kidneys: past, present and future. *Am J Kidney Dis* 2003;42:882–890.

Gebel HM, Bray RA, Nickerson P. Pre-transplant assessment of donor-reactive, HLA specific antibodies in renal transplantation: contradiction vs. risk. *Am J Transplant* 2003;3:1488–1500.

Hariharan S, Johnson CP, Bresnahan BA, et al. Improved graft survival after renal transplantation in the United States, 1988 to 1996. *N Engl J Med* 2000;342:605–612.

Hu H, Aizenstein BD, Puchalski A, et al. Elevation of CXCR3-binding chemokines in urine indicates acute renal allograft dysfunction. *Amer J Transplant* 2004;4:432–437.

Jordan S, Cunningham-Rundles C, McEwan R. Utility of intravenous immune globulin in kidney transplantation: efficacy, safety, and cost implications. *Am J Transplant* 2003;3:653–664.

Le Bas-Bernardet S, Hourmant M, Valentin N, et al. Identification of the antibodies involved in B-cell crossmatch positivity in renal transplantation. *Transplantation* 2003;75:477–482.

Li B, Hartono C, Ding R, et al. Noninvasive diagnosis of renal-allograft rejection by measurement of messenger RNA for perforin and granzyme B in urine. *N Engl J Med* 2001;344:947–954.

Marsh SGE, Albert ED, Bodmer WF, et al. Nomenclature for factors of the HLA system, 2002. *Tissue Antigens* 2002;60:407–464.

Metzger RA, Delmonico FL, Feng S, et al. Expanded criteria donors. *Am J Transplant* 2003;3(S4):114–125.

Pei R, Lee JH, Shih NJ, et al. Single human leukocyte antigen flow cytometry beads for accurate identification of human leukocyte antigen antibody specificities. *Transplantation* 2003;75:43–49.

Roberts JP, Wolfe RA, Bragg-Gresham MS, et al. Effect of changing the priority for HLA matching on the rates and outcomes of kidney transplantation in minority groups. *N Engl J Med* 2004;350:545–551.

Takemoto SK, Terasaki PI, Gjertson DW, et al. Twelve years experience with shipping HLA matched cadaver kidneys for transplantation. *N Engl J Med* 2000;343:1078–1084.

Terasaki PI, Ozawa M. Predicting kidney graft failure by HLA antibodies: a prospective trial. *Am J Transplant* 2004;4:438–443.

Williams M, Creger J, Belton A, et al. The Organ Center of the United Network for Organ Sharing and twenty years of organ sharing in the United States. *Transplantation* 2004;77:641–646.

Immunosuppressive Medications and Protocols for Kidney Transplantation

Gabriel M. Danovitch

A BRIEF HISTORY OF TRANSPLANT IMMUNOSUPPRESSION

To understand the construction of the immunosuppressive protocol and the use of immunosuppressive medications according to current standard transplant practice, it helps to follow the development of organ transplantation and, in particular, kidney transplantation, since the 1950s. Although sporadic attempts at kidney transplantation had been made throughout the first half of the twentieth century, the current era of transplantation was pioneered in the mid-1950s with live donor transplants from identical twins. The first attempts at immunosuppression used total-body irradiation; azathioprine was introduced in the early 1960s, and was soon routinely accompanied by prednisolone. The polyclonal antibody preparations antithymocyte globulin (ATG) and antilymphocyte globulin (ALG) became available in the mid-1970s. With azathioprine and prednisolone as the baseline regimen and ATG or ALG used for induction or for the treatment of steroid-resistant rejection, the success rate of kidney transplantation was approximately 50% at 1 year, and the mortality rate was typically 10% to 20%.

The situation was transformed in the early 1980s with the introduction of cyclosporine. Because the results of kidney transplantation were poor, it was not hard to recognize the dramatic benefit of cyclosporine that produced statistically significant improvement in graft survival rates to greater than 80% at 1 year. Mortality rates decreased with more effective immunosuppression, less use of corticosteroids, and overall improvements in surgical and medical care. The standard immunosuppressive regimen consisted of cyclosporine and prednisone, often combined with azathioprine, now used as an adjunctive agent in so-called triple therapy. Although the benefits of cyclosporine were clear-cut, its capacity to produce both acute and chronic nephrotoxicity was soon recognized to be a major detriment. In 1985, OKT3, the first monoclonal antibody used in clinical medicine, was introduced based on its capacity to treat first acute rejection episodes, although the toxicity of the drug tended to restrict its use to episodes of rejection that were resistant to high-dose steroids and, in some programs, to use as an induction agent. With this limited armamentarium of medications—cyclosporine, azathioprine, corticosteroids, and the antibody preparations—the transplant community entered the 1990s, achieving, with justifiable pride, success rates of up to 90% in many centers and minimal mortality. Because the number of available immunosuppressive medications was low, there was relatively little variation between the protocol options used in different programs.

Two major developments then followed. Tacrolimus was introduced into liver transplantation and eventually into kidney transplantation as an alternative to cyclosporine with respect to its capacity to produce equivalent patient and graft survival, and mycophenolate mofetil (MMF) was found to be a more effective agent than azathioprine by virtue of its capacity to reduce the incidence of acute rejection episodes when used with cyclosporine (and later with tacrolimus) and corticosteroids. Basiliximab and daclizumab, two humanized monoclonal antibodies, were approved for use after kidney transplantation, also based on their capacity to reduce the incidence of acute rejection episodes, and a polyclonal antibody, Thymoglobulin, available in Europe for several years, was approved for use in the United States for the treatment of acute rejection. In 1999, sirolimus was added to the immunosuppressive menu, and studies are in progress to evaluate several new chemical and biologic agents.

The therapeutic armamentarium for transplant immunosuppression thus continues to broaden and become more complex, as does the variety of potential drug combinations or protocols. To address this complexity, this chapter is divided into five sections. Part I reviews the drugs in current clinical use, emphasizing cyclosporine, tacrolimus, MMF, and sirolimus. Part II reviews the currently available biologic agents approved for use in transplantation. Part III discusses the clinical trial process used to develop new immunosuppressive agents and reviews available data on promising new agents at different stages of development. Part IV discusses combinations of these drugs in the form of clinically applied immunosuppressive protocols, both conventional and innovative. Part V discusses the treatment of the various forms kidney transplant rejection.

PART I. IMMUNOSUPPRESSIVE AGENTS IN CURRENT CLINICAL USE

MECHANISM OF ACTION OF IMMUNOSUPPRESSIVE DRUGS: THE THREE-SIGNAL MODEL

The molecular mechanisms that are the target of immunosuppressive drugs are discussed in detail in Chapter 2. The three-signal model of T-cell activation and subsequent cellular proliferation, illustrated in Fig. 4.1, is a valuable tool for understanding the sites of action of the agents discussed below. In brief, signal 1 is an antigen-specific signal provided by the triggering of the T-cell receptors by antigen-presenting cells (APCs) and is transduced through the CD3 complex. Signal 2 is a non–antigen-specific costimulatory signal provided by the engagement of B7 on the antigen-presenting cell with CD28 on the T cell. These two signals activate the intracellular pathways that lead to the expression of interleukin (IL)-2 and other growth-promoting cytokines. Stimulation of the IL-2 receptor (CD25) leads to activation of mTOR (mammalian target of rapamycin) and provides signal 3, which triggers cell proliferation. As each of the immunosuppressive agents is discussed below, it is useful to refer to Fig. 4.1 to review their relative sites of action.

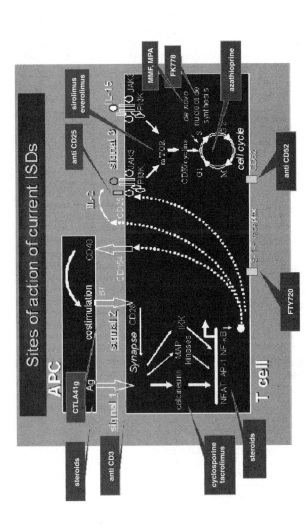

Fig. 4.1.   Sites of action of immunosuppressive drugs (ISDs) in the three-signal model. Abbreviations are detailed in the text. (From Halloran PF personal communication.)

THE CALCINEURIN INHIBITORS: CYCLOSPORINE AND TACROLIMUS

The term *calcineurin inhibitors* is a useful one because it emphasizes the similarity in the mechanism of action of the two drugs,
cyclosporine and *tacrolimus,* which have served as the backbone of
solid-organ transplant immunosuppression for the last 20 years.
Although they are biochemically distinct, they are remarkably
similar, not only in their mechanism of action, but also in their
clinical efficacy and side-effect profile. They are, therefore, considered together; discrete differences between them are discussed
in the text and summarized in Table 4.1. The choice of agent is
discussed in Part IV.

Cyclosporine is a small cyclic polypeptide of fungal origin. It
consists of 11 amino acids and has a molecular weight of 1,203.
It is neutral and insoluble in water, but soluble in organic sol-
vents and lipids. The amino acids at positions 11, 1, 2, and 3 form
the active immunosuppressive site, and the cyclic structure of the
drug is necessary for its immunosuppressive effect. Tacrolimus,
still often called by its nickname *Eff-Kay* from its laboratory designation *FK506,* is a macrolide antibiotic compound isolated from
Streptomyces tsukubaensis.

Mechanism of Action

The calcineurin inhibitors differ from their predecessor immunosuppressive drugs by virtue of their selective inhibition of the
immune response. They do not inhibit neutrophilic phagocytic
activity as corticosteroids do, nor are they myelosuppressive as
azathioprine is. Cell surface events and antigen recognition also
remain intact (see Chapter 2). Their immunosuppressive effect
depends on the formation of a complex with their cytoplasmic
receptor proteins, *cyclophilin* for cyclosporine and tacrolimus-
binding protein *(FKBP)* for tacrolimus (see Fig 4.1 and Plate 1).
This complex binds with *calcineurin,* whose normal function is
to act as a phosphatase that dephosphorylates certain nuclear
regulatory proteins (e.g., *nuclear factor of activated T cells*) and
hence facilitates their passage through the nuclear membrane
(see Chapter 2 and Fig. 2.5). Inhibition of calcineurin thereby
impairs the expression of several critical cytokine genes that promote T-cell activation, including those for IL-2, IL-4, interferon-
γ (IFN-γ), and tumor necrosis factor-α (TNF-α). The transcription of other genes, such as CD40 ligand and the protooncogenes
H-*ras* and c-*myc*, is also impaired. The importance of these factors in T-cell activation is discussed in more detail in Chapter 2,
but as a result of calcineurin inhibition, there is a quantitative
limitation of cytokine production and downstream lymphocyte
proliferation.

Cyclosporine enhances the expression of transforming growth
factor-β (TGF-β), which also inhibits IL-2 and the generation of
cytotoxic T lymphocytes, and may be responsible for the development of interstitial fibrosis, an important feature of calcineurin
inhibitor nephrotoxicity. TGF-β has also been implicated as an
important factor in the proliferation of tumor cells, which may be
relevant to the course of certain posttransplant neoplasias (see

Table 4.1. Some comparative features of cyclosporine and tacrolimus

	Cyclosporine	Tacrolimus
Mode of action	Inhibition of calcineurin	Inhibition of calcineurin
Daily maintenance dose	~3–5 mg/kg	~0.15–0.3 mg/kg
Administration	PO and IV	PO and IV[a]
Absorption bile dependent	Sandimmune, yes; Neoral, no	No
Oral dose available (capsules)	100 mg; 25 mg	5 mg; 1 mg; 0.5 mg
Drug interactions	Similar	Similar
Capacity to prevent rejection	+	++?
Use with MMF	+	+[b]
Use with sirolimus	+[c]	+[c]
Nephrotoxicity	+	+
Steroid sparing	+	++?
Hypertension and sodium retention	++	+
Pancreatic islet toxicity	+	++
Neurotoxicity	+	++
Hirsutism	+	−
Hair loss	−	+
Gum hypertrophy	+	−
Gastrointestinal side effects	−	+
Gastric motility	−	+
Hyperkalemia	+	+
Hypomagnesemia	+	+
Hypercholesterolemia	+	−
Hyperuricemia/gout	++	+

[a] IV rarely needed because oral absorption is good. [b]Dose of MMF may be less when used with tacrolimus. [c]Nephrotoxicity may be exaggerated when used in full dose.
Data are based on available literature and clinical experience. −, No or little effect; +, known effect; ++, effect more pronounced; ++?, probable greater effect; IV, intravenous; MMF, mycophenolate mofetil; PO, by mouth.

Chapter 9). The *in vivo* effects of cyclosporine are blocked by anti-TGF-β, indicating that TGF-β may be central to the mediation of both the beneficial and detrimental effects of the calcineurin inhibitors.

Patients receiving successful calcineurin inhibitor-based immunosuppression maintain a degree of immune responsiveness that is still sufficient to maintain host defenses. This relative immunosuppression may be a reflection of the fact that at therapeutic levels of these drugs calcineurin activity is reduced by only about 50%, permitting strong signals to trigger cytokine expression and generate an effective immune response. In stable patients receiving cyclosporine, CD4+ T cells have reduced IL-2 production to a degree that is inversely correlated to drug levels. The degree of inhibition of calcineurin activity and IL-2 production may be at the fulcrum of the delicate balance that exists between overimmunosuppression and underimmunosuppression.

Formulations and Pharmacokinetics

Cyclosporine

The original formulation of cyclosporine, the oil-based *Sandimmune,* has largely been replaced by the microemulsion formulation, *Neoral.* Both formulations are available in two forms: a 100-mg/mL solution that is drawn up by the patient into a graduated syringe and dispensed into orange juice or milk, or 25-mg and 100-mg soft-gelatin capsules. Patients usually prefer the convenience of the capsule that is typically administered twice daily. The absorption of Sandimmune cyclosporine from the gastrointestinal (GI) tract is bile dependent and may be unreliable for patients with diabetic gastroparesis, diarrhea, biliary diversion, cholestasis, and malabsorption. The absorption of cyclosporine after an oral dose can be represented graphically in the form of a concentration–time curve (Fig. 4.2). The time to peak concentration of Sandimmune cyclosporine (t_{max}) is variable but averages 4 hours. A substantial proportion of transplant recipients exhibit a second peak. The bioavailability of Neoral (F) is better than that of Sandimmune, and there is less variability in cyclosporine pharmacokinetics. Peak cyclosporine levels (C_{max}) of Neoral cyclosporine are higher, and the trough concentration (C_{min}) correlates better with the systemic exposure, as reflected by the *area under the curve* (AUC).

The improved GI absorption of the microemulsion and lesser dependence on bile for absorption may reduce the necessity for intravenous cyclosporine administration. Compared with intravenous infusion, the bioavailability of the orally administered drug is in the range of 30% to 45%. Conversion between the oral and intravenous forms of the drug perioperatively requires a 3:1 dose ratio. Bioavailability of oral cyclosporine increases with time, possibly as a result of improved absorption by the previously uremic GI tract. As a result, the amount of cyclosporine required to achieve a given blood level tends to fall with time and typically reaches a steady level within 4 to 8 weeks. Food tends to enhance the absorption of cyclosporine (see Chapter 18).

Some studies show a reduction in the incidence of acute rejection of up to 15% with Neoral than with Sandimmune, and the dose required to achieve an equivalent trough level may be reduced by about 10%. Chronic allograft loss appears similar for Sandimmune- and Neoral-treated patients.

The development of generic formulations of cyclosporine and other immunosuppressive agents is controversial because of the critical importance of these drugs to the success of transplantation and the corporate and financial implications of their introduction. Cyclosporine is regarded as a drug with a *narrow therapeutic index,* and the standards for proving the *bioequivalence* of

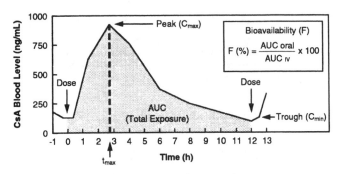

Fig. 4.2. Cyclosporine pharmacokinetic profile. AUC, the area under the concentration–time curve, which approximates a patient's total exposure to cyclosporine over a dosage interval; C_{max}, the maximum cyclosporine concentration; C_{min}, the minimum cyclosporine concentration, or trough level; F, percentage bioavailability of orally administered cyclosporine over a dosage interval; t_{max}, the time to reach maximum cyclosporine concentration. (From Grevel J, Kahan BD. Area under the curve monitoring of cyclosporine therapy: the early posttransplant period. *Ther Drug Monit* 1991;13:89–95, with permission.)

generic forms are more rigorous. Generic drugs, however, do not undergo the same extensive evaluation required of new drugs and information on discrete differences in their pharmacokinetics in different ethnic groups is not available. Generic formulations of cyclosporine, such as the capsule *cyclosporine USP* (Eon Labs), and the capsule *Gengraf,* are in widespread use in the United States; other generic formulations are available outside of the United States. The generic formulations are generally claimed to have an absorption profile that is very similar to that of Neoral. The capsules have received a so-called AB rating by the U.S. Food and Drug Administration (FDA), which means that they may be substituted for Neoral cyclosporine without the approval of the prescriber. If generic formulations are used, it is probably better to use them consistently and to avoid switching formulations. If conversions are made between the different formulations, it is wise to monitor drug levels and renal function (see Part IV).

Tacrolimus

Tacrolimus (Prograf) is available in an intravenous formulation and as 5-mg, 1-mg, and 0.5-mg capsules; there are currently no generic formulations. It is typically administered twice daily, a long-acting once-daily formulation is being developed. Gastrointestinal absorption is independent of bile salts. Because of the effectiveness and relative consistency of its absorption, it is rarely necessary to use the intravenous formulation, and if necessary, the drug can be administered through a nasogastric tube. It is absorbed primarily from the small intestine, and its oral bioavailability is approximately 25%, with large interpatient and intrapatient variability, particularly for patients with GI disease. Gastric emptying of solids is faster in patients taking tacrolimus than in those receiving cyclosporine, a property that may be beneficial for patients with gastric motility disorders.

Distribution and Metabolism

In the blood, one-third of absorbed and infused cyclosporine is found in plasma, bound primarily to lipoproteins. Most of the remaining drug is bound to erythrocytes. Whole-blood drug levels (see "Drug Level Monitoring," below) are thus typically threefold higher than plasma levels. The binding of cyclosporine to lipoproteins may be important in the transfer of the drug through plasma membranes, and the toxic effects of cyclosporine may be exaggerated by low cholesterol levels and reduced by high cholesterol levels.

The binding of cyclosporine to the low-density lipoprotein receptor may account for the hyperlipidemia associated with its use. Tacrolimus also has a high affinity for formed blood elements, but it differs from cyclosporine in that, although it is highly protein bound, it is not significantly associated with lipoproteins, and it has a less unfavorable effect on the cholesterol level than does cyclosporine.

Both parent drugs have a half-life of about 8 hours and are metabolized to multiple metabolites by the cytochrome P450 IIIA (CYP3A) found in the GI and liver microsomal enzyme systems. GI metabolism through CYP3A and p-glycoprotein produces a so-called first-pass metabolism, and the heterogeneity in intestinal CYP3A gene expression may explain some of the wide interpatient variability in drug kinetics. The liver is often considered the most important site of drug metabolism, but GI metabolism may account for up to half of cyclosporine metabolism. Gut metabolism of tacrolimus is also extensive. Some of the drug metabolites may have immunosuppressive and nephrotoxic potential, and the plasma levels of the most important cyclosporine metabolite, M17, may be similar to that of the parent compound.

Because both drugs are excreted in the bile with minimal renal excretion, drug doses do not need to be modified in the presence of kidney dysfunction. Neither drug is significantly dialyzed, and either can be administered during dialysis treatment without dose adjustment. The pharmacokinetic parameters of both drugs may vary among patient groups, and these variations may have clinical consequences. Pediatric and black transplant recipients may require relatively larger doses and short dosage intervals. Longer dosage intervals may be required in older patients and in the presence of liver disease.

Drug-Level Monitoring

The measurement of cyclosporine and tacrolimus levels is an intrinsic part of the management of transplant patients because of variation in interpatient and intrapatient metabolism. There is also a relationship, albeit an inconsistent one, between blood levels of the drug and episodes of rejection and toxicity. Drug-level monitoring is the source of much confusion because of the various assays available and the option of using different matrices (i.e., plasma or whole blood) for their measurement.

When Sandimmune was introduced, the trough level of cyclosporine (drawn immediately preceding the next dose), rather than the peak level, was measured because its timing was more consistent and appeared to correlate better with toxic complications. More sophisticated techniques of monitoring were suggested whereby a full, or abbreviated, pharmacokinetic profile is constructed to calculate the AUC, which reflects the bioavailability of the drug and may theoretically allow for more precise and individualized patient management. Although attractive, these techniques never proved popular because of their cost and inconvenience, and many centers continue to rely on trough levels. With the introduction of Neoral, this trend has continued, although there is considerable evidence to suggest that because of its more consistent absorption, its peak level (typically 2 hours after dosing; Fig. 4.2) may correlate better with drug exposure and clinical events than the trough level. So-called C2 monitoring is applied routinely in some centers and clinical trials. For tacrolimus, the trough level is used for monitoring, and this level appears to be an adequate approximation of drug exposure. Recommendations for target blood levels at different stages posttransplant are discussed in Part IV and Table 4.10.

Cyclosporine concentrations can be measured in plasma or whole blood. Whole blood [ethylenediaminetetraacetic acid (EDTA)-anticoagulated] is the recommended specimen type because the distribution of cyclosporine between plasma and erythrocytes is temperature dependent. The clinician cannot begin to assess the significance of a cyclosporine level without knowing what kind of assay is being used. Several methods are currently available to measure cyclosporine and each differs in specificity for parent compound. *High-performance liquid chromatography* (HPLC) is the most specific method for measuring unmetabolized parent cyclosporine and is considered the reference method. HPLC, however, is expensive and labor intensive and is not available at all centers. Immunoassays, which use monoclonal antibodies against cyclosporine, are commonly used and have largely replaced HPLC because they can be performed on automated chemistry analyzers. The two most commonly used immunoassays to measure cyclosporine in whole-blood samples are the Abbot (Chicago, IL) fluorescence polarization immunoassay (FPIA) and the Syva (Dade-Behring Inc., Cupertino, CA) enzyme-multiplied immunoassay technique (EMIT). Both assays have significant cross-reactivity with cyclosporine metabolites and overestimate cyclosporine levels by up to 45% and 15%, respectively. Peak cyclosporine level samples should be clearly identified when sent to the laboratory and should be reported as such. These samples may need to be diluted for accuracy of calibration. For monitoring of tacrolimus concentrations most laboratories use the Abbott monoclonal antibody-based *microparticle enzyme immunoassay* (MEIA) that can be performed on an automated instrument (IMx). This assay permits accurate estimation of tacrolimus levels as low as 2 ng/dL. Target cyclosporine (peak and trough) and tacrolimus (trough) levels are discussed in the section on immunosuppressive protocols.

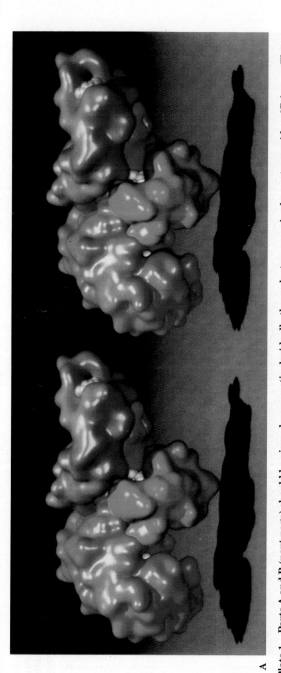

Plate 1. Parts A and B (next page) should be viewed consecutively, ideally through stereoscopic glasses to provide a 3D image. They show the x-ray structure at 2.5 Å resolution of the ternary complex of a calcineurin A fragment (CnA; blue), calcineurin B (CnB; green), tacrolimus-binding protein (FKBP; red), and tacrolimus (FK506; white). Note that the FKBP-FK506 complex does not directly contact the phosphatase active site on CnA that is more than 10 Å removed. Instead, the FKBP-FK506 complex is positioned so that it can inhibit the dephosphorylation of its substrates (e.g., nuclear factor of activated T cells [NFATpl]) by physically hindering their approach to the active site. (The bound phosphate in the phosphatase active site is shown in yellow). A. The solvent accessible surface of the ternary complex.

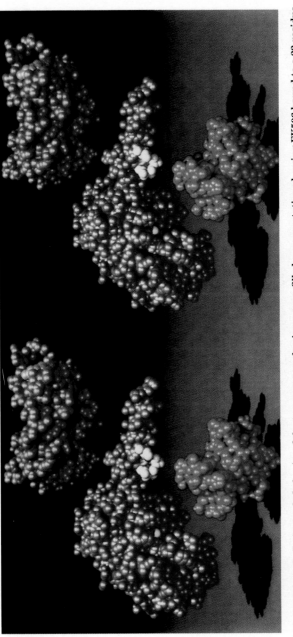

Plate 1 (continued). B. An exploded veiw of the ternary complex in a space-filled representation showing FK506 bound to a 22-residue alpha helix that is nearly 40 Å away from the surface of the phosphatase domain. (Reprinted with permission from Griffith JP, Kim JL, Kim EE et al. X-ray structure of calcineurin inhibited by the immunophilin-immunosuppressant FKBP12-FK506 complex. *Cell* 1995;82: 507–522.)

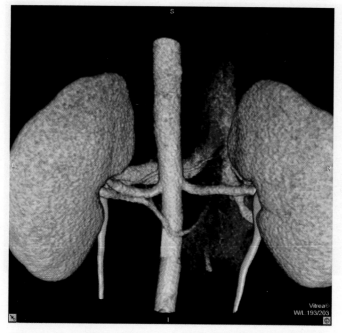

Plate 2.   CT angiogram of renal arteries with volume-rendered reformation. Posterior vantage with aorta on left, demonstrating two left renal arteries.

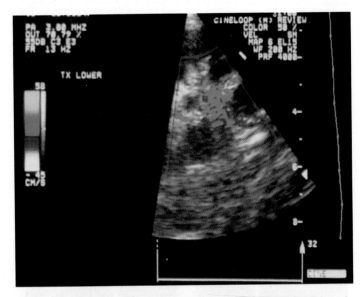

Plate 3. Postbiopsy arteriovenous fistula. Color Doppler image shows an area of random color assignment. Pulsed gate Doppler analysis revealed high-velocity, low-resistance arterial flow and arterialization of the venous waveform.

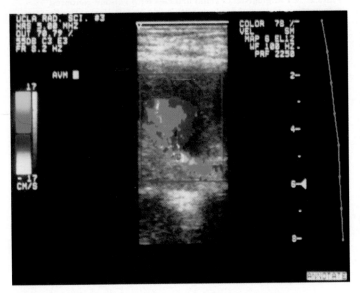

Plate 4. Pseudoaneurysm. Grayscale image demonstrated a cystic lesion and color Doppler image shows swirling internal flow.

Drug Interactions

The interaction of the calcineurin inhibitors with many commonly used drugs demands constant attention to drug regimens and cognizance of potential interactions. New drugs should be introduced with care, and patients should be warned to consult physicians familiar with the use of cyclosporine and tacrolimus before considering new pharmacologic therapy. Some of the drug interactions discussed below are consistent and well established (and are emphasized in **bold** lettering); others have been described in small series and case reports or are anticipated based on the pharmacologic properties of the agents. Any drug that impacts on P450 activity in the liver or intestinal tract, or that interacts with a drug that does, should be regarded as having a potential interaction with the calcineurin inhibitors. Some drugs affect calcineurin inhibitor levels when administered orally, but not intravenously, because the drug interaction is taking place at the intestine. In addition to their affect on P450, the calcineurin inhibitors inhibit multidrug resistance protein (MDR), and many of the interactions thought to be due to P450 are, in fact, due to an effect on MDR. The possibility that the calcineurin inhibitor is affecting the blood level of the interacting drug should also be considered.

Unless a comment is made to the contrary, the drug interactions noted below are common to both cyclosporine and tacrolimus, although more have been described with cyclosporine, which has been available longer. Drug interactions between calcineurin inhibitors and other immunosuppressive drugs are discussed in Part IV. Interactions with antibiotics are discussed below and in Chapter 10 and Table 10.7. Interactions with food are discussed in Chapter 18. Interactions with psychotropic drugs are discussed in more detail in Chapter 16. Drugs that cause impairment of graft function by virtue of their nephrotoxicity alone are not discussed here.

Drugs That Decrease Calcineurin Inhibitor Concentration by Induction of P450 Activity

ANTITUBERCULOUS DRUGS

Rifampin (and **rifabutin** to a lesser extent) markedly reduces cyclosporine and tacrolimus levels, and it may be difficult to achieve therapeutic levels in patients taking rifampin, the use of which should be avoided if at all possible. Isoniazid (INH) can be used with careful drug-level monitoring and is the preferred drug for tuberculosis prophylaxis if this proves essential (see Chapter 10).

ANTICONVULSANTS

Barbiturates markedly reduce cyclosporine and tacrolimus levels. Dose requirements may double or triple and three-times-a-day administration may be required under careful supervision. **Phenytoin** and primidone reduce levels and should be used with great care. The average requirement for cyclosporine or tacrolimus is about doubled for patients receiving phenytoin. **Carbamazepine** may also decrease cyclosporine levels, but the effect is less pronounced. Benzodiazepines and valproic acid do not affect drug levels, but the latter drug has been associated with hepatotoxicity. Modafinil can cause an up to 50% reduction in calcineurin inhibitor levels. Patients taking anticonvulsants before transplantation should have a neurologic assessment with a view toward discontinuing them when possible or exchanging them for one of the new generation of anticonvulsants that do not interact with calcineurin inhibitors.

OTHER DRUGS

There are isolated reports of several antibiotics, including nafcillin, intravenous trimethoprim, intravenous sulfadimidine, imipenem, cephalosporins, and terbinafine, reducing cyclosporine levels. An increased incidence of acute rejection episodes has been described after the introduction of ciprofloxacin. The antidepressant herbal preparation *Hypericum perforatum* (St. John's wort) may reduce cyclosporine levels by enzyme induction. Ticlopidine may reduce cyclosporine levels. Cholestyramine, GoLYTELY, and olestra may reduce levels by impairing gastrointestinal absorption. Corticosteroids are inducers of P450, an effect that needs to be considered if their administration is discontinued. Following cessation of concomitant corticosteroid therapy tacrolimus levels may increase by up to 25%. The serum creatinine level may increase as a result and lead to a confusing clinical picture.

PROLONGED USE

If prolonged use of a drug that induces P450 activity is required, addition of a drug that inhibits or competes with the P450 system (e.g., diltiazem, ketoconazole) may facilitate the achievement of therapeutic calcineurin inhibitor levels. Administration of the calcineurin inhibitor on a thrice-daily basis rather than the usual twice-daily basis may also be effective.

Drugs that Increase Calcineurin Inhibitor Levels by Inhibition of P450 or by Competition for its Pathways

CALCIUM CHANNEL BLOCKERS

Verapamil, diltiazem, amlodipine, and **nicardipine** may significantly increase calcineurin inhibitor levels. Diltiazem and verapamil are sometimes added routinely as adjuncts to the immunosuppressive regimen. Their use may safely permit up to a 40% reduction in the cyclosporine dose. Careful monitoring of drug levels is required when these calcium channel blockers are used for the management of hypertension or heart disease, and patients should be specifically warned that changing the dosage of these drugs is equivalent to changing the dosage of the calcineurin inhibitor. Brand-name and generic forms of these drugs (Cardizem, Dilacor, Tiazac, and Cartia are all forms of diltiazem) may have a different effect on calcineurin inhibitor levels. Nifedipine, isradipine, and felodipine have similar hemodynamic effects but have minimal effects on drug levels.

ANTIFUNGAL AGENTS

Ketoconazole, fluconazole, and **itraconazole** markedly elevate calcineurin inhibitor levels. The interaction with ketoconazole is a particularly potent one, which may permit a safe reduction of up to 80% in the cyclosporine or tacrolimus dose. Great care must be taken when stopping and starting these antifungal agents. An important interaction between ketoconazole and histamine blockers has also been described. The effective reabsorption of ketoconazole from the GI tract requires acidic gastric contents, and the addition of a histamine-2 receptor antagonist may reduce its absorption, indirectly producing a clinically significant fall in calcineurin inhibitor levels.

ANTIBIOTICS

Erythromycin, even in low doses, may increase calcineurin inhibitor levels. Other macrolide antibiotics (e.g., clarithromycin, josamycin, ponsinomycin) may also increase levels, although azithromycin does not. Because erythromycin is prescribed so ubiquitously, physicians, dentists, and patients should be warned about this interaction. Chloramphenicol may increase tacrolimus levels.

With the advent of highly active antiretrovirus therapy (HAART) selected HIV-positive patients may be deemed candidates for kidney transplantation (see Chapters 6 and 10). Some of the antiretroviral agents, particularly protease inhibitors, are potent inhibitors of P450. Ritonavir is the most potent inhibitor of P450 that is clinically available, and when used alone or in combination (kaletra-retonavir/lopinavir), very small doses of calcineurin inhibitor (e.g., 1 mg/week of tacrolimus) may maintain adequate drug levels.

HISTAMINE BLOCKERS

There are conflicting reports regarding the use of cimetidine, ranitidine, and omeprazole with calcineurin inhibitors. Cimetidine was initially reported to increase cyclosporine levels, but this effect has not been substantiated. These drugs may increase creatinine levels without reducing the glomerular filtration rate (GFR) by suppressing proximal tubular creatinine secretion. There may be increased hepatotoxicity when ranitidine and cyclosporine are used in combination.

HORMONES

Corticosteroids in high and low doses may decrease the clearance of cyclosporine metabolites. This effect may be particularly pronounced during "pulse" steroid therapy and may result in a confusing clinical picture if the drug levels are measured by a nonspecific assay. Oral contraceptives, anabolic steroids, testosterone, norethisterone, danazol, and somatostatin may also increase drug levels.

OTHER DRUGS

Amiodarone, carvedilol, allopurinol, bromocriptine, and chloroquine are reported to increase cyclosporine levels. Metoclopramide and grapefruit juice increase the absorption of calcineurin inhibitors (see Chapter 18).

Drugs that May Exaggerate Calcineurin Inhibitor Nephrotoxicity

Any potentially nephrotoxic drug should be used with caution in combination with the calcineurin inhibitors because the vasoconstrictive effect of the drug tends to potentiate other nephrotoxic mechanisms. Well-substantiated enhanced renal impairment has been described after the introduction of **amphotericin** and **aminoglycosides,** and renal impairment may occur earlier than anticipated. **Nonsteroidal antiinflammatory drugs** should be avoided if possible, but can be given for short periods under supervision. Calcineurin inhibitors may potentiate the hemodynamic renal dysfunction seen with **angiotensin-converting enzyme inhibitors** and **angiotensin receptor antagonists**. Metoclopramide may increase calcineurin inhibitor levels by increasing its intestinal reabsorption. A syndrome of diarrhea, hepatopathy, and renal dysfunction has been ascribed to the interaction between cyclosporine and colchicine, particularly when given to patients with familial Mediterranean fever.

LIPID-LOWERING AGENTS

The beta-hydroxy-β-methylglutaryl-coenzyme A (HMG-CoA) reductase inhibitors (HCRIs) are frequent accompaniments of the immunosuppressive protocol (see Part IV). **Lovastatin** has been implicated in several cases of acute renal failure. When used in full doses in combination with cyclosporine, lovastatin can cause rhabdomyolysis with elevated creatine phosphokinase levels and acute renal failure. Myopathy alone has been observed in up to 30% of recipients of the lovastatin–cyclosporine combination, with symptoms of muscle pain and tenderness developing 6 weeks to 16 months after commencement of therapy. The myopathic syndrome has not been observed when lovastatin is used in a daily dose of 20 mg or less. Even this dose should be used with caution, however, and patients should be made aware of the potential interaction. The coadministration of lovastatin with gemfibrozil further increases the likelihood of rhabdomyolysis. The newer HCRIs—pravastatin, fluvastatin, simvastatin, and atorvastatin—should be introduced at low doses and maximal doses avoided. Cyclosporine may increase the levels of ezetimibe but ezetimibe has not been reported to affect the levels of cyclosporine. Cholestyramine may interfere with cyclosporine absorption from the GI tract.

Side Effects

Nephrotoxicity

Nephrotoxicity is an important side effect of both calcineurin inhibitors and is the major detriment of these remarkable drugs. Theories linking the mechanism of immunosuppression and nephrotoxicity are discussed later. The terms *cyclosporine* and *FK toxicity* are often used loosely, and it is important to note that these terms encompass several distinct, overlapping syndromes

Table 4.2.   Syndromes of calcineurin-inhibitor nephrotoxicity

Exaggeration of early posttransplantation graft dysfunction
Acute reversible decrease in GFR
Acute microvascular disease
Chronic nonprogressive decrease in GFR
Chronic progressive decrease in GFR
Hypertension and electrolyte abnormalities
    Sodium retention and edema
    Hyperkalemia
    Hypomagnesemia
    Hyperchloremic acidosis
Hyperuricemia

GFR, glomerular filtration rate.

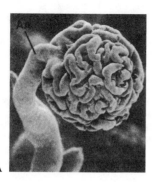 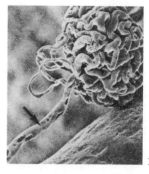

A   B

**Fig. 4.3.   Cyclosporine-induced afferent arteriolar vasoconstriction.
A: Control rat showing afferent arteriole (AA) and glomerular tuft.
B: Constricted afferent arteriole *(arrow)* and glomerular tuft after
14 days of cyclosporine at 50 mg/kg per day. (From English J, Evan A,
Houghton DC. Cyclosporine-induced acute renal dysfunction in the
rat. Evidence of arteriolar vasoconstriction with preservation of
tubular function. *Transplantation* 1987;44:135–141, with permission.)**

that are produced by both functional and morphologic changes
within the allograft (Table 4.2).

FUNCTIONAL DECREASE IN RENAL BLOOD FLOW AND FILTRATION RATE
The calcineurin inhibitors produce a dose-related, reversible, renal vasoconstriction that particularly affects the afferent arteriole (Fig. 4.3). The glomerular capillary ultrafiltration coefficient
(Kf) also decreases, possibly as a result of increased mesangial
cell contractility. The picture is reminiscent of "prerenal" dysfunction, and in the acute phase, tubular function is intact. Most of
the studies on the mechanism of this effect have used cyclosporine
rather than tacrolimus.

The normal regulation of the glomerular microcirculation depends on a complex, hormonally mediated balance between vasoconstriction and vasodilation. Cyclosporine-induced vasoconstriction is caused, at least in part, by alteration of arachidonic acid
metabolism in favor of the vasoconstrictor thromboxane. Cyclosporine is also a potential inducer of the powerful vasoconstrictor endothelin, and circulating endothelin levels are elevated in
its presence. Cyclosporine-induced changes in glomerular hemodynamics can be reversed by specific endothelin inhibitors and
by antiendothelin antibodies. The sympathetic nervous system is
also activated.

Several *in vivo* and *in vitro* studies have suggested that alterations in the L-arginine nitric oxide (NO) pathway may be involved in calcineurin-induced renal vasoconstriction. NO causes
relaxation of preglomerular arteries and improves renal blood
flow. The constitutive enzyme endothelial nitric oxide synthase
(NOS) is produced by renal endothelial cells and modulates
vascular tone. Both acute and chronic cyclosporine toxicity can
be enhanced by NOS inhibition with *N*-nitro-L-arginine-methyl
ester and ameliorated by supplementation with L-arginine.

Interestingly, sildenafil (Viagra) increases GFR in transplant patients, presumably by reversing this effect.

Calcineurin inhibitor-induced renal vasoconstriction may manifest clinically as delayed recovery of early malfunctioning grafts or as a transient, reversible, dose-dependent, blood level-dependent elevation in serum creatinine concentration that may be difficult to distinguish from other causes of graft dysfunction. Vasoconstriction may be a reversible component of chronic calcineurin inhibitor toxicity, which may amplify the functional severity of the chronic histologic changes seen with prolonged use. The vasoconstriction may be more pronounced with cyclosporine than with tacrolimus, and also helps to account for the hypertension and the tendency for sodium retention that are commonly associated with cyclosporine use.

CHRONIC INTERSTITIAL FIBROSIS

Interstitial fibrosis, which may be patchy or "striped" and associated with arteriolar lesions (see Chapter 13), is a common feature of long-term calcineurin inhibitor use. This lesion may produce chronic renal failure in recipients of organ transplants; however, several long-term studies show that in the dose regimens currently employed, kidney function may remain stable, although often impaired, for many years. The mechanism of calcineurin inhibitor-induced interstitial fibrosis remains poorly defined. Evidence from experimental models suggests that chronic nephropathy involves an angiotensin-dependent upregulation of molecules that are important in the scarring process, such as TGF-β and osteopontin. Enhanced production of TGF-β in normal T cells (see "Mechanism of Action" under "Calcineurin Inhibitors," above) may provide the link between the immunosuppressive effects of the calcineurin inhibitors and their nephrotoxicity (Fig. 4.4), and variation in fibrogenic gene expression may help explain the varying consistency of this effect. Calcineurin-inhibitor induced hypomagnesemia (see "Electrolyte Abnormalities and Hypertension," below) may induce interstitial inflammation and enhance the production of TGF-β thereby perpetuating chronic fibrotic lesions. Interstitial fibrosis may also be a reflection of intense and prolonged vasoconstriction of the renal microcirculation. Cyclosporine may also impair the regenerative capacity of microvascular endothelial cells and induce apoptosis. The resulting chronic renal ischemia may enhance the synthesis and accumulation of extracellular matrix proteins in the interstitium.

ACUTE MICROVASCULAR DISEASE

Thrombotic microangiopathy (TMA) (see Chapter 13 for pathology and Chapter 8 for clinical presentation and management) is a distinct form of calcineurin inhibitor vascular toxicity that may manifest as renal involvement alone or as a systemic illness. It produces a syndrome reminiscent of thrombotic thrombocytopenic purpura (TTP). In TTP, potentially pathogenic inhibitory antibodies against the von Willebrand factor (vWF)-cleaving protease ADAMTS13, a zinc metalloprotease, have been detected. A similar mechanism has been described in calcineurin inhibitor-induced TMA.

ELECTROLYTE ABNORMALITIES AND HYPERTENSION

Impaired sodium excretion is a reflection of the renal vasoconstrictive effect of the calcineurin inhibitors. Patients receiving

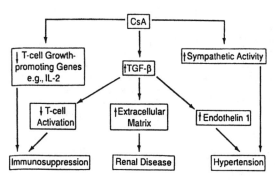

Fig. 4.4. **Potential sequelae of cyclosporine-mediated augmentation of TGF-β expression. In this scheme of events, the cyclosporine-associated increase in TGF-β expression is hypothesized to contribute to the following: immunosuppression (because TGF-β can prevent T-cell activation and generation of cytotoxic T cells); renal interstitial fibrosis (because TGF-β can enhance extracellular matrix accumulation); and hypertension (because TGF-β can increase endothelin production by vascular smooth-muscle cells). In this formulation, TGF-β represents the mechanistic link for the clinically desirable (immunosuppression) and deleterious (hypertension, fibrosis) consequences of cyclosporine use. CsA, cyclosporine-mediated augmentation. (From Khanna A, Li B, Stenzel KH, et al. Regulation of new DNA synthesis in mammalian cells by cyclosporine. Demonstration of a transforming growth factor beta-dependent mechanism of inhibition of cell growth.** *Transplantation* **1994;57:577–582, with permission.)**

long-term cyclosporine therapy tend to be hypertensive (see Chapter 9) and to retain fluid. Studies show activation of the renin–angiotensin–aldosterone system and sympathetic nervous system, and suppression of atrial natriuretic factor, which results in attenuation of the natriuretic and diuretic response to an acute volume load. NO production is also impaired. Hypertension tends to be less marked (or the need for antihypertensive drugs may be less) for patients receiving tacrolimus, possibly because it produces less peripheral vasoconstriction than does cyclosporine. *Hyperkalemia* is common and occasionally requires treatment, although it is rarely life-threatening as long as kidney function remains good. It is not uncommon for patients taking calcineurin inhibitors to have potassium levels in the mid-fives. Hyperkalemia is often associated with a mild *hyperchloremic acidosis* and an intact capacity to excrete acid urine. The clinical picture is thus reminiscent of type IV renal tubular acidosis. Patients receiving cyclosporine may have an impaired capacity to excrete an acute potassium load, and there is evidence to suggest impaired production of aldosterone, an acquired impaired renal response to its action, and inhibition of cortical collecting duct potassium secretory channels. Hyperkalemia may be exaggerated by concomitant administration of beta blockers, angiotensin-converting enzyme inhibitors, and angiotensin receptor blockers. A defect of collecting tubule hydrogen ion secretion has been described with tacrolimus.

Both cyclosporine and tacrolimus are magnesuric and hypercalciuric, and hypomagnesemia is commonly associated with their use. In liver transplantation, hypomagnesemia may predispose patients to seizures; this has been observed rarely in kidney allograft recipients. The urinary loss of Ca^{++} and Mg^{++} is due to downregulation of specific transport proteins. Magnesium supplements are often prescribed but may be ineffective because of a lowered renal magnesium threshold (see Chapter 18). Both cyclosporine and tacrolimus can produce hyperuricemia, although only cyclosporine had been associated with gout, which was reported to resolve when cyclosporine is switched to tacrolimus.

METHODS OF AMELIORATION

The vexing issue of calcineurin inhibitor nephrotoxicity has spawned a variety of clinical and experimental approaches designed to modify the renal effects of these drugs, particularly their capacity to produce vasoconstriction. Low-dose dopamine is used in some centers in the early postoperative period to "encourage" urine output. Various calcium channel blockers given to both the donor (see Chapter 5) and the recipient (see Part IV) may reduce the incidence and severity of delayed graft function. Omega-3 fatty acids in the form of 6 g of fish oil each day were initially thought to increase renal blood flow and GFR by reversing the cyclosporine-induced imbalance between the synthesis of vasodilator and vasoconstrictor prostaglandins, but long-term studies have shown no such benefit. The prostaglandin agonist misoprostol and thromboxane synthetase inhibitors may have a similar effect. Various protocol adjustments, discussed later in this chapter, can also be employed to minimize calcineurin inhibitor toxicity.

Nonrenal Calcineurin Inhibitor Toxicity

GASTROINTESTINAL

Episodes of hepatic dysfunction typically manifesting as subclinical, mild, self-limiting, dose-dependent elevations of serum aminotransferase levels with mild hyperbilirubinemia may occur in nearly half of all kidney transplant recipients taking cyclosporine and occur less frequently in those taking tacrolimus. No specific hepatic histologic lesion has been described in humans, and the hyperbilirubinemia is a reflection of disturbed bile secretion rather than hepatocellular damage. Cyclosporine does not itself produce progressive liver disease; other causes, most frequently one of the viral hepatitides, need to be considered when this occurs. Cyclosporine therapy is associated with an increased incidence of cholelithiasis, presumably resulting from an increased lithogenicity of cyclosporine-containing bile. Varying degrees of anorexia, nausea, vomiting, diarrhea, and abdominal discomfort occur in up to 75% of patients receiving tacrolimus, and less frequently in patients receiving cyclosporine.

COSMETIC

The cosmetic complications of cyclosporine, although not severe in a strict medical sense, must be treated seriously, particularly in women and adolescents, because of the misery they can produce and the temptation to resolve them through noncompliant behavior. Cosmetic complications are often exaggerated by concomitant use of corticosteroids. They are less prominent for patients receiving tacrolimus.

Hypertrichosis in varying degrees occurs in nearly all patients receiving cyclosporine and is particularly obvious in dark-haired girls and women. A coarsening of facial features is observed in children and young adults, with thickening of the skin and prominence of the brow. Tacrolimus may produce hair loss and frank alopecia. Gingival hyperplasia, which can be severe, may develop in patients receiving cyclosporine and is exaggerated by poor dental hygiene and possibly by concomitant use of calcium channel blockers. Azithromycin, a macrolide antibiotic that does not affect cyclosporine metabolism, may reduce gingival hyperplasia. Gingivectomy may occasionally be indicated, and switching from cyclosporine to tacrolimus is usually effective. Cosmetic complications tend to become less prominent with time. Sympathetic cosmetic counseling is required. Cyclosporine may increase prolactin levels, occasionally producing gynecomastia in men and breast enlargement in women.

HYPERLIPIDEMIA

Cyclosporine has been implicated as one of the various factors responsible for the generation of posttransplant hypercholesterolemia (see Chapter 9). The mechanism of this effect may be related to abnormal low-density lipoprotein feedback control by the liver, to altered bile acid synthesis, or to occupation of the low-density lipoprotein receptor by cyclosporine. Up to two-thirds of patients develop *de novo* hyperlipidemia in the first posttransplant year. The effect is less marked with tacrolimus, and lipid levels may decrease when patients are switched from cyclosporine to tacrolimus.

GLUCOSE INTOLERANCE

Posttransplant glucose intolerance and new-onset diabetes mellitus (NODM) are discussed in Chapter 9. Both calcineurin inhibitors are toxic to pancreatic islets, although tacrolimus is more so, possibly as a result of increased concentrations in islets of FKBP relative to cyclophilin. The affect is dose related and may be exaggerated by concomitant corticosteroid use. Morphologic changes in the islets include cytoplasmic swelling, vacuolization, and apoptosis, with abnormal immunostaining for insulin. Obesity, black and Hispanic ethnicity, family history of diabetes, and hepatitis C infection may predispose to NODM. Figure 4.5 shows the incidence of diabetes before and after transplantation by type of calcineurin inhibitor as reported to the United States Renal Data System.

NEUROTOXICITY

A spectrum of neurologic complications has been observed in patients receiving calcineurin inhibitors; they are generally more marked with tacrolimus. Coarse *tremor,* dysesthesias, headache, and insomnia are common and may be dose related. More severe complications are uncommon in kidney recipients, although isolated seizures may occur in 1% to 2% of patients, and full-blown leukoencephalopathy has been described. Patients receiving Neoral may complain of *headache* 1 to 2 hours after taking the drug, presumably because of high peak levels. Patients receiving cyclosporine may complain of *bone pain.*

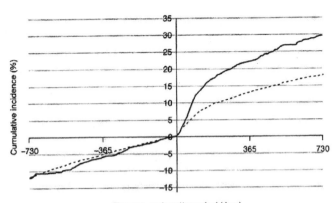

Time pre- and posttransplant (days)

Fig. 4.5. Incidence of diabetes before and after transplant by type of calcineurin inhibitor (solid line: tacrolimus; dashed line, cyclosporine). Note that the incremental incidence of diabetes for cyclosporine was 9.4% at 1 year and 8.4% at 2 years. The incremental incidence of diabetes for tacrolimus use was 15.4% at 1 year and 17.7% at 2 years. (From Woodward RS, Schnitzler MA, Baty J, et al. Incidence and cost of new onset diabetes mellitus among U.S. wait-listed and transplanted renal allograft recipients. *Am J Transplant* 2003;3:590–598, with permission.)

CARDIOTOXICITY
There are case reports of prolongation of the QT interval and potentially dangerous arrhythmias associated with tacrolimus use. A reversible hypertrophic cardiomyopathy was described in children receiving tacrolimus (see Chapter 15).

INFECTION AND MALIGNANCY
Infection and malignancy inevitably accompany immunosuppression and are discussed in detail in Chapters 9 and 10. Despite their immunosuppressive potency, the incidence of infections and most common *de novo* neoplasms has not significantly increased since the introduction of the calcineurin inhibitors, although the course of malignancies may be accelerated.

THROMBOEMBOLISM
In vitro, cyclosporine increases adenosine diphosphate-induced platelet aggregation, thromboplastin generation, and factor VII activity. It also reduces production of endothelial prostacyclin. These findings may be causally related to the somewhat increased incidence of thromboembolic events that have been observed in cyclosporine-treated kidney transplant recipients. The finding of glomerular microthrombi as part of calcineurin inhibitor-induced microangiopathy was discussed previously.

HYPERURICEMIA AND GOUT
Hyperuricemia, because of reduced renal uric acid clearance, is a common complication of calcineurin inhibitor therapy, particularly when diuretics are also employed. Episodes of gout are more common in patients receiving cyclosporine than tacrolimus and

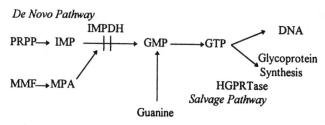

Fig. 4.6.   Mechanism of action of mycophenolate mofetil by inhibition of *de novo* purine synthesis. GMP, guanosine monophosphate; GTP, guanosine triphosphate; HGPRTase, hypoxanthine guanine phosphoribosyl transferase; IMP, inosine monophosphate; IMPDH, inosine monophosphate dehydrogenase; MPA, mycophenolic acid; PRPP, 5-phosphoribosyl-1-phosphate.

have been reported in up to 7% of patients. Treatment is discussed in Chapter 9.

MYCOPHENOLATE MOFETIL

MMF (CellCept) was introduced into clinical transplantation in 1995 after a series of clinical trials (see Part III) showed that it was more effective than azathioprine for the prevention of acute rejection in recipients of cadaveric kidney transplants when used in combination with cyclosporine and prednisone. MMF is a prodrug, the active compound of which is mycophenolic acid (MPA), a fermentation product of several *Penicillium* species; the mofetil moiety serves to markedly improve its oral bioavailability. An enteric-coated form of MPA (ERL-080, myfortic) became available in 2004. The role of MMF in clinical transplantation is discussed in Parts IV and V.

Mechanism of Action

MPA is a reversible inhibitor of the enzyme inosine monophosphate dehydrogenase (IMPDH). IMPDH is a critical, rate-limiting enzyme in the so-called *de novo* synthesis of purines and catalyzes the formation of guanosine nucleotides from inosine. Depletion of guanosine nucleotides by MPA has relatively selective antiproliferative effects on lymphocytes; lymphocytes appear to rely on *de novo* purine synthesis more than other cell types that have a "salvage" pathway for production of guanosine nucleotides from guanine (Figs. 4.1 and 4.6).

In principle, MMF is a more selective antimetabolite. It differs radically in its mode of action from the calcineurin inhibitors and sirolimus in that it does not affect cytokine production or the more proximal events following antigen recognition. It differs from azathioprine by virtue of its selective effect on lymphocytes. *In vitro*, MMF blocks the proliferation of T and B cells, inhibits antibody formation, and inhibits the generation of cytotoxic T cells. MMF also downregulates the expression of adhesion molecules on lymphocytes, thereby impairing their binding to vascular endothelial cells. The capacity of MMF to treat ongoing rejection (see Part IV) may be a reflection of its ability to inhibit the recruitment of mononuclear cells into rejection sites and the subsequent interaction of these cells with target cells. MMF may also exert a preventive effect on the development and progression of proliferative arteriolopathy, a critical pathologic lesion in chronic rejection (see Chapter 13). Retrospective analysis shows that MMF reduces the rate of late allograft loss by an effect that is both dependent and independent of its effect on the incidence of acute rejection.

Pharmacology and Toxicity

MMF is a generally well-tolerated and "user-friendly" compound that is available for clinical use in 250 mg and 500 mg capsules: the standard dose when used with cyclosporine is 1 g twice daily. For African American patients, a dose of 1.5 g twice daily may be required to produce the immunosuppressive benefit. The enteric-coated form is available in 180 mg and 360 mg capsules: the standard dose is 720 mg twice daily. An intravenous preparation is available but is usually not required in kidney transplant recipients. The pharmacokinetics of MMF are complex. Orally administered MMF is rapidly absorbed and hydrolyzed to MPA in the liver, producing a peak level in 1 to 2 hours. MPA is then glucuronidated to an inactive form (MPAG). Enterohepatic cycling of MPAG can occur producing a second peak occurs at 5 to 6 hours, which may account for some of its GI side effects. Bioavailability of MMF in the capsule form is 90%, with a half-life of 12 hours. The AUC of MPA is increased by renal impairment, although dose adjustments are not usually made. Neither MMF nor MPA is dialyzed.

Extensive safety data are available from the clinical trials of MMF. The most common adverse events are related to the GI tract, with diarrhea occurring in up to one-third of patients, and varying degrees of nausea, bloating, dyspepsia, and vomiting occurring in up to 20% of patients. Frank esophagitis and gastritis with occasional GI hemorrhage occur in approximately 5% of patients and may be associated with cytomegalovirus (CMV) infection. The incidence of GI side effects may be higher if the dosage is greater than 1 g twice daily. Most of these symptoms respond promptly to transient reduction of drug dosage. The total daily dose can also be split into three or four doses. The GI side affect profile of the enteric-coated formulation of MPA is not significantly different from the original formulation.

Despite the relatively specific action of MPA on lymphocytes, leukopenia, anemia, and thrombocytopenia occur with a frequency similar to that seen with azathioprine and may require dose adjustment. Prolonged leukocytosis may also occur. The incidence of lymphoproliferative disorders and opportunistic infections in all the various clinical trials of MMF is marginally greater than that seen in control groups and is a nonspecific reflection of its greater immunosuppressive potency. Nephrotoxicity, neurotoxicity, and hepatotoxicity have not been observed with MMF. Its safety in pregnancy has not yet been established.

A relationship has been described between the AUC for MPA and its clinical efficacy and side-effect profile. The relationship to random trough levels is less consistent. Therapeutic drug monitoring is generally not required for clinical management. In the event of side effects, the longer the period of drug-dose reduction or discontinuation, the greater is the subsequent incidence of episodes of acute rejection. Hence, the drug should be reintroduced as soon as possible and the clinical course carefully monitored.

Drug Interactions

MPA is not metabolized through the CYP3A enzyme system; thus, the multiple drug interactions seen with the calcineurin inhibitors do not occur. MMF and azathioprine should not be administered concomitantly because of the potential for combined hematologic toxicity. Standard hematologic parameters must be carefully followed when MMF is used with sirolimus (see Part IV). Cyclosporine lowers MPA concentrations by decreasing its enterohepatic recycling. Trough levels of MPA increase when cyclosporine administration is discontinued. This interaction is not seen with tacrolimus or sirolimus and the maintenance dosage of MMF, when used with standard doses and blood levels of these two drugs, is typically 500 mg to 750 mg twice daily. MMF should not be administered simultaneously with antacids, cholestyramine or oral ferrous sulfate all of which decrease intestinal absorption. MMF, as opposed to azathioprine, can be administered with allopurinol without dose adjustment.

THE "TOR INHIBITORS": SIROLIMUS AND EVEROLIMUS

TOR (target of rapamycin) is a key regulatory kinase in the process of cell division. The term "TOR inhibitor" refers to two similar immunosuppressant drugs whose mode of action (see "Mechanism of Action," below) is closely linked to inhibition of this kinase. Sirolimus (Rapamune), also known as *rapamycin,* is a macrolide antibiotic compound that is structurally related to tacrolimus. Everolimus (Certican), also known as *RAD,* is a similar compound with a shorter half-life. In heart transplant recipients, everolimus is more effective than azathioprine in reducing the severity and incidence of cardiac allograft vasculopathy. Most of the clinical experience with this class of immunosuppressants is with sirolimus.

Sirolimus was introduced into clinical transplantation in the United States in 1999, after a series of clinical trials (see Part III) demonstrated that, when used in combination with cyclosporine and prednisone, it produced a significant reduction in the incidence of acute rejection episodes in the early posttransplant period, when compared to either azathioprine or placebo. These trials were similar in design to those that led to the introduction of MMF in that full doses of cyclosporine were administered and therapeutic drug monitoring was not routinely performed. In Europe, its introduction was delayed because of concerns regarding impairment of kidney function documented in similar trials. It was eventually approved for use in Europe in a protocol based on withdrawal of cyclosporine starting at 3 months posttransplant (see Side Effects). Its use has since been approved in the United States for a similar indication. Sirolimus has also been used with tacrolimus, with prednisone without a calcineurin inhibitor, and with or without MMF, and has been claimed to be about equivalent in immunosuppressive potency to cyclosporine. It has not been formally approved for use in this manner. Sirolimus has not been rigorously compared with MMF; it is probably a more potent but also a more toxic immunosuppressant. The place of sirolimus in clinical transplantation and dosing recommendations are discussed in Part IV. Its potential future clinical use in tolerance-generating protocols is discussed in Part III.

Mechanism of Action

The immunosuppressive activity of the TOR inhibitors appears to be mediated through a mechanism distinct from that of the calcineurin inhibitors. Like the calcineurin inhibitors, they bind to a cytoplasm-binding protein (the same one that binds tacrolimus, FKBP). The resultant sirolimus–FKBP ligand, however, does not block calcineurin (see Chapter 2, Fig. 4.1, and "Mechanism of Action" under "Calcineurin Inhibitors," above); instead, it engages a protein designated *target of rapamycin* because its discovery was related to studies on the mechanism of action of rapamycin. TOR is a key regulatory kinase, and its inhibition reduces cytokine-dependent cellular proliferation at the G_1 to S phase of the cell-division cycle. Both hematopoietic and nonhematopoietic cells are affected. Because rapamycin occupies the same binding protein as tacrolimus, it was originally presumed that it would impair the action of tacrolimus; the drug was thus developed in clinical trials as an adjunctive agent with cyclosporine. It now appears that the abundance of FKBP *in vivo* makes it unlikely that there would be inhibitive competition of tacrolimus and sirolimus for their receptor, and trials of their concomitant use suggest that the combination is effective and safe.

Pharmacology

The original formulation of sirolimus was an oral solution available in a concentration of 1 mg/mL either in a multidose bottle or in fixed-dose pouches to be dispensed into water or orange juice. This formulation has been largely replaced by the more convenient 1 mg or 2 mg capsule. Sirolimus is rapidly absorbed from the GI tract, reaching peak concentrations in 1 to 2 hours. It has a long half-life, averaging 62 hours, and a steady-state trough concentration can be achieved in most patients within 24 hours by administering a loading dose three times the size of the maintenance dose. Everolimus has a half-life of 23 hours and is usually not administered with a loading dose. Both drugs are largely metabolized by the liver by both CYP3A and *p*-glycoprotein; the native compound is the major component in human blood and contributes most of the immunosuppressive activity. Renal excretion is minimal, and dose adjustment is not required in renal dysfunction but is required in hepatic dysfunction. Therapeutic drug level monitoring was not required in the initial labeling of sirolimus, but it has become an intrinsic part of its use now that it is administered in a manner different from that in the trials that led to its introduction (see Part IV). The target trough levels, using a HPLC assay, vary between 5 and 25 ng/dL, depending on the concomitant use of a calcineurin inhibitor and the clinical circumstances, and are a good reflection of drug exposure. Because sirolimus has a long half-life, levels should be checked several days after a dosage adjustment is made and once a steady state has been reached frequent monitoring is not required.

Drug Interactions

The TOR inhibitors and the calcineurin inhibitors are administered together and are metabolized by the same enzyme systems; therefore, the potential for interaction between them must be considered. In healthy volunteers, concomitant administration of sirolimus and the Neoral formulation of cyclosporine increased the AUC for sirolimus by 230%, when compared with administration of sirolimus alone; administration 4 hours after the cyclosporine dose increased the AUC by 80%. For this reason, it has been recommended that sirolimus be administered consistently 4 hours after the morning cyclosporine dose. In clinical practice, however, this recommendation is often ignored, which might account for some of the toxicity noted below (see "Side Effects"). The effect of sirolimus on cyclosporine metabolism is less marked, but over time, lower doses of cyclosporine are required to maintain target trough levels. The pharmacologic interaction between sirolimus and tacrolimus has not been rigorously studied Available information suggests, not surprisingly, that sirolimus interacts with calcium channel blockers, antifungal agents, anticonvulsants, and antituberculous agents in a manner similar to the calcineurin inhibitors. Careful surveillance for drug interactions with sirolimus will be required as the drug is introduced into clinical practice.

Side Effects

Nephrotoxicity

The TOR inhibitors, when administered alone, do not produce either the acute or chronic reductions in GFR that have been so consistently observed with calcineurin inhibitors. When administered with standard doses of calcineurin inhibitors, however, there appears to be a potentiation of nephrotoxicity that is not fully explained by their pharmacokinetic interaction. This phenomenon has been observed both in clinical trials and routine clinical use, and is the basis for the recommendation that when the drugs are used in combination the dose of the calcineurin inhibitor should be an attenuated one (see Part IV). The combined TOR inhibitor/calcineurin inhibitor toxicity is reversible. Figure 4.7, taken from the 3-year continuation study of the cyclosporine withdrawal trial that led to the introduction of sirolimus in Europe, shows that when cyclosporine is withdrawn from the cyclosporine/sirolimus combination at 3 months posttransplant, there is a consistent and persistent improvement in renal function. This is manifested not only in lower serum creatinine levels and higher GFR, but in lower uric acid levels and blood pressure, and less marked chronic histologic damage. The TOR inhibitor may be tubulotoxic and may produce hypokalemia and hypomagnesemia as a result of kaliuresis and magnesuria.

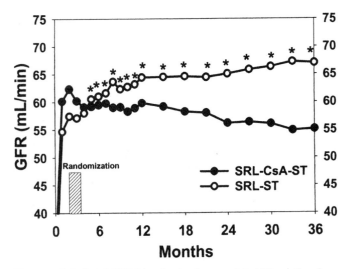

Fig. 4.7. Calculated GFR in patients who completed 36 months of therapy with either sirolimus and steroids alone (SRL-ST) or sirolimus, cyclosporine and steroids (SRL-CsA-ST). *p<0.001. (From Kreis H, Oberbauer R, Campistol JM et al. Long-term benefits with sirolimus-based therapy after early cyclosporine withdrawal. *J Am Soc Nephrol* 2004;15:809–817, with permission.)

Impaired Healing

The TOR inhibitors block a critical step in cell division and it is not surprising that their use would be associated with various manifestations of impaired healing and fibrogenesis. This property is exploited in the coating of coronary artery stents with sirolimus to reduce the incidence of restenosis and may theoretically be of benefit in slowing tumor progression (see Hematologic/Oncologic). Sirolimus may delay recovery from posttransplant delayed graft function by perpetuating "ATN." The combination of sirolimus and tacrolimus reportedly produces acute renal failure with a "cast nephropathy" as a consequence of tubular injury similar to that seen in myeloma. An increased incidence of lymphoceles and dehisced, poorly granulating wounds may occur when TOR inhibitors are used in the early postoperative period. Sirolimus is contraindicated in lung transplantation because of the risk of dehiscence at the bronchial anastomosis. Painful mouth ulcers may also occur that resolve when the drug is discontinued. A reversible oligospermia has been described during sirolimus administration and male patients should be informed accordingly.

Hyperlipidemia

Hyperlipidemia, hypercholesterolemia, and hypertriglyceridemia are common accompaniments of TOR inhibitor use and may occur in varying degrees in more than 50% of patients receiving these drugs. The effect has been ascribed to inhibition of lipoprotein lipase or to reduced catabolism of apoB100-containing lipoproteins. The hyperlipidemia is more pronounced for patients also receiving cyclosporine and tends to reach a peak at 2 to 3 months posttransplant. In most patients, the elevation is manageable with treatment with statins and, based on the Framingham risk model, the associated coronary heart disease (CHD) risk is small. In an animal model of aortic atherosclerosis, sirolimus was described as having a protective effect despite the hyperlipidemia, presumably because of an antiinflammatory effect. The overall impact of TOR inhibitors on clinical CHD has not been defined, but for the great majority of patients, the degree of hyperlipidemia does not contraindicate their use.

Pneumonia

In the early clinical trials of sirolimus, several case of fatal pneumocystis pneumonia were described in patients who did not receive prophylactic Bactrim. For this reason, it is recommended that Bactrim prophylaxis be continued for at least 1 year for patients receiving the drug (see Chapter 10). A noninfectious interstitial pneumonia has also been described, typically presenting as bilateral lower-lobe interstitial pneumonia. Pathologic features are similar to bronchiolitis obliterans organizing pneumonia with alveolar hemorrhage and lymphocytic infiltration. The diagnosis is one of exclusion and the pneumonia typically resolves with 2 to 3 weeks of drug discontinuation.

Hematologic/Oncologic

The TOR inhibitors can produce reversible "cytopenias" of a similar degree to that described with MMF and azathioprine, although the thrombocytopenia may be more pronounced. Hepatic artery thrombosis has been described in liver transplant recipients, but no increased thrombotic tendency has been described in kidney recipients. Thrombotic microangiopathy, well described with the calcineurin inhibitors (see "Acute Microvascular Disease" and Chapter 8), can occur when sirolimus is used in combination with calcineurin inhibitors, and occasional cases have been described when it is alone.

In the clinical trials and clinical experience of the TOR inhibitors, the incidence of malignancy and posttransplant lymphoproliferative disease has been small and no different from that expected from a potent immunosuppressive regimen. In animal models, sirolimus inhibits primary and metastatic tumors through antiangiogenesis and arrests malignant cell growth in the G_1/S phase. The potential of unlinking immunosuppression from tumor progression is clearly of critical importance in transplantation. Conversion from cyclosporine to sirolimus has been shown to be effective treatment for cases of Kaposi's sarcoma, but the broad clinical implication of the experimental antitumor effect of sirolimus is yet to be defined.

AZATHIOPRINE

Azathioprine (Imuran) is an antimetabolite, an imidazole derivative of 6-mercaptopurine. It has been used in clinical transplantation for more than 30 years. When cyclosporine was introduced, the role of azathioprine was largely relegated to that of an adjunctive agent in most circumstances (see Part IV), and with the introduction of MMF, its use has been discontinued in many programs.

Mode of Action

Azathioprine is a purine analogue that is incorporated into cellular deoxyribonucleic acid (DNA), where it inhibits purine nucleotide synthesis and interferes with the synthesis and metabolism of ribonucleic acid (RNA) (Fig. 4.1). Unlike cyclosporine, it does not prevent gene activation, but it inhibits gene replication and consequent T-cell activation.

Azathioprine is a broad myelocyte suppressant. It inhibits the proliferation of promyelocytes in the bone marrow and, as a result, it decreases the number of circulatory monocytes capable of differentiating into macrophages. Thus, it is a powerful inhibitor of the primary immune response and is valuable in preventing the onset of acute rejection. It is ineffective in the therapy of rejection episodes.

Side Effects

The most important side effects of azathioprine are hematologic. Patients first receiving the drug, particularly in higher dosages (2 mg/kg or more), should have complete blood counts performed, including a platelet count, at least weekly during the first month of therapy, and less frequently thereafter. Delayed hematologic suppression may occur. In the event of significant thrombocytopenia or leukopenia, the drug can be discontinued for long periods if the patient is also taking cyclosporine, without great danger of inducing acute rejection. It is unnecessary to maintain a low white blood cell count for the drug to be an effective immunosuppressant. The white blood cell count should be monitored with particular care when the corticosteroid dose is reduced or discontinued.

Azathioprine may occasionally cause hepatitis and cholestasis, which usually present as reversible elevations in transaminase and bilirubin levels. The azathioprine dose is usually reduced or stopped during episodes of significant hepatic dysfunction. Pancreatitis is a rare complication.

Azathioprine is converted to inactive 6-thiouric acid by xanthine oxidase. The inhibition of this enzyme by allopurinol demands that this drug combination be avoided or used with great care. When allopurinol is started, the azathioprine dose should be reduced to 25% to 50% of its initial level, and the white blood cell and platelet counts should be frequently monitored.

DOSE AND ADMINISTRATION

About half of orally administered azathioprine is absorbed; thus, the intravenous dose is equivalent to half the oral dose. Blood levels are not valuable clinically because its effectiveness is not blood-level dependent. The drug is not significantly dialyzed or excreted by the kidney. Dose reduction is often practiced during kidney dysfunction, although it may not be necessary. When used as the primary immunosuppressant, the daily oral dose is 2 to

3 mg/kg. When used as adjunctive therapy with a calcineurin inhibitor, the dose is 1 to 2 mg/kg.

CORTICOSTEROIDS

Corticosteroids have commanded a central position in clinical transplantation since they were first used to treat rejection in the 1960s. Despite this long experience, there remains only a general consensus on their best therapeutic use, and changing protocols often reflect both fear of prescribing them and fear of not prescribing them. The new generation of immunosuppressive drugs and protocols may permit avoidance or withdrawal of corticosteroids for many patients, although this goal has yet to be uniformly reached (see Part IV).

The diffuse effects of corticosteroids on the body reflect the fact that most mammalian tissues have glucocorticoid receptors within the cell cytoplasm and can serve as targets for the effects of corticosteroids. The immunosuppressive actions of corticosteroids can be somewhat simplistically divided into their specific actions on macrophages and T cells and their broad, nonspecific immunosuppressant and antiinflammatory actions.

Mechanism of Action

Blockade of Cytokine Gene Expression

Corticosteroids exert their most critical immunosuppressive effect by blocking T-cell-derived and antigen-presenting cell-derived cytokine and cytokine-receptor expression. They inhibit the function of dendritic cells, which are the most important of the antigen-presenting cells (see Chapter 2). They are hydrophobic and can diffuse intracellularly, where they bind to cytoplasmic receptors found in association with the 90-kDa heat shock protein. As a result, the heat shock protein becomes dissociated, and the steroid-receptor complex translocates to the nucleus, where it binds to DNA sequences referred to as *glucocorticoid response elements* (GREs). GRE sequences have been found in the critical promoter regions of several cytokine genes, and it is presumed that the binding of the steroid-receptor complex to the GRE inhibits the transcription of cytokine genes. Corticosteroids also inhibit the translocation to the nucleus of nuclear factor-κB, a transcription factor that plays a major role in the induction of genes encoding a wide variety of cytokines.

Corticosteroids inhibit the expression of IL-1, IL-2, IL-3, and IL-6, TNF-α, and γ-interferon. As a result, all stages of the T-cell activation process are inhibited. Cytokine release is responsible for the fever often associated with acute rejection. This fever typically resolves rapidly when high-dose corticosteroids are administered.

Nonspecific Immunosuppressive Effects

Glucocorticoids cause a lymphopenia that is a result of the redistribution of lymphocytes from the vascular compartment back to lymphoid tissue. The migration of monocytes to sites of inflammation is also inhibited. Steroids block the synthesis, release, and action of a series of chemokines, permeability-increasing agents, and vasodilators, although these antiinflammatory effects are a relatively minor aspect of their efficacy in the prevention and treatment of acute rejection. The total white blood cell count may rise several-fold during high-dose steroid administration.

Complications

The ubiquitous complications of corticosteroids are familiar to medical practitioners and are not reviewed here in detail. They are a reflection of their profound immunosuppressive, antiinflammatory, and hormonal action on numerous target tissues. The most important complications are cosmetic changes, growth impairment, osteonecrosis, osteoporosis, impaired wound healing and resistance to infection, cataracts, hyperlipidemia, glucose intolerance, and psychopathologic effects. There is marked variation in individual response to these drugs, presumably because of the varied concentration of tissue steroid receptors and individual variations in prednisone metabolism. In the dose regimens currently prescribed, untoward complications can be minimized but not totally prevented.

Commonly Used Preparations

In clinical transplantation, steroids are used in three ways: as a high-dose intravenous or oral pulse given over 3 to 5 days; as a steroid cycle or taper with a gradually decreasing oral dose over days or weeks; or as a steady low-dose daily or every-other-day maintenance regimen. Corticosteroid dosage is discussed in Part IV.

Prednisolone, its 11-keto metabolite *prednisone,* and *methylprednisolone* (Solu-Medrol) are the corticosteroid preparations most commonly used in clinical transplantation. Prednisolone is the most active circulating immunosuppressive corticosteroid. Prednisone is the oral preparation usually used in the United States, whereas prednisolone is often preferred in Europe. Methylprednisolone is the most commonly used intravenous corticosteroid. These preparations have a half-life that is measured in hours, but their capacity to inhibit lymphokine production persists for 24 hours; therefore, once-daily administration is adequate.

Corticosteroids are metabolized by hepatic microsomal enzyme systems. Drugs such as phenytoin, barbiturates, and rifampin, which induce these enzymes, may lower plasma prednisolone levels, whereas oral contraceptives and ketoconazole increase levels. Unfortunately, there is no readily available plasma prednisolone assay for clinical use, although empirical adjustments in dose may be advisable when potentially interacting drugs are administered.

PART II. BIOLOGIC IMMUNOSUPPRESSIVE AGENTS

MONOCLONAL AND POLYCLONAL ANTIBODIES

The antilymphocyte polyclonal antibodies are produced by immunizing either horses or rabbits with human lymphoid tissue and then harvesting the resultant immune sera to obtain gamma-globulin fractions. Various polyclonal antibodies—ALG,

Table 4.3.   Antibody preparations for renal transplant immunosuppression

| Treatment | Indication | | Mechanism of Action |
	Induction	Rejection	Lymphocyte Depletion
Monoclonal			
OKT3	(+)	+	Yes
Basiliximab	+*	—	No
Daclizumab	+*	—	No
Polyclonal			
Atgam	+	+	Yes
Thymoglobulin	(+)	+	Yes

+, Approved indication; (+) unapproved but commonly used indication; *, concomitant administration of calcineurin-inhibitor recommended.

antilymphoblast serum, and ATG—have been available for use in clinical transplantation since the 1970s. Currently, the only polyclonal antibodies widely available for clinical use are the antithymocyte globulins, Atgam and preparations of Thymoglobulin. The intravenous immune globulins (IVIG), which have been used in the treatment of antibody deficiency disorders for more than 25 years, are finding increasing relevance to current transplant therapeutics. They are made from pooled human plasma. The monoclonal antibody muromonab-CD3 (Orthoclone OKT3, referred to here as simply *OKT3*) has been available for clinical use since 1987, and the humanized anti-Tac (HAT) monoclonal antibody preparations daclizumab and basiliximab became available in 1998. Rituximab is an anti–B-cell monoclonal antibody developed for the treatment of hematologic malignancies that has proved useful in clinical transplantation. Alemtuzumab (Campath 1H) is an anti-CD52 humanized monoclonal antibody that is discussed in Part III, together with other monoclonal antibodies in clinical development. Biologic immunosuppressive agents can be used for induction immunosuppression and for the treatment of acute rejection; they are not used for maintenance immunosuppression. Table 4.3 reviews their major indications, which are discussed in detail in Part IV. The polyclonal antibodies (IVIG excluded), OKT3, and alemtuzumab cause varying degrees of T-cell depletion and are sometimes referred to as "depleting" antibodies; the HAT monoclonal antibodies cause T-cell dysfunction but are "nondepleting."

OKT3

Mode of Action

OKT3 is an immunoglobulin (Ig) G globulin—a monoclonal antibody produced by the hybridization of murine antibody-secreting B lymphocytes with a nonsecreting myeloma cell line whose neoplastic potential permits the secretion of antibody in perpetuity. Compared with the humanized monoclonal antibodies discussed later, OKT3 is *xenogeneic* because the whole antibody is of murine origin. OKT3 reacts with human T cells by binding to one of the 20-kDa subunits of the CD3 complex, an intrinsic part of the T-cell receptor (see Chapter 2 and Fig. 4.1). The subsequent deactivation of the CD3 complex causes the T-cell receptor to undergo endocytosis and be lost from the cell surface. The T cells become ineffectual, and within 1 hour, they become opsonized and are removed from the circulation into the reticuloendothelial system. OKT3 also blocks the function of killer T cells, which have an important role in generating the rejection response.

Concomitant with the initial depletion of CD3+ cells, there is depletion of T cells with other surface markers (CD4, CD8, CD11). Within a few days, T cells reappear in the circulation that carry CD4, CD8, and CD11 markers but are devoid of CD3 and are hence ineffectual, or so-called modulated, cells. CD3+ functional cells may reappear later in the course of OKT3 and during a second course, possibly because of the production of neutralizing antibodies. The clinical importance of this reappearance is discussed later.

Dosage and Administration

The standard dose of OKT3 is 5 mg given as an intravenous bolus through a Millipore filter. The standard course consists of a daily dose for 10 days, although shorter (5 to 7 days) or longer (14 days or more) courses are sometimes given. Protocols using lower doses of OKT3 may be just as effective but are less-well tested. OKT3 protocol recommendations are given in Table 4.4. The first few doses of OKT3 must be given in the hospital, preferably at an institution familiar with its use, side effects, and clinical indications. The first dose can be safely administered intraoperatively as long as the protocol recommendations are followed. If the drug is well tolerated, the course can be completed on an outpatient basis with substantial financial economy and patient convenience.

Monitoring

OKT3 monitoring refers to the repeated assessment of the effectiveness of the drug during a course because of the potential for the development of human antimurine antibodies, which may abrogate its action and allow for the reappearance of potent CD3+ T cells. Antibodies may be directed against the antibody site itself (antiidiotypic), against the IgG protein subclass (antiisotypic), and against the mouse protein of origin (antimurine).

During an effective course of OKT3, the percentage of CD3+ T cells decreases precipitously within 24 to 48 hours, from approximately 60% to less than 5%. The decrease may be somewhat slower in an effective second course. Failure of the CD3+ percentage to decrease or a decrease followed by a rapid rise indicates the appearance of blocking antibodies. The concomitant use of low-dose calcineurin inhibitor, MMF, or azathioprine during a course of OKT3 (Table 4.4) serves to minimize the antibody response.

Side Effects

Significant, potentially life-threatening adverse reactions may occur during the first days of treatment with OKT3. These adverse

Table 4.4.   Protocol recommendations for OKT3 use

1. Before administration of first dose, patient should be edema free, be within 3% of dry weight, and have a negative chest radiograph.
2. Use high-dose diuretics, dialysis, or ultrafiltration alone to achieve euvolemia in a volume-overloaded patient.
3. Administer premedication 15–60 minutes before the first and second doses. The premedication consists of methyl-prednisolone, 5–8 mg/kg; diphenhydramine hydrochloride (Benadryl), 50 mg IV; and acetaminophen, 500 mg PO.
4. Before the first and second doses, monitor vital signs every 15 minutes for 2 hours, then every 30 minutes for 2 hours.
5. Premedication is not required for remainder of the course; use acetaminophen p.r.n. for fever.
6. If OKT3 is stopped for more than one dose, repeat first-dose precautions.
7. Continue low dose of calcineurin-inhibitor, azathioprine, or MMF during the course.
8. If calcineurin-inhibitor is continued, use half dose; return to full dose 2 days before completion of the course and ensure therapeutic levels.
9. After the first two doses, continue prednisone according to the protocol schedule.
10. Use antiviral and antibacterial prophylaxis (see Chapter 10).
11. During second course of OKT3, monitor CD3 levels at least twice weekly.
12. After the first two doses, encourage hydration for patient diuresis.
13. Consider outpatient administration after third dose in stable patients.

reactions occur as the percentage of potent T cells plummets and a series of T-cell-derived cytokines, including TNF, IL-2, and γ-interferon, are released into the circulation. The term *cytokine release syndrome* has been used to describe the clinical events that follow. Immediate complement activation may also play an important etiologic role. The OKT3 administration protocol (Table 4.4) is designed to minimize the severity of this syndrome. Other proposed techniques include use of indomethacin, anti-TNF antibodies, pentoxifylline, and administration of OKT3 over 2 hours as an infusion rather than as a bolus injection. A double-blind, randomized study of pentoxifylline, however, showed no measurable benefit.

FEVER AND CHILLS

After the first exposure to OKT3, nearly all patients become febrile, and many suffer rigors. The fever and rigors often occur "like clockwork" 45 minutes after the injection, but may be delayed for hours. By the second or third dose, the fever typically abates, although some patients remain febrile for several days or throughout the whole course. Patients being treated with OKT3 are all immunosuppressed by definition; hence, infectious causes of fever should always be considered. If the fever is prolonged for more than two to three doses, a fever workup should be performed. The development of fever later in the course of OKT3 after an afebrile period is particularly suggestive of a infectious etiology (with CMV infection at the top of the differential diagnosis) and demands careful consideration of the wisdom of continuing the course.

PULMONARY EDEMA

A rapidly developing, potentially life-threatening noncardiogenic pulmonary edema may occur after the first or second dose of OKT3 if the patient is not euvolemic or is very close to his or her dry weight at the time of injection. Even euvolemic patients may wheeze and become dyspneic. Post-OKT3 pulmonary edema is a preventable syndrome as long as the precautions listed in Table 4.4 are adhered to rigidly. Clinical volume assessment is often unreliable, and patients may "hide" liters of fluid that are not clinically detectable. It is often wise and expeditious to dialyze or ultrafilter a patient before OKT3 administration to ensure that the required amount of fluid is removed.

After the first doses of OKT3, the fluid restrictions can be relaxed. Patients may, in fact, become hypotensive and dehydrated because of fever, diarrhea, and prior fluid restriction. The decision about whether to continue OKT3 in a hypotensive febrile patient may be difficult. In these circumstances, OKT3 can be continued safely as long as other causes of hypotension and fever are considered and excluded and hydration is maintained.

NEPHROTOXICITY

Renal function, as judged by serum creatinine levels, may deteriorate during the early days of an OKT3 course; a previously nonoliguric patient may even require dialysis. This deterioration of function is typically transient and is followed by a brisk diuresis. It may even be a harbinger of a successful course because it is presumably a manifestation of the hemodynamic abnormalities following cytokine release as the OKT3 takes its toll on the T cells. This transient nephrotoxicity probably accounts for the fact that the prophylactic use of OKT3 immediately after transplantation does not clearly reduce the frequency of delayed graft function when compared with postoperative use of calcineurin inhibitors, although the length of the oliguric period may be reduced. Occasional cases of irreversible graft thrombosis have been described after OKT3 administration and might be a result of OKT3-induced activation of the coagulation cascade.

NEUROLOGIC COMPLICATIONS

A spectrum of neurologic complications can occur during a course of OKT3, varying in severity from a commonly occurring mild headache to severe encephalopathy. The severe complications are more common when OKT3 is given for prophylaxis in patients with delayed graft function; diabetic patients may also be more susceptible.

The aseptic meningitis syndrome is self-limiting and typically resolves spontaneously without the necessity for discontinuing the OKT3 course. If a lumbar puncture is performed, a mild culture-negative leukocytosis with pleocytosis is often found. Clinicians may be more comfortable discontinuing the OKT3 for one or two doses while the results of lumbar puncture culture are awaited and the patient's clinical status is observed. About one-third of patients with a diagnosis of aseptic meningitis have coexisting evidence of encephalopathy. OKT3 should be discontinued in severely encephalopathic patients.

INFECTION
Infection, most commonly with CMV, may be a late adverse sequela of OKT3 use. The frequency of infection varies with the number of courses of OKT3 and the overall amount of immunosuppression given. Most programs routinely employ CMV prophylaxis before or during a course of OKT3, with recipients of CMV-positive allografts representing a particularly high-risk population. Techniques of CMV prophylaxis are discussed in Chapter 10.

REJECTION RECURRENCE
Episodes of rejection may occur after up to 60% of courses of OKT3. These episodes, which are typically mild, can usually be controlled with a low-dose prednisone pulse. They occur as potent CD3+ T cells reappear in the circulation. At the completion of a course of OKT3, it is important to ensure that calcineurin inhibitor blood levels are in the high therapeutic range (Table 4.4). It may be wise to increase the steroid dose routinely in the first 3 to 4 days after the course.

HEMATOLOGIC COMPLICATIONS
The development of lymphoma in transplant recipients is a well-recognized, although infrequent, consequence of effective immunosuppression. Use of repeat courses of OKT3 or polyclonal antibodies is associated with a particularly fulminant and typically rapidly fatal B-cell lymphoma that develops within the first few months after transplantation. Epstein-Barr virus (EBV) antibody-negative patients receiving a graft from an EBV-positive donor appear to be at greatest risk. The recognition, prevention, and management of posttransplant lymphoma are discussed in Chapters 9 and 10.

Administration of OKT3 may be associated with coagulopathy manifested by occasional cases of allograft thrombosis, thrombotic microangiopathy, and thrombocytopenia.

Polyclonal Antibodies

Mode of Action
Atgam, which is made by the immunization of horses with human lymphoid material, has been largely replaced by the more potent Thymoglobulin preparations. Thymoglobulin is made by immunization of rabbits with human lymphoid tissue. In the case of Thymoglobulin (Abbott), which is available in the United States, thymocytes are used; in the case of Anti-T-Lymphocyte Immune Globulin (ATG-Fresenius), which is available in Europe, an activated human T-cell line is used. The resultant gamma-globulin is then purified to remove irrelevant antibody material that may be responsible for some of the drugs' side effects. The precise mechanism of action of the polyclonal antibodies is not fully understood, but the immunosuppressive product contains cytotoxic antibodies directed against a variety of T-cell markers.

After their administration, there is depletion of peripheral blood lymphocytes. The lymphocytes, T cells in particular, are either lysed or cleared by the reticuloendothelial system, and their surface antigens may be masked by the antibody. With the use of Thymoglobulin, a prolonged lymphopenia can ensue, and the CD4 subset may be suppressed for several years. The prolonged immunosuppressive effect of these drugs may account for the relative infrequency of episodes of rejection recurrence when compared with OKT3 (see Part IV).

Dose and Administration

The standard dose of Thymoglobulin is 1.5 mg/kg given in a course lasting 4 to 10 days. When Thymoglobulin is used for induction, it is more effective when started intraoperatively (rather than postoperatively) in reducing the incidence of delayed graft function. Thymoglobulin may also be effectively dosed based on its impact on T-cell subsets. It is mixed in 500 mL of dextrose or saline and infused over 4 to 8 hours into a central vein or arteriovenous fistula. Use of a peripheral vein is sometimes followed by vein thrombosis or thrombophlebitis, although this may be prevented by adding hydrocortisone sodium succinate (Solu-Cortef), 20 mg, and heparin, 1,000 U, to the infusion solution.

To avoid allergic reactions, the patient should receive intravenous premedication consisting of methylprednisolone, 30 mg, and diphenhydramine hydrochloride (Benadryl), 50 mg, 30 minutes before injection. Acetaminophen should be given before and 4 hours after commencement of the infusion for fever control. Vital signs should be monitored every 15 minutes during the first hour of infusion and then hourly until the infusion is complete.

Azathioprine, MMF, and sirolimus should generally be discontinued during the course of treatment to avoid exacerbating hematologic side effects. Cyclosporine or tacrolimus can be omitted during the course or given in a low dose, and oral prednisone is replaced by the methylprednisolone given in the premedication.

Side Effects

Most of the side effects of polyclonal antibodies relate to the fact that foreign protein is administered. Chills, fever, and arthralgias are common, although the severe first-dose reactions seen with OKT3 do not occur. There have been occasional cases of anaphylaxis. Serum sickness occurs rarely because the continued immunosuppression that follows the treatment course reduces the production of antiidiotypic antibodies and the consequent immune complex deposition.

All the polyclonal antibody preparations can produce thrombocytopenia and leukopenia, necessitating reduction or curtailment of drug dosage. Leukopenia is more frequent with Thymoglobulin and occurs in up to half of patients. The drug dose is usually halved for patients with either a platelet count of 50,000 to 100,000 cells/mL or a white blood cell count of less than 3,000 cells/mL. Administration of the drugs should be stopped if the counts fall further. The infectious complications are similar to those described for OKT3. The incidence and severity of CMV infection is clearly more common with all of these agents, but

Table 4.5.   Clinical uses of immune globulin preparations in transplantation

1. To reduce high levels of preformed anti-HLA antibodies in sensitized patients awaiting deceased donor transplants (see Chapters 3 and 6).
2. To facilitate living donor transplants in the face of a positive cross-match or ABO incompatibility (see Chapters 3, 5, and 6).
3. To treat acute humoral rejection (see Part IV and Chapter 8).
4. To treat certain posttransplant viral infection (see chapter 10).

can be minimized with the prophylactic measures included in the protocol (see Chapter 10).

Intravenous Immune Globulins

Pooled human gamma-globulin preparations, which were initially developed for the treatment of humoral immune deficiency disorders, are now used for a variety of autoimmune and inflammatory disorders. They are proving to be invaluable in certain defined situations in clinical transplantation when used alone or in combination with plasmapheresis (Table 4.5). Immune globulin preparations are made from pooled plasma from thousands of blood donors in a tightly regulated manufacturing process that essentially removes the risk of transmission of infectious disease. Immune globulins may be unselected, in which case they contain IgG molecules with a subclass distribution corresponding to that in normal human serum; they may also be selected because of the high titer of desired antibody in the donor plasma. CMV hyperimmune globulin (CMVIG marketed in the United States as CytoGam), approved for CMV prophylaxis and treatment (see Chapter 10), is made from blood donors with a high titer of anti-CMV antibody.

Mechanism of Action

The mode of action of IVIG is complex (Table 4.6) and the broad range of its activities is a reflection of the importance of immunoglobulins in immune homeostasis in health. In highly sensitized patients, IVIG inhibits anti-HLA antibody and produces long-term suppression or elimination of anti-HLA reactive T cells and B cells. The cytokine signaling, critical for IgG synthesis, is inhibited and alloimmunization is inhibited through blockade of the T-cell receptor (see Chapter 2). Although discussed here in the context of immunosuppressant medications, IVIG is better regarded as immunomodulatory in its activity, and its use is not associated with the familiar complications of immunosuppression.

Dosage, Administration, and Side Effects

The dose of IVIG is protocol dependent and readers should consult the package insert and administration precautions of individual preparations prior to their use. All preparations are administered slowly over several hours. The standard dose of

Table 4.6. Immunoregulatory effects of immune globulin

Fc receptors
  Blockade of Fc receptors on macrophages and effector cells
  Induction of antibody-dependent cellular cytotoxicity
  Induction of inhibitory Fcγ receptor IIB
Inflammation
  Attenuation of complement-mediated damage
  Decrease in immune complex-mediated inflammation
  Induction of antiinflammatory cytokines
  Inhibition of activation of endothelial cells
  Neutralization of microbial toxins
  Reduction in corticosteroid requirements
B cells and antibodies
  Control of emergent bone marrow B-cell repertoires
  Negative signaling through the Fcγ receptors
  Selective downregulation and upregulation of antibody
    production
  Neutralization of circulating autoantibodies by antiidiotypes
T cells
  Regulation of the production of helper T-cell cytokines
  Neutralization of T-cell superantigens
Cell growth
  Inhibition of lymphocyte proliferation
  Regulation of apoptosis

From Kazatchkine MD, Kaveri SV. Immunomodulation of autoimmune and inflammatory diseases with intravenous immune globulin. *N Engl J Med* 2001; 345:747–755.

unselected IVIG used for the indications listed in Table 4.5 is 2 g/kg up to a maximum of 140 g in a single administration. The dose of CMVIG varies from 100 to 150 mg/kg and is given following plasmapheresis with one plasma volume exchange replaced by either 5% albumin or fresh-frozen plasma.

Minor reactions, such as flushing, chills, headache, nausea, myalgia, and arthralgia, occur in approximately 5% of patients soon after commencement of IVIG infusions. These symptoms resolve when the infusion is temporarily discontinued or its rate reduced. A spontaneously resolving aseptic meningitis, which can be prevented by the administration of nonsteroidal antiinflammatory agents, may occur in the first 72 hours following the infusion.

Of particular importance to transplant recipients is the development of acute renal failure following IVIG administration. Most preparations of IVIG contain carbohydrate additives such as sucrose or sorbitol, which can induce osmotic injury (so-called osmotic nephrosis) to the proximal tubular epithelium. Proximal tubular cells swell and are filled with isometric vacuoles. Patients with impaired baseline renal function may suffer further deterioration of function that may necessitate dialysis and may produce a confusing clinical picture. The tubular injury is self-limiting and typically resolves within several days. Patients should be warned of the possibility of transient graft dysfunction. The incidence of renal dysfunction can be minimized by slow infusion of IVIG or administration during dialysis.

Humanized Anti-CD25 Monoclonal Antibodies

Mechanism of Action

The anti-CD25 monoclonal antibodies basiliximab and daclizumab are targeted against the α chain (also referred to as CD25, or Tac) of the IL-2 receptor (Fig 4.1). The receptor is upregulated only on activated T cells (see Chapter 2), and as a result of the binding of the antibody, IL-2-mediated responses are blocked. The anti-CD25 monoclonal antibodies thus complement the effect of the calcineurin inhibitors, which reduce the production of IL-2. They are designed to prevent, but not treat, episodes of acute rejection.

Basiliximab (Simulect) and *daclizumab* (Zenapax) are two similar compounds that were introduced into clinical transplantation by virtue of their capacity to reduce the incidence of acute rejection episodes when used in combination with cyclosporine and corticosteroids (see Part III). They both originate as murine monoclonal antibodies, which are then genetically engineered so that large parts of the molecule are replaced by human IgG. The resulting compounds have low *immunogenicity* because they do not induce production of significant amounts of human antimurine antibody. As a result, they have a prolonged half-life in the peripheral blood, and they do not induce a first-dose reaction. The compounds thus differ from the fully xenogeneic OKT3, which has a short half-life, generates a strong antimurine response, and has a pronounced first-dose reaction.

In the case of basiliximab, the entire variable region of the murine antibody remains intact, whereas the constant region originates from human IgG; the resulting compound is strictly deemed *chimeric* and is of 75% human and 25% murine origin. In the case of daclizumab, only the antibody binding site is of murine origin, and the resulting compound is deemed *humanized* and is of 90% human and 10% murine origin. This discrete difference between the compounds accounts for the fact that the affinity of basiliximab for the IL-2 receptor is greater than the affinity of daclizumab for the receptor. This difference appears to have little clinical significance but explains why the dose of daclizumab is greater than the dose of basiliximab.

Dosage and Administration

The immunosuppressive potency of both drugs is presumed to be related to their capacity to produce complete and consistent binding to the IL-2 receptor α sites on T cells. Both drugs have a half-life of longer than 7 days, which permits a long dosage interval. The dosing protocols used in the clinical trials leading to their introduction into clinical transplantation were designed to produce binding of the receptor sites during the early posttransplant period when the incidence of acute rejection episodes is highest. In the case of basiliximab, two intravenous doses of 20 mg are given, the first dose preoperatively and the second dose on postoperative day 4; this regimen produces saturation of the IL-2α receptor sites for 30 to 45 days. In the case of daclizumab, five doses of 1 mg/kg are given, starting preoperatively and then at 2-week intervals, producing saturation of the IL-2α sites for up to 12 weeks. Two-dose courses of daclizumab have also been used effectively.

Side Effects

Both drugs are remarkable by virtue of the absence of significant side effects. Anaphylaxis or first-dose reactions are essentially absent with daclizumab but have occasionally been described with basiliximab. In the clinical trials leading to their introduction, the incidence of typical transplant-related side effects was not greater in the treatment groups than in the control groups.

PART III. CLINICAL TRIALS AND NEW IMMUNOSUPPRESSIVE AGENTS

During the 1990s, a series of promising new immunosuppressive agents underwent laboratory and clinical evaluation in a successful attempt to broaden and improve the immunosuppressive therapeutic armamentarium. This process continues apace, and several promising new immunosuppressive candidates are at various stages of development. The race for their introduction into clinical transplantation practice can be likened to an obstacle course. Some drugs have passed the finishing line (e.g., tacrolimus, MMF, sirolimus, the anti-CD25 monoclonal antibodies), some have already faltered and fallen from current clinical consideration in organ transplantation (e.g., brequinar sodium, cyclosporine G, deoxyspergualin, and the antiadhesion molecule antibodies), and some are still in the race with obstacles ahead (e.g., FTY720 and the new antibody preparations).

The great success of organ transplantation that was achieved in the 1990s with currently available agents is, paradoxically, making it exceedingly difficult (and enormously expensive) to prove the added benefit of new agents. In clinical trials of new agents, as discussed later, the use of the traditional marker of drug or protocol superiority—patient or graft survival—is now proving to be impractical and has largely been replaced by alternative end points.

CLINICAL TRIALS

Before any clinical trials can be performed with an investigational agent, an *investigational new drug* (IND) application has to be submitted to the FDA or to an equivalent regulatory body outside of the United States. Approval of the IND application is based on the evaluation of preclinical studies that suggest potential therapeutic benefits of a new agent and on the evaluation of studies in a variety of animals that suggest its safety.

Phase 1 clinical studies are performed in healthy human volunteers or patients to evaluate human metabolism, pharmacokinetics, dosage, safety, and, if possible, effectiveness. Phase 2 includes controlled, open-label, clinical studies conducted to evaluate the effectiveness of the drug for a particular indication(s) and to determine dose regimens, common side effects, and risks. Phase 3 studies are expanded trials based on preliminary evidence from the previous phases that suggest efficacy and safety. They are sometimes called *pivotal trials* because they are critical for

FDA-approved licensing. They typically involve large, usually *multicentered,* clinical trials that are *randomized* and, if possible, *double-blinded* using *placebo controls.* These studies serve to refine dosage, determine benefit, and further evaluate the overall risk-to-benefit ratio of the new drug. In organ transplantation, particular care has to be taken to ensure that any potential benefit of a new agent is not outweighed by the consequences of overimmunosuppression or by organ-specific toxicity. Successful completion of phase 3 should provide an adequate basis for product labeling and permit approval of the drug for its defined indications. Following introduction of a new drug into the clinical marketplace, phase 4 studies may be performed under the auspices of the manufacturer or of independent investigators or at the request of the FDA to further refine the role of the drug in clinical practice. For example, if a new immunosuppressant is introduced based on a protocol design that combines the drug with cyclosporine, a phase 4 study may test the safety and efficacy of the drug used in combination with tacrolimus.

Any human use of an experimental drug is strictly governed by the predetermined rules of the experimental protocol under which the drug is administered. Patients must read, understand, and sign an informed consent form that clearly defines the nature of the experiment in which they are involved and its potential risks and benefits. They must also receive a copy of the *patient's bill of rights,* which clearly defines the nature of their commitment and authorize the release of personal health information according to the provision of federal privacy laws [the Health Insurance Portability and Accountability Act (HIPAA)]. The experimental protocol and consent form must have been approved by an *institutional review board* (IRB) or *human subjects protection committee* (HSPC), and the medical staff administering the protocol must feel totally comfortable with it. After a drug is licensed, it is often used "off-label" for indications, or in doses, different from those precisely defined. Such use does not require a formal consent procedure, although it is wise to inform the patient that the drug is being given for an unapproved use.

Clinical Trial Design in Transplantation

Immunosuppressive practitioners must understand the way in which new agents are introduced because clinical trials of new immunosuppressive agents not only have led to their clinical use, but also have largely determined the way in which these agents are used. It is also particularly important to appreciate what primary *end points* were used to determine the efficacy of the new agents. The choice of primary end point, the frequency with which this end point occurs in the control population, and the anticipated capacity of the new agent to change the incidence of the end point (estimated from phase 2 studies), permits a statistical evaluation of the number of patients required to be enrolled in the study so that the study has sufficient statistical power to determine the effectiveness of the new agent. Secondary end points usually include side-effect comparisons, renal function estimations, and long-term effects on patient and graft survival. Studies may not have the *statistical power* to provide answers to the questions posed by the secondary end points.

When the clinical trials for cyclosporine use in kidney transplantation were designed in the late 1970s and early 1980s, the primary end point used was improvement of patient and graft survival, which cyclosporine indeed achieved. Tacrolimus was introduced based on its capacity to produce results equivalent to cyclosporine. OKT3 was introduced based on its superior capacity, when compared with corticosteroids, to reverse episodes of acute rejection, and Thymoglobulin was introduced for its superiority in reversing acute rejection when compared with Atgam. All the remaining available new drugs (MMF, sirolimus, anti-CD25 monoclonal antibodies) have been introduced based on their capacity, when combined with cyclosporine and prednisone, to reduce the incidence of acute rejection episodes.

Incidence of Acute Rejection Episodes as an End Point for Studies of New Immunosuppressive Drugs

The incidence of acute rejection episodes, typically biopsy-proven (see Chapter 13), has become the most frequently used marker of the effectiveness of new immunosuppressive drugs for the following reasons:

1. Because of the excellent results of kidney transplantation with currently available immunosuppressants, with 1-year graft survival of close to 90% in most centers and minimal mortality, it is statistically extremely difficult to prove the benefit of new agents or protocols in terms of patient or graft survival.
2. Acute rejection is a potent risk factor for the development of chronic allograft failure (see Chapter 9). In retrospective analyses, patients who have suffered episodes of acute rejection have a long-term graft survival rate that is 20% to 30% less than the graft survival rate of patients who have not suffered acute rejection.
3. Acute rejection episodes are morbid events in themselves, requiring intensification of immunosuppression and sometimes hospital admission.
4. Most acute rejection episodes take place within the first few months of transplantation, and their presence can be proved on biopsy. This permits a rapid evaluation of the effectiveness of a new agent or protocol (a "luxury" that is not available when immunosuppressive drug trials are performed in other clinical circumstances, such as systemic lupus erythematosus or rheumatoid arthritis).

Figure 4.8 provides an example of the way in which the incidence of biopsy-proven acute rejection episodes is used to show the effectiveness of a new agent from one of the pivotal trials leading to the introduction of MMF. This trial was a randomized, double-blind, placebo-controlled, multicenter, phase 3 study to evaluate the efficacy of MMF for the prevention of acute rejection episodes during the first 6 months after transplantation. In this trial, standard therapy consisted of cyclosporine, prednisone, and azathioprine. The study compared two doses of MMF (1.0 g given twice daily and 1.5 g given twice daily) or azathioprine in combination with cyclosporine and prednisone. In the United States, the study involved 500 recipients of a first deceased donor

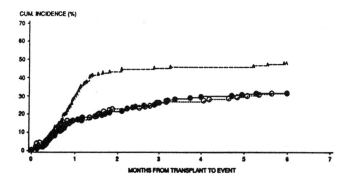

Fig. 4.8. Effects of mycophenolate mofetil on the cumulative incidence of biopsy-proved acute rejection and treatment failure during the first 6 months after transplantation. A, azathioprine group; O, mycophenolate mofetil, 1.0 g bid; •, mycophenolate mofetil, 1.5 g bid. (From Sollinger HW, for the U.S. Renal Transplant Mycophenolate Mofetil Study Group. Mycophenolate mofetil for the prevention of acute rejection in primary cadaveric renal allograft recipients. *Transplantation* 1995;60:225–232, with permission.)

transplant (very similar studies involving another 1,000 patients were performed in Europe, Canada, and Australia). Figure 4.8 illustrates the clear-cut benefit of MMF with respect to the primary end point. There was a statistically significant reduction in the incidence of acute rejection episodes from 41% in the azathioprine group to about 20% in both the MMF groups. Use of high-dose steroids and OKT3 was also markedly reduced in the MMF groups. In this particular study, however, there was no statistically significant benefit of MMF with respect to patient or graft survival when estimated at either 1 or 3 years.

A statistically significant reduction in the incidence of acute rejection episodes was also achieved in the pivotal clinical trials leading to the introduction of sirolimus, and the anti-CD25 monoclonal antibodies. A significant effect on patient and graft survival was not achieved, probably because the studies did not have the statistical power to show such an effect.

As new immunosuppressive drugs and protocols are introduced and the incidence of acute rejection decreases, it is becoming increasingly difficult to prove the statistically significant benefit of newer drugs. In the pivotal trials leading to the introduction of MMF, sirolimus, and the anti-CD25 monoclonal antibodies, the incidence of acute rejection in the patients receiving the experimental drug protocol was compared with the incidence of acute rejection in patients receiving *standard therapy* with cyclosporine, prednisone, and azathioprine. The success of MMF in reducing the incidence of acute rejection led to it becoming part of an updated standard therapy protocol in many centers (see Part IV). In the future, trials of newer agents, MMF, or possibly sirolimus, will represent standard therapy, and statistical proof of further reduction in the incidence of acute rejection will likely be more difficult to achieve. Similarly, it is becoming more difficult to introduce new drugs based on their capacity to reverse episodes of acute rejection because these episodes are becoming less frequent. In the future, new end points may be based on functional parameters such as estimates of renal function, on histologic parameters such as scores for chronic allograft nephropathy (see Chapter 13), on immune parameters (see Chapter 2), or on a composite of multiple end points.

NEW IMMUNOSUPPRESSIVE DRUGS

A variety of new immunosuppressive drugs are at different stages of development. Some of these may produce modest improvements of drugs that are already available (e.g., fewer side effects, better therapeutic index); some, if their clinical development proves successful, may radically alter the way immunosuppression is practiced in the near future; some have been approved for use in nontransplant situations and are being used off-label in clinical transplantation. Some of the new drugs are still known by their laboratory designations. The following is not intended to be a complete list of all the new immunosuppressive drugs in current clinical development but emphasizes those that appear most likely to be eventually introduced into clinical transplantation.

Modifications of Available Drugs

When effective drugs find a place in transplant therapeutics, attempts may be made to improve on them by making discrete alterations in their structure or mode of administration. Examples are *SDZ RAD* (Certican), a derivative of sirolimus with improved oral bioavailability, *ERL080A* (myfortic), an enteric-coated form of MMF, and tacrolimus MR a long-acting form of tacrolimus (see Part I).

FTY720

FTY720 is a novel immunosuppressive compound with a mechanism of action not previously encountered. It is a structural analogue of myricin, a metabolite of a traditional Chinese herb. FTY720 reduces the number of T and B cells in the peripheral blood while increasing their numbers in lymph nodes and Peyer patches. This redirected cell "homing" is thought to be a result of modification by FTY720 of chemokine receptors on lymphocytes. FTY720 activates cell mobility machinery via EDG-6, a G-protein-coupled membrane receptor of the endothelial differentiation gene (EDG) family. Several members of the EDG family share the same natural ligand, sphingosine-1-phosphate (S1P), a sphingolipid breakdown product with striking homology with FTY720 (Fig 4.1). S1P receptor agonists such as FTY720 restrict the egress of lymphocytes from lymphoid organs where they have been sequestered. The recirculation of lymphocytes through lymphoid organs, essential for the development of an effective immune response, is impaired.

Following administration of FTY720 there is suppression of lymphocyte infiltration into allografts and prolonged lymphopenia. Immunologic memory, however, is not impaired and granulocyte number and function are not affected. In phase 2 clinical trials a 2.5-mg dose of FTY720 in combination with cyclosporine was as effective and safe as a standard MMF/cyclosporine combination and a 5-mg dose of FTY720 seemed to permit a safe reduction in cyclosporine dose. The prolonged lymphopenia induced by FTY720 does not appear to increase the risk of opportunistic infections. Within 48 hours of the first dose, in up to 25% of patients, FTY720 may produce a reversible bradycardia without hemodynamic compromise. Phase 3 studies are in progress and their results will determine the place of this new form of immunosuppression in clinical transplantation.

Leflunomide

Leflunomide (Arava) is an immunosuppressive agent with a promising background in experimental transplantation, although its evaluation in clinical transplantation has not been pursued by its manufacturer. It is approved for use in the United States for the treatment of rheumatoid arthritis.

The active metabolite of leflunomide is a malononitrilamide (MNA) which blocks dihydro-orotate dehydrogenase (DHODH), an enzyme required for *de novo* pyrimidine synthesis in lymphocytes (Fig. 4.1). Tyrosine kinase activity is also blocked. Experimental data suggests that leflunomide may be effective in preventing and treating acute rejection and reversing established chronic rejection. It is not nephrotoxic and it has been used clinically to treat chronic allograft nephropathy. It does not appear to have pharmacokinetic interactions with other immunosuppressive agents. Leflunomide also has antiviral activity against herpes viruses and it has been used successfully in the treatment of polyomavirus nephropathy (see Chapter 10). Readers should consult the package insert for detailed prescribing information.

FK778 is an analogue of leflunomide with a shorter half-life that has been shown, in animal models, to have a vasculoprotective effect that is independent of its immunosuppressive activity. It inhibits neointima formation and has potential application for the treatment of chronic allograft failure.

New Biologic Agents

Alemtuzumab

"Lymphocyte depletion" is the term used to describe the strategy whereby the number of alloreactive T cells is radically reduced at the time of transplantation in order to make the host unresponsive to a mismatched allograft. Over time, there is a repopulation of the lymphoid compartment. The polyclonal antibodies and OKT3 described in Part II fall into this category, as do other techniques, such as whole-body irradiation. Alemtuzumab (Campath 1H) is an anti-CD52 monoclonal antibody (Fig. 4.1) approved for use in chronic lymphocytic leukemia that is a potentially valuable depletional agent in clinical transplantation. When used at the time of transplant as induction therapy (see Part IV), alemtuzumab induces a profound, rapid and effective depletion of peripheral and central lymphoid cells that may take months to return to pretransplant levels. Used as a single agent it does not induce tolerance and episodes of acute rejection can occur even in the absence of T cells. Its use facilitates minimization of maintenance immunosuppressive protocols and steroid sparing with monotherapy using sirolimus or low-dose calcineurin inhibitor. The term "prope tolerance," or "near tolerance," has been used to describe the immunologic balance that results.

Rituximab

Rituximab (Rituxan) is a monoclonal antibody directed against the CD20 antigen on B lymphocytes. A rapid and sustained depletion of circulating and tissue-based B cells follows its intravenous administration. B cell recovery begins approximately 6 months after completion of treatment. Rituximab is approved for use in the treatment of certain forms of non-Hodgkin lymphoma. It has also been used in a variety of presumed autoimmune diseases to suppress antibody formation. In clinical transplantation it has been used in a variety of ways: in an attempt to reduce high levels of preformed anti-HLA antigens; to facilitate living donor transplantation in the face of a positive cross-match or ABO incompatibility; to treat acute humoral rejection; and to treat posttransplant lymphoproliferative disease, which is usually CD20+ (see Chapter 9). The standard dosage is 375 mg/m^2 once weekly for four doses. Transient hypotension may occur during infusion. Premedication with acetaminophen and diphenhydramine is advisable. The reader should refer to the package insert for precise dosing and administration guidelines.

T-Cell Costimulatory Blockade

A promising approach to the induction of clinically relevant donor-specific graft tolerance comes from the studies manipulating the two major signals required for T-cell activation. Optimal and sustained T-cell response after antigen recognition (signal 1) requires costimulatory signals (signal 2) delivered through accessory T-cell surface molecules (see Chapter 2 and Fig. 4.1). The best understood of the costimulatory pathways are CD28:B7 and CD154:CD40. Cytotoxic T-lymphocyte antigen (CTLA)-4-Ig is a fusion protein, a homologue of CD28, which binds the B7 molecule with high affinity and blocks the interaction with CD28. Both CTLA-4-Ig and anti-CD154 antibodies, used alone or in combination, are effective in preventing rejection in small animal models. In nonhuman primates, a combination of the agents produced prolonged survival of kidney transplants without additional immunosuppression. In a randomized trial, CTLA-4-Ig combined with methotrexate was significantly more effective than placebo with methotrexate for the therapy of rheumatoid arthritis and is a promising new therapy for this disease. Clinical trials of using anti-CD154 antibodies were halted because of safety concerns relating to thromboembolic complications. BMS-224818 (LEA29Y) is an improved form of CTLA-4-Ig that binds with high affinity to the CD28 ligands, thereby preventing full T-cell activation. LEA29Y does not appear to be effective when used alone. Phase 2 studies of LEA29Y have shown that the drug, when used in combination with MMF, basiliximab, and corticosteroids, permits safe avoidance of calcineurin inhibitors. Renal function and metabolic parameters were improved for patients receiving LEA29Y compared to those receiving cyclosporine.

Other Monoclonal Antibodies

Infliximab (Remicade) is a chimeric monoclonal antibody that binds to TNF-α receptor sites and interferes with endogenous TNF-α activity. It is approved for use in the treatment of Crohn disease and rheumatoid arthritis. Potential transplant indications are being explored. HuM291 is a humanized form of OKT3 that may be as effective but is less toxic because it does not induce cytokine release. Clinical trials are in progress.

Antibodies targeted against adhesion molecules (see Chapter 2) have potential for both the prevention of rejection and the prevention of delayed graft function, presumably because of their capacity to reduce cell–cell interactions. Phase 3 trials of the antileukocyte factor antigen (-LFA) molecule *odulimomab* and the antiintercellular adhesion molecule (-ICAM)-1 molecule *enlimomab*, however, showed no significant reduction in the incidence of either acute rejection or delayed graft function, and further clinical development has been halted.

Chemokine Blockade

The process of allograft rejection requires recruitment of leukocytes into lymphoid compartments and their emigration into the allograft. The process of leukocyte recruitment is discussed in Chapter 2 (see Fig. 2.6). The steps of leukocyte recruitment are dependent on local concentrations of chemokines, a process that has become the subject of intensive scientific interest. The chemokine receptor CXCR3 has been linked to the development of acute rejection and patients with a deletion of the CCR5 chemokine receptor gene may have prolonged graft survival. Strategies to inhibit chemokine activity may have important applications in clinical transplantation.

Immune Modulation

Immune modulation is a somewhat vague term used to describe attempts to modify the immune response in a nonspecific fashion in order to facilitate allograft acceptance without impairing effector cells or mechanisms. Several techniques fall within this category.

Infusion of *donor-specific bone marrow,* in combination with short-term nonspecific immunosuppression, has produced long-term graft survival in the absence of immunosuppressive therapy in experimental and clinical organ allografts. The donor bone marrow provides an as yet unidentified signal for tolerance. *Blood transfusions* are known to exert beneficial effects on animal and human allograft survival through a variety of potential mechanisms. The tolerogenic effect of bone marrow and blood may also be a result of the development of a state of microchimerism (see Chapter 2). A randomized trial of perioperative donor-specific blood transfusions in live donor transplants showed no practical benefit.

Plasmapheresis has been used with inconsistent success to treat episodes of humoral rejection. It may be more effective in combination with CMVIG (see Part IV). *Photopheresis* is a new form of extracorporeal photochemotherapy used for the treatment of cutaneous T-cell lymphomas and a variety of autoimmune diseases. In a multicenter trial, it was effective in reducing the frequency of rejection in cardiac transplant recipients without increasing infection risk. Several case reports have shown benefits in the treatment of renal transplant rejection, although the results of large clinical trials are not yet available. Photopheresis may serve to downregulate autoreactive and alloreactive T-cell clones.

PART IV. IMMUNOSUPPRESSIVE PROTOCOLS

GENERAL PRINCIPLES OF PROTOCOL DESIGN

The variety of immunosuppressive drugs available for use in clinical transplantation permits permutations that make up immunosuppressive protocols. Transplant centers tend to be loyal to their own protocols, which have often been developed in response to local needs and experience. Protocols should be regarded as guides for therapy that need not necessarily be adhered to slavishly and may require modification from patient to patient and with new knowledge and experience. In an era in which short-term success rates for cadaveric transplantations of greater than 90% are commonplace, it may take experience with hundreds of patients followed for prolonged periods to prove the benefit of a new or modified approach. There is limited prospective data on the effects of different protocols on 5- and 10-year graft survival. Most of the data on long-term protocol design comes from retrospective analysis and analysis of large databases. Although valuable, these analyses bring with them intrinsic design flaws. For instance, in a prospective blinded study it is possible to ensure that the groups that are compared are demographically and clinically similar and that investigator bias in the choice of protocol is negated. In database analyses, such assurances are absent and analyses are limited by the reliability of the data that is entered. Database analyses, however, permit evaluation of a very large number of patients over a prolonged period and may permit recognition of trends and associations not noted in short-term prospective studies on a limited number of patients.

Table 4.7 lists the components of a conventional immunosuppressive protocol. These components are relevant to all recipients

**Table 4.7.   Components of the
conventional immunosuppressive protocol**

Class of Agent	Options
Calcineurin inhibitor	Cyclosporine, tacrolimus
Corticosteroids	Dose and regimen
Adjunctive agent	Azathioprine, MMF, sirolimus
Antibody induction	Lymphocyte depleting or nondepleting
Supplementary agents	CCB, HCRI
Infection prophylaxis	Bactrim, antivirals

CCB, calcium channel blocker; HCRI, HMG-CoA reductase inhibitor.

Table 4.8.   Conventional immunosuppressive protocols that can provide 90%–95% 1 year graft survival and 10%–20% incidence of acute rejection[a]

1. Cyclosporin/MMF/steroids
2. Tacrolimus/MMF/steroids
3. Cyclosporine/sirolimus/steroids
4. Tacrolimus/sirolimus/steroids

MMF, mycophenolate mofetil.
[a] Addition of antibody induction may further reduce incidence of acute rejection.

with the possible exception of two-haplotype-matched living-related donors. The broad range of immunosuppressive drugs now available has also led to the development of a series of innovative protocols. In some programs, innovative protocols have become the local standard of therapy. For all protocols, because the risk for acute rejection is highest in the first weeks and months after transplantation (*induction phase*) and diminishes thereafter (*maintenance phase*), immunosuppression should be at its highest level in this early period and should be reduced for long-term therapy. The most feared side effects of immunosuppression—opportunistic infection and malignancy—tend to reflect the total amount of immunosuppression given rather than the dose of a single drug. The total quantity of immunosuppression should thus be monitored and considered in all stages of the posttransplant course.

Conventional Immunosuppressive Protocols

Conventional immunosuppressive protocols consist of a calcineurin inhibitor, an adjunctive agent, corticosteroids, and the possible addition of antibody induction. With conventional protocols most programs are able to achieve 90% to 95% graft survival with an acute rejection rate of 10% to 20%. Table 4.8 lists the conventional protocols that have been evaluated in clinical trials. Readers are encouraged to refer to the reports of the clinical trials evaluating and comparing the various protocols.

Cyclosporine or Tacrolimus?

Calcineurin inhibitors remain the backbone of transplant immunosuppression. Although much has been made of discrete differences between cyclosporine and tacrolimus, the fact is that these drugs are remarkably similar, and both are highly effective. Table 4.1 summarizes their similarities and differences. These differences may guide the choice of agent in individual patients. For example, cyclosporine may be preferred in some centers for black patients because of the increased incidence of posttransplant glucose intolerance in patients who receive tacrolimus; tacrolimus may be preferred in adolescents and other patients who are concerned about cosmetics because of the more marked cosmetic changes associated with cyclosporine; cyclosporine may be preferred in some patients because of the generally milder neurologic side effects; tacrolimus may be preferred in recipients of simultaneous kidney and pancreas transplants because of its somewhat greater immunosuppressive potency despite its greater islet toxicity (see Chapter 14). Prospective data comparing the two drugs have tended to favor tacrolimus; however, these studies are often difficult to interpret because of the introduction of improved formulations and drug-level monitoring of cyclosporine. Long-term database analyses tend to show a trend in favor of tacrolimus-based therapy for deceased donor transplant recipients and for cyclosporine-based therapy for recipients of living donor transplants. In the United States, there has been a steady trend over the last decade to greater use of tacrolimus. As of 2001, 55% of patients were receiving tacrolimus at the time of discharge from hospital, and 39% were receiving cyclosporine.

Which Adjunctive Agent?

In this discussion, the term *adjunctive agent* is used to describe the immunosuppressive drugs that are used in combination with a calcineurin inhibitor to enhance the potency of the immunosuppressive protocol as reflected by a decreased incidence of acute rejection episodes. Most programs use an adjunctive agent for prophylactic purposes starting from the immediate posttransplant period. Azathioprine (used in combination with cyclosporine and prednisone in so-called triple therapy) has been replaced by MMF in most centers because of its superior capacity to reduce the incidence of acute rejection (Fig. 4.8) when compared with azathioprine. MMF can be used with great effect with tacrolimus and this combination is widely used. In the United States as of 2001, approximately 80% of patients received a calcineurin inhibitor/ MMF/corticosteroid combination during the first posttransplant year.

Sirolimus became available for clinical use in late 1999. It can be used, as per its initial U.S. package insert, in a manner similar to MMF, that is, with full-dose calcineurin inhibitor and fixed sirolimus dose. Most programs, however, prefer to exploit the potency of the drug to permit reduced calcineurin inhibitor dosage (see Innovative Transplant Protocols).

Antibody Induction

Antibody induction therapy refers to the use of the depleting antibodies, OKT3 or Thymoglobulin, or one of the nondepleting anti-CD25 monoclonal antibody in the first 2 weeks after transplantation. In the case of the depleting antibodies, the calcineurin inhibitor is withheld or its dose is kept to a minimum until 2 to 3 days before the antibody course is completed. Induction protocols with OKT3 or a polyclonal antibody represent the major alternative to the use of a calcineurin inhibitor in the early posttransplant period and are therefore different from induction using an HAT monoclonal antibody, in which concomitant use of a calcineurin inhibitor is recommended. In *sequential* therapy, OKT3 or the polyclonal antibody is administered and the calcineurin inhibitor is introduced only when renal function has reached a predetermined level (e.g., a plasma creatinine level of 3 mg/dL). The antibody is discontinued as soon as adequate calcineurin inhibitor levels are achieved. A patient with a well-functioning graft may thus receive only a few days of antibody treatment.

Table 4.9. Potential advantages and disadvantages of "depleting" antibody induction

Potential advantages

Improved graft survival for high-risk patients
Period of delayed graft function may be foreshortened
Onset of first rejection is delayed
Obviates early use of calcineurin inhibitor
May permit less-aggressive maintenance regimen

Potential disadvantages

Risk for first-dose reactions
May prolong hospital admission stay
Greater cost
Higher incidence of CMV infection
Increased short- and long-term mortality reported

Table 4.9 lists the advantages and disadvantages of depletional antibody induction. Thymoglobulin has essentially displaced Atgam and OKT3 is now rarely used for induction. There remains much discussion regarding the relative benefits of Thymoglobulin and the anti-CD25 monoclonals. It has been estimated that one rejection episode is avoided for every seven patients who receive either of the HAT monoclonals. For low-risk patients, they are as effective as the depletional agents. A prospective trial of the two forms of induction in high-risk recipients (see "High-Risk and Low-Risk Groups," below) was discontinued because of an apparent clearcut benefit of Thymoglobulin. This benefit, however, was not recognized in a retrospective analysis. Long-term retrospective studies have not shown significant benefit of routine induction therapy in terms of patient and graft survival, and some studies suggest that patient survival may be impaired as a result of increased early cardiovascular- and infection-related mortality, and a late increase in malignancy-related mortality. The availability of improved adjunctive therapy and the ease of administration of the anti-CD25 monoclonal antibodies has reduced the use of routine depletional antibody induction, and it is often reserved for immunologically high-risk recipients or for patients where delayed graft function is anticipated. Depletional antibody induction may also be indicated for patients requiring anticonvulsant drugs that may make it difficult to achieve therapeutic levels of calcineurin inhibitors in the early posttransplant period. In 2001 in the United States, approximately 60% of patients received some form of antibody induction.

High-Risk and Low-Risk Groups

All patients are not equal with respect to the chances of rejection or graft loss, and protocols should be individualized to take this into account. Patients undergoing simultaneous kidney–pancreas transplantation and patients with high levels of preformed antibodies or previously failed transplants may require more intense therapy. Patients with delayed graft function have an increased susceptibility to episodes of acute rejection. In several clinical trials, black patients have required higher doses of immunosuppressive drugs to achieve the same immunosuppressive benefit, and some programs take this into account routinely in protocol design. Young patients tend to be immunologically aggressive; protocol design for children is discussed in Chapter 15. Older patients may not tolerate heavy immunosuppression. Recipients of transplants from well-matched deceased donors or from living-related donors, particularly from two-haplotype-matched donors, may require less immunosuppression.

How Long to Continue Immunosuppression?

Kidney allografts have long memories! Immunosuppression is required for the functional life of the graft, even if it has lasted 20 years or more, and discontinuation of immunosuppressive drugs, even many years after transplantation, may lead to late acute rejection or accelerated chronic rejection. In stable patients, carefully monitored reduction or even discontinuation of individual components of the immunosuppressive protocol may be safe.

When to Stop Immunosuppression?

The minimal mortality that is now associated with kidney transplantation is to a large degree the result of an appreciation of when to minimize or stop immunosuppression and abandon a kidney. Discontinuation of immunosuppression may be necessary for patients with resistant opportunistic infection or malignancy (see Chapters 9 and 10). Patients with deteriorating graft function despite more than two or three appropriately treated rejections are better allowed to return to dialysis and seek another transplant. With the constant introduction of new immunosuppressive agents into clinical practice, great care and judgment is needed to avoid the temptation of excessively adding or exchanging new agents.

Specific Protocol Recommendations

Cyclosporine

Cyclosporine, 8 to 12 mg/kg per day orally (3 to 4 mg/kg per day intravenously), is given as a single dose or twice daily starting immediately before transplantation. The intravenous infusion is given over at least 4 hours or can be given as a constant infusion over 24 hours. Some programs prefer to omit the preoperative dose or avoid intravenous cyclosporine altogether. For patients who receive depleting antibody induction, oral cyclosporine is usually started several days before the completion of the course of therapy so that drug levels will be therapeutic at the time of the final antibody dose. Doses are then adjusted to maintain levels within the ranges given in Table 4.10. It is wise to continue to monitor levels of cyclosporine, although the degree of reliance on these levels and the frequency of their measurement varies from program to program. The desired dose and target levels are influenced by the concomitant use of adjunctive agents and history of rejections. By 3 months after transplantation, most patients are receiving cyclosporine in a dose of 3 to 5 mg/kg per day.

There is still no clear consensus regarding the best dose or drug level for long-term cyclosporine use, and it is unfortunate

Table 4.10. Approximate therapeutic ranges for cyclosporine

Posttransplant Month	HPLC and EMIT (ng/mL)	FPIA (ng/mL)	C2 levels[a] (μg/mL)
0–2[b]	150–350	250–450	1.5–2.0
2–6	100–250	175–350	1.1–1.5
>6	~100	~150	0.8–1.0

EMIT, emzyme-multiplied immunoassay technique; FPIA, fluorescent polar-ization immunoassay; HPLC, high-performance liquid chromatography.
[a]Drawn within 15 minutes of 2 hours postdose. For C2 levels, no change in target levels is required for different assay types.
[b]In the first few days post-transplant, the trough cyclosporine level should not fall below 300 ng/mL by HPLC.

that prospective randomized trials comparing cyclosporine dose ranges are not available. Drug-level monitoring with 2-hour (C2) peak levels may be more effective than trough-level monitoring. Peak-level monitoring, however, may be cumbersome in busy transplant clinics where many patients are being monitored with trough levels if they are receiving tacrolimus. Recommended peak levels have not been extensively validated with varied transplant populations and protocols, and the recommended levels noted in Table 4.10 should be considered accordingly. Fear of progressive nephrotoxicity has tempted many clinicians to permit low levels, yet such a policy may allow for the insidious development of chronic rejection. Retrospective studies show that continued use of cyclosporine is conducive to prolonged adequate graft function.

WHICH CYCLOSPORINE FORMULATION?

Most patients are started and maintained on Neoral. Although patients who were started on Sandimmune may choose to switch from Sandimmune to Neoral, there is no overriding medical rea-son to do so. The switch requires care because of the different pharmacokinetics of the two formulations (see "Cyclosporine" un-der "Formulations and Pharmacokinetics," above). Although a 1:1 dose ratio is recommended, some patients require somewhat less Neoral than Sandimmune. Even in stable patients, cyclosporine blood levels should be monitored more carefully in the month af-ter the switch and dose adjustments made. An elevation of the creatinine level soon after a switch is more likely to be a result of nephrotoxicity than of rejection. The decision to use a generic for-mulation is a financial rather than a medical one. Any switching of formulations requires careful monitoring because the pharma-cokinetic parameters of the generic formulations may differ.

Tacrolimus

The recommended starting dose of oral tacrolimus is 0.15 to 0.30 mg/kg per day administered in a split dose every 12 hours. Intravenous tacrolimus is rarely required in kidney transplan-tation. Doses are adjusted to maintain tacrolimus drug levels at between 10 and 20 ng/dL during the first few posttransplant months, and between 5 and 15 ng/dL thereafter. There is marked patient-to-patient variation in the dose of tacrolimus required to achieve these levels, with some patients receiving as little as 2 mg daily and some patients receiving ten times that dose. The relationship between drug levels and manifestations of toxicity varies considerably between patients.

Switching Calcineurin Inhibitors

If side effects develop with one of the calcineurin inhibitors it is quite reasonable to switch to the other agent. Common reasons for switching are cosmetic (tacrolimus to cyclosporine for hair loss and the converse for hirsutism; cyclosporine to tacrolimus for gingival hypertrophy). New-onset diabetes mellitus may respond to conversion from tacrolimus to cyclosporine. The dose chosen at the time of switching must be individualized. There is no need to overlap the drugs and steroid "coverage" is usually unnecessary. Patients should be monitored carefully after switching.

Corticosteroids

Methylprednisolone is typically given intraoperatively in a dose of up to 1 g. The dose is then reduced rapidly from 150 mg on day 1 to 20 to 30 mg on day 14. Some programs avoid the steroid cycle altogether, modifying it or starting at 30 mg daily or even less. The maximal oral dose of prednisone at 1 month should be 20 mg and 15 mg at 3 months. After a year, many patients tolerate an every-other-day regimen. The low long-term maintenance doses that patients typically receive (5 to 7.5 mg daily) should be regarded with great care and respect. Rejection episodes may occasionally occur when even very small dose reductions are made. High-maintenance-dose protocols of steroids sometimes used for collagen vascular disease and vasculitides are unnecessary and contraindicated in kidney transplantation.

Adjunctive Agents

The dose of azathioprine is 1 to 3 mg/kg. Drug levels are not measured, and the dose is usually fixed with adjustments made for hematologic toxicity. The standard dose of MMF in adults is 1,000 mg twice daily, although black patients may benefit from a higher dose (1,500 mg twice daily). Patients on full dose tacrolimus may require a lower dose. Some evidence suggests that measurement of mycophenolic acid AUC may be useful in predicting the effectiveness of MMF; however, blood levels are generally not measured. If the dose of MMF is reduced or held for short periods in the event of side effects, the dose of calcineurin inhibitor and prednisone should be maintained. The longer the MMF dose is reduced the greater is the risk of subsequent rejection and patients should be monitored accordingly. Most programs continue to administer MMF for prolonged periods; administration for at least 1 year has been shown, in retrospective studies, to produce measurable benefit in graft survival and to reduce the incidence of late acute rejections.

The maintenance dose of sirolimus is typically 2–5 mg daily with target blood levels similar to those described for tacrolimus (see Tacrolimus). If the accompanying calcineurin inhibitor is totally discontinued, the dose requirements of sirolimus to maintain adequate levels may increase markedly.

The standard recommended dose of sirolimus is 2 mg administered once daily 4 hours after the morning dose of cyclosporine. A loading dose of 6 mg is given on the first day of treatment. Black patients may benefit from a 5-mg per day maintenance dose with a 15-mg loading dose. Measurement of drug levels is not required when the drug is used according to the original FDA labeling. As has been noted, most programs do not use sirolimus in this manner and drug-level monitoring has become routine. In the clinical trials of sirolimus, the mean 24-hour whole-blood trough level for the 2-mg daily dose was 9 ng/mL, and a therapeutic trough level of 5 to 15 ng/mL (similar numbers as those for tacrolimus) is usually recommended.

The anti-CD25 monoclonal antibodies were developed for use with standard doses of cyclosporine and prednisone. They are now usually given with cyclosporine or tacrolimus and an adjunctive agent to produce a further reduction in the incidence of acute rejection. Their use is not associated with a significant increase in side effects; hence, the decision to use them is often based on an assessment of whether their extra cost can be justified.

Supplementary Agents

The inclusion of *calcium channel blockers,* usually either diltiazem or verapamil, in the standard immunosuppressive regimen has several potential advantages. In addition to their antihypertensive properties, both drugs may minimize calcineurin inhibitor-induced vasoconstriction and protect against ischemic graft injury and nephrotoxicity. Both drugs compete with the calcineurin inhibitors for excretion by the P450 enzyme system, raising drug levels and permitting safe administration of lower doses. Calcium channel blockers may also possess some intrinsic immunomodulatory activity of their own related to the role of cytosolic calcium levels or gene activation. The routine inclusion of calcium channel blockers in the posttransplant protocol may improve 1-year graft survival by 5% to 10%.

The statins lower cholesterol levels safely in transplant recipients and reduce the incidence of clinically severe rejection in cardiac transplant recipients. A similar beneficial effect has been observed in preliminary studies in kidney transplant recipients. The mechanism of this effect may be related to the ability of the statins to suppress the cytotoxic activity of natural killer cells (see Chapter 2). Statins may have benefits in the immunosuppressive regimen that are not directly related to their effect on the lipid profile.

Protocols for Living Donor Transplants

Excellent results were achieved for two-haplotype-matched living-related transplants immunosuppressed with azathioprine and prednisone alone before the introduction of cyclosporine into routine clinical practice. Despite this experience, most transplant programs now use calcineurin inhibitor-based protocols for these patients because of the lesser incidence of acute rejection. Two-haplotype-matched transplant recipients receiving calcineurin inhibitors may be good candidates for eventual steroid withdrawal. MMF or sirolimus could potentially be used to replace the calcineurin inhibitor. For all other living donor transplants conventional protocols are calcineurin inhibitor-based and are similar to those described for deceased donor transplants.

Innovative Transplant Protocols

The availability of multiple immunosuppressive agents has stimulated attempts to minimize or avoid the most toxic components of the standard protocol. The most obvious targets for such efforts are corticosteroids and the calcineurin inhibitors.

Steroid Withdrawal and Steroid Avoidance

Steroid withdrawal generally implies the discontinuation of steroid administration several months after transplantation and needs to be differentiated from steroid avoidance, in which steroids are not administered at all, or may be given for only 3 or 4 days postoperatively (rapid withdrawal). The difference between the two techniques is more than semantic and there is some evidence that steroid avoidance or early withdrawal may be safer than later steroid withdrawal. Because most of the side effects of steroids are a result of the high doses that are given in the early postoperative period rather than the small maintenance doses, there is good reason to focus efforts on avoiding their administration altogether.

Steroid withdrawal is a tempting ploy that may be considered in selected patients, although the anxiety associated with withdrawal (for both the patients and their physicians!) has tended to dampen its popularity. A randomized, blinded trial of steroid withdrawal 4 months after transplantation was performed in a group of patients with good graft function who had not suffered rejection episodes and who were receiving cyclosporine and MMF in standard doses. The trial was discontinued because of a 20% incidence of acute rejection in the withdrawn group compared with a 5% incidence in the control group. Most of the rejection episodes occurred in the black patients. Steroid withdrawal should thus be considered only at least several months after transplantation for patients who have not suffered recent or recurrent rejections and who have excellent graft function. Black patients may not be suitable candidates for withdrawal, and all patients should be warned of a small but finite increased incidence of rejection. A clear-cut benefit of withdrawal, in terms of certain steroid-related side effects (e.g., bone disease, hyperlipidemia), has not been demonstrated, presumably because most of the familiar steroid-related problems are produced by the high doses used in the early posttransplant period. There may be long-term deterioration in graft function patients after steroid withdrawal; these patients should be forewarned.

Steroid avoidance has been used in Europe for many years, although it was rarely practiced in the United States until recently. Most steroid-avoidance protocols administer Thymoglobulin postoperatively for several days, or use anti-CD25 monoclonal antibodies followed by combinations of a calcineurin inhibitor with sirolimus and/or MMF. Early evaluation of these protocols is encouraging and the rates of acute rejection and graft loss are comparable to standard protocols. Some programs now use them routinely for low-immunologic-risk patients. Long-term followup is required before a final verdict can be made on their more general application.

Calcineurin Inhibitor Avoidance, Withdrawal, and Dose Minimization

Avoidance, or at least minimization, of the nephrotoxic effects of the calcineurin inhibitors is indeed a worthy goal. It is a goal, however, that must be approached with great care. In low-risk patients, protocols avoiding calcineurin inhibitors by using combinations of anti-CD25 monoclonal antibodies, corticosteroids, and MMF, or by using rapamycin alone, reportedly permit excellent graft survival but with an unacceptably high incidence of acute rejection episodes. Some protocols effectively combine sirolimus, MMF, and corticosteroids. Sirolimus may increase the blood levels of MMF and dose adjustments resulting from hematologic toxicity are common. The greatest value of sirolimus may be in its capacity to permit safe withdrawal or minimization of the calcineurin inhibitor. Figure 4.6 well-illustrates the potential benefits of such an approach. It should be noted that although GFR improved after cyclosporine withdrawal in this study, there was a finite incidence of postwithdrawal acute rejection. Moreover, the patients selected for study were a low-risk group by virtue of their benign postoperative course. To avoid the risks of total calcineurin inhibitor withdrawal while reducing nephrotoxicity, it may be safer to continue to use them in low doses while maintaining adequate levels and doses of sirolimus or MMF.

Tolerogenic Protocols

The goal of complete donor-specific tolerance without the requirement for ongoing immunosuppression has yet to be consistently achieved. As noted in Part III, "prope" tolerance or "near" tolerance may be a more realistic goal. Tolerogenic strategies typically imply the use of potent perioperative lymphocyte depletion. Alemtuzumab has been used for this purpose, followed by sirolimus with or without low doses of calcineurin inhibitor. A protocol using high-dose Thymoglobulin followed by very-low-dose, or even discontinuation of, tacrolimus, has been reported to be effective in solid organ transplant recipients. Although the early results of these protocols are promising, they need extensive evaluation before their general applicability can be recommended.

PART V. TREATMENT OF KIDNEY TRANSPLANT REJECTION

ACUTE CELLULAR REJECTION

First Rejection

Pulse Steroids

High intravenous doses of steroids, typically referred to as "pulses," reverse approximately 75% of first acute rejections. There are numerous ways to pulse a patient, and there is no good evidence that the higher-dose pulses (500 to 1,000 mg methylprednisolone for 3 days) are more effective than the lower-dose pulses (120 to 250 mg oral prednisone or methylprednisolone for 3 to 5 days). Most programs still prefer to use intravenous methylprednisolone, which is given over 30 to 60 minutes into a peripheral vein. Pulse therapy is suitable for outpatient use when clinically indicated. The dose of prednisone can be continued at its previous level when the pulse is completed, although some programs elect to *recycle* the prednisone dose after the pulse has been completed.

Antibody Treatment

OKT3 is a highly effective therapy for the management of a first acute rejection, and approximately 90% of such rejections will be reversed. Similar results can be achieved with Thymoglobulin, which is more effective than Atgam. Despite the greater effectiveness of these agents, most programs still prefer to use pulse steroids as their first-line acute rejection therapy because of their convenience, lesser risks of side effects, and lower costs. OKT3 or Thymoglobulin may be a better first-line option for particularly severe or vascular rejections (Banff grade IIB or greater; see Chapter 13). The anti-CD25 monoclonal antibodies are not designed to be used in the treatment of established acute rejection.

Recurrent and Refractory Rejections

Repeated courses of pulse steroids may be effective in reversing acute rejections, but it is probably not wise to administer more than two courses of pulse therapy before resorting to OKT3 or Thymoglobulin. Many programs use antibody treatment for all second rejections unless the rejection is clinically mild or separated from the first by at least several weeks. Antibody treatment is particularly valuable for rejection episodes that are steroid resistant and may succeed in reversing a high percentage of such rejections. Some programs commence antibody treatment if there is not an immediate response to pulse therapy, whereas others wait several days. If renal function is deteriorating rapidly in the face of pulse steroids, it is probably wise to start antibody treatment early.

The term *refractory rejection* is not well defined. It usually refers to ongoing rejection despite treatment with pulse steroids and antibody. The management of these patients is problematic. Second courses of OKT3 or polyclonal antibodies can be given in selected patients, and long-term graft function can be achieved in 40% to 50% of such patients. When deciding whether to give a second course of an antibody preparation, the clinician should bear in mind the severity and potential reversibility of rejection on biopsy; the increased risk for infection and malignancy that ensues, particularly if two courses are given close together; and the possibility of generating high levels of anti-OKT3 antibodies that might limit treatment options for a future transplantation.

Switching from cyclosporine to tacrolimus, or adding MMF or sirolimus in patients who have not previously received it, may be effective treatments for refractory rejections. Approximately 75% of such rejections can be reversed in this manner.

Late Rejections

The terms *early* and *late rejection* are not well defined. The differentiation between early and late rejection is not just semantic; each may respond differently to therapy. For practical purposes, a late rejection is one that occurs more than 3 to 4 months after transplantation and may be a first, or more frequently, a recurrent rejection. Late rejections can also be divided into those that occur in the face of apparently adequate immunosuppression and those that occur as a result of inadequate immunosuppression, often in nonadherent patients. Late rejections are often a prelude to chronic rejection and accelerated graft loss.

The initial treatment of a late rejection is pulse steroids. The effectiveness of OKT3 for acute rejection treatment tends to diminish with time, so that by 3 to 4 months after transplantation, only 40% to 50% of episodes respond to OKT3 treatment. By 1 year after transplantation, this figure may be only approximately 20%, and at this stage, it may not be worth the risks associated with therapy. There is evidence that late rejections associated with noncompliance are more likely to respond to therapy. Use of Thymoglobulin for late steroid-resistant rejection has not been systematically studied.

Thus, there are limited therapeutic options for late steroid-resistant rejection, which often occurs in a background of chronic rejection. It may often be wiser to accept graft dysfunction or loss rather than use potent high-dose immunosuppression in an already chronically immunosuppressed patient.

ANTIBODY-MEDIATED REJECTION

The clinical and pathologic recognition of antibody-mediated rejection are discussed in Chapters 4 and 13, with particular emphasis on the role of the C4D immunostain. Two related treatment protocols are effective: high-dose IVIG or low-dose CMVIG combined with plasmapheresis. A dose of 2 g/kg of IVIG is usually adequate; plasmapheresis/CMVIG is usually performed every other day until levels of donor-specific antibodies are brought under control. In severe cases, for patients with high-titer donor-specific antibodies, rituximab or emergent splenectomy may reduce antibody burden and graft injury. Antibody-mediated rejection may recur and may be followed by episodes of acute cellular rejection. Patients must be monitored carefully in the weeks following treatment.

IMMUNOSUPPRESSIVE MANAGEMENT OF CHRONIC ALLOGRAFT NEPHROPATHY

The clinical course, pathology, and multifactorial etiology of chronic allograft nephropathy (CAN) are discussed in Chapters 9 and 13. Before making changes in the immunosuppressive protocol in a patient with CAN every effort must be made to rule out potentially reversible causes of graft dysfunction and it must be appreciated that many of the changes that take place in CAN are irreversible. Table 4.11 lists the issues that must be considered in all patients with presumed CAN before changes are made in the immunosuppressive protocol. The following general principles can serve to guide immunosuppressive management in CAN.

1. Intensification of calcineurin inhibitor dosage, or switching from one preparation to another, is generally not beneficial and may lead to exaggeration of nephrotoxicity.

Table 4.11. Steps to take before manipulating immunosuppression for patients with chronic allograft failure

1. Have reversible causes of deteriorating graft function been ruled out?
2. Is the patient clinically euvolemic?
3. Is there evidence of recurrent disease?
4. Have drug formulations been recently changed?
5. Have interfering drugs been introduced?
6. Is the patient (and physician!) adherent to the immunosuppressive regimen?
7. Have "nonimmune" intereventions been applied?

2. Consideration should be given to reduction or even discontinuation of calcineurin inhibitor therapy. Such a therapeutic maneuver requires careful followup to screen for episodes of deteriorating graft function.
3. Reduction of calcineurin inhibitor dosage is generally accompanied by addition of, or continuation of, a nonnephrotoxic immunosuppressant. There is most experience and documented benefit with MMF in these circumstances, although sirolimus may be an appropriate alternative.
4. Patients with CAN that have deposition of C4D as a marker of ongoing humoral injury may represent of separate category that may benefit from intensification of immunosuppression.
5. Introduction of a new immunosuppressive agent in previously immunosuppressed patients has potentially dangerous consequences. Patients should be monitored carefully and consideration given to prophylaxis to prevent development of infectious complications.
6. High baseline doses of corticosteroids are not indicated. "Pulse" steroid therapy may be valuable for episodes of deteriorating function but repeated treatment should be avoided. Ideally, use of pulse steroids in these circumstances should follow histologic confirmation of an element of acute rejection.
7. Because repeated pulse steroid therapy should be avoided, it is rarely indicated to repeatedly biopsy patients with established CAN.
8. If graft function continues to deteriorate despite the above measures plans should be made to prepare for end-stage renal disease treatment options and immunosuppression should be withdrawn in a stepwise fashion as when dialysis commences.

SELECTED READINGS

Part I

Alloway RR, Isaacs R, Lake K, et al. Report of the American Society of Transplantation conference on immunosuppressive drugs and the use of generic immunosuppressants. *Am J Transplant* 2003;3: 1211–1215.

Bennett W. Immunosuppression with mycophenolic acid: one size does not fit all. *J Am Soc Nephrol* 2003;14:2414–2418.

Boots J, Van Duijnhoven E, Christiaans M, et al. Glucose metabolism in renal transplant recipients on tacrolimus: the effect of steroid withdrawal and tacrolimus trough level reduction. *J Am Soc Nephrol* 2002;13:221–227.

Cho S, Danovitch G, Deierhoi M, et al. Mycophenolate mofetil in cadaveric renal transplantation. *Am J Kidney Dis* 1999;34:296–302.

Danovitch GM. Immunosuppressant induced metabolic toxicities. *Transplant Rev* 2000;14:65–72.

Heisel O, Heisel R, Balshaw R, et al. New onset diabetes mellitus in patients receiving calcineurin inhibitors: a systemic review and meta-analysis. *Am J Transplant* 2004;4:583–595.

Johnson RWG. How should sirolimus be used in clinical practice? *Transplant Proc* 2003;35[Suppl 3A]:79–85.

Kahan B, Camardo J. Rapamycin: clinical results and future opportunities. *Transplantation* 2001;72:1181–1193.

Kasiske B, Snyder J, Gilbertson D, et al. Diabetes mellitus after kidney transplantation in the United States. *Am J Transplant* 2003;3:178–185.

Luan F, Hojo M, Maluccio M, et al. Rapamycin blocks tumor progression: unlinking immunosuppression from antitumor efficacy. *Transplantation* 2002;73:1565–1572.

Maluccio M, Sharma V, Lagman M, et al. Tacrolimus enhances transforming growth factor-beta1 expression and promotes tumor progression. *Transplantation* 2003;76:597–602.

Miller L. Cardiovascular toxicities of immunosuppressive agents. *Transplantation* 2002;2:807–902.

Perico N, Ruggenenti P, Gotti E, et al. In renal transplantation blood cyclosporine levels soon after surgery act as a major determinant of rejection: insight from the M.Y.S.S. trial. *Kidney Int* 2004;65:1084–1090.

Pham PT, Danovitch GM, Wilkinson AW, et al. Inhibitors of ADAMTS13: a potential factor in the cause of thrombotic microangiopathy in a renal allograft recipient. *Transplantation* 2002;74:1077–1081.

Pham PT, Pham PC, Danovitch G, et al. Sirolimus-associated pulmonary toxicity. *Transplantation* 2004;77:1215–1220.

Sabatini S, Ferguson RM, Helderman JH, et al. Drug substitution in transplantation: a National Kidney Foundation white paper. *Am J Kidney Dis* 1999;33:389–393.

Smith K, Wrenshall L, Nicosia R, et al. Delayed function and cast nephropathy associated with tacrolimus plus rapamycin use. *J Am Soc Nephrol* 2003;14:1037–1041.

Thervet E, Pfeffer P, Scolari M, et al. Clinical outcomes during the first three months posttransplant in renal allograft recipients managed by C2 monitoring of cyclosporine microemulsion. *Transplantation* 2003;76:903–907.

Part II

Brennan DC. Faith supported by reason: mechanistic support for the use of polyclonal antibodies in transplantation. *Transplantation* 2003;75:577–582.

Ducloux D, Challier B, Saas P, et al. CD4 cell lymphopenia and atherosclerosis in renal transplant recipients. *J Am Soc Nephrol* 2003;14:767–771.

Gaber AO, First MR, Tesi RJ, et al. Results of the double-blind, randomized, multicenter, phase III clinical trial of Thymoglobulin versus ATGAM in the treatment of acute graft rejection episodes after renal transplantation. *Transplantation* 1998;66:29–36.

Goggins WC, Pascual MA, Powelson JA, et al. A prospective, randomized trial of intraoperative versus postoperative Thymoglobulin in adult cadaveric renal transplant recipients. *Transplantation* 2003;76:798–803.

Jordan SC, Bunnapradist S, Toyoda M, et al. Intravenous immune globulin treatment inhibits crossmatch positivity and allows for successful transplantation of incompatible organs in living donor and cadaveric recipients. *Transplantation* 2003;76:631–636.

Michallet MC, Preville X, Flacher M, et al. Functional antibodies to leukocyte adhesion molecules in antithymocyte globulins. *Transplantation* 2003;75(5):657–662.

Müller TF, Grebe SO, Neuman MC, et al. Persistent long-term changes in lymphocyte subsets induced by polyclonal antibodies. *Transplantation* 1997;64:1432–1437.

Tsinalis D, Dickenmann M, Brunner F, et al. Acute renal failure in a renal allograft recipient treated with intravenous immunoglobulin. *Am J Kidney Dis* 2002;40:667–671.

Vincenti F, Pace D, Birnbaum J, et al. Pharmacokinetic and pharmacodynamic studies of one or two doses of daclizumab in renal transplantation. *Am J Transplant* 2003;3:50–52.

Webster AC, Playford EG, Higgins G, et al. Interleukin 2 receptor antagonist for renal transplant recipients: a meta-analysis of randomized trials. *Transplantation* 2004;77:166–176.

Part III

Budde K, Schmouder R, Brunkhorst R, et al. First human trial of FTY720, a novel immunomodulator, in stable renal transplant patients. *J Am Soc Nephrol* 2002;13:1073–1078.

Eisen H, Tuzcu M, Dorent R, et al, Everolimus for the prevention of allograft rejection and vasculopathy in cardiac-transplant recipients. *N Engl J Med* 2003;349:847–851.

Haanstra KG, Ringers J, Sick EA, et al. Prevention of kidney allograft rejection using anti-CD40 and anti-CD86 in primates. *Transplantation* 2003;75:637–641.

Kanmaz T, Knechtle S. Novel agents or strategies for immunosuppression after renal. transplantation. *Transplantation* 2003;8:172–175.

Kasiske BL. Endpoint or turning point. *Am J Transplant* 2003;3:1463–1464.

Kremer J, Westhovens R, Leon M, et al. Treatment of rheumatoid arthritis by selective inhibition of T-cell activation with fusion protein CTLA4Ig. *N Engl J Med* 2003;349:1907–1911.

Lachenbruch P, Rosenberg A, Bonvini E, et al. Biomarkers and surrogate end-points in renal transplantation: present status and considerations in clinical trial design. *Am J Transplant* 2004;4:451–457.

Li Y, Li XC, Zheng XX, et al. Blocking both signal 1 and signal 2 of T-cell activation prevents apoptosis of alloreactive T cells and induction of peripheral allograft tolerance. *Nat Med* 1999;5:1298–1301.

Knechtle SJ, Pirsch JD, H Flechner J Jr, et al. Campath-1H induction plus rapamycin monotherapy for renal transplantation: results of a pilot study. *Am J Transplant* 2003;3:722–726.

Matloubian M, Lo CG, Cinamon G, et al. Lymphocyte egress from the thymus and peripheral lymphocyte organs is dependent on S1P receptor 1. *Nature* 2004;427:355–360.

Savikko J, Von Willebrand E, Hayry P, et al. Leflunomide analogue FK778 is vasculoprotective independent of its immunosuppressive effect: potential applications for restenosis and chronic rejection. *Transplantation* 2003;76:455–458.

Tyden G, Kumlein G, Fehrman I. Successful ABO-incompatible kidney transplantations without splenectomy using antigen-specific immunoadsorption and rituximab. *Transplantation* 2003;76:730–734.

Williams JW, Mital D, Chong A, et al. Experiences with leflunomide in solid organ transplantation. *Transplantation* 2002;73:358–362.

Yilmaz S, Tomlanovich S, Mathew T, et al. Protocol core needle biopsy and histologic chronic allograft damage index (CADI) as surrogate end point for long-term graft survival in multicenter studies. *J Am Soc Nephrol* 2003;14:773–777.

Parts IV and V

Artz MA, Boots JM, Ligtenberg G, et al. Improved cardiovascular risk profile and renal function in renal transplant patients after randomized conversion from cyclosporine to tacrolimus. *J Am Soc Nephrol* 2003;14:1880–1884.

Blanco-Colio LM, Tunon J, Martin-Ventura JL, et al. Anti-inflammatory and immunomodulatory effects of statins. *Kidney Int* 2003;63:12–23.

Bodziak K, Hricik D. Minimizing the side effects of immunosuppression in kidney transplant recipients. *Transplantation* 2003;8:160–165.

Bunnapradist S, Daswani A, Takemoto SK, et al. Graft survival following living-donor renal transplantation: a comparison of tacrolimus and cyclosporine microemulsion with mycophenolate mofetil and steroids. *Transplantation* 2003;76:10–15.

Cianco G, Burke GW, Gatnor J, et al. A randomized long-term trial of tacrolimus and sirolimus versus tacrolimus and mycophenolate mofetil versus cyclosporine (Neoral) and sirolimus in renal transplantation. I. Drug interactions and rejection at one year. *Transplantation* 2004;77:244.

Cole E, Midtvedt K, Johnston A, et al. Recommendations for implementation of Neoral C_2 monitoring in clinical practice. *Transplantation* 2002;73:S19.

Danovitch GM. Immunosuppressive medications for renal transplantation: a multiple choice question. *Kidney Int* 2001;59:388.

Danovitch GM. Management of immunosuppression in patients with chronic allograft nephropathy. *Kidney Int* 2002;61, S 80:68.

Gill JS, Tonelli M, Mix C, et al. The effect of maintenance immunosuppression medication on the change in kidney allograft function. *Kidney Int* 2004;65:692.

Gonwa T, Johnson C, Ahsan N, et al. Randomized trial of tacrolimus plus mycophenolate mofetil or azathioprine versus cyclosporine plus mycophenolate mofetil after cadaveric kidney transplantation: results at three years. *Transplantation* 2003;75:2048.

Gotti E, Perico N, Perna A, et al. Renal transplantation: can we reduce calcineurin inhibitor/stop steroids? Evidence based on protocol biopsy findings. *J Am Soc Nephrol* 2003;14:755.

Helderman J, Bennett W, Cibrick D, et al. Immunosuppression: practice and trends. *Transplantation* 2003;3[Suppl 4]:41.

Helderman JH, Goral S. Gastrointestinal complications of transplant immunosuppression. *J Am Soc Nephrol* 2002;13:277.

Johnson DW, Nicol DL, Purdie DM, et al. Is mycophenolate mofetil less safe than azathioprine in elderly renal transplant recipients? *Transplantation* 2002;73:1158.

Kirk A. Less is more: maintenance minimization as a step toward tolerance. *Transplantation* 2003;3:643.

Knoll G, Macdonald I, Khan A. Mycophenolate mofetil dose reduction and the risk of acute rejection after renal transplantation. *J Am Soc Nephrol* 2003;14:2381.

Lemieux I, Houde I, Pascot A, et al. Effects of prednisone withdrawal on the new metabolic triad in cyclosporine-treated kidney transplant patients. *Kidney Int* 2002;62:1839.

Margreiter R. Efficacy and safety of tacrolimus compared with ciclosporin microemulsion in renal transplantation: a randomised multicentre study. *Lancet* 2002;359:7.

Meier-Kriesche HU, Arndorfer JA, Kaplan B, et al. Association of antibody induction with short- and long-term cause-specific mortality in renal transplant recipients. *J Am Soc Nephrol* 2002;13:769.

Meier-Kriesche HU, Steffen B, Gordon R, et al. Long-term use of mycophenolate mofetil is associated with a reduction in the incidence and risk of late rejection. *Transplantation* 2003;3:68.

Molina MG, Seron D, del Moral R, et al. Mycophenolate mofetil reduces deterioration of renal function in patients with chronic allograft nephropathy. A follow-up study by the Spanish Cooperative Study Group of Chronic Allograft Nephropathy. *Transplantation* 2004;77:215.

Pascual M, Curtis J, Delmonico FL, et al. A prospective, randomized clinical trial of cyclosporine reduction in stable patients greater than 12 months after renal transplantation. *Transplantation* 2003;75:1501.

Shaw L, Korecka M, Venkataramanan R, et al. Mycophenolic acid pharmacodynamics and pharmacokinetics provide a basis for rational monitoring strategies. *Transplantation* 2003;3:534–542.

Starzl TE, Murase N, Abu Elmagid K, et al. Tolerogenic immunosuppression for organ transplantation. *Lancet* 2003;361:1502.

Vincenti F, Jensik SC, Filo RS, et al. A long-term comparison of tacrolimus (FK506) and cyclosporine in kidney transplantation: evidence for improved allograft survival at five years. *Transplantation* 2002;73:775.

Vinceti F. Immunosuppression minimization: current and future trends in transplant immunosuppression. *J Am Soc Nephrol* 2003; 14:1940.

Medical and Surgical Aspects of Kidney Donation

Elizabeth Kendrick, Jennifer Singer, H. Albin Gritsch, and J. Thomas Rosenthal

Kidney transplantation cannot proceed without kidney donors, and although much emphasis is justifiably given to posttransplant patient management, the appropriate identification and preparation of donors contribute critically to the success of the transplant endeavor on both the individual and the national levels. As of 2004, living donors accounted for 27% of all kidney transplants performed in the United States, where most transplant centers regard them as the preferred donation modality. Since 2001, more donors in the United States have been living than deceased. There are wide variations in the use of living and deceased kidney donors around the world (see Chapter 1, Fig. 1.3). These differences reflect varying medical and societal cultural values, and varying realities in the availability of sophisticated care for patients with advanced kidney disease (see Chapter 1, Fig. 1.2). Differences can also be driven by the availability of deceased donor organs relative to the number of patients waiting for transplants, attitudes of local physicians regarding the risk of living donation, as well as the degree of government oversight. In Spain, for example, where a highly effective mechanism for identifying deceased donors has helped keep waiting lists short, living donation accounts for less than 5% of all transplants. In most European countries, living donation accounts for less than 10% of transplants. In Japan, strong cultural and, till recently, legal barriers have limited deceased donor transplants and living donation is the most common form of transplantation. Although illegal throughout the industrialized world (see Chapter 17) and proscribed by national and international professional transplant organizations, paid living donation is a common practice in many parts of the world. The transplant community finds itself critically reexamining some long-held tenets regarding the suitability of certain types of living and deceased donors, and carefully reevaluating the manner in which potential donors and their loved ones are approached.

To address the various aspects of kidney donation, this chapter is divided into two parts. Part I addresses the selection and evaluation of living donors, and the surgical techniques of living donor nephrectomy. Part II addresses these issues for deceased kidney donors.

PART I. LIVING DONOR KIDNEY TRANSPLANTATION

The steady increase in both the percentage and absolute numbers of living donor transplants in the United States (see Chapter 1, Fig. 1.1) has been driven by several factors. While the number of patients listed for a kidney transplant per year has increased, the number of deceased donor kidneys available has remained relatively flat. Despite persistent efforts to increase the numbers of deceased donor organs, wait times for these organs have increased to 5 or 6 years in many areas of the country. There has been increasing recognition that the length of time on dialysis has a major impact on patient morbidity and survival, which contributes to the desire to transplant the patient in a more timely fashion. Living donor transplantation may represent the only realistic hope of avoiding dialysis.

With the increase in living donation, the demographics of living kidney donors has also evolved. The first living donor transplants were performed using identical twins without immunosuppression. Well-matched living-related kidney donors were then used because it was believed that with a limited capacity for safe immunosuppression, lesser-matched donors should not be used because of the risk of rejection. Although patients who receive a "perfect match" related donor kidney still enjoy a better graft survival than lesser matched related donor kidneys, the kidney graft survival of even nonmatched related donor kidneys is now only marginally less good (see Chapter 3, Fig. 3.4). Moreover, the survival of kidneys from living-unrelated donors has been demonstrated to be superior to well-matched deceased donor kidneys and approaches that of related donor kidneys. Donors who are not biologically related to the recipient account for more than 25% of living kidney donors in the United States.

EVALUATION OF LIVING KIDNEY DONORS

There are discrete differences in opinion and practice of evaluation and acceptance of living kidney donors between different transplant programs. In the medical assessment of every potential living kidney donor, however, three basic questions are always to be considered:

1. Is the potential donor at higher risk to undergo the actual surgical procedure than what would be expected?
2. Are there recipient issues, such as risk of cancer or infectious disease transmission via the donor organ, or factors that would lead to an unacceptable risk of early graft loss, such as recurrent disease?
3. What is the degree of risk of developing medical problems in the future as a result of having a single kidney?

The first and second questions may be easier to answer than the third. The third question for the most part pertains to determining whether there is an increased future risk of developing hypertension or kidney disease, where often the family history deserves careful consideration and the existing medical literature is at best an imperfect guide.

Informed Consent

An extremely important part of the assessment of a potential donor involves informed consent (Table 5.1). Living donor consent is also discussed in Chapters 16 and 19. Emphasis on the adequacy of the consent process is particularly important because

Table 5.1. Suggested elements for consent in the living donor evaluation process

The potential donor should understand that:

Undergoing evaluation is not a commitment to donate.

I can stop at any time.

The physicians may turn me down as a donor, and will inform me why.

I will be evaluated by an independent donor evaluation doctor or team to protect my interests.

The information obtained during the course of the evaluation is confidential.

I will be tested for AIDS, hepatitis, and other infectious diseases.

I may get unexpected information during the evaluation process that may have implications for my future health and insurability.

There may be risks and discomfort associated with some of the testing (blood draws, intravenous contrast).

There are potential financial costs to me related to time off work, travel expenses, and the like that might not be reimbursed.

There are potential study uses to the information obtained during the evaluation. I may be asked to participate in a living donor registry.

It may be suggested to me that I have routine long-term medical followup after kidney donation.

There are alternative treatments available to the recipient other than my donating a kidney to him or her.

Modified from a personal communication from D. Cohen, MD.

unlike standard medical procedures, living donation is not specifically designed to help the donor or advance the donor's health. Moreover living donation has the potential for contravening that basic tenet of medical ethics *primum non nocere.* The person who gives consent to donate an organ must be competent (possessing decision-making capacity); willing to donate; free from coercion; medically and psychosocially suitable; fully informed of the risks and benefits of donation; and fully informed of alternative treatments available to the recipient (i.e., the donor must understand that in the absence of the donation the patient can, in most circumstances, continue dialysis and is unlikely to die). Two other principles of living donor consent have been endorsed: that of "equipoise"—the benefits to both the donor and recipient must outweigh the risks associated with the donation and the transplantation of the live donor organ—and that it is clear to the potential donor that his participation is completely voluntary and may be withdrawn at any time.

It has also been suggested, although not routinely implemented, that a separate consent be obtained for the donor evaluation itself. This would ensure that, in addition to being informed of the risks of donation, the donor is informed about all aspects of organ donation and the implications of the evaluation process itself.

Table 5.2.   Recommended evaluation of a living donor

Required

Complete history and physical
Psychologic evaluation
Measurement of BMI (body mass index)
Blood pressure measurements on three separate occasions
Complete blood count, prothrombin time, partial thromboplastin
    time, chemistry panel, urinalysis
Fasting blood sugar; fasting cholesterol and triglycerides
Timed urine collection to measure creatinine clearance or
    measurement of GFR using a radiolabelled filtration marker
24-Hour urine collection to measure protein
Chest x-ray
Electrocardiogram
Pap smear
Viral serologies: HIV, hepatitis B and C, HTLV-1, CMV, EBV
RPR or VDRL
Renal imaging: helical CT, CT angiogram, or MR angiogram

Optional

(These tests are performed to further evaluate abnormalities of
    initial studies or age/history appropriate screening.)
Ambulatory blood pressure monitoring
Echocardiogram
24-Hour urine albumin excretion or spot urine albumin:creatinine
    ratio
Colonoscopy
Mammogram
Prostate-specific antigen
2-Hour oral glucose tolerance test
Screening for hypercoagulability
Skin testing for tuberculosis
Infectious disease screening if endemic exposure (e.g., malaria,
    trypanosomiasis, schistosomiasis, strongyloides)
Cardiac stress testing
Cystoscopy
Renal biopsy

CMV, cytomegalovirus; CT, computed tomography; EBV, Epstein-Barrvirus;
GFR, glomerular filtration rate; HIV, human immunodeficiency virus; HTLV-1,
human T-lymphotropic virus1; MR, magnetic resonance; RPR, rapid plasma
reagent test; VDRL, Venereal disease research laboratory test.

The Evaluation Process

Table 5.2 outlines the general recommendations for donor evaluation. Initial determinations include whether the recipient is
prepared to accept the offer of a living donor kidney (most often
whether a parent is prepared to accept a kidney from an adult
child). A particular patient may not want another person to be
put at risk, however small that risk, on their behalf. ABO compatibility between the donor and the recipient is determined, as
well as exclusion of the presence of preformed antibodies against

the donor (negative cross-match). Some programs provide options for transplantation against incompatible blood group and positive cross-matching barriers (see Chapter 3). Although these options do not add medical risk to the donor, they may impact on the success of the transplant venture and the donor should be informed accordingly. There are some characteristics of the donor that would confer such significant risk to either the donor or the recipient as to contraindicate donation (Table 5.3). A woman should not be evaluated further while she is pregnant or if she is planning to get pregnant in the near future, although how long she should wait after delivery before donating has not been determined. Desire for future pregnancy does not contraindicate donation. Obvious contraindications should be determined at the beginning of the donor assessment so as to not perform unnecessary tests on an unqualified donors.

Which Donor to Choose?

If there is more than one donor in a family, it is logical to commence workup on the relative who is best matched (i.e., a two-haplotype match versus a one-haplotype match). If the donors are of the same match grade (i.e., a one-haplotype-matched parent and a one-haplotype-matched sibling), it may be advisable to choose the older donor with the thought that the younger donor would still be available for donation if the first kidney eventually fails. When more than one one-haplotype-matched sibling is available, it may be worthwhile to check the tissue typing of one parent to determine which sibling shares the noninherited maternal antigens (see Chapter 3). Such sharing may improve long-term graft survival. Women of childbearing age are not at increased risk for obstetric problems after donation. Biologically related donors are generally preferred over unrelated donors.

It is often a good prognostic sign when the donor accompanies the recipient to the recipient's pretransplant evaluation appointments. The first approach to the potential donor should ideally come from the patient and not from the patient's nephrologist, transplant physician, or surgeon. Some patients find it difficult to approach family members, and the nephrologist and transplant team should be prepared to facilitate the discussion of donation. Written material explaining the donation process can often help to alleviate the fears and anxiety of potential donors.

Psychosocial Evaluation

The psychosocial evaluation is an important initial step in the evaluation of the potential donor (see also Chapters 16 and 19). It also presents a valuable forum for fulfilling the tenets of informed consent, exploring donor motivation, excluding coercion. Significant psychiatric problems that would either impair the person's ability to give informed consent or that might be negatively impacted by the stress of surgery are considered contraindications to living donation. The social support of the potential donor should be deemed adequate. Monetary or nonmonetary remuneration provided to a donor in perceived exchange for an organ disqualifies a potential donor (except for compensation for expenses directly related to donation such as travel, housing, lost

Table 5.3.   Exclusion criteria for living kidney donors

Absolute

Cognitive deficit severe enough to cause inability to comprehend
    risk of donation
Inadequately treated psychiatric disease
Active drug or alcohol abuse
Evidence of renal disease (low GFR, albuminuria/proteinuria,
    unexplained hematuria and pyuria)
Significantly abnormal renal anatomy
Recurrent nephrolithiasis or bilateral kidney stones
Collagen vascular disease
Diabetes
Hypertension
Prior myocardial infarction or treated coronary artery disease
Moderate to severe pulmonary disease
Current neoplasm (unless *in situ* nonmelanoma skin cancer,
    cervical or colon—excludes *in situ* bladder carcinoma)
History of cancer (lung, breast, renal or urologic, melanoma,
    gastrointestinal, hematologic)
Familial history of renal cell cancer
Active infection
Chronic active viral infection (hepatitis B or C, HIV, HTLV)
Significant chronic liver disease
Significant neurologic disease
Disorders requiring anticoagulation
Current pregnancy
History of thrombotic disease with risk factors for future events
    (such as anticardiolipin antibody, factor V Leiden mutation)

Relative

ABO incompatibility
Age <18 or >65 years
Obesity (especially BMI >35)
Mild or easily treated hypertension
Single prior episode of nephrolithiasis
Borderline urinary abnormalities
Younger donor with more than one first-degree relative with
    diabetes, or family history of renal disease
History of gestational diabetes
Current tobacco use
Jehovah's Witness

GFR, glomerular infiltration rate; HIV, human immunodeficiency virus; HTLV,
human T-lymphotropic virus.

wages). The psychosocial evaluation of so-called altruistic donors
(see Biologically Unrelated Donors) and donors who do not have
significant personal relationship with the recipient is particularly
important because these donors may not enjoy the psychologic
gain of seeing the recipient benefit from their altruism. Covert
depression may be present in such potential donors, and long-
term data on their psychologic well-being is not available.

Risks of Donation

The short-term risks of undergoing donor nephrectomy are low. The risk of mortality as a result of donor nephrectomy is estimated to be 0.03%. Between 1999 and 2002 there were more than 15,000 living donors reported to the United Network for Organ Sharing (UNOS) and 2 reported deaths before discharge from hospital. The reoperation rate and the readmission rate are both less than 1%, and approximately 1.5% of donors require blood transfusion. The incidence of other postoperative complications, such as wound infection, pneumonia, deep venous thrombosis, and pulmonary embolism, approximates 3%. The incidence of complications is marginally higher for laparoscopic donor nephrectomy than for open nephrectomy.

Fear of the development of chronic renal failure in the remaining kidney is a concern that is the focus of much of the evaluation process. Although such a morbid complication has been described, it is very rare. Between 1987 and 2001, 48,000 living kidney donors were reported to UNOS and 20 (0.04%) previous donors, mostly siblings, were listed for transplantation. A followup of more than 356 donors for at least 20 years reported one case of chronic renal failure in an aged patient. This favorable data also needs to be viewed in the context of the lifetime incidence of chronic renal failure in the general population, which is estimated to be approximately 2% for whites and 7.5% for African Americans.

Donor Age

Advanced age also can increase the risk of perioperative complications, and while the majority of transplant centers have an upper age limit beyond which the person is not accepted as a donor, this is highly variable between centers. In a survey by UNOS of approved transplant centers, 27% of programs had no defined age exclusion, 6% used 55 years of age, 13% used 60 years of age, 70% used 70 years of age, 3% used 75 to 80 years of age. One consideration in using older living donors is that these kidneys have a shorter life span than kidneys from younger donors. An absolute younger age cut off of 18 years appears to be more consistent between centers; crossing below this is rare because of consent issues. Donors in their late teens and early twenties must be carefully evaluated for the maturity of their understanding of the donation process and to ensure they are not being subjected to overt or covert pressure.

Assessment of Surgical Risks

Certain characteristics and/or medical problems in potential donors potentially increase the risk of postoperative complications to the point where they no longer become acceptable. In general, underlying problems such as coronary artery disease (even if corrected), cerebrovascular disease, and significant chronic pulmonary disease increase the risk of having perioperative morbid events and contraindicate donation. Potential donors with multiple risk factors for coronary artery disease warrant noninvasive screening. Potential donors who smoke should be instructed to stop for 8 weeks prior to surgery to decrease pulmonary complications, and strongly urged to quit permanently to decrease future health risks. Some transplant centers will not accept a potential donor if the donor continues to smoke.

Because obesity can increase the risk of wound and thrombotic complications, these need to be carefully considered in the evaluation of a potential donor. The future impact in these donors of having a single kidney should not be ignored (see Obesity). A history of hypercoagulability significantly increases the risk of perioperative thrombotic complications and contraindicates donation. Persons with a family history of thrombotic disease, or a personal history of one episode of venous thrombosis or recurrent miscarriage, should be screened for the presence of underlying factors that would increase the risk of thrombotic complications, such as factor V Leiden mutation or anticardiolipin antibody. A person heterozygous for factor V Leiden mutation without previous thrombotic disease is not necessarily excluded from donation because the risk of complications is still low. Appropriate perioperative prophylaxis to prevent thrombotic complications, as well as discussion of the significance of this abnormality, is advised.

Risk of Disease Transmission to the Recipient

The presence of chronic viral infections, such as human immunodeficiency virus (HIV), hepatitis B, and hepatitis C, in a donor, is associated with a significant risk of transmission of disease to the recipient and contraindicates donation (see Chapter 10). The risk of associated renal disease in the donor associated with these infections is an additional consideration. Transmission of human T-cell lymphotropic virus (HTLV) and human herpesvirus (HHV)-8 to the recipient has been associated with development of T-cell leukemia and spastic paraparesis, and Kaposi sarcoma, respectively. Living donation is contraindicated in the face of active infection. Fully treated syphilis and tuberculosis and latent cytomegalovirus (CMV) do not need to prevent donation.

Potential kidney donors should be screened for both a personal and family history of cancer. They should undergo standard age-related screening tests as recommended by the American Cancer Society. There are some types of cancers that have characteristics that would exclude any person with a prior history from donation. These cancers would either not be considered a curable malignancy, may be known to have a lengthy disease-free interval before possible recurrence, or may have the potential for increased virulence in the immunocompromised patient. A history of melanoma, renal cell carcinoma, breast cancer, most hematologic malignancies, gastric cancer, and Kaposi sarcoma would contraindicate donation. The effect of prior treatment of a malignancy on renal reserve of the potential donor (as well as potential nephrotoxicity of future treatment if there is a recurrence) is an additional concern. Kidney donation is not contraindicated in the presence of *in situ* carcinomas that have been treated, such as squamous cell skin cancer or cervical carcinoma. *In situ* bladder cancer contraindicates donation.

Evaluation of Future Risk to Donor

An important part of the evaluation of potential donors is determining whether a medical condition is present that could adversely affect the health of the donor in the presence of a single kidney: namely, is there an increased risk of developing renal failure or significant renal impairment as a result of kidney donation. Avoiding increased risk of even moderate renal impairment takes on more importance in light of the evidence of increased risk of cardiovascular disease associated with impaired renal function. Studies following living kidney donors for 20 years or more seem to demonstrate long-term safety of the procedure and, in general, do not show significant increases in kidney disease or hypertension. However, the demographics of living donors has changed so that we can no longer count on all persons being evaluated being young with absolutely no medical issues to consider. While the welfare of the donor both in the long- and short-term is the primary concern, a somewhat wider net is cast than in the past. Surveys of transplant centers show a fair amount of variability in reporting of acceptance criteria for living donors. While some centers have reported acceptable short-term followup of donors with mild, treated hypertension, for example, there is little documentation as to the long-term effects of such donation. The following sections address some common coexisting problems in potential donors and how they relate to the evaluation process.

Assessment of Renal Function

GLOMERULAR FILTRATION RATE
The majority of transplant centers use either 24-hour urine collections to measure creatinine clearance or iothalamate or diethylenetriamine pentaacetic acid (DTPA) clearance (see Chapter 12) to more directly measure glomerular filtration rate (GFR). An iothalamate GFR is more accurate than a urine collection, but considerably more expensive. Many centers use urine collection initially and a more accurate test such as iothalamate clearance if there is concern over borderline renal function. Creatinine-based prediction equations are not reliable in this population, and should not be used as the sole estimate of GFR. A urine collection has the advantage of also being able to measure urine protein in the same specimen. There is no agreed specified level of renal function below which a person would not be considered an acceptable donor. Older donors, women with low muscle mass, and vegetarians may have a low GFR without intrinsic renal disease. It has been suggested that GFR should be higher for younger donors. The lower limit of renal function acceptable to donate needs to take into account not only that the GFR after donation will be approximately 75% of the predonation level, but also the normal decrease in renal function with aging. Taking this into account, a lower limit of GFR of 80 cc per minute per 1.73 m^2 has been proposed.

PROTEINURIA
Proteinuria, in general, is a sign of renal disease and, therefore, in general, a person with significant fixed proteinuria would not be considered to be a kidney donor. A 24-hour urine protein of greater than 250 mg is considered abnormal. There are transient causes of proteinuria that should be excluded, such as fever, urinary tract infection, or intense exercise. A repeat urine protein in the absence of these factors should be normal. Orthostatic

proteinuria, defined as elevated urine protein when the person is active and no elevated protein excretion during recumbency, should be ruled out. This usually occurs in younger age groups and has been shown to follow a benign course. It does not need to preclude donation. Borderline elevations in urine protein can be further evaluated with assessment of microalbuminuria, which may have more significance in terms of association with renal abnormalities.

HEMATURIA

Hematuria as defined by greater than five red cells per high-power field, can be associated with abnormalities throughout the urinary tract. Examination of the urine sediment for casts or dysmorphic red cells with or without proteinuria would indicate underlying intrinsic renal disease. Anatomic causes, such a stones and tumors, should be excluded; cystoscopy may be indicated to exclude bladder pathology. In the absence of any specific abnormalities, microscopic hematuria could be associated with the Alport carrier state or thin basement membrane disease (the former with a potentially worse future prognosis); consequently, the family history and other associated problems, such as ocular abnormalities and deafness, need to be carefully considered before proceeding with donor nephrectomy. If a workup is negative and there is no associated proteinuria, the risk of progressive renal disease is very small.

Hypertension

In general, it is recommended that a potential donor with clinically significant hypertension be excluded from donating. The rationale behind this recommendation is that hypertension is associated with development of chronic renal disease and that hyperfiltration in a single kidney could increase the risk of developing renal dysfunction in the remaining kidney, or make it more difficult to control the blood pressure. Unfortunately, the long-term risk of renal dysfunction after nephrectomy in the presence of mild hypertension is not well documented. However, because only a very small proportion of the population with mild hypertension are expected to develop renal disease, potential donors who do not have associated risk factors that would be expected to contribute to an increased risk of renal disease after donating may be considered as donors at some centers. Hence, it may not be unreasonable to consider a donor with mild hypertension if the age is older than 50 years, the GFR is greater than 80 cc per minute, the ethnicity is white, and the blood pressure is easily controlled. The mildly hypertensive donor should not have microalbuminuria or other end-organ involvement. Recommended screening for hypertension in a potential donor includes blood pressure readings on three separate occasions using criteria of the Joint National Committee (JNC 7) for the diagnosis of hypertension, as well as a chest x-ray and electrocardiogram to look for evidence of ventricular hypertrophy, GFR estimation, and urinary albumin excretion to exclude hypertensive renal disease. High blood pressure readings can be further evaluated using ambulatory blood pressure monitoring to exclude "white coat" hypertension. Arterial blood pressure tends to increase with age and older patients can be misclassified as hypertensive. An echocardiogram may be considered to further assess borderline high blood pressure or abnormalities on chest x-ray or electrocardiogram.

Diabetes

The concern over donation in diabetics, prediabetics, and those at high risk of becoming diabetic relates to the possibility that donation might induce the development of diabetic nephropathy or that diabetic nephropathy, if it develops, might progress more rapidly with a single kidney. The latter is a more relevant concern. There is no question that a person with evidence of incipient diabetic renal disease (i.e., low-grade proteinuria or microalbuminuria) should not donate; however, there is little evidence that removing a kidney in a person without evidence of renal involvement increases their risk of renal disease in the future. Tight control of blood sugars and use of angiotensin-converting enzyme inhibitors or receptor blockers would be expected to further decrease any risk. Most transplant centers do not accept persons with diabetes as living kidney donors and many centers exclude persons deemed at high risk. Some centers have used carefully selected diabetics—their diabetes being well controlled on oral agents—as donors and have not reported adverse outcomes.

All persons considered as living donors should have a fasting plasma glucose to exclude undiagnosed diabetes or glucose intolerance. A fasting plasma glucose of greater than 126 mg/dL defines the presence of diabetes; a fasting blood sugar of between 100 and 126 mg/dL should be evaluated further with a 75-g 2-hour oral glucose tolerance test (OGTT). Persons with risk factors for the development of diabetes in the absence of an abnormal fasting blood sugar should also receive an OGTT [this includes persons with a first-degree relative with diabetes, a history of gestational diabetes or babies greater than 9 pounds at delivery; obesity, i.e., body mass index (BMI) >30; fasting hypertriglyceridemia greater than 250 mg/dL; high-density lipoprotein (HDL) level less than 35 mg/dL; blood pressure greater than 140/90 mm Hg]. A blood sugar of more than 200 mg/dL at 2 hours in an OGTT defines the diabetic state. Persons with glucose intolerance on OGTT should be assessed in light of other potential risk factors for development of frank diabetes and future risk of nephropathy. Modification of risk factors, such as weight loss and exercise, should be emphasized.

Women with a history of gestational diabetes have a high lifetime risk of developing type II diabetes—as high as 50% to 70% in some series. Most women who are destined to develop diabetes do so within the first 5 years after delivery; the risk appears to be negligible beyond 10 years. Therefore, acceptance for donation and counseling for future risk can be dictated by these time frames. An OGTT in conjunction with stimulated insulin levels may be more helpful in determining risk than an OGTT alone because some women with a history of gestational diabetes who have a normal OGTT may have evidence of insulin resistance that may, in fact, portend a higher risk of diabetes in the future.

Obesity

Obesity, defined by a BMI greater than 30, is associated with increased risk of surgical complications. Obese persons have a higher risk of medical problems that are relevant in their evaluation as donors. There is a higher risk of development of diabetes and hypertension, as well as glomerular disease with associated albuminuria separate from the presence of hypertension and diabetes. Moreover, an increased risk of proteinuria and renal insufficiency has been reported in obese patients after unilateral nephrectomy. The impact of other medical issues that may be present in this group (e.g., cardiovascular disease, sleep apnea, hepatosteatosis) should also be considered. Ideally, obese potential donors will lose weight prior to donation. Most programs regard a BMI greater than 35 as a contraindication to donation.

Nephrolithiasis

The concern over performing a nephrectomy in a person with a prior history of kidney stones is that a recurrent episode may cause ureteral obstruction in a single kidney, or otherwise contribute to renal dysfunction. However, persons with a single stone episode more than 10 years previously without metabolic abnormalities associated with a higher recurrence rate (e.g., hypercalcemia, metabolic acidosis) are at low risk for stone recurrence and may be acceptable as living donors. The presence of underlying medical disorders associated with a high risk of recurrent stones, such as cystinuria, primary or enteric hyperoxaluria, inflammatory bowel disease, and sarcoid, contraindicates donation. A history of struvite stones contraindicates donation because these stones are associated with infection that is difficult to eradicate. Persons with bilateral stones, nephrocalcinosis, or stone recurrence on preventative therapy should not donate. A history of a single stone episode associated with treated primary hyperparathyroidism and normocalcemia need not contraindicate donation.

Spiral computed tomography (CT) of the kidneys should be used to detect the current presence of stones or nephrocalcinosis in persons with a history of stone disease. Radiolucent stones and small stones will not be adequately assessed by plain films and ultrasound can miss small stones. Timed urine collections to look metabolic abnormalities are not as predictive of the risk of recurrent stones as clinical parameters such as age and amount of time passed since an initial stone episode, but may be helpful to assess the need for treatment and dietary counseling. A stone initially detected in a person older than age 50 years is unlikely to recur. The risk is higher younger patients age 25 to 35 years, and needs to be considered when evaluating these persons as donors.

Inherited Renal Disease

Potential kidney donors, particularly related donors, need to be assessed for hereditary kidney disease. The presence of renal disease in a first-degree relative increases the risk of renal disease several fold, and when there is more than one first-degree relative with kidney disease, the risk is very high. Knowledge of the recipient's renal disease is a critical part of donor evaluation. For some hereditary renal diseases, the family history may be obvious; for others, biopsy documentation may be lacking, and other family information, such as others with renal failure or urinary abnormalities, or ocular or hearing abnormalities, may gain added importance.

AUTOSOMAL DOMINANT POLYCYSTIC KIDNEY DISEASE

Persons contemplating kidney donation with a first degree relative with autosomal dominant polycystic kidney disease (ADPKD) need to be screened by ultrasound. The diagnosis of ADPKD in a person at risk is defined by specific age-dependent criteria: the presence of one cyst in each kidney or two or more cysts in one kidney for those younger than age 30 years; two or more cysts in each kidney for those age 30 to 59 years; and four or more cysts in each kidney for those older than age 60 years. Ultrasound is a sensitive, relatively inexpensive, and noninvasive method of screening, but can miss cysts smaller than 1 cm. Renal ultrasound is 100% sensitive in excluding presence of ADPKD in persons age 30 years or older, but it is less reliable for those younger than age 30 years. Genetic testing, either by linkage analysis or direct deoxyribonucleic acid (DNA) sequencing can reliably exclude the presence of ADPKD in a younger donor but is not routinely available. A person at risk for ADPKD who is younger than age 30 years should not be accepted as a donor without this confirmation. It has been suggested that the greater sensitivity of heavily T2-weighted magnetic resonance imaging (MRI) in detecting smaller cysts may reliably exclude ADPKD at younger ages and allow donation.

ALPORT SYNDROME

Most cases of Alport syndrome are transmitted as an X-linked recessive trait. In 15% of cases, the transmission is autosomal recessive. There are many different mutations that can lead to Alport syndrome, but they all cause a defect in the α_5 chain of type IV collagen in the glomerular basement membrane, which can lead to glomerulosclerosis and eventual renal failure. The mutation can be associated with basement membrane abnormalities in the eye and sensorineural part of the ear causing ocular abnormalities such as lenticonus and deafness. Persons being evaluated as kidney donors with a family history of Alport syndrome need to be carefully screened for hematuria, hypertension, and hearing and eye abnormalities. An adult male relative of a patient with Alport syndrome who has a normal urinalysis can be presumed not to have the genetic defect and can safely donate. Female relatives with a normal urinalysis have a low risk of being carriers and are acceptable as donors. Female relatives with persistent hematuria are most likely carriers of the mutation. They have an elevated risk of developing chronic renal failure (approximately 10% to 15%) and should not donate.

Potential donors who may have had a kidney biopsy to evaluate hematuria or a have a family history of hematuria or kidney disease may be found to have thin basement membrane disease (TBMD). This disease generally has a benign prognosis, although the impact of hyperfiltration after uninephrectomy is may increase the risk of renal complications. TBMD needs to be carefully differentiated from female carriers of X-linked Alport syndrome as early biopsy findings may be similar. Persons with TBMD may be considered as living donors, particularly if they are older than 40 years of age. The presence of hypertension, proteinuria, and other biopsy findings of renal disease such as focal segmental glomerulosclerosis, immunoglobulin (Ig) A, or more significant basement membrane abnormalities suggestive of Alport syndrome would contraindicate donation.

FAMILIAL PRIMARY GLOMERULONEPHRITIS

There are some familial forms of the primary glomerulonephritides. Familial forms of idiopathic steroid-resistant focal segmental glomerulosclerosis are probably the best described and are associated with mutations of proteins related to podocyte function. Genetic testing may be helpful if the family history of a potential donor is of concern. Other forms of familial glomerulonephritis such as IgA, and membranoproliferative glomerulonephritis have also been described and should be considered whenever there is more than one family member affected with renal disease.

SYSTEMIC LUPUS ERYTHEMATOSUS

There is an approximately 12% incidence of lupus in first-degree relatives of patients with systemic lupus erythematosus (SLE), so that potential donors who are closely related to patients with SLE should undergo laboratory screening to exclude an abnormal antinuclear antibody (ANA), abnormal complement levels, and abnormal urinary findings. They should be questioned regarding a history of pregnancy-related complications and thrombotic events that might suggest an anticardiolipin syndrome. A family member of a patient with SLE who has a positive ANA has an approximately 40-fold increased risk of developing lupus and should be excluded from donation.

Surgical Evaluation of the Living Kidney Donor

The term "surgical evaluation" is used here narrowly to refer to the assessment of the anatomic features of the donor kidneys to determine if nephrectomy can safely be performed, to determine which kidney should be removed, and to determine which nephrectomy technique is to be employed. Preoperative spiral CT urography provides both functional and sufficiently sensitive anatomic detail to detect most polar renal arteries. This less-invasive imaging modality has replaced intravenous urography and renal arteriography in most centers (see Chapter 12). Usually, the left kidney is selected for donation because the left renal vein is longer than the right vein and thus easier to transplant, particularly in laparoscopic procedures. If there are multiple arteries to the left kidney and a single artery to the right kidney, the right kidney can usually be used. If there are two arteries bilaterally, a kidney may still be used, employing one of several surgical techniques to handle multiple renal arteries. Occasionally, the donor has minor unilateral renal abnormalities, such as renal cysts, or even more severe problems, such as ureteropelvic junction obstruction. In these situations, the most prudent approach, if such abnormalities are not too severe, is to transplant the abnormal kidney, leaving the donor with the normal one. The unexpected finding of unilateral or bilateral fibromuscular dysplasia in a normotensive potential donor presents a difficult dilemma. In the absence of definitive data regarding natural history of this condition, most programs have avoided using such donors.

SURGICAL TECHNIQUES FOR LIVING DONOR NEPHRECTOMY

The introduction of laparoscopic or endoscopically assisted living kidney donation has been a major advance in organ donation. First introduced with some trepidation in selected centers in the mid-1990s these procedures are now performed in most large transplant programs. The relative advantages and disadvantages of laparoscopic nephrectomy compared to conventional open nephrectomy are summarized in Tables 5.4 and 5.5, and should be discussed with all potential donors. The major impetus for the development of the laparoscopic techniques has been the pain and discomfort suffered after standard open nephrectomy. By reducing convalescence time and facilitating an early return to work, laparoscopic donor nephrectomy has been responsible for an expanding pool of living donors. Long-term renal function is not different between open nephrectomy and laparoscopic nephrectomy. Laparoscopic donation accounts for much of the increased "popularity" and frequency of living donation. As of 2003, approximately 70% of living donor transplant nephrectomies performed in the United States employed laparoscopic techniques.

Open Nephrectomy

The traditional method for removing a kidney from a living donor has been through an open surgical technique, using a modified flank incision. Most donor surgeons use an extrapleural and extraperitoneal approach, just above or below the twelfth rib. The kidney must be carefully dissected to preserve all renal arteries, renal veins, and the periureteral blood supply. Excessive traction on the renal artery should be avoided to prevent vasospasm. The donor should be well hydrated, and intraoperative mannitol is administered to ensure a brisk diuresis. After the renal vessels are securely ligated and divided, the kidney is removed and placed in a basin of frozen saline slush to decrease renal metabolism. The renal arteries are cannulated and flushed with cold heparinized

Table 5.4. Advantages and disadvantages of open nephrectomy

Advantages

Long-term international record of safety
Less-sophisticated equipment requirements
Retroperitoneal approach minimizes potential abdominal complications
Shorter operative time
Minimal warm ischemia time to remove kidney
Excellent early graft function

Disadvantages

Postoperative pain, occasionally persistent
Requires 6–8 weeks of recovery to return to work
Long surgical scar with potential for hernia and abdominal wall asymmetry

**Table 5.5.   Advantages and disadvantages
of laparoscopic nephrectomy**

Advantages

Less postoperative pain
Minimal surgical scarring
Rapid return to full activities and work (approximately 4 weeks)
Shorter hospital stay
Magnified view of renal vessels

Disadvantages

Impaired early graft function
Graft loss or damage during "learning curve"
Pneumoperitoneum may compromise renal blood flow
Longer operative time
Tendency to have shorter renal vessels and multiple arteries
Added expense of specialized instrumentation
Slight increase in donor mortality

normal saline or lactated Ringer solution in lieu of using systemic heparinization in the donor.

Laparoscopic Nephrectomy

Laparoscopic or endoscopically assisted nephrectomy techniques are used preferentially in many centers except in select cases of complex donor anatomy, donor obesity, or in some centers where right nephrectomy is required. Laparoscopic techniques require specially trained surgical staff and a capacity for sophisticated renal imaging (see Chapter 12). For a full laparoscopic nephrectomy, the donor is placed in the flank position and the abdominal cavity is insufflated with carbon dioxide gas. Four ports are established through small incisions in the abdominal wall, and a miniature video camera and instruments are then manipulated through these ports (Fig. 5.1). The surgical procedure is visualized on a video monitor. First, the colon is reflected medially, away from the kidney and Gerota fascia. Next, the spleen (for left-sided nephrectomy) or the liver (for right-sided nephrectomy) is mobilized and retracted away from the upper pole of the kidney. The perinephric tissues are then freed and the ureter and periureteral tissues are then mobilized. The renal artery and vein are then carefully identified and isolated, and any remaining surrounding attachments are ligated. Next the ureter, renal arteries and veins are divided with a vascular stapler, and the kidney is placed in a plastic sack. An incision (either Pfannenstiel or midline below the umbilicus) is made just large enough to remove the kidney and sack. After removal, the kidney is then placed in frozen saline slush, the vascular staples are removed, and the renal artery is flushed with heparinized solution, as for open nephrectomy. The hand-assisted laparoscopic technique employs a relatively small abdominal incision to allow the introduction of the surgeon's hand to supplement the laparoscopic procedure and permit

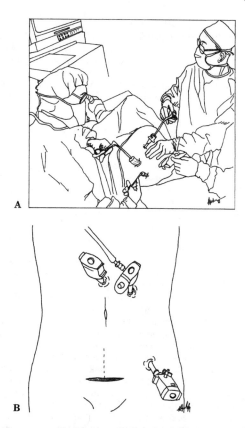

Fig. 5.1. Laparoscopic donor nephrectomy. A: The surgeon and assistants perform the operation by using a miniature television camera to view instruments placed through the abdominal wall. B: After the kidney has been completely mobilized and the ureter and renal vessels have been divided, the kidney is removed through a small incision in the lower abdomen.

rapid, atraumatic removal of the kidney. Laparoscopic techniques can be rapidly converted to open nephrectomy in the event of uncontrolled bleeding or unforeseen anatomic abnormalities.

Postoperative Management

A chest radiograph is obtained in the recovery room if a pneumothorax is suspected, and, if necessary, the air is evacuated or a chest tube is placed. A nasogastric tube is not routinely inserted. Most patients are able to eat 24 to 48 hours after open surgery. Early ambulation is encouraged, as is aggressive pulmonary toilet. The use of ketorolac as an analgesic in postoperative management protocol reduces the postoperative discomfort of both open and laparoscopic donation. The average hospital stay is 2 to 4 days. Most donors can return to all but the most strenuous exercise or work by 3 to 4 weeks. Complete recovery takes 6 to 8 weeks, although some donors complain of incisional pain for 2 to 3 months. Laparoscopic procedures are associated with a faster recovery. These donors are usually in the hospital for 1 to 2 days and report less postoperative pain and a full recovery in 4 to 5 weeks.

LONG-TERM POSTNEPHRECTOMY ISSUES

Renal Function

Within days to weeks after uninephrectomy, hyperfiltration in the remaining kidney causes GFR to increase to approximately 75% to 80% of the previous two-kidney value. The amount of compensation is dictated by age-related renal reserve. Follow-up studies of donors up to 35 years postnephrectomy attest to the long-term safety of the procedure. Decline in renal function parallels that of age-related declines in persons with two kidneys. Urine albumin excretion, attributable to hyperfiltration, may be elevated, but is usually low grade, and is not associated with a higher risk of renal dysfunction. The incidence of treatment for hypertension increases with length of time after nephrectomy, but in most studies is not different from an age-matched population. Living kidney donation has no apparent adverse effect on survival that may actually be better than national mortality rates. Better survival is most likely attributable to the fact that only healthy persons are accepted as donors.

It should be noted that the apparent long-term safety of donor nephrectomy and lack of increased risk of medical complications is based upon the demographics of the donor population 10 to 20 or more years ago. That was an era when there was less pressure to find a living kidney donor and the criteria by which donors were accepted may have been stricter than is now applied at some centers. Ultimately, accepting donors with relatively minor medical problems, such as mild hypertension, needs to be done in a setting where there can be a reasonable expectation that the future risk to the donor is not greatly increased, as well as a clear understanding by the donor of the potential risk. More widespread prospective followup of donors will be provided by the establishment of a "Living Donor Registry" to provide better documentation of long-term safety.

Pregnancy

Women of childbearing age should be told that there is no evidence that kidney donation has a deleterious effect on either fertility or the course of pregnancy. They should be counseled to delay pregnancy at least 2 to 3 months postdonation to allow for maximum compensatory hypertrophy of the single kidney. Because the diagnosis of toxemia depends on the lack of prior hypertension, they should receive early prenatal care with screening for hypertension and urinary abnormalities, as well as assessment of renal function. There is no evidence to support an increased risk of renal-related complications as a consequence of obstruction from a gravid uterus if a donor of childbearing age is left with a solitary right kidney. Therefore, the desire for future pregnancy does not need to dictate the selection of which kidney to use for donation.

Employment and Insurance

Most donors can return to their prior employment without limitation. In the United States, the federal government provides its employees with up to 30 paid working days after organ donation and many private employers do the same. Donors engaged in heavy physical labor may have some difficulty after open nephrectomy; this possibility should be discussed with them before the procedure. In general, kidney donors do not have insurability issues in terms of higher rates or an inability to obtain insurance. Problems they might experience are most likely attributable to incomplete knowledge regarding kidney donor outcome on the part of the insurance company and should prompt contact and education by the transplant program. Most branches of the military will allow a person on active duty to donate a kidney and remain in the service, but it may impact the future ability to participate in all aspects of the military and should be discussed prior to donation. A person cannot initially join the military after donating; therefore, future career plans should be discussed prior to kidney donation.

Long-Term Medical Care

Recommendations for future medical care and risk modification for a kidney donor are not much different than those for the general population; that is, routine check-ups and cancer screening appropriate for age, and smoking and excessive alcohol abstinence. Persons who are accepted as donors with issues such as mild hypertension, a history of stones, or obesity would likely benefit from more regular followup, and data relating to the followup of these and certain other groups of patients would add to current knowledge about the safety of donation. Donors should be discouraged from using high-protein diets for weight loss or protein supplements for body building, because they may contribute to hyperfiltration injury. They should be advised to avoid long-term regular use of nonsteroidal antiinflammatory drugs or acetaminophen, because both these types of drugs have an association with renal insufficiency and hypertension. They should avoid potentially nephrotoxic herbal medications.

CONTROVERSIES AND INNOVATIONS IN LIVING KIDNEY DONOR PRACTICE

Biologically Unrelated Donors

The number of living-unrelated donor transplants performed in the United States is steadily increasing. Centers in other countries, such as Australia and Germany, also report an increasing experience in living-unrelated donor transplantation, mostly driven by spousal kidney donation. The majority of biologically unrelated donors are "emotionally related" and have an apparent or easily documented close and long-standing relationship with the recipient (spouse, significant other, close friend, adopted sibling). Spousal donation can be particularly gratifying because the health of the couple, not just the recipient, is being improved. France and the United Kingdom have government oversight of living donation. In the case of France, living donation is restricted to competent adults giving to a parent, sibling, or child; spousal donation is restricted to emergency situations only.

While transplants from unrelated donors with a much more casual relationship with the recipient are performed commonly in the United States (e.g., from coworkers, acquaintances, church members), these situations usually undergo close scrutiny. The concern is that there is a greater possibility of illegal payment, monetary or otherwise, in exchange for the organ. Despite investigation, it still may be difficult to determine whether this is occurring covertly, and realistically, it probably occurs with higher frequency than is recognized by transplant centers despite safeguards against it. When the motive of the donor is not readily apparent there may concern that there is some form of coercion on the part of the recipient or the donor.

The term "altruistic donors" refers to donors who have absolutely no personal relationship with the potential recipient, but who have the desire to donate a kidney "to benefit mankind" or, more specifically, to improve one person's life even though they do not know the recipient. These donors may never meet the recipient and therefore may not observe or enjoy the recipient's return to health. The motives of the altruistic donor are sometimes looked upon with skepticism or suspicion. Surveys demonstrate, however, that up to 50% of individuals would be willing, in principle, to donate a kidney to a stranger while alive. Some transplant centers in the United States have well-developed protocols that the potential donor has to go through to ensure that there is full understanding of the risks they are undertaking and that there is no "commerce" involved. This involves a careful psychosocial examination to fully explore the motivation for wishing to donate a kidney—unrealistic expectations and misperceptions need to be identified. Practical and ethical guidelines for the triage and evaluation of potential altruistic donors have been developed (see Adams et al. in Part I of "Selected Readings"). Less than 10% of persons engaging in altruistic donation who contact transplant programs actually become donors. Generally, the recipient of a kidney from an altruistic donor would be a patient on the deceased donor waiting list with a compatible blood type, the most wait time, and negative cross-matching.

Incompatible Donor and Recipient

There are several innovative options available in some centers for healthy donors who are incompatible to their potential recipients because of blood group type or positive cross-matching. Intravenous immunoglobulins, often combined with plasmapheresis, may be used to abrogate a positive cross-match (see Chapters 3 and 4). A similar technique that is often combined with splenectomy may be used for ABO-incompatible donors. Donation from blood group A2 or A2B to blood group O or B may be performed with or without plasmapheresis, depending on anti-A titers (see Chapter 3). The most experience with ABO-incompatible transplantation is from Japan, where cultural barriers to deceased donor transplantation have made achieving living donation all the more urgent.

So-called paired donor exchange (e.g., an A to B couple "swaps" with a B to A couple) has been proposed as a solution for donor–recipient pairs for whom there is ABO incompatibility. Although seemingly attractive, the logistical problems with this approach have limited its applicability. UNOS has introduced a variance to the standard deceased donor allocation algorithm (see Chapter 3) whereby an incompatible donor may donate a kidney to the next suitable, compatible, long-waiting recipient on the wait-list, while the initially intended but incompatible recipient takes the place of the actual recipient on the wait-list, thereby reducing their anticipated waiting time for a deceased donor organ. These innovative solutions provide potential options for motivated but incompatible donors, although the practical difficulties with them mandate that whenever possible a compatible donor be found.

Paid Donation

In the United States, the direct payment of money in exchange for organ donation violates the National Organ Transplant Act (NOTA) (see Chapter 17). Similar legislation is in place internationally, and all the major professional transplant organizations prohibit such payment. Reimbursement for expenses related to donation incurred by the donor, such as for travel and lodging, is generally not prohibited. Despite these regulations, commerce in kidney transplantation, although officially condemned, is a common phenomenon in many parts of the world, and in some cases, has been associated with criminal activity. The donors are typically poor, or under great financial stress; recipients are often wealthy or come from other wealthier countries; and "middlemen" are often involved. Arguments against paid donation express concern for the exploitation of the poor, the commodification of the human body, and the negative impact of paid donation on the altruism that is a gratifying feature of both living and deceased donation. Arguments made for allowing paid donation claim that the money paid to poor donors would have a significant positive impact on their quality of life, that paid donors are entitled to use their bodies as they see fit, that the risks of the procedure are small, and that there is no other way to address the organ donor shortage. A study of Turkish patients who received kidney transplants from paid donors in Iran, Iraq, and India showed a higher rate of unconventional complications, mainly infectious, in the recipients. In India, most paid donors ended up back in debt and with a lower family income than before donation. Most reported deterioration in health after donation.

Living Donor Registry

Long-term followup of transplant recipients is one of the responsibilities of transplant programs. Followup data are submitted to UNOS and are available for scientific analysis and to the general public. No such followup is mandated after living donation. In the past, living donors have all been kidney donors and criteria for donation have been very strict. Concern over a perceived trend to liberalization of current kidney donor criteria, together with reports of morbid experiences in donors of nonrenal solid organs, has generated a consensus that formal followup of living donors should be instigated. Such followup might permit more substantive answers to questions over the safety of donor evaluation and acceptance practices. The logistics of such national and international living donor registries have yet to be finalized.

Risk Assessment

Donors have typically been accepted or rejected based on the perception of safety on the part of the evaluating physician. The most common reasons for declaring an otherwise acceptable donor as "unsafe" are mild hypertension and asymptomatic urinary abnormalities. It is the fear of the evaluator that these patients are at particular risk of developing chronic renal failure. In fact, however, no donor, or, for that matter, no person, can be told that there is no risk of developing chronic renal failure. All risk is relative and the risk of developing chronic renal failure in the face of mild hypertension or isolated microscopic hematuria is actually very small (somewhere between 1/100 and 1/10,000 donations), and considerably smaller than for the general population. Rather than declining such "borderline" patients outright, it has been suggested that an attempt be made, based on available data on the demographics of renal disease, to give the potential donor an estimate of their risk and to permit them, within rational limits, after careful education, to decide what degree of risk is acceptable to them. Risk assessment is not absolute: the finding of mild hypertension or a kidney stone in a 20-year-old person will clearly be of greater concern than such findings in a 60-year-old person.

PART II. DECEASED DONOR KIDNEY TRANSPLANTATION

Figure 1.1 (Chapter 1) illustrates graphically the inexorably widening gap between the demand for deceased donor kidneys and their supply. The number of deceased donors has remained steady in recent years, whereas the number of potential recipients has risen steadily each year. The inevitable effect of this discrepancy is an increase in the waiting time for deceased donor kidneys, which is now measured in years (see Chapter 3).

Surveys suggest that almost all Americans are aware that kidney transplants are performed and as many as 75% of Americans express a willingness to donate an organ after death. Review of hospital medical records of deaths occurring in intensive care units in the United States between 1997 and 1999 predict an annual number of brain-dead potential organ donors of between 10,500 and 13,800. In this period, the overall *consent rate* (the number of families agreeing to donate divided by the number of families asked to donate) was 54%; the overall *conversion rate* (the number of actual donors divided by the number of potential donors) was 42%. Some possible reasons for these discrepancies are discussed below.

The process of deceased donor transplantation, from identification of a potential donor to the operation itself, is complex

Table 5.6. Sequence of events preceding deceased donor transplantation[a]

1. Identification of potential donor (see Table 5.7)
2. Notification of organ procurement organization
3. Diagnosis of brain death made by attending physicians; family informed
4. Suitability of donor ascertained
5. Permission for organ donation obtained from family
6. Tissue typing and ABO blood typing of donor[b]
7. Kidneys removed and stored
8. Local and national computer listing of all potential recipients reviewed
9. Top recipient selected by ABO blood type and United Network for Organ Sharing scoring system[b]
10. Transplantation program to review clinical indication for transplantation for recipients of marginal kidneys
11. Top recipient patient notified and admitted to hospital
12. "Backup" recipient prepared when recipient's panel-reactive antibodies are high
13. Donor lymphocytes and recipient serum cross-matched[b]
14. Preoperative history and physical examination
15. Preoperative chest radiograph, electrocardiogram, ABO blood typing, and routine chemistry
16. Dialysis performed if necessary
17. Transplantation performed

[a] The precise sequence may vary in individual cases.
[b] See Chapter 3.

(Table 5.6). It represents the epitome of coordinated teamwork and institutional cooperation. It is orchestrated by regional *organ procurement organizations* (OPOs) (see Chapter 3) that provide a nationally integrated 24-hour service. The quality of the deceased donor kidneys that are recovered by this process has a major effect on the short- and long-term outcome of the whole transplant endeavor (see Chapters 8 and 9).

The responsibility for identifying potential donors and notifying the OPOs belongs to every health professional and hospital involved in acute patient care; it has been legally established in *required request legislation* (see Chapter 17). The benefits of this legislation have been less than expected. Trained organ procurement professionals should handle the most difficult and sensitive part of the donation process, the approach to the recently bereaved family. Family members are more likely to permit donation if they are given time to accept the fact that their relative is brain dead before organ donation is discussed. *Uncoupling* of the discussion of death and donation significantly increases the likelihood of family consent. Although organ donor cards are in themselves valid legal documents, OPOs generally request specific permission from families to maintain a high degree of public trust and acceptance. Discussion among family members of their attitudes toward organ donation should be encouraged so that the wishes of the deceased can be respected in the event of a catastrophe. Ongoing education by the transplant community of both healthcare professionals and the lay public is central to the maintenance of the deceased donor organ supply.

The country with the most effective organ recovery network is Spain. The Spanish model differs from that applied in the United States in that paid medical personnel are available at trauma centers to approach bereaved family members. The approach is based on a presumption of consent for organ donation and to ensure that no specific denial of consent had been made.

WHO IS A DONOR?

Most solid-organ donors are brain-dead cadavers whose hearts are still beating; these are often victims of head trauma, vascular catastrophes, cerebral anoxia, and nonmetastasizing brain tumors. It is best to regard all such patients as potential donors and then to exclude inappropriate candidates (Table 5.7). Many governmental agencies have implemented legislation to increase awareness of the need for organ donation. In the United States, current law requires hospitals to report all deaths to the local OPO; the OPO staff can then determine the potential for organ donation and approach the family for consent. The criteria for donor acceptance are not all absolute, and some are controversial. The next stage in the process—the decision to offer a given kidney to a specific patient, particularly if the features of that

Table 5.7.   **Contraindications to deceased donor donation**

Absolute

Chronic renal disease
Age >70 years
Potentially metastasizing malignancy
Severe hypertension
Untreated bacterial sepsis
Current intravenous drug abuse
Hepatitis B surface antigen (HBsAg) positive
Human immunodeficiency virus (HIV) positive
Prolonged warm ischemia
Oliguric acute renal failure

Relative

Age >60 years
Age <5 years
Mild hypertension
Treated infection
Nonoliguric acute tubular necrosis
Positive hepatitis B and C serology
Donor medical disease (diabetes, systemic lupus erythematosus)
Intestinal perforation with spillage
Prolonged cold ischemia
High-risk behavior

kidney suggest that it is not "ideal," and the decision by the patient to accept it—may be one of the most difficult in clinical transplantation. A discussion of the principles that can guide these decisions is found in Chapter 6.

Donor Age

Young Donors

In response to the organ donor shortage, there has been a broadening in the age limits traditionally applied to organ donors. The use of kidneys from donors younger than 5 years of age is associated with an increased risk for surgical complications and impaired tolerance to episodes of graft dysfunction. Some programs have reported favorable results by transplanting both infant kidneys with their attachment to the great vessels, so-called *pediatric en bloc* transplantation. The decision to split pediatric kidneys or use them *en bloc* is made based on donor age and kidney size (see Chapter 7, Fig. 7.4). With advances in immunosuppression, the success of pediatric donor kidney transplantation has improved. If rejection can be avoided, the pediatric kidney will grow to nearly adult size within the first year.

Older Donors/Marginal Donors/Expanded Criteria Donors

There is a consistent trend to use organs from older donors, and as of 2002, about one-third of all kidney donors were older than 50 years of age. Donor age is an important determinant of long-term graft function. The 5-year graft survival of donors in their mid-twenties compared to donors in their mid-sixties falls by approximately 5% each decade. It should be noted, however, that this data is not corrected for the fact that there is a trend to put older donor kidneys into older recipients whose survival is impaired. The long-term outcome of older donor kidneys may be further impaired if the cause of the death was vascular rather than traumatic, if the donor had a history of hypertension, and if there was impaired kidney function at the time of death. Older kidneys may be more susceptible to delayed graft function, particularly if the cold ischemia time is prolonged (see Chapter 8).

The terms "marginal kidney" or "borderline kidney" are imprecise and are used to describe kidneys with one or more of a variety of unfavorable characteristics, such as advanced age, prolonged warm or cold ischemia time, and impaired kidney function at the time of organ harvest. The term "expanded criteria donor" (ECD) is a more precise term that has been introduced in the United States as part of a concerted effort to increase the use of kidneys that might otherwise have been discarded, and to attempt to minimize the length of cold ischemia to which they are subjected. ECD kidneys are defined by donor characteristics that are associated with a 70% greater risk of graft failure at 2 years posttransplant when compared to an "ideal" reference group (nonhypertensive donors age 10 to 39 years whose cause of death was not cerebrovascular accident and whose terminal creatinine was less than or equal to 1.5 mg/dL). The matrix shown in Table 5.8 displays the factors that define ECDs. Thus, all kidneys from donors older than age 60 years are, by definition, ECD kidneys. Donors between the ages of 50 and 60 years are defined as ECD kidneys

Table 5.8.   Definition of expanded criteria donors

Donor Condition	Age 50–59 Years	Age 60 Years or Older
CVA + HTN + Creat >1.5	X	X
CVA + HTN	X	X
CVA + Creat >1.5	X	X
HTN + Creat >1.5	X	X
CVA		X
HTN		X
Creat >1.5		X
None of the above		X

Creat >1.5, terminal serum creatinine greater than 1.5 mg/dL; CVA, cerebrovascular accident as cause of death; HTN, history of hypertension; X, expanded criteria donor.

if other risk factors are present. It should be noted that the definition of an ECD kidney is based on information that is available at the time of organ recovery. In 2003, 24% of all deceased donors in the United States were from ECD donors.

The definition of ECD kidneys in terms of the relative risk of graft loss compared to an ideal reference group may suggest an overly pessimistic outcome. Thus, a 70% increased relative risk of graft loss still reflects an excellent chance of graft survival; for example, if the 2-year survival of the "ideal" kidney was 90%, that of the ECD kidney would still be close to 80%. It should be emphasized that the relative mortality risk for recipients of ECD kidneys is still considerably greater than remaining on dialysis (see Chapter 1, Figs. 1.5 and 1.6). The decision as to who should receive an ECD or otherwise marginal kidney is discussed in Chapter 6.

Donor Biopsy

A biopsy of the potential allograft can be performed to aid in the decision to transplant it. The degree of glomerular sclerosis is relatively easy to measure. If more than 20% of glomeruli are sclerosed, the functional prognosis of the graft is poor and these kidneys are usually discarded or both kidneys are transplanted into a single recipient. Although the numeric percentage of glomerulosclerosis is often emphasized in the decision process to accept a kidney, the extent of interstitial fibrosis and atrophy and vascular changes may be more important (see Chapter 13). Because of the rapid processing techniques that are required, the diagnostic value of donor biopsy is quite limited. A biopsy should only be requested and performed if it is likely that its result will have a significant impact on the decision-making process to accept an organ.

Nephron Dose

Kidneys from donors who are male, nonblack, of intermediate age, with immediate postoperative function, and a good tissue match may be less susceptible to chronic allograft failure than kidneys from poorly matched, female, black donors who are older than 60 years of age or younger than 3 years of age with delayed initial function (see Chapter 9). The common factor explaining these findings may be the relative "nephron dose" that is transplanted (see Chapter 3). No systematic attempt is made to match the kidney size and nephron number to the size of the patient, and retrospective analysis suggests that such a policy would not necessarily be beneficial.

Contraindications to Donation

Table 5.7 summarizes the contraindications to deceased donor transplantation. Positive serology for HIV is a contraindication to the use of a deceased donor kidney. Concern regarding transmission of HIV and the possibility of a false-negative HIV test result is such that HIV-negative donors are often excluded if they are deemed to be at high risk for HIV infection because of intravenous drug use or because of high-risk sexual behavior. If a decision is made to offer such a kidney to a patient, explicit consent must be obtained. The use of donors with serologic evidence of hepatitis B or C infections is discussed in Chapter 11.

Cancer can be transmitted by donor organs and, other than for some specific exceptions, is a contraindication to donation. Rare, but well-documented, cases of transplanted cancer have been described as a result of covert malignancy in the donor. Most primary brain tumors are generally not regarded as a contraindication to transplantation because, in the absence of a systemic shunt, they rarely metastasize. Highly malignant primary brain tumors (aggressive astrocytomas, medulloblastomas, and glioblastoma multiforme) do present a small but finite risk of recurrence in the recipient, and kidneys from these donors should be transplanted only under special circumstances (see Chapter 6). Confirmation of histology is mandatory to ensure that the tumors are not metastases.

Ideally, donors have excellent graft function at the time of harvesting, but nonoliguric acute renal failure is common. In such cases, it is crucial to review the clinical circumstances carefully to determine whether the cause of acute renal failure is consistent with reversible renal failure, usually *acute tubular necrosis* (ATN). The kidney function of young donors with ATN typically recovers rapidly after transplantation, whereas with older donors, recovery may be delayed or incomplete. The combination of donor ATN and prolonged cold ischemia time may be particularly unfavorable, and it may be wise to discard such kidneys.

Donation After Cardiac Death

The term "donation after cardiac death" (DACD) is preferred to the more familiar term "non-heart-beating donor" (NHBD) because of the parallel to the more common donation after brain death. Before the acceptance of criteria for the declaration of brain death (see Table 5.9), all deceased donor organs were recovered from patients with cardiac arrest. With the acceptance of brain death criteria, recovery of these organs decreased substantially because of the fear of irreparable ischemic damage. The organ donor shortage has led to a reevaluation of this policy.

Table 5.9.   Clinical criteria for diagnosis of brain death

Irreversibility

No sedating, paralyzing, or toxic drugs
No gross electrolyte or endocrine disturbances
No profound hypothermia

Absent cerebral function

No seizures or posturing
No response to pain in cranial nerve distribution[a]
Absent brainstem function
Apnea in response to acidosis or hypercarbia
No pupillary or corneal reflexes
No oculocephalic or vestibular reflexes
No tracheobronchial reflex

[a] Spinal reflexes may be present.

Potential DACD donors fall into two major categories. "Uncontrolled" DACD donors are pulseless and asystolic after adequate but failed attempts at resuscitation. Some trauma centers have developed protocols to minimize ischemia in these circumstances by rapid placement of intravenous cannulas to cool the organs after death has been declared. The option to donate is preserved until the family can be informed of the death and then counseled by the organ procurement staff. If consent to donate is obtained, the organs are recovered quickly to prevent further ischemic injury. Uncontrolled DACD is infrequent in the United States, but is the most common form of DACD in Europe and Japan. "Controlled" DACD donors are deeply comatose, irreversibly brain damaged, "vegetative," and respirator dependent, but are not brain dead by strict definition. In these circumstances, the decision to withdraw supportive care is made by the family and primary medical team, and appropriate consent is obtained. Ventilator support is discontinued either in the operating room or in an intensive care unit, cardiac function is monitored, and death is pronounced by standard cardiac criteria after a predetermined (usually 10 minutes) period of asystole. Organ recovery then proceeds expeditiously.

Controlled DACD is more common in the United States where it accounts for 4% of all deceased donors. It has been estimated that if DACD protocols were maximized, the supply of deceased donor organs could increase by up to 25%. DACD is associated with an increased rate of delayed graft function, but long-term graft survival is similar to that of brain-dead donors. It is critical that protocols for DACD be ethically sound, respect the feelings of donor families and medical staff, and avoid any appearance of conflict of interest.

DIAGNOSIS OF BRAIN DEATH

Deceased donor transplantation requires that the organ to be transplanted be maintained in a state of good function until the moment of recovery. Somatic death and cardiac standstill tend to follow brain death by 2 to 3 days; by this time, organ function is often irreversibly impaired. Societal acceptance and the legal and medical establishment of brain-death criteria are essential components of deceased donor transplantation (see Chapter 17); countries that do not have such criteria do not have well-developed deceased donor transplant programs.

The diagnosis of brain death should be made by a physician who is independent of the transplant team and thus free of conflict of interest. Clinically, the diagnosis requires irrefutable documentation of the irreversible absence of cerebral and brainstem function (Table 5.9). Electroencephalogram and isotope or dye angiography can be used to support the diagnosis, but they are not mandatory. After the diagnosis of brain death has been made in a potential donor, steps must be taken to maintain adequate circulatory and respiratory function until permission for donation is given. Organ recovery should then be performed as expeditiously as possible.

Management of the Brain-Dead Donor

Maintenance of cardiovascular stability becomes more difficult the longer the period of brain death. At the time of diagnosis, patients are often relatively hypovolemic because of prior therapeutic attempts to minimize brain swelling by inducing dehydration. A diabetes insipidus-like state may accompany head injuries and brain death, resulting in obligatory urine outputs of up to 1 L per hour. Brain death is associated with a massive release of cytokines, a so-called cytokine storm, which has the potential to injure the donated kidney and make it more susceptible to ischemic and immunologic injury (see Chapter 8).

Blood pressure should be maintained at greater than 100 mm Hg by aggressive administration of crystalloids, colloids, or blood products. Central venous pressure should be monitored and maintained at greater than 10 mm Hg. If urine output decreases to less than about 40 mL per hour in a well-hydrated donor, furosemide or mannitol may be given. Insulin administration may be necessary to minimize hyperglycemia and glycosuria. If, despite good hydration, blood pressure remains low, low-dose dopamine and other inotropic agents, such as dobutamine or norepinephrine, are sometimes required. If a hypotonic diuresis ensues, suggesting a diagnosis of diabetes insipidus, a hypotonic infusion should be used to replace the urine output. Dextrose infusion, which may induce an additional osmotic diuresis, should be avoided; a vasopressin infusion may be required if the hypotonic urine volume is massive (more than 500 mL per hour). Hormonal resuscitation with methylprednisolone, triiodothyronine (T3), and arginine vasopressin (so-called 3HR treatment) may improve the quality of recovered organs.

TECHNIQUE OF DECEASED DONOR ORGAN RETRIEVAL

The principles of the retrieval operation are similar regardless of the organs to be removed. Wide surgical exposure is obtained. Each organ to be removed is dissected with its vasculature intact. To avoid damage to the vasculature and to prevent delayed

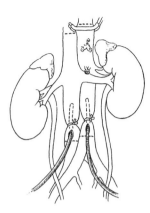

Fig. 5.2. *En bloc* **dissection for deceased donor kidney donation with cannulas in place for *in situ* perfusion. Perihilar and periureteral fat are left in place.**

graft function caused by vasospasm, there is no dissection into the renal hilum. Cannulas are placed for *in situ* cooling. At the time of aortic cross-clamping, flush and surface cooling is begun. The organs are removed in an orderly fashion. The kidneys are removed *en bloc* with the aorta and vena cava (Fig. 5.2). If multiple organs are to be removed, the preferred sequence is heart or lung first, liver or pancreas second, and kidneys last. The kidneys are protected against ischemia by the cold flush and surface cooling during the 10 to 15 minutes that it takes to remove the other organs.

One variation of this approach is a rapid infusion technique whereby cannulas are placed immediately, the aorta is cross-clamped, and the dissection is completed under cold infusion. This technique is used primarily when the donor is hemodynamically unstable.

Kidneys Alone
Fewer than 5% of all organ donations are for kidneys only. In these circumstances, either a long midline incision from pubic notch to sternal notch can be used, splitting the sternum, or a cruciate midline incision can be made. The right colon and duodenum are mobilized, exposing the great vessels. The aortic bifurcation is isolated. The inferior mesenteric artery and vein are ligated. The aorta is controlled above the take-off of the celiac trunk. Exposure can be achieved either by mass ligation of the porta hepatis to expose the superior mesenteric and celiac arteries, or by mobilization of the left lateral segment of the liver, splitting the diaphragmatic crus, controlling the aorta, and mass-clamping the superior mesenteric and celiac arteries. The supraceliac aorta can also be controlled in the left chest behind the heart before the thoracic aorta enters the abdomen. The ureters are divided deep in the

pelvis, maintaining a long segment and leaving all periureteral tissue. The aorta is cannulated at the bifurcation of the iliac arteries, and the proximal aorta is cross-clamped. An ice flush solution is begun. The kidneys are then widely mobilized, leaving Gerota capsule intact, and removed *en bloc* with the abdominal aorta and vena cava.

If the heart and kidneys are being donated, the procurement is similar, except that the heart team mobilizes the heart before cross-clamping the aorta, and the heart is removed first. The kidneys are separated in slush on a back table. The left renal vein is taken off the cava with a small cuff of vena cava. The remainder of the vena cava is left with the right kidney. The aorta is divided longitudinally, leaving the renal arteries attached to cuffs of aorta on each side.

Kidneys with Other Abdominal Organs

If the liver and pancreas are removed, their removal precedes kidney removal. The lower border of their dissection is the vena cava, just above the insertion of the renal veins, and the aorta, at or just below the take-off of the superior mesenteric artery. After their removal, the abdominal landmarks are usually obscured. *En bloc* kidney removal, as described in the previous section on kidneys alone, is carried out by dissecting widely around the kidneys to avoid damage to the important hilar structures.

Pharmacologic Adjuncts

Most deceased donors are given large doses of corticosteroids to deplete circulating donor lymphocytes. Mannitol, in doses of up to 1 g/kg, is also given to ensure diuresis and possibly to minimize ischemic injury. There is some evidence that alpha blockers or calcium channel blockers given intravenously before kidney manipulation may lower the rate of delayed graft function. If Thymoglobulin is to be the form of antibody induction that is prescribed, it should be administered during the procedure. Phentolamine (Regitine), 10 to 15 mg, may be used just before cross-clamping of the aorta; earlier use would cause significant hypotension. Systemic heparinization is carried out at the time of cannula placement with doses of 10,000 to 30,000 units.

Ischemia Times

Warm ischemia time refers to the period between circulatory arrest and commencement of cold storage. With modern *in situ* perfusion techniques, the warm ischemia time is essentially zero, although there is warm ischemia if hemodynamic deterioration or cardiac arrest occurs before harvest. A kidney may function after up to 20 minutes of warm ischemia, but rates of delayed function and nonfunction increase markedly thereafter.

Cold ischemia time refers to the period of cold storage or machine perfusion (see "Cold Storage Versus Machine Perfusion," below). *Rewarm time* is the period from removal of the kidney from cold storage or perfusion to completion of the renal arterial anastomosis. Rewarm time can be minimized by cooling the kidney during surgery (see Chapter 7).

DECEASED DONOR KIDNEY PRESERVATION

Cold Storage Versus Machine Perfusion

Recovered kidneys must be stored for a period of time before transplantation, either by cold storage on ice or by machine perfusion. For cold storage, the kidneys are flushed and separated and then placed on ice in sterile containers for transport. For machine perfusion, they are flushed and separated and then placed on specially designed perfusion machines that pump a cold colloid solution continuously through the renal artery until the time of transplantation. Machine perfusion may allow a longer preservation time. Rates of delayed graft function of approximately 25% are obtained with simple static cold storage with cold ischemia times of up to 30 hours. After 30 hours, the rate of delayed graft function increases significantly. Most centers prefer not to use kidneys that have been in cold storage for longer than 48 hours. Delayed graft function rates of approximately 25% are obtainable with up to 48 hours of machine perfusion. Machine preservation is expensive and complex, and most transplant centers prefer simple static cold preservation, attempting to keep cold ischemia times under 30 hours.

Collins Solution Versus University of Wisconsin Solution

For many years, kidneys have been flushed with modifications of a solution called *Collins solution* during recovery to achieve rapid cooling and blood washout. This solution is high in potassium, is hyperosmolar, and has an intracellular-like composition to stabilize cell membranes and prevent cell swelling.

The University of Wisconsin (UW) solution for flushing deceased donor organs is clearly superior to Collins solution for liver and pancreas preservation. It may also be preferable for kidneys with prolonged preservation times. UW solution contains a number of components, and the importance of each has not been fully resolved (Table 5.10). Glutathione may serve to facilitate the regeneration of cellular adenosine triphosphate (ATP) and

Table 5.10.   Comparison of contents of flush solutions for kidney preservation

University of Wisconsin Solution	Collins Solution	HTK-Custodial
Modified hydroxyethyl starch	Potassium phosphate	Histidine
Lactobionic acid	Potassium chloride	Tryptophan
Potassium phosphate	Sodium bicarbonate	Low potassium
Magnesium sulfate	Glucose	Ketoglutarate
Raffinose	Magnesium sulfate	Calcium
Adenosine		Magnesium
Allopurinol		Mannitol
Glutathione		

maintain membrane integrity, and adenosine may provide the substrate for regeneration of ATP during reperfusion. The introduction of UW solution has had a major effect on nonrenal solid-organ transplantation by allowing much longer cold ischemia times. HTK-Custodial is a low viscosity preservation solution that is suitable for all solid organs and widely used in Europe.

SELECTED READINGS
Part I

Adams P, Cohen DJ, Danovitch GM, et al. The nondirected live-kidney donor: ethical considerations and practice guidelines: a national conference report. *Transplantation* 2002;74:582–587.

Authors for the Live Organ Donor Consensus Group. Consensus statement on the live organ donor. *JAMA* 2000;284:2919–2921.

Davis CL. Evaluation of the living kidney donor: current perspectives. *Kidney Dis* 2004;43:508–530.

Delmonico FL. Exchanging kidneys—advances in living donor transplantation. *N Engl J Med* 2004;350:1812–1815.

Delmonico F, Susman O. Is this live organ donor your patient? *Transplantation* 2003;76:1257–1260.

Ellison M, McBride M, Taranto SE, et al. Living kidney donors in need of kidney transplants: a report from the Organ Procurement and Transplantation Network. *Transplantation* 2002;74:1349–1353.

Goyal M, Mehta RL, Schneiderman LJ, et al. Economic and health consequences of selling a kidney in India. *JAMA* 2002;288:1589–1592.

Henderson AJ, Landolt MA, McDonald MF, et al. The living anonymous kidney donor: lunatic or saint? *Am J Transplant* 2003;3:203.

Kahn JP, Delmonico FL. The consequences of public policy to buy and sell organs for transplantation. *Am J Transplant* 2004;4:178–180.

Kasiske B, Ravenscraft M, Ramos EL, et al. The evaluation of living renal transplant donors: clinical practice guidelines. *J Am Soc Nephrol* 1996;7:2288–2300.

Kavoussi L. Laparoscopic donor nephrectomy. *Kidney Int* 2000;57:2175–2180.

Matas AJ, Bartlett ST, Leichtman AB, et al. Morbidity and mortality after living kidney donation, 1999–2001: survey of United States transplant centers. *Am J Transplant* 2003;3:830.

Ramcharan T, Kasiske B, Matas AJ. Living donor kidney transplants: the difficult decisions. *Transplant Rev* 2003;17:3–8.

Ramcharan T, Matas A. Long-term (20–37 years) follow-up of living kidney donors. *Am J Transplant* 2002;2:959–963.

Rule AD, Gussak HM, Pond G, et al. Measured and estimated GFR in healthy potential kidney donors. *Am J Kidney Dis* 2004;43:112–119.

Steiner RW, Danovitch GM. The medical evaluation and risk estimation of end-stage renal disease for living kidney donors. In: Steiner RW, ed. *Educating, evaluating, and selecting living kidney donors.* Philadelphia: Kluwer Academic Publishers, 2004:49.

Textor S, Taler S, Larson T, et al. Blood pressure evaluation among older living kidney donors. *J Am Soc Nephrol* 2003;14:2159.

Part II

Beasley CL. Maximizing donation. *Transplant Rev* 1999;13:31–36.

Brook NR, Waller JR, Nicholson ML. Nonheart-beating kidney donation: current practice and future developments. *Kidney Int* 2003;74:1657–1661.

Feng S, Buell JF, Cherikh WS, et al. Organ donors with positive viral serology or malignancy: risk of disease transmission by transplantation. *Transplantation* 2002;74:1657–1662.

Lu CY. Management of the cadaveric donor of a renal transplant: more than optimizing renal perfusion. *Kidney Int* 1999;56:756–761.

Matas AJ, Gillingham K, Payne WD, et al. Should I accept this kidney? *Clin Transplant* 2000;14:90–94.

Metzger RA, Delmonico FL, Feng S, et al. Expanded criteria donors for kidney transplantation. *Am J Transplant* 2003;3[Suppl 4]:114–125.

Potts JT. *Non-heart-beating organ transplantation: medical and ethical issues in procurement.* Washington, DC: National Academy Press, 1998.

Pratschke J, Wilhelm MJ, Kusaka M, et al. Brain death and its influence on donor organ quality and outcome after transplantation. *Transplantation* 1999;67:343.

Randhawa PS, Minervini MI, Lombardeno M, et al. Biopsy of marginal donor kidneys: correlation of histologic findings with graft dysfunction. *Transplantation* 2000;69:1352.

Rosendale J, Chabalewski F, McBride M, et al. Increased transplanted organs from the use of a standardized donor management protocol. *Am J Transplant* 2002;2:701–708.

Rosengard BR, Feng S, Alfrey EF, et al. Report of the Crystal City meeting to maximize the use of organs recovered from cadaveric donors. *Am J Transplant* 2002;2:701–711.

Salahudeen A, Haider N, May W. Cold ischemia and reduced long-term survival of cadaveric renal allograft. *Kidney Int* 2004;65:713–718.

Siminoff LA, Arnold RM, Caplan AL, et al. Public policy governing organ and tissue procurement in the United States. *Ann Intern Med* 1995;123:10–15.

Terasaki PI, Cecka JM, Gjertson DW, et al. High survival rates of kidney transplants from spousal and living unrelated donors. *N Engl J Med* 1995;333:333–336.

Veller MG, Botha JR, Britz RS, et al. Renal allograft preservation: a comparison of University of Wisconsin solution and of hypothermic continuous pulsatile perfusion. *Clin Transplant* 1994;8:97–101.

Evaluation and Preparation of Renal Transplant Candidates

Nauman Siddqi, Sundaram Hariharan, and Gabriel Danovitch

The preparation of patients with end-stage renal disease for renal transplantation should start from the time of recognition of progressive chronic kidney disease (CKD). The improved life expectancy and quality-of-life benefits of transplantation over dialysis therapy has attracted an increasing number of patients to the transplantation option; ideally, these patients are evaluated for transplantation before the initiation of dialysis treatment. The management of these patients consists of an initial evaluation followed, if they are appropriate transplant candidates, by their supervision while awaiting transplantation. Initial evaluation is aimed not only toward assessing the chances of recovery from surgery, but also toward short- and long-term patient survival. The limited number of organs available has changed the focus of the transplant evaluation toward better long-term outcome over short-term benefits. Moreover, although transplant outcome is related to recipient and donor factors, physicians are largely restricted to recipient factors because deceased donor factors will be known only at the time of transplantation.

In the United States, the wait for a deceased donor kidney, once measured in weeks and months, is now measured in years, and may soon approach a decade or more (see Chapter 1). The mean annual mortality of dialysis patients waiting for a transplant is greater than 6% (10% for diabetics) so that a patient waiting for a deceased donor transplant may well die before an organ becomes available. In the absence of a living donor transplant, the traditional algorithm that has guided the care of patients with advanced renal disease (progressive CKD–chronic dialysis–transplantation), has changed to progressive CKD–chronic dialysis–more and more chronic dialysis–to be followed, eventually, if patients are fortunate and survive the long wait, by a deceased donor transplant.

To address the major stages of pretransplant patient preparation this chapter is divided into two parts. Part I focuses on the initial recipient evaluation and Part II focuses on the management of the waiting list for deceased donor transplantation. Several topics critical to the evaluation process are discussed in detail elsewhere in this book. The immunologic evaluation of transplant recipients is discussed in Chapter 3; recommendations for the screening of candidates for infectious disease are discussed in Chapter 10; the evaluation of candidates with viral hepatitis and liver disease is discussed in Chapter 11; the evaluation of diabetic candidates and the various options for pancreatic transplantation are discussed in Chapter 14; the evaluation of children is discussed in Chapter 15; psychiatric evaluation is discussed in Chapter 16; and psychosocial and financial issues and assessment of compliance are discussed in Chapter 19.

The process of referral, evaluation, and preparation of patients for transplantation has been extensively reviewed in the professional literature. Guidelines for the referral and management of patients eligible for solid-organ transplantation have been proposed by the Clinical Practice Committee of the American Society of Transplantation (see Steinman et al. in "Selected Readings," below). For a detailed algorithmic approach to the evaluation of renal transplant candidates the reader is referred to the clinical practice guidelines developed by the American Society of Transplantation (see Kasiske et al. in "Selected Readings," below). For a detailed discussion of the of the deceased donor transplant waiting list, the reader is referred to *The Report of a National Conference on the Wait List for Kidney Transplantation* (see Gaston et al. in "Selected Readings," below).

PART I.   EVALUATION OF TRANSPLANT CANDIDATES

THE TRANSPLANT REFERRAL PROCESS

The Benefits of Early Referral

In ideal circumstances, preparation for transplantation begins as soon as progressive CKD is recognized. Chronic renal disease care, care on dialysis, and transplant care are interdependent. Increased cardiovascular risk, which is a major determinant of posttransplant morbidity and mortality, can be recognized as soon as the serum creatinine is elevated. The various aspects of the care of patients with CKD are beyond the scope of this text. Better-managed patients with CKD, both before and after commencement of chronic dialysis, make better transplant candidates.

Early referral of patients to nephrologic care during the course of CKD permits better preparation for dialysis and transplantation. Patients who are referred to the care of a nephrologist at least 1 year before commencement of renal replacement therapy are documented to have decreased morbidity and mortality. Unfortunately, 25% to 50% of CKD patients are unaware of their problem until end-stage renal disease (ESRD) develops. Transplantation before the commencement of dialysis, so-called preemptive transplantation has been convincingly shown to improve posttransplant graft and patient survival. Five- and 10-year graft survival is 20% to 30% better in patients who either received no dialysis or less than 6 months of dialysis, than it is for those who received more than 2 years of dialysis. The benefit of preemptive transplantation is likely largely a result of the avoidance of the cardiovascular consequences of long-term dialysis (see Chapter 1).

In the United States, patients may begin to accrue points on the deceased donor transplant waiting list when the glomerular filtration rate (GFR) is estimated to be 20 mL per minute or less. However, less than 3% of patients added to the waiting list are predialysis. Because of the long wait anticipated for a deceased donor transplant, preemptive transplantation is infrequent in these patients, unless they are allocated a "zero-mismatch" kidney from the national pool (see Chapter 3). The great advantage of early referral is that it permits recognition and evaluation of potential living donors and the elective timing of the transplant so as to avoid dialysis and the necessity for placement of dialysis access. Avoidance of access placement is a great and tempting benefit but it is one that must be considered carefully. If there is a reasonable doubt that a living donor is available, or that the workup of the donor can be completed expeditiously, it may be wiser to place a permanent access so as to avoid reliance on temporary access techniques that bring with them added morbidity.

Because of the varied course of advanced CKD, it is hard to provide a precise point when referral for transplant should be made. Patients with diabetic nephropathy typically progress rapidly through the advanced stages of CKD, whereas patients with interstitial nephritis, for example, may progress slowly. Patients with a GFR in the twenties, and patients whose course suggests they will become dialysis dependent in 1 to 2 years, should be referred.

Delays to Referral

All dialysis centers in the United States are mandated to be associated with transplant centers and all Medicare patients are legally entitled to referral for transplant evaluation. Unfortunately, there are wide variation in access to transplantation because of delays in the referral process that tend to disadvantage ethnic minorities and other vulnerable population groups. It is the responsibility of nephrologists, dialysis unit staff, transplant program staff, and, most importantly, the patients themselves, to minimize these delays.

THE EVALUATION PROCESS

Patient Education

Figure 6.1 illustrates the structure of the evaluation process. Patient education is at the core of the process. Transplant evaluation not only implies the medical assessment of the potential recipient by the transplant team, but the assessment by the patient of transplant option and its relevance to their well-being. The evaluation process is an opportunity to counsel patients as to their ESRD options and to advocate for their welfare. It should not be an obstacle course for patients to pass or fail!

All potential transplant candidates should be encouraged to attend an information session, preferably accompanied by family members and friends. At the informational meeting, the risks of the operation, as well as the side effects and risks of immunosuppression, should be explained to the patient and family members. The surgical procedure and its complications should also be discussed. The relative benefits of living donor and deceased donor transplantations should be compared and contrasted in the context of the prolonged wait that is anticipated for a deceased donor transplant in the event that a living donor is not available. Graft survival and morbidity statistics should be shared with the patient and family members. The nature of rejection should be explained and discussed along with the increased risk of infection, posttransplant tissue malignancy, and mortality. Patients should

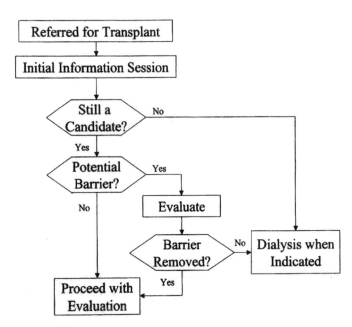

Fig. 6.1.   The renal transplant candidate evaluation process. (From Kasiske BL, Cangro CB, Hariharan S, et al. The evaluation of renal transplant candidates: clinical practice guidelines. *Am J Transplant* 2001;1(Suppl 2):1–95.)

be warned that even a successful transplant may not last forever and that at some point they may be required to return to dialysis. The importance of compliance with dialysis and dietary prescription while waiting for transplant, and with immunosuppressive therapy posttransplant, should be emphasized. The possibility of posttransplant pregnancy should be discussed with women of childbearing age.

Candidates for Extended Criteria Donor Kidneys

The precise definition of extended criteria donor (ECD) kidneys and the rationale for their use is described in Chapter 5. The regulations for the allocation of ECD kidneys mandate that transplant candidates be informed as to the benefits (shortening of waiting time) and risk (impaired long-term graft function) associated with their use. They should sign an informed consent document. A useful guiding principle when counseling patients is to compare the relatively small additional risk of accepting an ECD kidney with the risk of remaining on dialysis for a prolonged period while waiting for an "ideal" kidney. Candidates for ECD kidneys are usually older than age 60 years, or younger if they are diabetic or have coronary heart disease, or have failing dialysis access, or are particularly intolerant of dialysis. Patients in their sixties

Table 6.1. Major contraindications to kidney transplantation

Recent or metastatic malignancy[a]
Untreated current infection
Severe irreversible extrarenal disease
Recalcitrant treatment nonadherence
Psychiatric illness impairing consent and adherence
Current recreational drug abuse
Recurrent native kidney disease
Limited, irreversible rehabilitative potential
Primary oxalosis

[a]See Table 6.2.

who have been on the wait-list for several years may do better to wait for an ideal kidney because they should not have to wait long. Patients going on the list in their sixties may not survive long enough to enjoy an ideal kidney and would be well advised to accept an ECD kidney if they are offered one.

Educational Resources

Transplant patients and family members should be encouraged to seek out educational material that is available in the United States in printed and electronic form from the American Society of Transplantation (www.a-s-t.org), the National Kidney Foundation (www.kidney.org) and the United Network for Organ Sharing (UNOS) (www.unos.org). The UNOS web site also provides detailed information on the performance of individual transplant programs, so-called center-specific data, that can assist patients who have the opportunity to elect the program to which they wish to be referred. Information on living donation and ECD kidneys is also available on the UNOS web site.

Who Is Not a Transplant Candidate?

The risks and benefits of transplantation should be explained during the initial session because some patients may decide that they do not want to proceed with the evaluation, thus avoiding the need for costly evaluation. Table 6.1 lists the major contraindications to transplantation. Although some contraindications to transplantation are absolute, many are relative and are determined by local policy and experience. For example, some programs but not others, exclude patients who are morbidly obese, or who continue to smoke despite being requested to stop. Attitudes vary as to transplantation in the aged or the extent of cardiovascular disease deemed "acceptable" for transplant candidates. It should be noted that of the nearly 300,000 patients on dialysis in the United States as of early 2004, only approximately 60,000 are on the transplant waiting list (see Chapter 1). Most of the unlisted patients are aged and/or have multiple medical morbidities, but many patients are potential candidates who have yet to be referred for transplantation or who have encountered delay in the process. Patients should be presumed to be transplant candidates until shown otherwise. If there is any question regarding a transplant contraindication, the patient should be referred to the transplant program to make that determination. Patients should be entitled to a second opinion if they find the recommendation of the transplant program to be unacceptable to them.

THE ROUTINE EVALUATION

History and Physical Examination

A detailed medical history at the time of initial evaluation should be obtained and efforts should be made to determine the cause of underlying renal disease. Estimation of urine output is important because it might help to determine the significance of the urine output in the early postoperative period and because it helps in determining the need for further urologic evaluation. If a kidney biopsy has been performed, the report should be sought out and reviewed. Family history is extremely important because it may provide information regarding the cause of the renal failure and may also allow the physician to initiate discussion regarding living-related donor donation. The evaluation of patients with potentially recurring renal diseases posttransplant are discussed in the section "Relevance of the Etiology of Renal Disease to the Transplant Evaluation."

A detailed cardiovascular history is mandatory for all recipients, and patients should be instructed about symptoms of cardiac disease while awaiting transplantation. Risk factors for coronary artery disease should be sought in the history, including a history of diabetes, smoking, family history of coronary artery disease, and previous cardiac events. Exercise tolerance should be assessed. A history of claudication warrants an evaluation for peripheral vascular disease and may also point toward a higher chance of ischemic heart disease. A full physical examination must be performed, including evaluation for evidence of congestive heart failure, carotid artery disease, and peripheral vascular disease. The presence of femoral bruits and poor peripheral pulses, may warrant further evaluation of the pelvic vasculature with either a Doppler ultrasound or a magnetic resonance angiogram. The presence of strong femoral and peripheral pulses are a valuable indicator to the transplant surgeon that the pelvic vessels will be adequate for the transplant vascular anastomosis (see Chapter 7).

A detailed history of infectious disease should be obtained (see Chapter 10). This should include assessment for possible exposure to tuberculosis, such as history of residence or travel to endemic areas, prior exposure, and any prior treatment and its duration. Evidence of other possible infections including hepatitis and endemic fungal infections should be sought.

Male patients older than age 40 years should undergo a rectal examination with a digital prostate exam and a prostate-specific antigen (PSA) estimation. All adult female patients should have a Papanicolaou (Pap) smear and a pelvic examination. Women older than 40 years of age should have a mammogram to evaluate for malignancy. All patients older than 50 years of age, and those younger than 50 years with guaiac-positive stools, should undergo colonoscopy.

Laboratory Studies

A complete blood count and a chemistry panel should be obtained along with a prothrombin time and partial prothrombin time. Blood should be sent for blood and tissue typing. Patients should be screened for evidence of hepatitis B and C, syphilis, human immunodeficiency virus (HIV) and cytomegalovirus (CMV). A screening purified protein derivative (PPD) and a screening chest x-ray may be required for certain population to assess for evidence of prior tuberculosis exposure or infection. Patients with a positive skin test or abnormal chest x-ray, or who are allergic to tuberculin and who have risk factors for tuberculosis infection, may require preventive therapy with isoniazid. The risk of isoniazid therapy needs to be evaluated alongside the risk of occurrence of tuberculosis. An infectious disease consult might be needed. A urinalysis and urine culture should be performed on all urinating patients. In the event of proteinuria, a 24-hour urine collection for protein should be obtained, which may reflect the cause of primary kidney disease and be a guide for further management.

EVALUATION OF SPECIFIC TRANSPLANT RISK FACTORS RELATED TO ORGAN SYSTEM DISEASE

Cardiovascular Disease

The cardiovascular evaluation of diabetic transplant candidates is discussed in Chapter 14, and of patients on the deceased donor transplant waiting list in Part II of this chapter. Most transplant teams include a designated cardiologist to assist in the evaluation of the often complex issues of assessing and managing cardiovascular disease in the CKD population.

Cardiovascular disease is the leading cause of death after renal transplantation. Almost half of the deaths with functioning graft occurring within 30 days after transplantation are as a consequence of cardiovascular disease, primarily acute myocardial infarction. Cardiovascular disease is the major cause of long-term mortality and death with graft function, most frequently as a result of cardiovascular disease is the major cause of late graft loss (see Chapter 9). All patients with CKD are at high cardiac risk, although for some the risk is particularly high. Diabetic patients, older patients, patients on dialysis for prolonged periods, and patients with multiple Framingham risk factors for coronary artery disease, should undergo noninvasive cardiac testing.

Because many dialysis patients are unable to exercise adequately, noninvasive testing usually takes the form of chemical stress echocardiography or scintography. Patients with a positive stress test should proceed to a coronary angiogram. A prior history of ischemic heart disease is a major risk factor for posttransplant ischemic events, so that all patients with a history of myocardial infarction and/or congestive heart failure should undergo cardiac stress testing, or possibly angiography, even if the stress test is negative. Risk factors associated with posttransplant ischemic heart disease include age greater than 50 years, diabetes, and an abnormal electrocardiogram. Most transplant programs use noninvasive testing as their initial mode of screening for coronary artery disease, although some prefer to go directly to the coronary angiogram. Data is unavailable to test the effectiveness of more expensive screening techniques such as using single-photon emission computed tomography (SPECT)/positron emission tomography (PET) or electron beam computed tomography (CT). Both dobutamine stress echocardiogram and dipyridamole sestamibi have similar sensitivities in detecting coronary artery disease in the non-ESRD population. Specific sensitivities and sensitivities for the ESRD population are lacking. Patients who have critical lesions should probably undergo correction with either coronary artery bypass surgery, angioplasty, or stent placement prior to transplantation.

Calcific aortic stenosis and valvular heart disease is common in transplant candidates, and when suspected it is important to perform an echocardiogram to elicit systolic or diastolic dysfunction because this may have important prognostic implications. Reversible myocardial dysfunction should be treated. Irreversible heart failure should probably preclude renal transplantation unless heart transplantation is also considered. However, many patients with mild to moderate cardiac dysfunction may respond to renal transplantation with an improvement in myocardial function. In many cases, an improvement in the ejection fraction can been documented after transplantation.

Cerebrovascular and Peripheral Vascular Disease

Signs and symptoms of cerebrovascular disease in transplant candidates must be evaluated. Risk factors identified for posttransplant cerebrovascular disease include a history of pretransplant cerebrovascular disease, age, smoking, diabetes, hypertension, and hyperlipidemia. There is no evidence that routine screening of asymptomatic renal transplant candidates for cerebrovascular disease is beneficial. In the general population, asymptomatic carotid artery stenosis does not correlate with posttransplant cerebrovascular disease. Patients who have suffered cerebral vascular events and have significant and fixed neurologic deficits may be poor candidates in terms of their perioperative risk and rehabilitative potential. Patients who have had recent transient ischemic attacks or other cerebrovascular events should be assessed by a neurologist. Patients receiving anticonvulsant medications for a seizure disorder should undergo neurologic assessment to determine if these medications can be safely discontinued. If anticonvulsants are required, it is preferable to use those that do not have a pharmacologic interaction with the calcineurin inhibitors (see Chapter 4).

Peripheral vascular disease is important as a cause of both allograft ischemia and lower-extremity amputation. There is a high incidence of peripheral vascular disease in diabetic recipients. Patients who have undergone lower-extremity amputations have a significantly higher mortality rate within the ensuing 2 years. Males, diabetics, patients with hypertension, lipid abnormalities, a history of vascular disease elsewhere, and who smoke cigarettes are at higher risk for peripheral vascular disease. Patients with diabetes and history of ischemic ulceration in the lower extremity, or patients with claudication, should, at the very least, have a noninvasive evaluation of the peripheral vasculature. Angiography should be considered if noninvasive studies suggest the presence of large-vessel disease. Asymptomatic patients should not be subjected to routine angiography. Patients who have significant aortoiliac disease, or who required intraabdominal reconstructive arterial surgery, represent a formidable surgical challenge and transplantation may be contraindicated.

Malignancy

Patients undergoing ESRD have a higher risk of cancer than does the general population. This relative risk is greatest for patients younger than 35 years of age and decreases gradually with increasing age. CKD patients who required immunosuppressive treatment as part of the therapy of their underlying renal disease, or who failed prior renal transplants, or who required other solid-organ transplants, pose an additional risk of malignancy. All posttransplant patients are at increased risk of malignancy (see Chapter 9) and transplant candidates should be forewarned.

Patients who have been successfully treated for a pretransplant malignancy may be deemed suitable transplant candidates. Much of the data for advice and recommendations regarding transplant candidacy in cancer survivors comes from the Israel Penn International Transplant Tumor Registry (www.ipittr.uc.edu), an invaluable resource of information on malignancies and solid-organ transplant recipients. Most, but not all, cancer survivors benefit from a disease-free waiting period, which in most cases is a minimum of 2 years, although in some circumstances a 5-year waiting period is safer. The precise waiting period, however, should be determined on an individual basis by the type of tumor, its staging, and its response to therapy. An oncologic consultation may be wise. Table 6.2 lists broad guidelines for screening and waiting periods for commonly encountered tumors in potential transplant patient recipients.

Infections

Pretransplant screening for infectious disease and recommendations for specific infections are discussed in Chapter 10. Whenever possible, all treatable infections should be eradicated. The presence of chronic infection precludes transplantation and the use of immunosuppressive therapy. Whenever possible, transplant candidates should receive immunization for infections that are prevalent, preferably before the development of ESRD. Osteomyelitis should be treated and, if necessary, the infected parts should be removed surgically to prepare the patient for transplantation. Diabetic foot ulcers must be healed before transplantation.

An important change has taken place with respect to the candidacy of patients with HIV infection. Patients with HIV/acquired immune deficiency syndrome (AIDS) were long regarded as inappropriate transplant candidates because of the fear of immunosuppressant-induced opportunistic infection and the anticipation of a short life span. The onset of effective antiviral therapy has radically altered the prognosis of infected patients. Patients who are consistently receiving and tolerating an effective antiviral regimen (with an undetectable viral load and normal T-cell counts) can be considered as candidates after completing their evaluation together with education with respect to their high-risk status.

Table 6.2.   Recommendations for minimum tumor-free waiting periods for common pretransplant malignancies[a]

Tumor Type	Minimal Wait Time
Renal	
Wilm	2 years
Renal cell carcinoma	None (incidental tumors)
	2 years (< 5 cm)
	5 years (> 5 cm)
Bladder	
In situ	None
Invasive	2 years
Prostate	2 years
Uterus	
Cervix (*in situ*)	None
Cervical invasive	2–5 years
Uterine body	2 years
Breast	2–5 years
Colorectal	2–5 years
Lymphoma	2–5 years
Skin (local)	
Basal cell	None
Squamous cell	Surveillance
Melanoma	5 years

[a]The broad recommendations must be individualized based on specific clinical and oncologic information.

Gastrointestinal Disease

Diverticulitis

Diverticulitis is the most frequent cause of colonic perforation in renal transplant recipients. This may be related to the high prevalence of diverticulosis in patients on dialysis, especially patients with adult polycystic kidney disease. Mortality from colonic perforation is very high, but the incidence of colonic perforation after renal transplantation has remained stable over many years. It seems reasonable that patients with a history of diverticulitis should be evaluated by a barium enema or a colonoscopy with consideration for resection of extensive disease if symptomatic diverticulitis persists.

Peptic Ulcer Disease

Peptic ulcer disease was once a frequent and potentially lethal posttransplant complication that required pretransplant screening in all patients and surgery in a selected few. With the use of histamine antagonists, antacids, and proton pump inhibitors, the incidence of peptic ulcer disease has declined significantly. Transplantation is considered safe even in patients with a history of peptic ulcer disease, although active disease should be treated medically prior to transplantation. The role of *Helicobacter pylori* infection should be recognized, although routine screening for this organism is generally not recommended.

Cholelithiasis

Patients with a history of cholecystitis and cholelithiasis should undergo pretransplant evaluation using ultrasound to identify the presence of cholelithiasis and should be considered for cholecystectomy. Some programs recommend cholecystectomy for asymptomatic diabetic patients with cholelithiasis.

Pancreatitis

A pretransplant history of pancreatitis increases the risk of posttransplant pancreatitis. Posttransplant pancreatitis has a high morbidity. Patients who have suffered episodes of pancreatitis may be more likely to develop posttransplant diabetes mellitus and should be forewarned. Both prednisone and azathioprine have been implicated in the etiology of pancreatitis. Hyperparathyroidism should be excluded as a possible factor. Other possible contributing factors, such as lipid disturbances, cholelithiasis, and alcohol, should be addressed before transplantation.

Pulmonary Disease

Surgical risks associated with severe lung disease include fluid overload, ventilator dependency, and infection. All patients should be screened with a history, physical evaluation, and chest x-ray to identify lung disease that may increase the risk for major postoperative pulmonary complications. Formal pulmonary function testing may be required to assess surgical risk for patients with known lung disease and patients with signs and symptoms suggesting active lung disease. Chronic lung disease may preclude safe general anesthesia. Chronic obstructive lung disease and restrictive lung disease recipients have increased posttransplant infectious complications and mortality. Patients with evidence of chronic lung disease who continue to smoke must stop before transplantation. They should be directed to smoking cessation programs.

Urologic Evaluation

Ideally, the lower urinary tract should be sterile, continent, and compliant before transplantation. Urinalysis and urine culture should be performed on all urinating patients. Most patients will have undergone renal imaging studies as part of the evaluation of their underlying renal disease and the studies themselves, or reports thereof, should be available at the time of the transplant evaluation. Dialysis patients who have not had an imaging study within the previous 3 years should have a renal ultrasound because of the risk of adenocarcinoma associated with acquired cystic disease.

A voiding cystourethrogram (VCUG) and other urologic procedures are unnecessary unless there is a history of bladder dysfunction. Patients with a history of genitourinary abnormalities and individuals younger than 20 years of age may require a full evaluation, including a VCUG, cystoscopy, and urodynamic studies. Patients with bladder dysfunction secondary to neurogenic bladder and those who have chronic infection can often be managed without urinary diversion or bladder augmentation procedures. Self-catheterization may be an acceptable option for some

Table 6.3. Indications for pretransplantation native nephrectomy

Chronic renal parenchymal infection
Infected stones
Heavy proteinuria
Intractable hypertension
Polycystic kidney disease[a]
Acquired renal cystic disease[b]
Infected reflux[c]

---

[a]Only when the kidneys are massive, recurrently infected, or bleeding.
[b]When there is suspicion of adenocarcinoma.
[c]Uninfected reflux does not require nephrectomy.

patients, infection being a major complication. Graft implantation into the native bladder is always preferred. Diverted urinary tracts should be undiverted where possible to make the lower urinary tract functional before transplantation. Even a very small bladder may develop normal compliance and capacity after transplantation. Transplantation is possible for patients whose urinary tracts have been diverted into ileal conduits and cannot be undiverted. The rate of urologic complications is high, but the overall patient and graft survival is not different from patients with intact urinary tracts.

Older men frequently have prostatic enlargement and may develop outflow tract obstruction posttransplant. In general, if patients are still passing sufficient volumes of urine, the prostate should be resected preoperatively. Otherwise, the operation should be postponed until after the transplantation has been successfully performed. These patients may require an indwelling bladder catheter, or be prepared to self-catheterize, until the prostate has been resected.

Patients with adult polycystic kidney disease (PKD) may benefit from unilateral or bilateral nephrectomy to reduce symptomatic bleeding or recurrent infection or for the discomfort suffered because of their massive size. Occasionally, polycystic kidneys are so large that they reach deep into the lower abdominal quadrants and may need to be removed to make room for the transplant. Pretransplant nephrectomy may be indicated for patients with chronic renal infections, infectious renal stones, or obstructive uropathy complicated by chronic infections. Patients with uncomplicated recurrent urinary tract infection do not usually require pretransplant nephrectomy. Bilateral nephrectomy may be recommended in patients with congenic nephrotic syndrome, and in patients with persistent nephrotic syndrome despite optimal medical management. Adenocarcinoma of the native kidneys may manifest posttransplant and is associated with considerable morbidity and mortality. Table 6.3 lists the major indications for pretransplant native kidney nephrectomy. If nephrectomy is required, it should be done 6 weeks to 3 months before transplantation. Occasionally, unilateral transplant nephrectomy is performed at the time of the transplant surgery.

Renal Osteodystrophy and Metabolic Bone Disease

Patients with ESRD suffer from multiple bone disorders, including secondary hyperparathyroidism, osteomalacia, and dialysis-related amyloid bone disease (see Chapter 1). Successful renal transplantation is the best treatment for most cases of osteomalacia and dialysis-related amyloid bone disease. Persistence of hyperparathyroidism after renal transplantation is common. The majority of renal transplant recipients have elevated parathyroid hormone (PTH) levels at the time of transplantation and more than 30% of these patients persist to have elevated levels up to 3 years after transplantation. The duration of time on dialysis and the intensity of hyperparathyroidism prior to transplantation correlates with the severity of posttransplant hyperparathyroidism (see Chapter 9). Hypercalcemia is the most common marker of hyperparathyroidism posttransplant. Every attempt should be made to minimize the effect of impaired calcium metabolism, metabolic acidosis, and secondary hyperparathyroidism in the pretransplant period. Patients with persistent hyperparathyroidism that is unresponsive to medical therapy may need pretransplant parathyroidectomy. Females and diabetics are at an exaggerated risk for osteopenia and pathologic fractures. These patients may benefit from early diagnosis of bone loss.

Hypercoagulable States

There appears to be an increased prevalence of several prothrombotic factors in renal transplant candidates and thrombophilic patients are at a higher risk of early graft loss. All transplant candidates should have routine coagulation studies performed. Patients who have had a history of thrombosis, including recurrent thrombosis of arteriovenous grafts and fistulas, should have a more extensive coagulation profile performed. This should include screening for activated protein C (APC) resistance; factor V and prothrombin gene mutations; anticardiolipin antibody; lupus anticoagulant; proteins C and S; and antithrombin III and homocystine levels. Approximately 6% of whites have APC resistance, usually as a result of heterozygosity for the factor V Leiden mutation. They are prone to thrombotic complications and graft loss. All renal transplant candidates with systemic lupus erythematosus should have antiphospholipid antibodies measured.

Thrombophilia is rarely a contraindication to transplantation. Rather, its recognition should initiate preventive strategies. Perioperative anticoagulation is discussed in Chapter 7. Therapeutic decisions for long-term anticoagulation need to be individualized with respect to the agent used and the length of treatment. Chronic anticoagulation of dialysis patients with recurrent access thrombosis but without an underlying coagulopathy is often ineffective and should be avoided. Long-standing warfarin administration is associated with accelerated vascular calcification.

EVALUATION OF RISK FACTORS RELATED TO SPECIFIC PATIENT CHARACTERISTICS

Transplantation in the Aged

There is no formal upper age limit at which patients may no longer be accepted for transplant. Nearly 10% of all patients on the waiting list for renal transplantation are 65 years of age or older. There has been a marked increase in the number of renal transplants performed in older patients in the last 10 years. As a group, patients age 60 years or older who receive a renal transplant have a better survival rate than patients who remain on the transplant waiting list. Older transplant recipients have an increased risk of death as a consequence of cardiovascular disease in the few months after renal transplantation. They also tend to have longer initial hospitalizations, but fewer acute rejection episodes, because their immune system may be less aggressive. Older patients may be at increased risk of infection and malignancy related to immunosuppression. The metabolism of immunosuppressive drugs may be slowed in aging.

The possibility of covert coronary artery disease should be routinely evaluated with stress testing and the need for assessment of cerebrovascular and peripheral vascular disease should be considered. Older patients with significant vascular disease may be inappropriate transplant candidates. Standard malignancy screening recommendations should be applied compulsively in older patients. The assessment of older patients should also take into account their cognitive abilities and their capacity to ambulate and care for themselves in the posttransplant period. Clearly there are sprightly patients in their early seventies who are excellent transplant candidates, while many patients of this age would do better to remain on dialysis.

Most of the published data on transplantation in older patients relates to patients older than age 60 years. Data on patients older than age 70 years is more limited. The available data also tends to relate to the "dry" statistics of patient and graft survival. Most older patients seek improved quality of life in their later years, which they may resent spending on dialysis. Older patients may have also have unrealistic expectations about their quality of life after transplantation—the transplant will not make them younger! The waiting time for a deceased donor transplant in the United States is such that older patients may not survive to be allocated a kidney by the standard algorithm; consequently, to benefit from transplantation, they should be encouraged to accept an ECD kidney. Prolonged waiting times dramatically decrease the clinical benefits and economic attractiveness of transplantation. Older patients are often reluctant to accept living donor kidneys from their children, although these kidneys offer them the best chance of meaningful improved survival and quality of life. Even devoted family members may have reservations about living donation for family members with an intrinsically limited life span. These issues must be discussed with older patients and their families with particular care and compassion so as to optimize the chance of a satisfactory outcome.

Obesity

Malnutrition at the time of dialysis is a strong predictor of short- and long-term mortality, whereas a high body mass index (BMI) is associated with reduced mortality among hemodialysis patients. In contrast, obesity is an important risk factor for renal transplant recipients and is considered by some transplant centers to be an exclusion criteria. Approximately 20% of transplant recipients have a pretransplant BMI of more than 30 kg/m^2, and this percentage is increasing. Obese renal transplant recipients have a higher risk of delayed graft function and suffer from more surgical complications, including more wound infections. Obesity is also associated with a prolonged posttransplant hospital stay, an increased cost of transplantation, and a higher incidence of posttransplant diabetes and cardiovascular disease (see Chapter 9). Obese recipients of combined kidney–pancreas transplantation have also reported decreased pancreas and renal graft survival rates.

It is prudent to recommend weight reduction to a BMI of less than 30 kg/m^2 for renal transplant candidates, although for many patients this is an unachievable goal. Some authorities have recommended excluding patients with a BMI of greater than 35 kg/m^2 from transplantation, although the available patient and graft survival data in this group is not significantly less than for nonobese patients. Special attention should be given to the cardiac evaluation of obese renal transplant candidates. Aged, obese patients and those with concomitant coronary heart disease may have a worse prognosis; these patients may be better served by remaining on dialysis. It is better to individualize transplant recommendations rather than make broad exclusionary rules base on an arbitrary BMI.

Highly Sensitized Patients

The immunologic challenge faced by highly sensitized patients is discussed in Chapter 3. Approximately 40% of the national pool of patients awaiting deceased donor transplants have high levels of preformed cytotoxic antibodies that may prevent them from receiving a kidney or might prolong their wait considerably. Cytotoxic antibodies result from failed prior transplants, multiple pregnancies, and multiple blood transfusions. Attempts have been made to reduce the antibody levels by infusion of intravenous immunoglobulins (IVIGs), plasma exchange with cyclophosphamide and immunoabsorption, and rituximab (see Chapter 4). Use of IVIG in these circumstances appears to be the most promising. After three to four IVIG treatments, the average level of preformed antibodies falls to approximately 50% of the initial level, although it tends to return to baseline in the ensuing months if treatment is not continued. Patients with high levels of antibodies should be warned of the probability of a prolonged wait for a kidney. The widespread use of erythropoietin in dialysis patients may serve to lower the level of preformed antibodies by minimizing blood transfusion requirements.

Previously Transplanted Candidates

The fate of second and multiple transplants is dependent to a considerable extent on the rate and etiology of the prior transplant loss. Patients who lost kidneys because of surgical complications, or who have kidneys that functioned for more than a year, have a prognosis that is not significantly different from that of patients with primary transplants. If the primary transplant is lost to early rejection, the prognosis for another transplant is impaired, and the patient will do best with a highly matched deceased donor transplant or a two-haplotype-matched living-related transplant if a suitable donor is available. Patients must be made aware of their impaired prognosis.

The process of evaluating a patient for a repeat transplant is the same as for a primary transplant. For patients whose first transplant life was prolonged, special attention should be paid to the possibility of covert coronary artery disease or malignancy. Patients with a failing transplant should be referred early for retransplantation in the hope of avoiding the need to return to dialysis. Multiple transplanted patients are at an increased risk of suffering immunosuppressant-related malignancy and infection and should be forewarned.

Candidates for Double-Organ Transplants

Patients with end-stage liver disease (ESLD) who are candidates for orthotopic liver transplantation (OLT) frequently have impaired renal function as a result of hepatorenal syndrome, "prerenal" dysfunction, acute tubular necrosis, or nephrotoxicity. In the great majority of cases, renal function will improve following successful OLT, despite what is often a prolonged period of dialysis dependence. Consequently, concomitant renal transplantation is not indicated when it is anticipated that native renal function will improve.

Irreversible renal dysfunction may accompany ESLD; in these cases, it is logical to consider a combined procedure. The addition of a kidney transplant adds relatively little to the considerable morbidity of an OLT, but a well-functioning kidney may facilitate posttransplant management. The indications for combined kidney and liver transplantation are discussed further in Chapter 11 and are listed in Table 11.3.

Experience with combined heart and kidney transplants is more limited, but many of these procedures have been performed successfully. The same principles regarding reversibility of renal dysfunction apply.

RELEVANCE OF THE ETIOLOGY OF RENAL DISEASE TO THE TRANSPLANT EVALUATION

The cause of CKD is important for prognosticating transplant outcome. This information may also be critical in selecting a suitable living donor for transplantation. The risk of recurrence of the native kidney disease in the transplant is summarized in Table 6.4, which can be used as a guide to counsel patients. The effects of recurrent renal disease on the posttransplant course are discussed in Chapter 9.

Diabetes Mellitus

The special considerations related to the evaluation of diabetic transplant candidates who account for approximately 40% of the ESRD population in the United States are considered in Chapter 14. Diabetic transplant recipients can develop histologic features of diabetic nephropathy as soon as 3 years after transplantation. However, patients should be informed that recurrent diabetic nephropathy is an uncommon cause of graft failure and its possibility should not be used as a reason to seek out the more complex simultaneous kidney and pancreas transplant. Optimal management of diabetes while on dialysis is critical factor in the

Table 6.4. Risk of recurrent disease after renal transplantation

Focal and segmental glomerulosclerosis	30%–50%
IgA nephropathy	40%–60%
MPGN-I	30%–50%
MPGN-II	80%–100%
Membranous nephropathy	10%–30%
Diabetic nephropathy	80%–100% (by histology)
HUS/TTP	50%–75%
Oxalosis	80%–100%
Wegener disease	<20%
Fabry disease	<5%
Systemic lupus erythematosus	3–10%

HUS, hemolytic uremic syndrome; MPGN, membranoproliferative glomerulonephritis; TTP, thrombotic thrombocytopenic purpura.

prevention of posttransplant diabetic complications. Reinforcement of diabetic education should be considered at the time of transplant evaluation.

Focal and Segmental Glomerulosclerosis

This discussion relates to primary focal and segmental glomerulosclerosis (FSGS). FSGS that is secondary to reflux nephropathy and obesity, for example, does not recur posttransplant. Evidence of focal sclerosis is often found on histologic evaluation of patients with hypertensive renal disease and other causes of CKD, and should be differentiated from the primary disorder. Presumably as a result of an unidentified serum factor that effects the permeability of the glomerular basement membrane (GBM), transplant candidates with primary FSGS have a 20% to 40% incidence of recurrence after transplantation. The odds of recurrence are increased in patients who are younger, those who had a rapid progression to ESRD, those with the collapsing variant, and those whose initial biopsy showed residual hypertrophy. The strongest predictor of recurrence is a history of recurrence in a previous transplant. Patient should be forewarned of the possibility of recurrence. If a living donor is being considered, both the transplant candidate and the potential donor should be aware that nearly 40% to 50% of grafts may be lost with recurrent FSGS. Plasma exchange before transplantation has been suggested to reduce the risk for recurrent disease. Some patients with FSGS continue to have heavy proteinuria while on dialysis. In these cases, native kidney nephrectomy may be indicated both for nutritional consideration and because persistent native kidney proteinuria makes the evaluation of posttransplant proteinuria very difficult. Posttransplant management and prevention of recurrent FSGS is discussed in Chapter 9. Patients who lost a prior transplant to recurrent FSGS are a high risk of re-recurrence, which is an important consideration in assessing their candidacy for a repeat transplant. Many programs avoid living donor transplantation in these circumstances.

Recurrent Glomerulonephritis

Table 6.4 shows the recurrence rate of the most common primary glomerulopathies. These figures are imprecise estimates because only approximately 20% of CKD patients have a specific histologic diagnosis at the time of presentation for transplant evaluation. The rate of recurrence of the glomerulopathies continues to increase with longer duration of followup after transplantation and may be more common in recipients of living-related donor transplants. Evidence of histologic recurrence of immunoglobulin (Ig) A nephropathy is very common, however. In the largest reported series, graft loss as a consequence of recurrent IgA nephropathy was reported in 12% of patients. Recurrent IgA nephropathy in a prior transplant is generally not a contraindication for repeat transplantation and re-recurrence is not inevitable. IgA nephropathy may be familial in some cases and donors should be carefully screened (see Chapter 5).

Thrombotic Thrombocytopenic Purpura

There is a high rate of recurrence of the nondiarrheal form of thrombotic thrombocytopenic purpura (TTP), and a nearly 50% graft failure from that recurrence (see Chapter 15). Older age at onset, a shorter interval between onset of ESRD and transplantation, the use of living donors, and the use of calcineurin inhibitors are all associated with recurrence. Both of the calcineurin inhibitor drugs may induce a TTP-like syndrome (see Chapter 4), although its severity is typically less than the recurrent form. Patients and living donors should be counseled regarding risks of recurrence for patients with a history of TTP and consideration should be given to a calcineurin-inhibitor-free regimen. Patients should be advised to avoid oral contraceptives.

Systemic Lupus Erythematosus and Vasculitis

Recurrence of systemic lupus erythematosus (SLE) can occasionally lead to graft failure. Clinical activity of SLE should be quiescent prior to transplantation. The patient should require no more than 10 mg of prednisone before transplantation to maintain quiescence. Clinically active SLE typically improves with the development of renal failure but may not do so in some patients, particularly black women. Some patients are clinically quiescent but maintain persistently abnormal levels of serologic markers of disease activity while on dialysis. It is the degree of clinical activity that should determine transplant candidacy.

Patients with antineutrophil cytoplasmic antibody (ANCA)-associated systemic vasculitis are at risk for recurrence. However, pretransplant ANCA levels are not predictive of recurrence for asymptomatic patients. Successful transplantation has been reported in active disease, but it is probably wise to wait until the disease is quiescent before transplantation.

Patients who are heavily immunosuppressed during the course of their native kidney disease may be at increased risk of posttransplant opportunistic infections and lymphoma. The risk of avascular necrosis is higher in patients with SLE, most of whom have received high doses of corticosteroids during the course of their illness.

Oxalosis and Oxaluria

Primary oxalosis is rare cause of renal failure. It is an autosomal recessive disorder caused by a deficiency of the hepatic enzyme alanine glycoxylate aminotransferase. The presence of this enzyme leads to increased urinary secretion of calcium oxalate and nephrocalcinosis, which leads to renal failure. Accumulation of oxalate occurs throughout the body. Failure of the graft usually occurs after transplantation with rapid deposition of oxalate in the graft. Failure of the graft usually occurs despite intensive therapy with perioperative intensive dialysis and oral phosphates which are designed to minimize oxalate deposition. All reduce renal calcium oxalate deposition. Oxalate production can be reduced by high dose oral pyridoxine which is a coenzyme that converts glycoxylate to glycine rather than oxalate. Combined liver and kidney transplantation is the best option for patients with primary oxalosis (see Chapter 11). The transplanted liver provides the absent enzyme. Because the usual parameters of hepatic function are normal in these patients, the patients may require a prolonged wait for a transplant. It has been suggested that isolated kidney transplantation is a reasonable first option for patients with oxalosis as long as the precautions listed above are adhered to rigorously and patients are adequately warned of the recurrence risk.

Secondary hyperoxaluria is most commonly of intestinal origin and may also lead to recurrence in the allograft. Patients have usually suffered from inflammatory bowel disease or morbid obesity. If the underlying defect is reversible (e.g., intestinal bypass for obesity), consideration should be given to surgical reversal pretransplant.

Fabry Disease

Fabry disease is caused by a deficiency of α-galactosidase enzyme, which results in accumulation of glycosphingolipid in the kidney and other organs. It was initially hoped that kidney transplantation would provide enough enzyme to prevent disease progression, but this has not proven to be the case and Fabry disease may recur and progress in the transplanted kidney. Recurrence is slow and death is usually a result of sepsis and other systemic complications. Renal transplantation is treatment of choice for patients with Fabry disease who do not have severe systemic disease. Fabrazyme is a newly available recombinant form of the deficient human enzyme; it may have a major beneficial impact on the course of the disease.

Alport Syndrome

Patients with Alport syndrome have a genetic abnormality of type 4 collagen that is X-linked in 80% of patients. Autosomal recessive (15%) and autosomal dominant (5%) forms also occur. The introduction of normal collagen in the basal membrane of the transplanted kidney may induce antibody formation to donor kidney collagen found in the GBM. The precise incidence of anti-GBM antibody formation is unknown. Patients should be warned that there is a potential to develop clinically significant anti-GBM disease, which may occur in 3–4% of grafts and may reoccur in a subsequent transplant graft. The presence of inherited kidney disease always requires intensive family screening before consideration of living-related donor donation.

Sickle Cell Disease

Sickle cell disease often leads to ESRD, probably by causing chronic intestinal fibrosis, but FSGS and nephrotic syndrome also do occur. Short-term patient and graft survival are not any different than for patients without sickle cell disease; however, long-term mortality is increased about 2.5-fold. There is an increased incidence of severe, and potentially lethal, sickling crisis after transplantation, presumably related to the improving hematocrit. Exchange transfusions may be an effective treatment. There is a trend toward improved survival for transplanted patients with sickle cell disease when compared to sickle cell disease patients left on the waiting list. Renal transplantation appears to be the treatment of choice for patients without severe systemic complications.

Amyloidosis and Plasma Cell Dyscrasias

Patients with primary amyloidosis are high-risk transplant candidates. Their mortality rate after transplantation has been reported to be as high as 50% at 1 year. Infectious and cardiac complications are common. In general, patients with primary amyloidosis should be discouraged from renal transplantation, although some patients without severe extrarenal disease may be considered acceptable candidates. Patients with secondary amyloidosis are more likely to be acceptable candidates. An echocardiogram should be performed to assess the extent of myocardial infiltration. The subgroup of patients with amyloidosis complicating familial Mediterranean fever may not tolerate the combination of colchicine and cyclosporine therapy as a consequence of systemic and gastrointestinal symptoms. Recurrence of amyloid deposition in the allograft is common. Light chain disease also has a high rate of recurrence and associated morbidity, although some patients are reported to do well for long periods of time following transplantation.

The pretransplant evaluation of all patients older than age 60 years should include plasma immunoelectrophoresis to screen for paraproteins. The rate of conversion from benign monoclonal gammopathy to frank multiple myeloma is approximately 1% per year. If a monoclonal gammopathy is of long-standing duration and is stable, transplantation can be performed. Transplantation should be delayed for at least 12 months in other cases to exclude the development of myeloma or microglobulinanemia. If, after followup there is no evidence of progression to myeloma, it is reasonable to progress with transplantation. Patients should be instructed about higher morbidity risk in the posttransplant period. Occasional cases of successful transplantation for patients with myeloma have been reported, although this disease is usually regarded as a contraindication to transplantation. Patients with myeloma who have been successfully treated by bone marrow transplantation may be considered to be transplant candidates. Extraordinary cases have been reported of simultaneous bone marrow and kidney transplantation from the same fully matched living donor.

Polycystic Kidney Disease

Patients with PKD are excellent potential transplant candidates. The graft and patient survival rates are not any different from those of other low-risk groups. The necessity for pretransplant or posttransplant nephrectomy is discussed above. There may be an increased risk of gastrointestinal complications after transplantation, which is usually related to diverticular disease. Patients with headaches or other symptoms of the central nervous system or with a family history of aneurysm should undergo noninvasive screening for cerebral aneurysm. The possibility of living-related donation in families with polycystic kidney is discussed in Chapter 5.

PART II. MANAGEMENT OF THE DECEASED DONOR TRANSPLANT LIST

Once patients are placed on the deceased donor transplant waiting list, they are likely to face a prolonged wait until a kidney becomes available to them. During the years they spend waiting, their health, particularly their cardiovascular health, may deteriorate and the conclusions drawn from the initial evaluation may no longer apply. For this reason, it is critical that there be ongoing communication between dialysis units, patients, and transplant programs regarding health and demographic issues that may be relevant to the transplant candidacy. All dialysis patients, but particularly patients awaiting transplantation, should receive optimal care according to accepted guidelines during their prolonged wait for a transplant so as to minimize posttransplant morbidity. Performance of preventive health measures recommended in the general population (e.g., mammography, lower endoscopy) should be decided on an individual basis because the risk to benefit ratio of such testing may be less favorable in a population whose intrinsic life span is limited.

Most transplant programs attempt to reassess each patient's candidacy on an annual basis. In addition to updating the patient's medical status, this reassessment also provides an opportunity to review the availability of living donors and to educate patients with regard to changes in allocation rules that may be relevant to them.

Patients and family members who may have been reluctant to consider living donation when the transplant evaluation process began, may wish to reconsider after a prolonged period on dialysis. For older patients, the advantages and disadvantages of receiving an ECD kidney should be addressed. There is widespread agreement among transplant programs that repeated cardiovascular surveillance is required for many patients while awaiting a transplant and that in high-risk patients this surveillance should be more intense. Table 6.5 suggests a protocol for this followup. For recommendations regarding repetition of screening tests for infectious diseases and HLA antibody reactivity see Gaston et al. in the "Selected Readings," below.

**Table 6.5.   Recommendations for cardiac
surveillance of wait-listed patients**

Initial evaluation negative:
  Diabetic ESRD—annually
  Nondiabetic "high-risk"[a]—biannually
  "Low-risk"—every 3 years
Initial evaluation positive:
  No prior revascularization—annually
  Prior percutaneous coronary intervention—annually
  Postcoronary artery bypass: successful[b]—every 3 years, then
    annually; incomplete—annually
  Asymptomatic moderate or worse aortic stenosis—
    echocardiogram annually

[a]High-risk (more than 20% per 10 years cardiovascular event rate risk) according to Framingham data includes those with two or more "traditional" risk factors, a known history of coronary disease, left ventricular ejection fraction <40%, or peripheral vascular disease.
[b]Complete revascularization of all target vessels.
From Gaston RS, Danovitch GM, Adams PL, et al. The report of a national conference on the wait list for kidney transplantation. *Am J Transplant* 2003;3:775–785, with permission.

Relevance of the Allocation Algorithm to the Predictability of Transplantation

Deceased donor transplantation is unique among surgical procedures in that it is an urgent procedure performed in an elective population. Because of the inclusion of histocompatability matching in the allocation algorithm in the United States, it has not been possible to anticipate with any degree of accuracy when a given patient will be called for his or her long-awaited transplant. This unpredictability has presented transplant programs with the formidable challenge of attempting to ensure that large numbers of patients, most of who are not under their direct care, are medically cleared for transplantation at all times. A consequence of a patient not being cleared is that the transplant may need to be canceled, resulting in prolongation of ischemic injury to the allograft, or a decision may be made to proceed with the transplant, placing the patient at unnecessary or unrecognized risk. Unpredictability has, in fact, been implicated as a cause of death in the first posttransplant year, particularly in older patients, diabetics, and patients with vascular disease.

The greater the number of points for human leukocyte antigen (HLA) matching in the allocation algorithm, the greater is the degree of unpredictability. Because one point is given for each year on the waiting list, the system that was in place in the United States up until May 2003, whereby seven points were given to matching, exposed the patients in the top 7 years of the list to the likelihood of being allocated a kidney. Now that two points are given for matching, it is the patients in the top 2 years of the list who are likely to be allocated a kidney (see Chapter 3 and Table 3.4). For kidneys allocated based on waiting time alone, it is easy to predict which patient in each blood group category is likely to be allocated a kidney and to ensure that they are ready to safely proceed.

In the United States, the policy on national sharing of zero-mismatched kidneys means that, in principle, any patient can be offered a kidney at any time because the allocation of these kidneys takes priority over other determinants of allocation. Close to 20% of kidneys are allocated in this fashion. In practice, close to 80% of zero-mismatched kidneys are allocated within the first 2 years after patients are placed on the list. This is because recipients with common HLA types rapidly receive kidneys from donors with common HLA types. Patients who have undergone a thorough workup at the time of listing should still be prepared to accept these kidney offers. If a patient is not allocated such a kidney, the patient is likely to require a prolonged wait until the patient reaches the top 2 years of the list, at which time the patient's waiting-time points, together with any additional points for DR matching, will lead to allocation of a kidney.

SELECTED READINGS

Alexander GC, Sehgal A. Variation in access to kidney transplantation across dialysis facilities: using process of care measures for quality improvement. *Am J Kidney Dis* 2002;40:824–831.

Cibrik DM, Kaplan B, Campbell DA, et al. Renal allograft survival in transplant patients with focal segmental glomerulosclerosis. *Am J Transplant* 2003;3:64–67.

Fleisher LA, Eagle KA. Lowering cardiac risk in noncardiac surgery. *N Engl J Med* 2001;345:1677–1682.

Gaston RS, Danovitch GM, Adams PL, et al. The report of a national conference on the wait list for kidney transplantation. *Am J Transplant* 2003;3:775–785.

Gertz MA, Lacy MQ, Dispenzieri A. Immunoglobulin light chain amyloidosis and the kidney. *Kidney Int* 2002;61:1–9.

Heidenreich S, Junker R, Wolters H, et al. Outcome of transplantation in patients with inherited thrombophilia: data of a prospective study. *J Am Soc Nephrol* 2003;14:234–239.

Howard RJ, Thai VB, Patton PR, et al. Obesity does not portend a bad outcome for kidney transplant recipients. *Transplantation* 2002;73:53–55.

Jassal S, Krahn MD, Naglie G. Kidney transplantation in the elderly: a decision analysis. *J Am Soc Nephrol* 2003;14:187–196.

Kasiske BL, Cangro CB, Hariharan S, et al. The evaluation of renal transplant candidates: clinical practice guidelines. *Am J Transplant* 2001;1[Suppl 2]:1–95.

Kiberd BA, Keough-Ryan T, Clase CM. Screening for prostate, breast and colorectal cancer in renal transplant recipients. *Am J Transplant* 2003;3:619–625.

Mange KC, Weir M. Preemptive renal transplantation: why not? *Am J Transplant* 2003;3:1336–1340.

Ponticelli C, Traversi L, Feliciani A, et al. Kidney transplantation in patients with IgA mesangial glomerulonephritis. *Kidney Int* 2001;60:1948–1954.

Sorrell VL. Diagnostic tools and management strategies for coronary artery disease in patients with end stage kidney disease. *Semin Nephrol* 2001;21:13–24.

Steinman TI, Becker BN, Frost AE, et al. Guidelines for the referral and management of patients eligible for solid organ transplantation. *Transplantation* 2001;71:1189–1204.

Sung RS, Althoen M, Howell TA, et al. Peripheral vascular occlusive disease in renal transplant recipients: risk factors and impact on kidney allograft survival. *Transplantation* 2000;70:1049–1054.

Sung RS, Althoen M, Howell TA, et al. Excess risk of renal allograft loss associated with cigarette smoking. *Transplantation* 2001;71:1752–1757.

The Transplant Operation and Its Surgical Complications

Jennifer Singer, H. Albin Gritsch, and
J. Thomas Rosenthal

Kidney transplantation is an elective or semielective surgical procedure performed in patients who have undergone careful preoperative assessment and preparation. Chronic dialysis enables patients to be maintained in optimal condition and provides time to address potentially complicating medical and surgical issues. Chapter 6 describes these preparations. In this respect, kidney transplantation differs from heart or liver transplantation, in which the condition of the patient is often deteriorating rapidly in the pretransplant period.

TRANSPLANTATION OPERATION

Immediate Preoperative Preparations

Chapter 5 describes the process of kidney transplant donation and provides a standard preoperative checklist (see Chapter 5, Table 5.6). If transplantation candidates have been well prepared, it is rarely necessary to call off surgery because of last-minute findings. Occasionally, cancellation of surgery is required because of recent events, such as new onset of chest pain or cardiographic changes, diabetic foot ulcers, peritonitis, pneumonia, or gastrointestinal (GI) bleeding. Perioperative anticoagulation is discussed later in the chapter.

The decision to dialyze a patient before transplantation depends on the timing of the previous dialysis, clinical assessment of volume status, and serum electrolyte levels, particularly potassium. Pretransplant dialysis is associated with an increased incidence of delayed graft function. Because of the danger of intraoperative or postoperative hyperkalemia in oliguric patients, it is wise to dialyze patients with a serum potassium level of more than 5.5 mEq/L. In well-dialyzed patients, preoperative dialysis for fluid removal is usually unnecessary. If fluid is removed, it should be done with care to maintain the patient at or somewhat above dry weight to facilitate postoperative diuresis. If time constraints demand it, a brief preoperative dialysis lasting 1 to 2 hours may be all that is necessary to reduce potassium levels and to optimize the hemodynamic status.

Operative Technique

Because all kidney transplant recipients receive immunosuppressive drugs and because many are anemic or malnourished at the time of surgery, wound healing is potentially compromised. Meticulous surgical technique, attention to detail, strict aseptic technique, and perfect hemostasis are essential. Drains

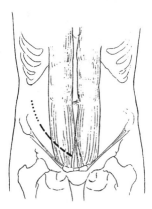

Fig. 7.1. Standard incision for adult kidney transplantation. An oblique incision is made from the symphysis in the midline curving in a lateral and superior direction to the iliac crest.

should be closed systems and should be removed as quickly as possible.

Incision

An oblique incision is made from the symphysis in the midline curving in a lateral superior direction to the iliac crest (Fig. 7.1). It can be extended into the flank, or as high as the tip of the twelfth rib, if more exposure is needed. In a first transplantation, the incision site may be in either lower quadrant. There are different approaches to the decision regarding which side to use. One approach is to always use the right side, regardless of the side of origin of the donor kidney, because the accessibility of the iliac vein makes the operation easier than on the left side. Another approach is to use the side contralateral to the side of the donor kidney; that is, a right kidney is put on the left side, and vice versa. This technique was used when the hypogastric artery was routinely used for the anastomosis because the vessels lie in a convenient position and the renal pelvis is always anterior, making it accessible if ureteral repair is needed. The third approach is to use the side ipsilateral to the donor kidney; that is, a right kidney is put on the right side, and vice versa. This choice is best when the external iliac artery is used for the arterial anastomosis. The vessels then lie without kinking when the kidney is placed in position. In repeat transplantations, the side opposite the original transplant is generally used. In further transplants, the decision regarding where to place the kidney is more complex; a transabdominal incision may be necessary, and more proximal vessels may be used.

The retroperitoneal space is entered, and a pocket is made for the kidney. In patients with type 1 diabetes who may be eventual candidates for pancreas transplant, the kidney is preferentially

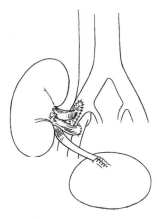

Fig. 7.2.   The standard hook-up. The donor renal artery is shown anastomosed end-to-end on a Carrel aortic patch to the recipient external iliac artery. The donor renal vein is anastomosed to the recipient external iliac vein. The donor ureter is anastomosed to the recipient bladder with an antireflux technique.

placed in the left iliac fossa to facilitate a possible pancreas transplant on the right side (see Chapter 14).

Vascular Connections

Figure 7.2 shows the vascular connections for a kidney transplant.

RENAL VEIN

The renal vein is sewn to the external iliac vein. Suture material similar to that used for the arterial anastomosis is usually chosen. If there are multiple renal veins, the largest may be used; the others can be ligated safely because of internal collateralization of the renal venous drainage. With deceased donor renal transplants, the donor vena cava may be used as an extension graft for the short, right renal vein. The venous anastomosis is usually done first to minimize ischemia to the leg.

RENAL ARTERY

The donor renal artery may be sewn to the external iliac artery in an end-to-side fashion or to the hypogastric artery in an end-to-end fashion. In a deceased donor kidney transplantation, the donor renal artery or arteries are usually kept in continuity with a patch of donor aorta called a *Carrel patch,* which makes the end-to-side anastomosis much easier and safer, and facilitates the anastomosis of multiple renal arteries. In a living-related donor transplant, a Carrel patch is not available, and the renal artery itself is sewn to the recipient artery. If an end-to-side anastomosis is chosen, a 2.7-mm aortic punch is useful in creating the recipient arteriotomy. A fine, nonabsorbent, monofilament suture, such as 5-0 or 6-0 polypropylene, is usually chosen. In small children and in patients undergoing repeat transplantation on the same side, it may be necessary to use arteries other than the external iliac or hypogastric. The common iliac artery or even the aorta may sometimes be used. During the anastomosis time, the kidney is wrapped in a gauze pad with crushed ice saline to minimize warm ischemia.

MULTIPLE ARTERIES

A variety of techniques have been proposed for handling donors with multiple renal arteries. In deceased donor transplants, it is best to keep them all on a single large Carrel patch, which minimizes the likelihood of damage to a small polar artery. In no case should polar arteries be sacrificed. Ligation of a lower-pole artery may lead to ureteral necrosis. There may be visible capsular vessels that supply a tiny part of the cortical surface of the kidney. These vessels may be ligated, and tiny superficial ischemic areas on the surface of the kidney may result. If there are multiple arteries in a living donor transplant, or if a Carrel patch is not available, the donor arteries can be anastomosed individually or anastomosed to each other before being anastomosed to the recipient vessel. Occasionally, a small lower-pole branch may be anastomosed end-to-end to the inferior epigastric artery.

Ureter Anastomosis

The ureter can be anastomosed to the recipient bladder or into the ipsilateral native ureter as a ureterostomy. The native ureter may also be brought up to the allograft renal pelvis as a ureteropyelostomy. Most surgeons use the bladder whenever possible. Preferably, the recipient's bladder will have been shown to be functional before the transplantation; however, even small, contracted bladders that have not "seen" urine for prolonged periods can function well. If necessary, the ureter can be connected to a previously fashioned ileal or colonic conduit.

There are several ways of reimplanting the ureter into the bladder. Each attempts to establish an antireflux mechanism in order to prevent posttransplant pyelonephritis. In a *Leadbetter-Politano* type reimplantation, the bladder is opened, the ureter is brought into the bladder by a separate opening posteriorly, and a submucosal tunnel is created laterally. The ureter is sewn into the bladder from within, and the bladder is then closed.

A more common approach is one in which the ureter is reimplanted extravesically, the *Lich-Gregoir* technique. First, the bladder is distended with saline and the extravesical tissues are dissected from the detrusor muscle. A muscular tunnel is then created by separating the detrusor muscle from the bladder mucosa for a length of approximately 2 to 4 cm. The ureter is prepared by removing redundant ureteral length, preserving adequate distal blood supply, and spatulating posteriorly. A mucosal opening is created, and interrupted or running biodegradable suture, preferentially polydioxanone surgical suture, is used to approximate the ureteral and bladder mucosa. Finally, the detrusor muscle is closed exteriorly to create an antireflux mechanism (Fig. 7.3). Absorbable suture is used to prevent stone formation. Foley catheter drainage of the bladder is required for about 4 days, unless there are bladder abnormalities that may necessitate longer drainage.

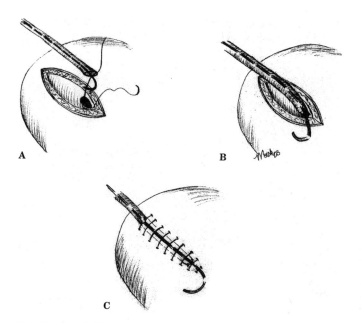

Fig. 7.3. A Lich-Gregoir reimplantation. A single, small opening is made in the bladder (A), and the ureter is sewn in from the outside (B). Bladder muscle is used to create an antireflux mechanism (C).

A third approach is the more simple, double-stitch *Taguchi* or single-stitch *Shanfield* reimplantation technique. A detrusor tunnel is created and the ureter is fashioned as in the Lich-Gregoir technique. An absorbable U stitch is placed on the anterior aspect of the ureter and an orifice is created in the bladder mucosa. The ureteral sutures are then brought out through the bladder wall, approximately 2 cm distal to the caudal edge of the ureteral orifice, and are tied. The detrusor is closed exteriorly as in the Lich-Gregoir technique. While this method is technically simpler and more time efficient, postoperative hematuria, requiring endoscopic clot evacuation or fulguration, may occur from the intravesical stump of the ureter. Rarely, the adventitial tissue of the ureter can calcify. A fourth approach described by *Barry,* uses two parallel incisions 3 to 4 cm apart in the bladder muscle. An antireflux tunnel is created between them and the spatulated ureter tip is pulled through and anastomosed to the bladder mucosa with interrupted sutures.

Whatever technique is used for the ureteral anastomosis an indwelling stent may be placed at the discretion of the transplant surgeon. Routine stenting may not be necessary for patients at low risk for urologic complications. If a stent is placed, it should be removed within 4 weeks of transplantation. Clear notation of stent placement and its subsequent removal must be made to prevent inadvertent stent retention. A retained stent may be very difficult to remove intact and may be a source of recurrent urinary tract infections and ureteral stones.

Drains

Drains may be placed through a separate small incision into the perirenal space to drain blood, urine, or lymph. Some surgeons routinely place drains, while others do not. Closed drains, such as the Jackson-Pratt type, are preferred over the open Penrose-type drains because of a lower risk for wound infection. When drains are used, they should be removed as soon as there is no longer significant drainage, typically 24 to 48 hours after transplantation. Placement of a drain may reduce the incidence of lymphoceles.

Surgical Considerations in Young Children

Urologic disease is the cause of renal failure in nearly half of children with end-stage renal disease (see Chapter 15). It is therefore important to study bladder function in children with a history of urinary tract infections or voiding abnormalities. Reconstructive surgery must be coordinated with possible renal transplantation. The parent(s) and child must be psychologically prepared for intermittent catheterization, which may be necessary postoperatively.

The transplantation procedure for children who weigh more than 20 to 25 kg is the same as the procedure for adults. In smaller children, comparatively large adult-size kidneys are implanted because kidneys from equivalently sized infant donors are more prone to technical complications. A larger incision and more proximal blood vessels are used for implantation. The common iliac artery and vein, or even the aorta and vena cava, can be used. In children who weigh more than 10 to 12 kg, an extraperitoneal approach can still be used. The right side is almost always preferable because of the easy exposure of the common iliac vein. In children who weigh less than 10 to 12 kg, a midline transabdominal approach is necessary. The great vessels are approached by mobilizing the cecum, and the kidney is placed behind the cecum. To provide room for a large kidney in the right flank, a right native nephrectomy is sometimes necessary at the time of the transplantation to create room for the allograft. Careful intraoperative fluid management is crucial to prevent thrombosis of large kidneys in small children.

Intraoperative Fluid Management

Adequate perfusion of the newly transplanted kidney is critical for the establishment of an immediate postoperative diuresis and the avoidance of delayed graft function (see Chapter 8). Volume contraction should be avoided and mild volume expansion maintained, conducive to the recipient's cardiac status. Central venous pressure should be maintained at about 10 mm Hg with the use of isotonic saline and albumin infusions, and systolic blood pressure should be kept above 120 mm Hg. If blood is required, cytomegalovirus-negative units should be used.

Before the release of the vascular clamps, a large dose of methylprednisolone is usually given (up to 1 g in some programs; see Chapter 4). If thymoglobulin is administered (see Chapter 4)

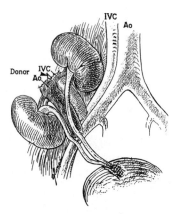

Fig. 7.4. Pediatric *en bloc* kidney transplantation. The donor aorta (*Ao*) and inferior vena cava (*IVC*) are anastomosed to the external iliac vessels. The ureters are anastomosed to the bladder using pediatric stents. (From Bretan PN, Koyle M, Singh K, et al. Improved survival of en bloc renal allografts from pediatric donors. *J Urol* 1997;157:1592–1595, with permission.)

it should be commenced at this time. Mannitol (12.5 g) and furosemide (up to 200 mg) are also given, and fluid replacement is maintained accordingly. Direct injection of verapamil 5 mg, a calcium channel blocker, into the renal artery reduces capillary spasm and improves renal blood flow. This medication must be administered with caution in patients taking beta-blocker anti-hypertensive medications to avoid complete heart block. Postoperative management is discussed in Chapter 8.

Dual-Kidney Transplantation

At the extremes of donor age, both donor kidneys are sometimes transplanted into a single recipient. The simultaneous use of both kidneys entails some additional risks to the recipient. It is a reflection of the donor shortage and reluctance to discard potentially functional organs.

For donors younger than 2 years of age, both kidneys are usually transplanted *en bloc* with the donor aorta and vena cava (Fig. 7.4); for donors between the ages of 2 and 5 years, the decision to transplant the kidneys separately or together is made by the transplant surgeon after assessing the size of the organs. For the *en bloc* procedure, the aorta and vena cava superior to the renal vessels must be of adequate length to allow closure without compromising the lumen of the renal vessels. All of the other branches of the great vessels are carefully ligated, the aorta is then anastomosed to the external iliac artery, and the vena cava is anastomosed to the external iliac vein. Both ureters are then anastomosed to the bladder. The kidneys must be carefully positioned to avoid kinking of the blood vessels and tension on the ureteral anastomoses. If the ureters are implanted into the bladder

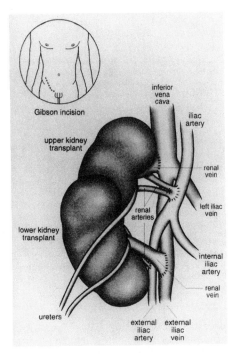

Fig. 7.5.   Dual transplantation of adult kidneys into a single recipient. (From Masson D, Hefty T. A technique for the transplantation of 2 adult cadaver kidney grafts into 1 recipient. *J Urol* 1998;160:1779–1780, with permission.)

separately, the risk for injury to the second kidney in case of vascular thrombosis is reduced. The rate of technical complications, most typically urine leaks and vascular thrombosis, varies between 10% and 20% with young donor kidneys transplanted individually or *en bloc*. The rate of thrombosis may be reduced by using a very low dose of an anticoagulant, such as intravenous (IV) heparin at 100 to 200 units per hour or oral aspirin. Excessive anticoagulation carries a significant risk of bleeding.

Kidneys from older "marginal" donors are sometimes discarded for fear they will not provide adequate renal function for their recipients. To avoid this waste, some centers now advocate the use of two kidneys from donors age 60 years or older, if the calculated creatinine clearance is less than 90 mL per minute at the time of admission, or if there is evidence of significant histologic damage on the biopsy specimen taken at the time of organ retrieval. These kidneys are typically placed into older recipients whose metabolic requirements may be less. One kidney can be placed in each iliac fossa by using a preperitoneal midline incision or separate lower abdominal incisions. Alternatively, both kidneys can be placed on one side, with anastomosis of the vessels of one kidney to the common iliac artery and the vena cava (Fig. 7.5). The survival rate of double marginal kidneys is approximately 7% less than that for single kidneys, although when compared to the survival rate of single kidneys from donors older than age 55 years their outcome is similar.

SURGICAL COMPLICATIONS OF KIDNEY TRANSPLANTATION

The clinical presentation of surgical and nonsurgical complications of kidney transplantation may be similar. Graft dysfunction may reflect an acute rejection or a urine leak; fever and graft tenderness may reflect wound infection or rejection. Posttransplantation events have a broad differential diagnosis that must include technical complications of surgery, as well as immunologic and other causes.

The fundamental algorithm in the management of posttransplantation graft dysfunction requires that vascular and urologic causes of graft dysfunction be ruled out before concluding that an event is a result of a medical cause such as rejection or cyclosporine toxicity. The differential diagnosis of postoperative graft dysfunction is discussed in Chapter 8, and the radiologic diagnostic tools are discussed in Chapter 12. Doppler ultrasound is invaluable in the differentiation of medical and surgical postoperative complications.

Wound Infection

In the 1960s and 1970s, wound infection rates after kidney transplantation were as high as 25%. Wound infections should now occur in less than 1% of cases. This improvement is a result of several factors: patients receiving transplants are healthier; lower steroid doses are used for both maintenance and treatment of rejection; and perioperative antibiotics are routinely used. In most cases, a first-generation cephalosporin is sufficient (see Chapter 10). Obviously, strict aseptic technique in the operating room is essential to prevent wound infection. If infections do occur, they should be treated with drainage and systemic antibiotics to avoid contamination of the vascular suture line and possible mycotic aneurysm formation. The risk of infection or other wound problems is significantly higher in obese patients.

Lymphocele

Presentation

Lymphoceles are collections of lymph caused by leakage from severed lymphatics that overlie the iliac vessels. They may develop and present within weeks after transplantation. The incidence of lymphoceles reported in the literature ranges varies widely. Some lymphoceles are small and asymptomatic. Others are large and produce symptoms. Usually, the larger the lymphocele, the more likely it is to produce symptoms and require treatment, although there are some cases of very small but strategically placed lymphoceles producing ureteral obstruction. Lymphoceles may present by producing ureteral obstruction; by compressing the iliac vein, leading to deep vein thrombosis or leg swelling; or as an abdominal mass. Lymphoceles occasionally produce incontinence secondary to bladder compression, scrotal masses secondary to spontaneous drainage into the scrotum, or vena cava obstruction. Lymphoceles can be avoided by minimizing the dissection of the iliac vessels and by ligating all lymphatics. The use of the immunosuppressant agent sirolimus in the early posttransplant period reportedly increases their incidence from approximately 18% to 38% (see Chapter 4).

Diagnosis

Lymphoceles are usually diagnosed by ultrasound (see Chapter 12). The characteristic ultrasound finding is a roundish, sonolucent, septated mass. Hydronephrosis may be present, and the ureter may be seen adjacent to and compressed by the lymphocele. More complex internal echoes may signal an infected lymphocele. Usually, the clinical situation and ultrasound appearance distinguish a lymphocele from other types of perirenal fluid collections, such as hematoma or urine leak. Simple needle aspiration of the fluid using sterile technique makes the diagnosis. The fluid obtained is clear and has a high protein content, and the creatinine concentration is equal to that of serum.

Treatment

No therapy is necessary for the common, small, asymptomatic lymphocele. Percutaneous aspiration should be performed if there is suspicion of a ureteral leak, obstruction, or infection. The most common indication for treatment is ureteral obstruction. If the cause of the obstruction is simple compression caused by the mass effect of the lymphocele, drainage alone will resolve the problem. The ureter itself is often narrowed and may need to be reimplanted because of its involvement in the inflammatory reaction in the wall of the lymphocele. Repeated percutaneous aspirations are not advised because they seldom lead to dissolution of the lymphocele and often result in infection.

Infected or obstructing lymphoceles can be drained externally using either a closed or an open system. Closed systems are superior because they control the fluid and are less susceptible to infection. Sclerosing agents, such as povidone iodine (Betadine), tetracycline, or fibrin glue, can be instilled into the cavity with good results. Lymphoceles can also be drained internally by marsupialization into the peritoneal cavity, where the fluid is resorbed. Marsupialization can be done as an open surgical procedure or laparoscopically. It is important to ensure that the opening in the lymphocele is large enough to prevent peritoneal closure, which can produce recurrence or bowel entrapment and incarceration. Omentum is often interposed in the opening to prevent closure. Care must be taken to avoid injury to the ureter, which may lie in the wall of the lymphocele. On rare occasions, the actual site of lymph leak can be identified and ligated.

Bleeding

The risk for postoperative bleeding can be minimized by close attention to pretransplant coagulation parameters, which should be considered during the pretransplantation workup (see Chapter 6). Aspirin and anticoagulant medications should be discontinued before transplantation, and well-dialyzed patients may have improvement of the platelet dysfunction and abnormal bleeding time associated with uremia. Postoperative bleeding seldom arises from the vascular anastomoses unless a mycotic aneurysm ruptures or the graft itself ruptures. These events are not likely to occur until a few days after transplantation and are associated with exsanguinating hemorrhage. Early postoperative bleeding can occur from small vessels in the renal hilum, which may not have been apparent before closure because of vasospasm. After surgery, when perfusion improves, these hilar vessels can then bleed. Meticulous preparation of the allograft and hemostasis during the operation minimizes this risk. Close observation of vital signs and serial hematocrits is necessary for the first several postoperative hours to recognize this type of bleeding. Ultrasound can confirm the presence of perigraft hematoma. Surgical exploration may be necessary. If bleeding occurs, coagulation parameters should be studied to ensure that there is no occult coagulopathy. Administration of blood, efficient dialysis, estrogen infusions, and vasopressin all improve platelet function and reduce bleeding time in uremic patients.

Late hemorrhage can result from the rupture of a mycotic aneurysm. The bleeding may be profound. Nephrectomy and repair of the artery are usually required. Rarely, the external iliac artery may have to be ligated and blood supply to the ipsilateral leg provided by extraanatomic bypass.

Graft Thrombosis

Arterial or venous thrombosis occurs most often within the first 2 to 3 days after transplantation, although it may occur as long as 2 months after transplantation. The reported incidence varies widely, from 0.5% to as high as 8%. The incidence of thrombosis may be increased in patients with a prior thrombotic tendency, anticardiolipin antibodies, or high platelet counts (more than 350×10^9/L). The early variety of thrombosis is most often a reflection of surgical technique; the later variety is most often associated with acute rejection. If the kidney has been functioning well, thrombosis is heralded by a sudden cessation of urine output and rapid rise in serum creatinine, often with graft swelling and local pain. Platelets may be consumed, and thrombocytopenia and hyperkalemia may develop. Venous thrombosis may present with severe graft swelling, tenderness, and gross hematuria. If a patient's native kidneys were a source of significant quantities of urine, however, the only sign of thrombosis may be the rising creatinine level; if the allograft had not been functioning, there may be no overt signs of thrombosis at all. For this reason, grafts that are not functioning are routinely imaged radiologically to ensure ongoing blood flow to the graft. Diagnosis of thrombosis is by a Doppler ultrasound or isotope flow scan (see Chapter 12). These techniques help distinguish thrombosis from other causes of acute anuria, such as rejection or obstruction. Confirmed thrombosis usually requires graft nephrectomy.

The transplanted kidney has no collateral blood supply, and its tolerance for warm ischemia is short. Unless the problem can be diagnosed quickly and repair carried out immediately, the kidney will be lost. Although there are a few case reports of kidney salvage after thrombosis, most grafts sustaining either arterial or venous thrombosis are lost. Successful graft salvage by intraarterial fibrinolysis within 24 hours of thrombosis has been described.

Perioperative Anticoagulation

Anticoagulation is required for patients with mechanical cardiac valves, atrial fibrillation, or a history of coagulopathy. Hemodialysis patients are often treated with anticoagulation to prevent vascular access thrombosis though the effectiveness of this treatment has been questioned. The risk of operating on anticoagulated patients is an increased tendency to postoperative bleeding, most frequently at the operative site. This risk has to be balanced against the thromboembolic risk on an individual basis. Living donor recipients should, whenever possible, discontinue aspirin, clopidogrel, or warfarin therapy 1 week prior to transplant. For patients admitted for deceased donor transplantation, attempts should be made to bring the international normalized ratio (INR) to less than 2.0 at the time of operation. For those patients deemed at particular risk for allograft thrombosis (preoperatively identified hypercoagulable states, multiple or small renal arteries requiring complex repair), some form of perioperative anticoagulation is prudent. Such patients must be observed intraoperatively for adequacy of hemostasis. If satisfactory, a small bolus dose of intravenous heparin, usually 1,000 units, is given, followed postoperatively by a heparin infusion at 100 units per hour for 24 hours. If no bleeding is observed at the operative site, and if the hemoglobin concentration remains stable, the heparin infusion is increased to 300 units per hour. If still no bleeding complications are observed, oral warfarin is commenced after 48 hours. The heparin infusion is maintained at 300 units per hour until oral anticoagulation with warfarin achieves a predetermined therapeutic level. Blood counts are checked every 6 hours for the first 24 hours and then daily thereafter. Should the hemoglobin or hematocrit decline markedly, the heparin infusion is discontinued until stabilization of the blood count is achieved. At this point, heparin infusion is resumed pending therapeutic oral anticoagulation. Although theoretically a heparin infusion of 100 units per hour should not alter the partial thromboplastin time (PTT), this dose, in addition to the relative anticoagulant effect of uremic platelet dysfunction, achieves a level of anticoagulation adequate to avoid thrombotic complications in the first 24 hours after surgery. At this dose, it is generally not necessary to follow postoperative PTT. For patients at risk for thrombosis because of complex renal arterial anatomy, without a predisposing thrombotic tendency, a daily aspirin can be used in lieu of warfarin. Low-molecular-weight heparin should be avoided in patients with uremia because the degree of anticoagulation may be unpredictable and difficult to monitor.

Renal Artery Stenosis

Renal artery stenosis is a late complication that usually occurs 3 months to 2 years posttransplant with a prevalence of 1–23% in different series. Its presentation, diagnosis, and management are discussed in Chapters 9 and 12. Two major types of stenosis are seen. One is a discrete, suture line stenosis, which is most often seen after end-to-end anastomosis. The other type is a more

Table 7.1.   Potential causes of renal artery stenosis

Rejection of the donor artery.

Atherosclerosis of the recipient vessel.

Clamp injury to the recipient or donor vascular endothelium.

Perfusion pump cannulation injury of the donor vessel.

Faulty suture technique: purse-string effect, lumen encroachment by the suture, improper suture material, fibrotic inflammatory reaction to polypropylene in the setting of abnormal hemodynamics.

End-to-end anastomosis with abnormal fluid dynamics.

Angulation as a consequence of disproportionate length between graft artery and iliac artery.

End-to-end anastomosis with vessel size disproportion.

Pseudorenal artery stenosis by critical iliac atherosclerotic lesion.

Kinking of the renal artery.

---

diffuse, postanastomotic stenosis, which can occur after any type of arterial anastomosis. The term *pseudorenal artery stenosis* has been used to describe the situation that can occur if an atherosclerotic plaque in the iliac vessels impairs blood flow to the transplant renal artery. Table 7.1 lists potential causes of stenosis. The postulate that rejection can cause renal artery stenosis has not been conclusively proved.

When technically feasible, percutaneous transluminal angioplasty, often with the placement of intraarterial stents, offers the safest mode of treatment, with a high rate of success as judged by reversal of the hemodynamic effects of the stenosis. Stenosis may recur in up to 20% of cases. Doppler ultrasound is a reliable way of monitoring the functional response (see Chapter 12). If angioplasty is not technically feasible, or if it fails as a primary form of therapy, surgical repair may be necessary. Graft loss after surgical repair has been reported in up to 30% of cases and is a reflection of the difficulty in directly approaching the vascular anastomosis in a noncollateralized kidney.

Urine Leaks

Etiology and Diagnosis

Urine leaks may occur at the level of the bladder, ureter, or renal calyx. They typically occur within the first few days after transplantation or at the onset of posttransplantation diuresis in patients with delayed graft function. Urine leaks may be technical in etiology as a result of a nonwatertight ureteral reimplantation or bladder closure. They may also be the result of ureteral slough secondary to disruption of ureteral blood supply; the blood supply to the distal donor ureter is the most endangered by the harvesting procedure. Leaks can also occur as a result of a tight ureteral stenosis that leads to forniceal rupture in the presence of a high urine volume.

If the transplantation incision is drained, a urine leak may present with copious drainage. Any excess fluid drainage from the incision should be sent urgently for creatinine estimation. Any significant elevation in concentration over that of plasma confirms that the fluid is urine (occasionally, at a time of a falling serum creatinine level, serous fluid may be trapped at a slightly higher creatinine level than the current plasma level). If the wound is not drained, a urine leak may present with agonizing pain, rising plasma creatinine level as a result of the reabsorption of urine, and a fluid density mass on ultrasound. This clinical picture may be confused with rejection, although the pain of a urine leak is typically much more severe than the aching pain of an acute rejection. Fluid leaking from the incision line may have a typical uriniferous odor. If ultrasound shows a fluid collection, the fluid should be tapped under sterile conditions and sent urgently for creatinine estimation. A renal scan will often identify the leak by showing radioisotope outside the urinary tract. A cystogram may show leakage of contrast outside of the bladder (see Chapter 12).

Treatment

There should be no delay in instituting therapy. A Foley catheter should be immediately placed if there is clinical suspicion of a leak. The catheter reduces intravesical pressure and occasionally may reduce or stop leakage altogether. Percutaneous antegrade nephrostomy may be used to diagnose the leak and control the flow of urine. Some leaks can be managed definitively with external drainage and stent placement alone. It may be difficult, however, to access the collecting system percutaneously because there is often not enough hydronephrosis present. If the leak is caused by a ureteral slough, percutaneous treatment will never work and only delays definitive treatment. For these reasons, when leaks occur, early surgical exploration and repair are usually required.

The type of surgical repair depends on the level of leak and the viability of the tissues. Bladder fistulas should be closed primarily. A calyceal leak that is the result of obstruction is treated by removal of the obstruction. If a ureteral leak is a simple anastomotic leak, resection of the distal ureter and reimplantation is the easiest solution. If the ureter is nonviable because of inadequate length of blood supply, ureteropyelostomy using the ipsilateral or contralateral native ureter is a good option. Cystopyelostomy has also been done to replace a sloughed ureter. Here, the bladder is mobilized and brought directly to the allograft renal pelvis without an intervening ureter. The advantage of using the native ureter over direct anastomosis of the bladder to the renal pelvis is that the native ureter is antirefluxing, which may result in a lower incidence of pyelonephritis.

An indwelling double-J stent is usually left in place after repair of a urine leak. Nephrostomy drainage is not essential, although if a prior percutaneous nephrostomy has been done, it is wise to leave it in place for several days after surgery. It should be removed only after a trial of nephrostomy occlusion to ensure continuity of distal drainage. The double-J stent can be removed cystoscopically several weeks later, followed by ultrasound to ensure that urine is not recollecting.

Ureteral Obstruction

Diagnosis

Ureteral obstruction is usually manifested by impairment of graft function. Obstruction may be painless because of the absence of innervation. Hydronephrosis may be seen on ultrasound; increasing hydronephrosis is good evidence of obstruction. Low-grade dilation of the collecting system secondary to edema at the implantation site is often seen on early posttransplant ultrasound examinations and should not necessarily lead to the conclusion that there is obstruction present. Confirmation of the obstruction and identification of the site can be made by intravenous pyelogram, although often graft function is inadequate to allow good visualization. Obstruction can be confirmed by retrograde pyelogram, although the ureteral orifice may be difficult to catheterize. Renal scan with furosemide wash-out is a good screening test, but does not provide clear anatomic detail. The most effective way to visualize the collecting system is by percutaneous antegrade pyelography.

Etiology and Treatment

Acute postoperative obstruction usually requires surgical repair. Blood clots, a technically poor reimplantation, and ureteral slough are the common causes of early acute obstruction after transplantation. Ureteral fibrosis secondary to either ischemia or rejection can cause an intrinsic obstruction, and obstruction associated with polyomavirus BK has also been described (see Chapters 10 and 13). Extrinsic obstruction can be caused by ureteral kinking or periureteral fibrosis from lymphoceles or graft rejection. Calculi are rare causes of transplant obstruction.

Intrinsic ureteral scars can be treated effectively by endourologic techniques in an antegrade (Fig. 7.6) or retrograde approach. If graft dysfunction is associated with significant or increasing hydronephrosis, obstruction is confirmed with a fine-needle percutaneous nephrostogram (step A in Fig. 7.6; see Chapter 12). If obstruction is confirmed, a guidewire is passed endoscopically through the stricture (step B in Fig. 7.6). If the stricture is short (i.e., less than 2 cm), balloon dilation allows a working element to be passed, and under direct vision, the stricture is incised with a cold knife (step C in Fig. 7.6). The stricture can also be approached retrograde through the bladder cystoscopically. A stent is left indwelling (step D in Fig. 7.6) and removed cystoscopically after 2 to 6 weeks. The nephrostomy is removed after an antegrade nephrostogram has confirmed that the urinary tract is unobstructed. Early reports suggest success rates of 70% to 80% with these techniques. Endourologic techniques can also be used to remove calculi, which can also be destroyed by extracorporeal shock wave lithotripsy.

Extrinsic strictures or strictures that are longer than 2 cm are less likely to be amenable to percutaneous techniques and require surgical treatment than are those strictures that fail endourologic incision. The same surgical options are used as for ureteral leaks: direct reimplantation of the ureter above the stricture, or anastomosis of the native ureter or bladder to the renal pelvis if the stricture is high.

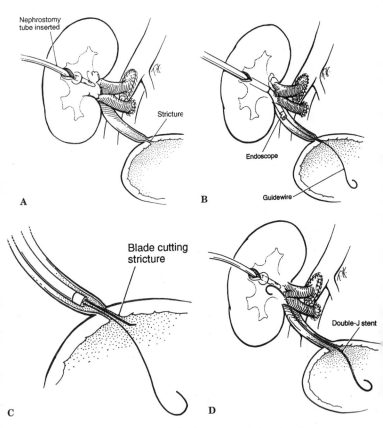

Fig. 7.6. Stages in the endourologic treatment of ureteral structure. See text for description of steps.

Gastrointestinal Complications

Gastrointestinal complications of renal transplantation are not uncommon. Nausea and vomiting may simply be related to the multiple medications these patients require, but more serious conditions, such as bowel obstruction, cholecystitis, infectious gastritis, pancreatitis, gastric ulceration, and colonic perforation, may occur. A high degree of suspicion is crucial because immunosuppressed patients may not present with typical symptoms of peritonitis. Timely diagnosis and surgical treatment are essential to avoid significant mortality. Sodium polystyrene sulfonate (Kayexalate)-sorbitol enemas should not be administered to uremic patients because they have been associated with colonic necrosis. Constipation is a common postoperative problem; sodium phosphate (Fleet) enemas should be avoided in patients with poor renal function because of the high phosphate load.

ALLOGRAFT NEPHRECTOMY

Indications

Kidneys that have failed either for technical reasons or because of rejection may need to be removed. Indications for allograft nephrectomy are symptoms and signs that typically occur when immunosuppression is withdrawn but may be delayed by weeks or months. These can include low-grade fever, graft tenderness and swelling, malaise, thrombocytopenia, and hematuria. It may be possible to lessen the symptoms and avoid nephrectomy by temporary reinstitution of small doses of steroids. Avoidance of nephrectomy is preferred because the procedure may have an unfavorable effect on the prognosis of a future transplant and may cause a steep elevation in the percentage of preformed cytotoxic antibodies (see Chapter 3). If the graft loss is acute and occurs within 1 year of transplantation, nephrectomy may be necessary in up to 90% of cases. Graft loss from chronic rejection after 1 year results in nephrectomy in up to 50% of cases. The rejected graft that remains *in situ* typically becomes a small, fibrotic mass. Acquired cystic disease may develop as described in chronically diseased native kidneys.

Procedure

The removal of a failed allograft may be technically more difficult than the transplantation itself because of the inflammatory response and scarring as a consequence of rejection. For this reason, the procedure should be performed at centers with appropriate experience. Usually, the old incision is reopened. Care must be taken to avoid the peritoneum, which may have become draped across the surface of the kidney. If the nephrectomy is performed soon after transplantation, especially if there has not been a great amount of rejection, the kidney can be removed entirely because it is not very adherent to surrounding structures. If there has been recurrent rejection, the kidney usually adheres to surrounding structures and needs to be removed subcapsularly. The hilar vessels are friable and should be ligated and suture ligated. It is almost always safe to leave a small amount of donor vessel in the recipient so that repair of the recipient iliac vessels is not necessary.

Hemostasis should be meticulous. Some dead space is always left after nephrectomy. If this fills with blood, abscess formation is more likely. Although a closed drain may be used, it may inadequately drain the blood and create the potential for infection by its presence. Electrocoagulation of the entire raw surface of the capsule should be performed, and spraying thrombin topically may improve hemostasis. Topical and parenteral antibiotics are routinely used.

Complications

Although there are few series in the literature, the reported morbidity for allograft nephrectomy is high. The potential complications include acute bleeding during surgery secondary to injury to the iliac artery or vein; injury to other surrounding structures, such as the bowel; infection; and lymph leaks. Leaving small segments of the allograft renal artery or vein does not usually cause

Table 7.2. Precautions for kidney transplant recipients undergoing posttransplant surgical procedures

Maintain hydration.
Use nonnephrotoxic prophylactic antibiotics.
Give calcineurin inhibitor by mouth when possible.
Modify intravenous calcineurin inhibitor dose when necessary.
Provide perioperative steroid coverage.
Adjunctive immunosuppressants can be held for several days.
Avoid nephrotoxic antibiotics and analgesics.
Monitor graft function and plasma potassium and acid–base status.
Consider wound healing impairment.

long-term problems, although rupture can occur if they become secondarily infected. Likewise, leaving a small amount of allograft ureter in place can result in some gross hematuria after the allograft nephrectomy; the hematuria is almost always limited and usually does not require reoperation.

NONTRANSPLANT-RELATED SURGERY

Immunosuppressed transplant recipients may occasionally require significant surgical intervention not directly related to the transplantation, such as coronary artery bypass, cholecystectomy, or hip replacement. Nephrologists or members of the transplantation team are often requested to aid in the perioperative management of such patients, and certain precautions are required (Table 7.2).

The renal function of many transplant recipients is impaired to varying degrees, and the capacity to concentrate urine and lower urinary sodium concentration may be limited. Maintenance of hydration is, therefore, particularly important perioperatively to avoid further reduction in renal function. If a patient will be unable to take immunosuppressive medications orally for more than 24 hours, calcineurin inhibitors should be given intravenously in a dose that is about one-third of the total daily oral dose (see Chapter 4) over 4 to 8 hours. Although functional adrenal suppression in patients taking 10 mg per day or less of prednisone is uncommon, 100 mg of hydrocortisone is typically given every 8 hours postoperatively until the patient can return to the preoperative oral prednisone dose. Additional agents, such as mycophenolate mofetil or rapamycin, can be safely withheld for 2 to 3 days. Nonnephrotoxic antibiotics should be given prophylactically, and if intravenous contrast is required for radiologic studies, a saline diuresis should be maintained. In patients with markedly impaired graft function, careful monitoring of postoperative plasma potassium levels and acid–base status is mandatory.

SELECTED READINGS

Aslam S, Salifu M, Ghali H, et al. Common iliac artery stenosis presenting as renal artery dysfunction in two diabetic patients. *Transplantation* 2001;71:814–817.

Barry JM, Hatch DA. Parallel incision, unstented extravesical ureteroneocystostomy: followup of 203 kidney transplants. *J Urol* 1985;134:249–251.

Bruno S, Remuzzi G, Ruggenenti P. Transplant renal artery stenosis. *J Am Soc Nephrol* 2004;15:134–141.

Bunnapradist S, Gritsch HA, Peng A, et al. Dual kidneys from marginal adult donors as a source for cadaveric renal transplantation in the United States. *J Am Soc Nephrol* 2003;14:1031–1036.

Churchill BM, Steckler RE, McKenna PH, et al. Renal transplantation and the abnormal urinary tract. *Transplant Rev* 1993;7:21–25.

Dominguez J, Clase CM, Mahalati K, et al. Is routine ureteric stenting needed in kidney transplantation? A randomized trial. *Transplantation* 2000;70:597–601.

Gruessner RW, Fasola C, Benedetti E, et al. Laparoscopic drainage of lymphocele after kidney transplantation, indications and limitations. *Surgery* 1995;117:288–295.

Hobart MG, Modlin CS, Kapoor A, et al. Transplantation of pediatric en bloc cadaver kidneys into adult recipients. *Transplantation* 1998;66:1689–1694.

Langer R, Kahan BD. Incidence, therapy, and consequences of lymphocele after sirolimus-cyclosporine-prednisone immunosuppression in renal transplant recipients. *Transplantation* 2002;74:804–808.

Nargund VH, Cranston D. Urologic complications after renal transplantation. *Transplant Rev* 1996;10:24.

Remuzzi G, Grinyo J, Ruggenenti P, et al. Early experience with dual kidney transplantation in adults using expanded donor criteria. *J Am Soc Nephrol* 1999;10:2591–2598.

Rouviere O, Berger P, Beziat C, et al. Acute thrombosis of renal transplant artery. *Transplantation* 2002;73:403–409.

Ruggenenti P, Mosconi L, Bruno S, et al. Posttransplant renal artery stenosis: the hemodynamic response to revascularization. *Kidney Int* 2001;60:309–318.

Satterthwaite R, Aswad S, Sunga V, et al. Outcome of *en bloc* and single kidney transplantation from very young cadaver donors. *Transplantation* 1997;63:1405–1410.

The First Three Posttransplant Months

William J. C. Amend, Jr., Flavio Vincenti, and Stephen J. Tomlanovich

The early posttransplant period refers to the first 3 posttransplant months. It is useful to further divide this period to enable consideration of diagnostic and therapeutic issues that impact on both routine and complicated transplant management that tend to change with time. Generally, surgical issues tend to predominate in the first posttransplant days and medical and immunologic issues tend to predominate thereafter. During this entire period, patients should ideally be followed by a combined surgical and medical team. In this chapter, patient management on the first posttransplant day, the first week, and the first 3 months are considered separately. This separation is not totally arbitrary. Postoperative surgical issues predominate on the first day; uncomplicated patients typically leave the hospital by the first week; most episodes of acute rejection occur during the first 3 months (see Fig. 4.8). Patients who successfully navigate their way through these first 3 months can usually look forward to prolonged graft function. Immunosuppressive therapy during this period is discussed in Chapter 4.

THE FIRST POSTOPERATIVE DAY

Recovery Room Assessment

Patients are evaluated by the transplant team immediately on arrival from the operating room. Familiarity with the patient's preoperative course and workup and preoperative urine output is critical. The initial assessment should first address routine postoperative issues such as hemodynamic and respiratory stability. Most patients will be extubated and awake. The operative record should be reviewed to assess fluid and blood loss and fluid replacement. Intraoperative immunosuppressive protocols should have been fulfilled (e.g., corticosteroids, antibody induction; see Chapter 4). The surgeon should report any untoward intraoperative events and the appearance of the transplanted organ after completion of the anastomosis and release of vascular clamps. The surgeon can often anticipate early graft function based on the intraoperative perfusion characteristics of the kidney, the firmness or turgidity of the allograft, and the intraoperative urine volume. Details of the surgery (e.g., multiple donor vessels, recipient vascular condition, type of ureteral anastomosis, presence or absence of ureteral stent) are documented.

Table 8.1 reviews routine postoperative orders. The length of time a patient remains in recovery will depend on both medical and logistical factors. The postoperative nursing unit must allow for close hemodynamic and fluid management. This environment

Table 8.1. Suggested postoperative orders on transfer of kidney transplant recipient from the recovery room

Postoperative Nursing Orders

1. Vital signs checked every hour for 24 h, then every 4 h when patient is stable
2. Intake and output every hour for 24 h, then every 4 h
3. Intravenous fluids per physician
4. Daily weight
5. Turn, cough, deep breathe every hour; encourage incentive spirometry every hour while awake
6. Out of bed first postoperative; ambulate daily thereafter
7. Head of bed at 30 degrees
8. Dressing changes every 4 h for 24 h, then every 8 h and p.r.n.
9. Check dialysis access for function every 4 h
10. No blood pressure; venipuncture in extremity with fistula or shunt
11. Foley catheter to bedside drainage, irrigate gently with 30 mL normal saline p.r.n. for clots
12. Catheter care every 8 h
13. Notify physician if urine output drops to less than 50 mL/h or if greater than 200 mL/h
14. Notify physician if temperature is >180 mm Hg or <110 mm Hg
15. NPO until changed by surgical team
16. Chest radiograph in the morning
17. Electrocardiogram in the morning

Postoperative Laboratory Orders

1. Complete blood count with platelets, electrolyte, creatinine, glucose, and blood urea nitrogen every 6 h for 24 h, then every morning
2. Calcineurin inhibitor level each morning
3. Chemistry panel, urine culture, and sensitivity twice a week

can be an intensive care unit or a surgical "step-down" unit, depending on the facilities available in a given institution and on the patient's postoperative condition. Postoperative management of diabetic patients is discussed in Chapter 13.

Hemodynamic Evaluation

Postoperative hemodynamic evaluation is critical for several reasons: for routine postsurgical management; to optimize graft function; to assess the significance of the urine output or lack thereof; and to undertake prompt therapeutic intervention.

Hemodynamic evaluation may be somewhat difficult in patients with chronic renal failure and dialysis access. Vascular sclerosis is frequent in uremic patients, especially in elderly and diabetic patients, such that systolic hypertension is frequent. The clinician should be familiar with the patient's pretransplant blood pressure and antihypertensive medications. A review of the operative course with the transplant surgeon may be useful for blood pressure management decisions, because the initial blood flow to the allograft is primarily dependent on mean systemic arterial blood pressure. There is little extrinsic or intrinsic autoregulation of early allograft vascular reactivity. The surgeon can report on the optimum intraoperative level of mean arterial blood pressure that provided the best observed allograft turgor and urine output. Excessive postoperative arterial hypertension may increase the risk of anastomotic leak and cerebrovascular catastrophes. Reduced mean arterial pressures, on the other hand, increase the risk of postoperative acute tubular necrosis (ATN) or irreversible vascular thrombosis (especially with a fresh venous anastomosis). Oral nifedipine or clonidine is effective and convenient for management of postoperative systolic hypertension. Intravenous labetalol or hydralazine can be used in resistant cases where the systolic blood pressure is consistently over 180 mm Hg.

Many kidney transplant units use venous pressure or pulmonary artery and pulmonary wedge pressure measurements in the first 24 to 48 hours posttransplant. These measurements can be useful especially when the clinical team is not sure of the need for or amount of fluid resuscitation. Because many kidney transplant recipients have degrees of heart failure (as a result of uremic cardiomyopathy, hypertensive cardiomyopathy, and coronary artery disease), preload monitoring techniques may be invaluable. Clinical judgment, however, should supersede slavish commitment to venous pressure parameters. Thus, a normotensive patient with a good urine output may have a low recorded central venous pressure and yet not need fluid resuscitation.

Intravenous Fluid Replacement

Several factors need to be assessed to determine the rate and form of posttransplant fluid replacement. In general, the patient should be kept euvolemic or mildly hypervolemic, and repeated hemodynamic assessment is required. Insensible fluid losses are typically 30 to 60 mL per hour. Intravascular volume contractions as a consequence of "third-spacing" over the first 12 to 24 postoperative hours needs to be corrected. Volume losses at the operative site must be considered, especially if there are concomitant changes in urine volume and hemodynamic status. Urine volume must be monitored hourly and replaced accordingly (see "Urine Output," below).

Which Intravenous Fluid?

Insensible fluid loss is essentially water loss and is replaced by a 5% dextrose solution at approximately 30 mL per hour. If the patient is deemed to be hypervolemic, it may be wise not to replace this fluid and allow the patient to reach his or her postoperative dry weight over the ensuing days. Hourly urine output (and nasogastric losses if present) is replaced with half-normal saline on an "milliliter-for-milliliter" basis. Half-normal saline is used for urine replacement because the sodium concentration of the urine of a newly transplanted diuresing kidney is typically 60 to 80 mEq/L. If the patient is deemed to be hypovolemic, or if an attempt is being made to increase urine volume (see "Urine Output," below), isotonic saline boluses are given after bedside clinical and hemodynamic evaluation.

Potassium replacement is usually not required unless urine volumes are very high and should be given with great care in oliguric patients. Lactated Ringer solution and other premixed intravenous fluids are unnecessary. Their potassium and bicarbonate content is inadequate if replacement is indeed required, and it is better to supplement saline infusions with potassium, bicarbonate, and calcium on an as-needed basis. The necessity for blood transfusion is discussed in the section on "Early Postoperative Bleeding," below.

Urine Output

The initial urine volumes can range from anuria to oliguria, "nonoliguria," or polyuria, and may shift from one to the other based on parenchymal, urologic, or perfusion factors. A background knowledge of the patient's native urine output is important to assess the significance of the postoperative urine output. Patients who are fortunate to have received a transplant before they started dialysis typically pass 1,500 to 2,000 mL of urine daily from their native kidneys in order to maintain osmolar balance with urine that is close to isotonic. Information about the donor kidney itself is critical. When the transplant is from a living donor, postoperative oliguria is unusual because of the short ischemia time (see Chapter 5) and, if it occurs, must raise immediate concern regarding the vascularization of the graft. On the other hand, when a patient receives a deceased donor kidney with a prolonged ischemia time or preharvesting ATN, postoperative oliguria can be anticipated.

Various techniques and protocol modifications have been made to encourage postoperative diuresis (see Chapter 4). Some protocols do not permit the use of intravenous cyclosporine or tacrolimus in the early postoperative period. Dopamine or fenoldopam infusions at "renal-dose" levels of 1 to 5 μg/kg per hour are used routinely at some centers to promote renal blood flow and counteract calcineurin inhibitor-induced renal vasoconstriction.

The Anuric and Oliguric Patient

Anuria is easy to define; oliguria is relative, and in the posttransplant situation usually refers to urine outputs of less than approximately 50 mL per hour. Before addressing a low posttransplant urine output, the patient's volume status and fluid balance must be assessed, and the Foley catheter irrigated to ensure patency. If there are clots and an associated ball–valve effect, the catheter should be removed while applying gentle suction in an attempt to capture the offending clot. Thereafter, a larger-size catheter may be required. If the Foley catheter is patent and the patient is clearly hypervolemic (i.e., edematous, with congested pulmonary vasculature on chest x-ray, or with elevated venous or wedge pressures), then up to 160 mg of furosemide should be given intravenously. If there is no response, dialysis with ultrafiltration may be necessary. If the patient with oliguria is judged to be hypovolemic, then isotonic saline should be given in boluses of 250 to 500 mL and the response assessed and the infusion repeated if necessary. If the patient is judged to be euvolemic, or a confident clinical assessment cannot be made, then a judicious

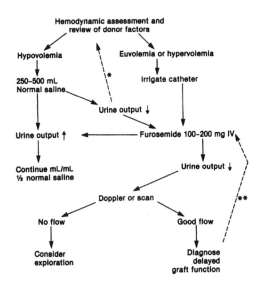

Fig. 8.1. Algorithmic approach to posttransplantation oliguria.
*The volume challenge can be repeated, but only after careful
reassessment of the volume status an fluid balance. **Repeated
doses of intravenous furosemide or furosemide "drips" may be
valuable in patients whose urine output fluctuates. Persistent
oliguria usually does not respond to a repeat dose.

isotonic saline challenge should be given, followed by a high dose
of furosemide.

If a diuresis follows these maneuvers, then urine output is
again replaced milliliter for milliliter with half-normal saline.
The volume challenge and furosemide dose may be repeated if
urine volume falls, but only after careful hemodynamic assessment. A constant infusion of furosemide in a dose of 5 to 10 mg
per hour is employed in some centers. Figure 8.1 suggests an algorithmic approach to the management of postoperative oliguria.

Diagnostic Studies in Persistent Oliguria or Anuria

If the volume challenge, furosemide dose, and volume replacement have no significant impact on the posttransplant urinary
output, then diagnostic studies should be carried out to determine
the cause of the early posttransplant oliguric state (see Chapter
12). The urgency of this workup depends somewhat on the clinical circumstances. If diuresis is anticipated, such as after a living
donor kidney transplant, diagnostic studies, should be performed
immediately—in the recovery room if necessary. If oliguria is anticipated, then studies can usually be safely delayed by several
hours. Patients who pass significant amounts of urine from their
native kidneys may be oliguric from their transplant and this
may be difficult to recognize. In this circumstance, if a transplant

diuresis is anticipated, imaging studies should be performed to ensure that there is blood flow to the allograft.

The purpose of diagnostic studies is to establish the presence of blood flow to the graft and the absence of a urine leak or obstruction. Blood flow studies are performed scintigraphically with diethylenetriamine pentaacetic acid (DTPA) or by Doppler ultrasound. Doppler ultrasound can usually be performed more expeditiously. If the flow study reveals no demonstrable blood flow, a prompt surgical reexploration is necessary to attempt to repair any vascular technical problem and diagnose hyperacute rejection.

If adequate blood flow is visible with the DTPA scan or Doppler studies, additional investigation with an isotope scan or renal ultrasound is necessary to rule out ureteral obstruction or urinary leak. In the first 24 hours posttransplant, as long as the Foley catheter has been providing good bladder drainage, the obstruction or leak is almost always at the ureterovesical junction and represents a technical problem that needs surgical correction. To avoid this complication, some surgeons place a ureteral stent at the time of transplantation. Stent removal occurs in the subsequent weeks.

The Polyuric Patient

Occasionally patients, usually recipients of living donor transplants, have massive amounts of urine (greater than 500 mL per hour) in the early posttransplant period. Generally, these patients are hypervolemic, and urine replacement can be reduced to less than milliliter-for-milliliter replacement. If a negative fluid balance is permitted, then the volume status must be reassessed at frequent intervals and the fluid replacement returned to milliliter for milliliter when the urine volume becomes more manageable. Evidence of rebound hypotension during this phase may prompt fluid boluses. Potassium and calcium may need to be replaced in the polyuric patient.

Early Postoperative Bleeding

The possibility of surgical postoperative bleeding must be considered in any patient with a rapidly falling hematocrit and saline-resistant hypotension. A perigraft Jackson-Pratt drain may repeatedly fill with blood, and there may be a palpable or visible perinephric hematoma. Most hematomas will spontaneously tamponade and do not require reoperation as long as the patient can be maintained hemodynamically stable with crystalloid, colloid, or blood. The threshold for postoperative blood transfusion will depend on the clinical circumstances. Older or diabetic patients who may have coronary artery disease should be transfused more liberally. If possible, blood from cytomegalovirus-negative donors should be given. At reoperation, an identifiable bleeding site is not uniformly discovered (see Chapter 7).

Postoperative Hemodialysis

If the patient is well-dialyzed preoperatively and enters the operation normokalemic, then early postoperative dialysis is usually not required. Oliguric patients with falling hematocrit levels may develop dangerous hyperkalemia and may require urgent therapy with intravenous calcium, bicarbonate, or insulin and glucose combinations. Sodium polystyrene sulfonate (Kayexalate) enemas should be avoided in the early postoperative period as they may cause colonic injury. Patients with persistent hyperkalemia should be dialyzed. A no-heparin protocol should be used; a bicarbonate bath is preferred; and ultrafiltration should be avoided to prevent hypotension. A 2- or 3-hour dialysis is usually adequate.

THE FIRST POSTOPERATIVE WEEK

The first postoperative week is generally characterized by progressive improvement in the patient's overall condition in conjunction with steady improvement in kidney function. Continued close observation of the urine output is still indicated, but fluid replacement need not be adjusted on an hourly basis and can be ordered on a 4- to 8-hour record of urine output. The urine volume is a useful indicator of kidney allograft function but may be misleading in those patients who had appreciable urine output from their native kidneys. Mild fluctuation in urine volumes are acceptable, but a persistent drop in urine volume of greater than 50% or the sudden onset of oliguria or anuria must be promptly investigated (see "Patients with Delayed Graft Function," below). The Foley catheter can usually be removed after 2 to 4 days. Patients should void frequently after catheter removal to avoid overdistention of the bladder with resulting tension on bladder surgical sites. If there is concern regarding inadequate bladder emptying, the postvoid residual volume should be checked, and the Foley catheter may need to be replaced. Older men, and patients with prolonged anuria while on dialysis, are particularly susceptible to postoperative voiding problems.

Patients should be encouraged to ambulate within 24 hours of surgery and are usually started within 48 hours on a liquid diet and progressed thereafter as tolerated. Abdominal distention and pain and the prolonged absence of bowel sounds require investigation by abdominal x-rays to diagnose the occasional occurrence of intraabdominal catastrophes. Incisional pain may persist throughout the first postoperative week but is usually mild. Severe pain or a change in the pain pattern should be thoroughly investigated to rule out rejection, perinephric hematoma, or a urine leak. Fever is not uncommon in the first week and is most commonly due to postoperative atelectasis or drug reaction. Opportunistic infections do not occur at this time, and extensive workup of fever is usually not indicated. Persistent fever with no obvious infectious source may be a manifestation of unrecognized rejection.

The early management of the transplant patient is largely determined by the quality of function of the allograft. Patients typically exhibit one of three patterns of function: excellent graft function, moderate graft dysfunction, or delayed graft function. At the time of discharge from the hospital, usually at the end of the first week, the most powerful predictor of long-term graft function is the serum creatinine level. This reflects the relevance of early events on long-term outcome (see Chapter 9).

Patients with Excellent Graft Function

In ideal circumstances, graft function and diuresis is excellent postoperatively, dialysis is not required, and the serum creatinine level declines rapidly so that patients achieve stable kidney function within the first posttransplant week (the serum creatinine level may reach less than 2.5 mg/dL). Almost all the recipients of kidneys from living donors will enjoy such a postoperative course, as will 30% to 50% of deceased donor kidney recipients. For patients with excellent early function, both the urine volume and serum creatinine levels are useful markers to monitor the occurrence of early rejection, calcineurin inhibitor toxicity, or other underlying pathologic events in the allograft.

If the course of these patients remains uneventful, then it is not mandatory to routinely perform imaging studies. Some transplant centers elect to perform renal ultrasound and isotope scans to provide baseline data.

Patients with Moderate Graft Dysfunction

Patients with moderate graft dysfunction are nonoliguric and exhibit modest daily declines in serum creatinine levels. These patients do not usually require dialysis but will not normalize their kidney function within the first postoperative week. In these patients, the urine volume and the daily serum creatinine concentration are useful markers to monitor the development of complications. Depending on the rate of decline in the serum creatinine concentration, it may be wise to obtain imaging studies to rule out the possibility that urine leak or partial obstruction is accounting for the slow improvement of function. Studies should be performed if the serum creatinine concentration plateaus at a high level or begins to rise. The pathophysiology of the slow improvement in function in these patients is usually ATN, which may be exaggerated by cyclosporine or tacrolimus toxicity (see Chapter 4). "Slow graft function" in the early posttransplant period has a similar impact on long-term function as does delayed graft function, which is discussed next.

Patients with Delayed Graft Function

Any newly transplanted kidney that does not function well can be said to be suffering from delayed graft function. Most, but not all, of these patients will be oliguric and, in this regard, it is important to consider the patient's preoperative urine output which, if large, can be a source of confusion because it cannot easily be differentiated from urine output from the transplant. Most, but not all, patients with delayed graft function require dialysis; however, using the need for dialysis alone to define delayed graft function may lead to underdiagnosis, particularly if there is some residual native kidney function. The frequency of delayed graft function may be as low as 10% and as high as 50% in some programs. In recipients of transplants from living donors, this occurrence is exceptional and almost always portends a serious complication. Table 8.2 lists potential causes of delayed graft function.

Because two kidneys are usually transplanted from the same deceased donor, the first few days of allograft function are often similar in both recipients. Knowledge of the initial clinical

Table 8.2. Differential diagnosis of delayed graft function

Acute tabular necrosis
Intravascular volume contraction
Arterial occlusion
Venous thrombosis
Ureteric obstruction
Catheter obstruction
Urine leak
Hyperacute rejection
Nephrotoxicity
Thrombotic microangiopathy (TMA)

outcome of the other deceased donor kidney recipient may be valuable in evaluating the cause of delayed graft function. Early allograft dysfunction usually stems from factors originating in the donor and during the procurement surgery or the preservation period, and it usually occurs in both recipients. The preservation period may be especially prolonged by delays in transport from procurement to implantation. When there is a disparity in the clinical courses and one recipient has much more kidney dysfunction in the early postoperative period than the other, then causes of dysfunction originating in the recipient become more likely.

Posttransplant Acute Tubular Necrosis

The terms delayed graft function and ATN are often used interchangeably. It is wise to differentiate them. Not all delayed graft function is caused by ATN, and covert accelerated acute rejection and technical complications such as vascular thrombosis will account for some of the cases and cause permanent or so-called primary nonfunction. Posttransplant ATN, as in ATN in the nontransplant situation, is essentially a diagnosis of exclusion. When differentiated from other causes of delayed graft function and when uncomplicated by the development of rejection, ATN appears, at least in the short-term, to be a relatively benign condition that resolves spontaneously over days and sometimes weeks. Recovery is usually first recognized by the patient and is heralded by a steady increase in urine output, diminution in intradialytic rise in creatinine concentration, and eventual steady improvement in kidney function.

The deceased donor kidney is subject to injury at every step along the path from donor death to organ procurement to surgical reanastomosis and the postoperative course (Table 8.3). Posttransplant ATN is essentially an ischemic injury that may be exaggerated by synergistically acting immunologic and nephrotoxic insults. The transplanted kidney is particularly susceptible to so-called ischemia–reperfusion injury as a result of the reintroduction of oxygen into tissues with a high concentration of oxygen free radical radicals resulting from anaerobic metabolism. Superoxide anion and hydrogen peroxide are produced, which lead to lipid peroxidation of cell membranes. This process may be responsible for the commonly occurring clinical sequence whereby an early

**Table 8.3. Preoperative factors promoting
ischemic injury in cadaveric renal transplantation**

Premorbid factors
  Donor age
  Donor hypertension
  Donor cause of death
  Donor acute renal dysfunction
Preoperative donor management
  Brain-death stress
  Cardiac arrest
  Circulating catecholes
  Nephrotoxins
  Catabolic state
Procurement surgery
  Hypotension
  Traction on renal vessels
  Inadequate flushing and cooling
  Flushing solution
Kidney storage
  Prolonged cold storage
  Cold storage versus machine perfusion
  Prolonged anastomosis time
Recipient status
  Preoperative dialysis
  Recipient volume contraction
  Pelvic atherosclerosis
  Preformed antidonor antibodies
  Poor cardiac output

Modified from Shoskes DA, Halloran PF. Delayed graft function in renal transplantation: etiology, management and long-term significance. *J Urol* 1996; 155:1831–1840, with permission.

posttransplant diuresis is followed within hours by oliguria. In animal models of ischemia–reperfusion injury, gene transfer-induced overexpression of heme oxygenase-1 (HO-1, heat shock protein) protects against renal injury, and strategies that increase expression of HO-1 may prove to be useful therapeutically.

The oliguria of ATN is caused by a combination of diminished glomerular filtration rate (GFR), tubular obstruction with cellular debris, backleak of tubular fluid through damaged proximal tubular membranes, and increased interstitial pressure. Although blood flow to the renal cortex is reduced, there is a relatively greater reduction in GFR and tubular function that accounts for the commonly encountered radiologic find of "good flow and poor excretion" on scintigraphic studies. The alterations in vascular resistance and increased intracapsular pressure produce the increased "resistive index" and reduced or reversed diastolic flow found on Doppler ultrasound (see Chapter12).

ATN may have significant immunologic implications that largely determine its impact on short- and long-term graft prognosis (see Chapter 9). The ischemia reperfusion injury may cause upregulation and exposure of histocompatability antigens, costimulatory molecules, and adhesion molecules (see Chapter 2). Nitric oxide, produced by the nitric oxide synthase enzymes, may provide the link between injury and immune activation. Activation of inflammatory cytokines and growth factors (epidermal growth factor and transforming growth factor β) may facilitate the development of low-grade inflammation, which, in turn, facilitates acute and chronic immune injury, the sequence thus being *injury–inflammation–immune response–further injury*. Immunologic factors may also make the kidney more susceptible to injury as illustrated by the observation that patients receiving a second transplant with high levels of preformed antibodies are more likely to develop ATN.

Prevention and Management

Prevention is better than cure! Assiduous attention to pretransplant donor care and intraoperative hemodynamic management (see Chapter 5) with minimization of cold ischemia time may reduce the incidence of delayed graft function, particularly for older donors. Pretransplant dialysis should be avoided when possible. Delayed graft function complicates management because it masks clinical detection of posttransplant events. Graft thrombosis and acute rejection are difficult to detect in an anuric or oliguric patient, and a urine leak will not manifest itself if the kidney does not make urine. Thus, in this situation, there must be greater reliance on noninvasive imaging studies to assess the status of the allograft. Doppler ultrasound or scintigraphic scanning should be performed at regular intervals to ensure maintenance of blood flow and to rule out urine leak and obstruction (see Chapter 12). Core biopsy should be performed at 7- to 10-day intervals to ensure that the diagnosis is indeed ATN and not early acute rejection.

The fact that ATN is unusual in recipients of living donor transplant emphasizes the factors, listed in Table 8.3, that need to be addressed if ATN is to be prevented in recipients of deceased donor kidneys. Programs that avoid the use of "marginal kidneys" (see Chapter 5) and insist on short cold ischemia times can reduce their incidence of ATN to less than 5%. Many programs accept a higher incidence as an unavoidable consequence of the pressure to provide kidneys to the growing population of patients in need (see Chapter 1). There are also important financial implications to the development of posttransplant ATN because the hospital stay is often prolonged and the immunosuppressive protocol used may be more expensive.

Some transplant programs modify their immunosuppressive protocols in the presence of ATN, or in its anticipation, usually on the premise that the calcineurin inhibitors should be avoided or minimized in these situations (see Chapter 4, Part IV). Their avoidance may reduce the length of the oliguric period, but the incidence of delayed graft function is not clearly lower with alternative protocols. Some programs routinely use depleting antibodies in the presence of anticipated or established delayed graft function and there is evidence that commencing the antibody infusion prior to the graft reperfusion may be beneficial, presumably because of suppression of adhesion and costimulatory molecule expression. Clinical trials of oxygen free radical scavengers, prostaglandin E analogues, pentoxyphylline, and monoclonal antibodies against the intercellular adhesion molecule (ICAM)-1 have not shown benefit. Sirolimus may delay recovery from ATN by inhibiting the regenerative response of tubular cells, and some programs avoid its administration in the presence of ATN (see Chapter 4, Part I).

Prognostic Implications

The reported impact of delayed graft function on long-term graft survival and function has been the subject of much controversy. Some studies report little or no impact, while others report a greater than 20% reduction in 1-year graft survival when early graft function is impaired. Much of the discrepancy can be probably accounted for by failure to differentiate between ATN and other causes of delayed function. There are also degrees of ATN severity and patients who require prolonged posttransplant dialysis are clearly at increased risk of early graft loss. Kidneys with ATN that do not develop rejection appear to do as well in the short-term as kidneys without ATN that do not develop rejection. Rejection is more likely to occur "silently" in patients with ATN, and delay in diagnosis of rejection may be help explain the impact of ATN on long-term function. Hence it is the immunologic consequences of ATN that appear to be responsible for its prognostic significance. Highly matched kidneys may be less susceptible to the harmful affects of delayed graft function presumably because ATN exposes the mismatched kidney to a more aggressive immune attack. In addition to any acute or chronic repercussions of ATN, it also complicates patient management, and every attempt should be made to minimize its frequency and severity.

Early Transplant Rejection

Accelerated Acute Rejection

Accelerated acute rejection is caused by presensitization and is mediated by antibodies to donor human leukocyte antigens (HLAs). The rejection occurs after an anamnestic response, and a critical level of antibodies is produced that results in an irreversible vascular rejection. Accelerated rejection can occur immediately posttransplant (hyperacute rejection), or it may be delayed by several days. Because of assiduous attention to the pretransplant cross-match (see Chapter 3), it occurs rarely. Patients are usually anuric or oliguric and often have fever and graft tenderness. The renal scan shows little or no uptake, and there may be evidence of intravascular coagulation. The differential diagnosis in this setting includes both arterial and venous thrombosis; however, patients with these vascular complications are frequently asymptomatic. Prompt surgical exploration of the allograft is indicated, and when in doubt an intraoperative biopsy is performed to determine its viability. The pathology of accelerated acute rejection is described in Chapter 13.

Early Cell-Mediated Rejection

Classic cell-mediated rejection can be detected in the latter part of the first transplant week, although it typically occurs somewhat later. Patients who have had recent blood transfusions, especially those patients who have donor-specific blood transfusions, may develop a typical reversible cell-mediated rejection very early in the first posttransplant week. These cell-mediated rejections can be differentiated from accelerated rejection by a renal scan or Doppler ultrasound, which show decreased but persistent perfusion. The differential diagnosis of acute rejection is discussed below (see "Antibody-Mediated Rejection"). At this early stage, kidney biopsy is mandatory for diagnosis. Treatment of acute rejection is discussed in Chapter 4, and pathology is discussed in Chapter 12.

Antibody-Mediated Rejection

The availability of the C4d stain as a marker of humoral injury has permitted the recognition of a form of antibody-mediated rejection or humoral rejection that is more discrete in its clinical and pathologic manifestations than the accelerated acute rejection described above (see "Accelerated Acute Rejection"). This form of antibody-mediated rejection usually occurs in the first few weeks posttransplant, and often, but not always, in the presence of presensitization. It typically presents as an asymptomatic elevation in the serum creatinine level and transplant biopsy is required for diagnosis. Morphologic features may be minimal with tubular injury being the only manifestation in some cases. The diagnosis requires the finding of diffuse C4d staining. The full range of morphologic features are discussed in Chapter 13. Where possible, the donor–recipient cross-match should be repeated; in most cases, donor-specific antibodies can be detected.

The diagnosis of antibody-mediated rejection is easy to miss and the clinical events ascribed to ATN if appropriate pathologic expertise is not available. Diagnosis is critical because this form of rejection does not typically respond to high-dose steroids. It does respond to treatment with intravenous immune globulin (IVIG) that may be combined with plasmapheresis in some protocols (see Chapter 4, Part V). Cell-mediated rejection may accompany or follow the antibody-mediated process and needs to be treated accordingly.

Nonimmunologic Causes of Graft Dysfunction

There are a variety of nonimmunologic causes of graft dysfunction in the early posttransplant period. Technical vascular complications such as renal artery or renal vein thrombosis may result in abrupt loss of function. Urologic complications such as obstruction, urine leaks from the ureteroneocystostomy, or necrosis of the ureter can present with deterioration in kidney function, increased pain over the allograft, or drainage of fluid through the wound. The combination of Doppler ultrasound and renal scan can be extremely useful in determining the diagnosis. In cases of obstruction, an antegrade pyelogram provides the most accurate localization of the obstruction (see Chapter 11). In patients with a suspected urine leak associated with wound drainage, a prompt diagnosis can be made if after the intravenous infusion of indigo carmine, the drainage turns blue, or if the creatinine concentration of the fluid is greater than the simultaneously measured plasma level. Heavy or persistent drainage should always raise the possibility of a urine leak and checking the creatinine concentration in the drain fluid is a rapid way to exclude the diagnosis.

The use of the calcineurin inhibitors during the first week after transplantation may result in abnormalities in graft function (see Chapter 4). The recovery from ATN may be delayed, and even in patients with excellent graft function, these drugs, on occasion, cause an abrupt deterioration in function that needs to be differentiated from early rejection or graft thrombosis. This response is most likely caused by renal vasoconstriction and can be reversed by decreasing the calcineurin inhibitor dose. Patients with thrombogenic tendencies, typically those with systemic lupus erythematosus, must be diagnosed in the pretransplant setting and prompt anticoagulation is begun early posttransplant (see Chapter 7). The failure to do so can result early posttransplant thrombosis and graft loss.

Posttransplant Thrombotic Microangiopathy

Both calcineurin inhibitors may induce a de novo thrombotic microangiopathy (TMA). The pathogenesis and morphologic findings are discussed in Chapter 4, Part I, and in Chapter 13. TMA may be localized within the kidney transplant or be associated with a full-blown hemolytic uremic syndrome (HUS). A C4d stain should always be performed since TMA may also be a manifestation antibody mediated rejection. Cases of TMA have also been described in patients receiving OKT3 and sirolimus used alone or in combination with calcineurin inhibitor. The frequency varies depending on how it is defined. Evidence of intrarenal TMA has been described in approximately 15% of transplants, with HUS occurring in up to 3% of cases. HUS may be evident clinically by virtue of the typical laboratory findings of varying degrees of renal impairment with evidence of intravascular coagulation (e.g., thrombocytopenia, distorted erythrocytes, elevated lactic dehydrogenase levels) accompanied by an arteriolopathy and intravascular thrombi on transplant biopsy. Development of calcineurin inhibitor-induced TMA may be covert, however, and the laboratory findings may be minimal and inconsistent. The syndrome may occur soon after the introduction of the calcineurin inhibitor, but it also may be delayed; blood levels of cyclosporine and tacrolimus are not necessarily elevated. The initial transplant biopsy may also be misleading, so that a high level of clinical suspicion is required. Full-blown posttransplant HUS can lead to dialysis dependence and graft loss. It is critical to make the diagnosis early because improvement in transplant function may follow discontinuation or reduction of calcineurin inhibitor and institution of plasmapheresis.

Medical Management in the First Week

Cardiovascular and hemodynamic stability remain extremely important during the first week following transplantation to ensure adequate perfusion of the allograft. While control of hypertension during the first week following transplantation is important, tight control should be avoided to prevent episodes of orthostatic hypotension. Calcium channel blockers are effective and well-tolerated antihypertensive agents, and they have some theoretical and practical advantages over other agents (see

Chapters 4 and 9). Angiotensin-converting enzyme (ACE) inhibitors are effective and can be used safely in the early posttransplant period, although some programs prefer to avoid them for fear of inducing graft disfunction.

Changes in immunosuppressive strategy during the first week following transplantation should be based as much as possible on the results of diagnostic studies. Combined therapeutic and diagnostic maneuvers can be useful on a short-term basis; for example, a decrease in graft function after institution of cyclosporine or tacrolimus can be managed by withholding or reducing the dose for a day or two. Other causes of kidney dysfunction must be ruled out by noninvasive studies. More aggressive pursuit of a definitive diagnosis with core kidney biopsy should be considered in patients with significant risk factors, including highly sensitized individuals, patients who have had a previous, rapidly rejected kidney transplant, and patients who have native kidney diseases with a high risk of early recurrence. Generally speaking, core kidney biopsies are riskier in the first week because there may be a greater incidence of bleeding.

The Surgical Incision

With modern surgical techniques and prophylactic perioperative antibiotics, significant wound infections and problems have become infrequent following transplantation. Obese patients are more susceptible to wound dehiscence and infection, especially if treated with high-dose sirolimus, a potent antiproliferative immunosuppressive drug. A serosanguineous incisional ooze is not uncommon posttransplant and, if it is profuse enough that it can be collected into a syringe, its creatinine concentration should be measured to ensure that it is not a urine leak. Staples and sutures are usually removed at 14 to 21 days.

THE FIRST THREE POSTOPERATIVE MONTHS

The 2-month period is characterized by the transition from inpatient to outpatient management. Most stable patients are discharged 4 to 10 days postoperatively. Transplant centers vary with respect to their enthusiasm for early discharge, and logistical issues, such as travel distance to the transplant center and the availability of a helpmate, need to be considered. Before discharge, it is critical to counsel the patient about his or her medications. The patient should be familiar with the medication names, doses, and purposes, as well as their side effects and possible drug interactions, especially with cyclosporine. Diet, exercise, and wound care are discussed. The patient can be encouraged to ambulate and to begin light aerobic exercise by walking or exercise biking. Premenopausal, sexually active female patients must receive contraceptive counseling because many women presume, often mistakenly, that they are still infertile. Patients must be taught to recognize the symptoms and signs of infection and rejection. It is wise to instruct patients to maintain a diary of their vital signs, urine output, and medications. Patients should be warned and prepared for the possibility of readmission to the hospital.

Discharge from the hospital often engenders anxious anticipation in both the patient and family members, and empathic counseling should be available on an informal and formal level.

Clinical Course

By the second posttransplant week, the graft function of most patients with delayed graft function caused by ATN begins to improve. Some patients remain oliguric for several weeks, and constant surveillance for covert rejection and urologic complications is required (see "Patients with Delayed Graft Function," above). Patients who still require dialysis can receive it on an outpatient basis.

Because many of the patients are at home during this period, close attention to the development of allograft pain, fever, weight gain, or decreased urine output is important. If any of these signs or symptoms occur, patients are instructed to contact the transplant team, whose representatives must be available on a 24-hour basis. Optimally, patients without complications should be seen as outpatients at least twice weekly for the first month and weekly for the following month. During each outpatient visit, a routine physical examination is required to assess the volume status, adjust blood pressure medications, and examine the allograft to detect enlargement, tenderness, or the presence of a new bruit. Routine laboratory work should include a urinalysis, complete blood count, plasma creatinine and blood urea nitrogen levels, and an electrolyte panel that includes phosphate and calcium levels. Hepatic enzyme levels should be checked regularly.

At each clinic visit, the medications should be carefully reviewed with the patient, and changes, particularly of critical immunosuppressive medications, should be explained with great care. At this stage, the patient is often taking a multitude of medications—immunosuppressives, antihypertensives, and infection prophylactic agents. Every attempt should be made to simplify the therapeutic regimen and to reemphasize the importance of adherence. Meticulous attention to detail is crucial in this posttransplant period, and early intervention is necessary to minimize morbidity and mortality.

Well patients should gradually return to normal activity, and some patients will wish to return to work after 4 to 6 weeks. A 3-month leave of absence from work is legitimate. Regular, graduated aerobic exercise should be encouraged, and normal social and family life should resume.

The Differentiation of Infection, Rejection, and Cyclosporine Toxicity

The accurate recognition and treatment of infection, rejection, and drug toxicity and their differentiation from surgical posttransplant complications is a constant concern in the early posttransplant period. The treatment of common posttransplant infections is discussed in Chapter 10, and the treatment of rejection is discussed in Chapter 4, Part V.

Fever

Fever may indicate either rejection or infection, although in the current era of potent immunosuppression, rejection is usually not associated with fever. Infection during the first month is occasionally caused by opportunistic organisms, but usually results from bacterial pathogens in the wound, urinary tract, or respiratory tract. Cytomegalovirus (CMV) infection may mimic acute rejection; it occurs in approximately 20% to 30% of patients 1 to 3 months posttransplantation (see Chapter 10), and its possible presence needs to be constantly considered, particularly in recipients of kidneys from CMV-positive donors.

Posttransplant fever must always be taken seriously. Acute rejection will often be present with seemingly innocuous flu-like symptoms or upper respiratory tract infection. The fever and the symptoms consistently, and usually rapidly, resolve when the rejecting patient receives antirejection therapy (see Chapter 4). Febrile patients should have a chest x-ray and be fully cultured. They usually require readmission to the hospital or very close outpatient followup.

The Elevated Creatinine Level

Measurement of the serum creatinine level is a simple, inexpensive diagnostic test that lies at the core of early posttransplant management. Its significance is not lost on patients, who often wait in trepidation at each clinic visit for their creatinine "verdict." Large elevations in plasma creatinine concentration (i.e., greater than 25% from baseline) almost always indicate a significant, potentially graft-endangering event. Smaller elevations may represent laboratory variability, and recognition of their significance is sometimes more of an art form than a science. If there is any question regarding a small asymptomatic rise in the plasma creatinine concentration, the test should be repeated within 48 hours, and the directional change will usually facilitate its clinical evaluation.

Potential anatomic or surgical cause of graft dysfunction must be ruled out before "medical" diagnoses are made to explain deteriorating graft function. Doppler ultrasound is an invaluable noninvasive diagnostic tool (see Chapter 12), and it should be performed before any major therapeutic intervention. Isotope scans are nonspecific in the setting of ATN, rejection, or calcineurin inhibitor toxicity, and the test is of limited diagnostic value at this stage. Clinical differentiation between acute rejection and other causes of graft dysfunction is notoriously unreliable even in experienced hands. The gold-standard diagnostic tool is the kidney biopsy (see Chapter 12). The timing and frequency of kidney biopsies vary between centers. One clinical approach to graft dysfunction is to make a therapeutic intervention empirically based on the clinical presentation and laboratory values. A favorable response confirms the diagnosis, but a lack of a response will likely require a tissue diagnosis.

The safety of renal transplant biopsy and reluctance to employ empiric therapy has popularized a more aggressive approach to graft dysfunction whereby a kidney biopsy is performed when the serum creatinine rises by approximately 25% over the baseline value or fails to fall from a high baseline level. Therapy is then based on the histologic findings. This approach should always be taken for patients deemed to be at high immunologic risk because of high levels of panel reactive antibodies, retransplant, combined kidney–pancreas transplantation, or kidney diseases associated with early recurrence. In each transplant center, a protocol should be developed that logically incorporates both non-invasive and invasive techniques to evaluate allograft dysfunction during this time period.

Cyclosporine and Tacrolimus Levels

Guidelines for trough and peak levels of cyclosporine and trough levels of tacrolimus are provided in Chapter 4, Part IV. It is clear that high blood levels do not preclude a diagnosis of rejection and that nephrotoxicity may occur at apparently low levels. This form of drug nephrotoxicity is caused by intense, yet reversible, arteriolar vasoconstriction (see Chapter 4, Fig. 4.3). Nephrotoxicity and rejection may also coexist. With these provisos, however, it is fair to initially presume that a patient with deteriorating graft function and a very high cyclosporine or tacrolimus level is probably toxic, and that a patient with deteriorating graft function and very low levels is probably rejecting. If the appropriate empiric clinical therapeutic response does not have a salutary effect on graft function, the clinical premise needs to be reconsidered. Drug toxicity usually resolves within 24 to 48 hours of a dose reduction. Progressive elevation of the plasma creatinine level even in the face of persistently high drug levels is highly suggestive of rejection. A greater than 50% increase in the creatinine level is more likely to be caused by rejection than by drug toxicity.

Graft Tenderness

Graft tenderness on palpation in the first few days posttransplant is usually an innocuous finding related to recent surgery. In a stable patient, it is important to regularly palpate the graft to provide a clinical baseline for future changes. The development of graft tenderness in a previously pain-free, stable patient is a significant symptom that needs to be evaluated. A tender, swollen graft in a patient with a rising creatinine concentration and fever usually indicates rejection, or acute pyelonephritis. Drug toxicity and CMV infection do not produce graft tenderness. Excruciating localized perinephric pain is usually caused by a urine leak.

Fluid Retention and Oliguria

Both rejection and calcineurin inhibitor toxicity may produce weight gain and edema as a result of GFR and avid tubular sodium reabsorption. Rejection episodes may be preceded by hypertension, possibly because of concomitant salt retention. Mild peripheral edema is common in stable patients receiving calcineurin inhibitors and usually responds to oral furosemide. Both acute rejection and calcineurin inhibitor toxicity can produce graft dysfunction in the absence of oliguria. Oliguria is common in acute rejection but makes a diagnosis of calcineurin inhibitor toxicity unlikely.

Unexpected Causes of Graft Dysfunction

After anatomic and hemodynamic causes of graft dysfunction have been excluded, there is an understandable tendency to presume that an elevated creatinine level is always due to acute cellular rejection, as calcineurin inhibitor toxicity. The critical advantage of a histologic diagnosis is that it permits diagnoses of other causes of graft dysfunction that may present solely as an elevated creatinine. These diagnoses include polyoma virus infection (see Chapters 10 and 13), TMA, posttransplant lymphoma (see Chapter 9), antibody mediated rejection, recurrent renal disease (see Chapter 9), and acute pyelonephritis (see Chapters 10 and 13). Each of these diagnoses requires radically different forms of therapeutic intervention, and histologic guidance is mandatory.

Innovative Techniques for the Diagnosis of Rejection

Although reliance on repeated estimations of the serum creatinine level and waiting for the level to rise is a timeworn and invaluable clinical technique of diagnosing allograft rejection, it is intellectually unsatisfying. Clearly there must be potentially recognizable intragraft events that precede the fall in GFR and the rise in creatinine level. The ability to reliably diagnose rejection in its early stages would represent a major step forward in transplant diagnostics and therapeutics.

Protocol Biopsies

Up to 30% of clinically stable patients may experience so-called subclinical rejection episodes that do not produce overt renal dysfunction or elevation in serum creatinine values. Subclinical rejections are typically mild by pathologic criteria (Banff type 1, see Chapter 13). Recognition of subclinical rejection requires uniform performance of protocol biopsies at prespecified posttransplant intervals. The approach to treatment and long-term impact of these episodes is unresolved, although a prospective study has shown that treatment with corticosteroids may lead to a reduction in the incidence of clinical rejections and improvement in long-term function and histology. Protocol biopsies performed for clinical purposes have not yet become standard practice in most transplant centers although they represent a potentially valuable approach to management.

Immune Monitoring

The potential clinical uses of immune monitoring are discussed in Chapters 2 and 3. Measurement of urinary perforins and granzymes are the most promising available techniques. Validation of their reliability in large populations, and their capacity to clearly differentiate between immune activation as a result of rejection and other causes of inflammation, remain to be determined before these techniques are widely employed clinically.

Common Laboratory Abnormalities in the Early Posttransplant Period

Urinalysis

Examination of the urine for the presence of red and white blood cells, bacteria, and protein should be part of the routine outpatient visit. Pyuria can indicate either rejection or infection, and the urine should be cultured. The presence of proteinuria may herald the early recurrence of the primary kidney disease or chronic rejection. Trace or "one-plus" proteinuria, amounting to less than 500 mg daily, is usually not a morbid finding. Transient microscopic hematuria is common posttransplant, but requires urologic evaluation if it is persistent.

Hyperkalemia and Hypokalemia

Elevated serum potassium levels are not uncommon in the first few posttransplant months in patients receiving calcineurin inhibitors. As long as the patient is not oliguric and kidney function is good, this hyperkalemia is rarely dangerous and can usually be managed safely with dietary potassium restriction and diuretics. Occasionally, Florinef use can be effective. Care should be taken to avoid concomitant use of drugs that may further exaggerate hyperkalemia such as ACE inhibitors, beta blockers, and phosphate supplements. Hypokalemia is usually caused by diuretic administration, and it may be exaggerated by hypomagnesemia. Sirolimus use has been associated with hypokalemia.

Hypophosphatemia, Hypercalcemia, and Hypomagnesemia

The mechanisms of posttransplant hypophosphatemia and abnormalities of divalent ion metabolism are discussed in Chapter 9. Profound hypophosphatemia may develop in the first few weeks posttransplant, particularly in patients with excellent graft function, and up to 25% of patients develop some degree of hypophosphatemia within the first 3 posttransplant months. Phosphate supplements, usually in the form of Neutra-Phos, in a dose of 250 to 500 mg three times daily should be given if the serum phosphate levels fall below 2.5 mg/dL (see Chapter 17). Phosphate supplementation is usually adequate to control mild posttransplant hypercalcemia, which is usually a manifestation of residual hyperparathyroidism. Magnesium supplements should be given for calcineurin inhibitor-induced hypomagnesemia if the serum magnesium level falls below 1.5 mg/dL.

Hyperchloremic Metabolic Acidosis

Proximal, distal, and type IV renal tubular acidosis have been described to occur posttransplant; mild hyperchloremia and hypobicarbonatemia are also common. Renal tubular acidosis may be a manifestation of immune-mediated impairment of hydrogen ion secretion; of acute or chronic interstitial renal disease impairing tubular ammonia secretion; of parathyroid hormone-induced reduction in proximal tubular bicarbonate reabsorption; or of calcineurin inhibitor-induced impairment in tubular aldosterone responsiveness. The ensuing metabolic acidosis is usually not so severe that it requires therapeutic intervention, and the finding is too nonspecific to be of much diagnostic value.

Anemia, Leukopenia, and Thrombocytopenia

Cytopenias are common in the posttransplant period. Profound anemia at the time of transplantation is much less common in the present erythropoietin era. Erythropoietin is usually discontinued at the time of transplantation, and the hematocrit level may fall posttransplant and then rise toward normal over weeks and months. The posttransplant fall may sometimes be so rapid as to suggest bleeding. Resistant anemia needs to be evaluated, with the possibility of gastrointestinal bleeding high on the differential diagnosis. Patients may be iron deficient and intravenous iron replacement is often required to replete iron stores. In anticipation of a rising hematocrit as renal function improves, there may be a temptation to permit patients to remain anemic unnecessarily. Patients whose baseline graft function is impaired should be regarded to have a degree of chronic kidney disease and should be treated with adequate doses of erythropoietin. Posttransplant infection with parvovirus should be considered in iron replete patients with severe resistant anemia. ACE inhibitors and angiotensin-receptor blockers may contribute to anemia.

Patients receiving azathioprine often develop macrocytosis, and all the antiproliferative drugs (azathioprine, mycophenolate mofetil, sirolimus) may produce varying degrees of pancytopenia (see Chapter 4). A complete blood count should be performed at least weekly in the early posttransplant period and less frequently with time. In the absence of clinical evidence of infection, thrombocytopenia and leukopenia are usually drug related. Because the calcineurin inhibitors generally do not cause hematologic abnormalities, it is usually safe to continue them and to reduce the dose or discontinue other components of the immunosuppressive regimen for a short time, until the abnormality resolves. If leukopenia is severe, granulocyte-stimulating factor can be given; it appears to be safe in the posttransplant period. Posttransplant polycythemia is discussed in Chapter 9.

Transaminitis

Elevation of the levels of the hepatic transaminases associated with discrete alterations in hepatic function is common posttransplant and is usually a transient and self-limiting manifestation of drug toxicity. More severe manifestations of liver disease may require further investigation and modification of the immunosuppressive regimen (see Chapter 11).

EARLY POSTTRANSPLANT MORTALITY

The overall mortality in the first posttransplant year is approximately 5% and approximately two-thirds of this mortality takes place within the first 3 months. Mortality rates are several-fold higher in older patients than in younger patients, and are higher in recipients of deceased donor kidneys and "marginal" kidneys (see Chapter 5). Approximately 40% of the mortality has been ascribed to cardiovascular disease and close to 30% to infectious disease. Particular care must be taken to optimize standard cardioprotective therapy in high cardiac risk patients with perioperative cardiac monitoring and appropriate use of beta blockers, ACE inhibitors, aspirin, and statins.

SELECTED READINGS

Blydt-Hansen T, Katori M, Lassman C, et al. Gene transfer-induced local heme oxygenase-1 overexpression protects rat kidney transplants from ischemia/reperfusion injury. *J Am Soc Nephrol* 2003;14:745–754.

Cosio FG, Pelletier R, Pesavento TE, et al. Elevated blood pressure predicts the risk of acute rejection in renal allograft recipients. *Kidney Int* 2001;59:1158–1164.

Dragun D, Hoff U, Park JK. Ischemia-reperfusion injury in renal transplantation is independent of the immunologic background. *Kidney Int* 2000;58:2166–2177.

Gill JS, Periera BJ. Death in the first year post-transplant: implications for patients on the transplant waiting list. *Transplantation* 2003;75:113–118.

Jani A, Polhemus C Corrigan G, et al. Determinants of hypofiltration during acute renal allograft rejection. *J Am Soc Nephrol* 2002;13:773–778.

McGilvray I, Lajoie G, Humar A, et a1. Polyoma virus infection and acute vascular rejection in a kidney allograft: coincidence or mimicry? *Am J Transplant* 2003;3:501–504.

McTaggart RA, Gottlieb D, Brooks J, et al. Sirolimus prolongs recovery from delayed graft function after cadaveric renal transplantation. *Am J Transplant* 2003;3:416–423.

Morrissey PE, Ramirez PJ, Gohh RY, et al. Management of thrombophilia in renal transplant patients. *Am J Transplant* 2002;2:872–876.

Ojo AO, Wolfe RA, Held PJ, et al. Delayed graft function: risk factors and implications for renal allograft survival. *Transplantation* 1997;63:968–974.

Qureshi F, Rabb H, Kasiske B. Silent acute rejection during prolonged delayed graft function reduces kidney allograft survival. *Transplantation* 2002;74:1400–1404.

Rush D. Protocol biopsies should be part of the routine management of kidney transplant recipients. *Am J Kidney Dis* 2002;40:671–673.

Sayegh MH, Colvin RB. Case record of the Massachusetts General Hospital. Weekly clinicopathological exercises. Case 8-2003. A 35-year-old man with early dysfunction of a second renal transplant. *N Engl J Med* 2003;348:1033–1044.

Shoskes DA, Halloran P. Delayed graft function in renal transplantation: etiology, management and long-term significance. *J Urology* 1996;155:1831–1840.

Schwimmer J, Nadasdy T, Spitalnik PF. *De novo* thrombotic microangiopathy in renal transplant recipients: a comparison of hemolytic uremic syndrome with localized renal thrombotic microangiopathy. *Am J Kidney Dis* 2003;41:471–479.

Woo YM, Jardine AG, Clark AF, et al. Early graft function and patient survival following cadaveric renal transplantation. *Kidney Int* 1999;55:692–699.

Long-Term Posttransplant Management and Complications

Meena Sahadevan and Bertram L. Kasiske

CURRENT SUCCESS AND FUTURE CHALLENGE

The care of renal transplant recipients can be roughly divided into early and late posttransplant periods. This division, although somewhat arbitrary, is justified by the fact that episodes of acute allograft rejection are most common in the first few months after transplantation when relatively large amounts of immunosuppressive medications, with their potential for complications, must be administered. For patients who survive the first few months with a functioning allograft, doses of immunosuppression can then usually be reduced. Most statistical analyses use 12 months to define the onset of the late posttransplant period. For example, the United Network for Organ Sharing (UNOS) Scientific Registry usually reports short-term survival and graft survival beyond the first year separately as major posttransplant outcomes.

The incidence of acute rejection and early graft failure has declined dramatically as a result of new immunosuppressive medications (see Chapter 4). One-year graft survival is now close to 90% in most transplant centers. There is also evidence that there was an improvement in the long-term stability of renal function in the decade between 1990 and 2000. This success has occurred despite the fact that the risk of graft failure has increased with the acceptance of transplant candidates who are older and who have more cardiovascular disease and other risk factors (see Chapter 6). In addition, the shortage of deceased donor organs has encouraged centers to accept older, "expanded criteria" donors that also add to the risk for graft failure (see "Expanded Criteria Donors" in Chapters 3 and 5). It would appear, therefore, that the new immunosuppressive regimens have helped to overcome this increased risk, reducing the rate of graft failure.

The rate of late renal allograft failure is often measured by graft half-life. Allograft half-life is the time that 50% of the patients who survive beyond the first year posttransplant are still alive with a functioning kidney. Therefore, half-life is determined by both the rate of death and return to dialysis (or retransplantation). There has been an increase in renal allograft half-life in the past several years (see Chapter 3). For patients receiving deceased donor renal transplants in 1988, the half-life was 7.6 years, whereas for those receiving deceased donor renal transplants in 1995, the half-life had increased to 11.6 years. However, the half-life of two-haplotype-matched living-related kidney recipients over this same time period was 22.8 years. This suggests that there remains a long way to go before the half-life for deceased donor renal transplants can be considered optimal.

This chapter is divided into two main sections. Part I reviews the causes and pathogenesis of late renal allograft failure. Part II offers a practical guide to the prevention of graft failure and other major complications of the late posttransplant period. Important topics in long-term management are discussed elsewhere in this book. Long-term immunosuppressive therapy and the immunosuppressive management of chronic allograft failure is discussed in Chapter 4, Part V; posttransplant infectious disease is discussed in Chapter 10; posttransplant liver disease is discussed in Chapter 11; and medication noncompliance is discussed in Chapter 19. Readers are also referred to the American Society of Transplantation's *Guidelines on the Outpatient Surveillance of Renal Allograft Recipients* (see Kasiske et al. in Part II of "Selected Readings," below).

PART I. CAUSES OF LATE ALLOGRAFT FAILURE

DEFINING THE CAUSE OF ALLOGRAFT FAILURE

It is more difficult to define the cause of allograft failure than it may seem. Allograft failure is usually defined either by the patient's death or by the patient's need to undertake new treatment for end-stage renal disease (ESRD) (i.e., chronic dialysis or retransplantation). Making a distinction between these two categories of allograft failure may have important implications for understanding how to prevent allograft failure. However, making the distinction may sometimes be difficult. For example, a patient with severe acute rejection may require dialysis support and may die of complications of immunosuppression before the rejection can be reversed. Did this patient die with a functioning graft, or was the graft loss because of acute rejection? Studies show, however, that most patients who die with a functioning graft have good allograft function (so-called death with graft function). In these cases, attempts to understand the pathogenesis of allograft failure should focus on understanding the cause of death and its pathogenesis.

In the United States, death with graft function accounts for 40% to 50% of all graft losses (Fig. 9.1). The goal of renal transplantation should be to have every patient who dies do so with a kidney that functions well. Unfortunately, most deaths that now occur with a functioning allograft are premature and are potentially preventable. Most of the premature deaths that occur in the late posttransplant period can be directly or indirectly attributed to the events that initially led to ESRD and the consequences thereof (see Chapter 1), and to allograft dysfunction or the immunosuppression used to prevent or treat allograft rejection. The three most commonly defined causes of death in the late posttransplant period are *cardiovascular disease* (CVD), *infection,* and *malignancy.*

CAUSES OF DEATH AFTER TRANSPLANTATION

Cardiovascular Disease

Atherosclerotic CVD kills patients by causing myocardial infarction, congestive heart failure, stroke, ischemic colitis, and peripheral vascular disease. In the case of ischemic colitis and

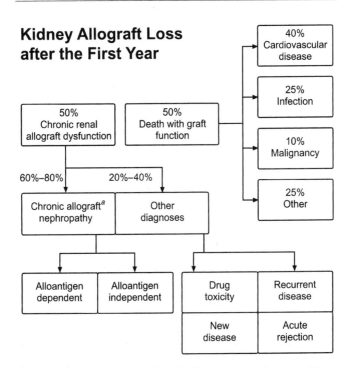

Fig. 9.1. Cause of graft loss after the first posttransplant year. Note that the percentages are approximations based on data from the United States Renal Data Systems report of 2003. [a]See Table 9.2. (Modified from Pascual M, Theruvath T, Kawai T, et al. Strategies to improve long-term outcomes after renal transplantation. *N Engl J Med* 2002;346:580–590, with permission.)

peripheral vascular disease, the terminal event may be infection (e.g., sepsis from a perforated cecum or cellulitis). To understand how to prevent posttransplant CVD deaths and complications, it is crucial to define the etiologic risk factors (Table 9.1). Identifying risk factors is important for two reasons. Some risk factors can be modified, and for some of these, there is strong evidence from studies in the general population that intervention improves survival. It is also important, however, to identify risk factors that cannot be modified because these risk factors help to identify high-risk patients who can be targeted for screening and possibly intervention, as well as for treatment of other modifiable risk factors.

Patients with pretransplant CVD are at increased risk for posttransplant CVD complications. Such patients should be targeted for aggressive management of modifiable CVD risk factors. Because atherosclerosis is often diffuse, it should not be surprising that patients with a history of cerebral vascular disease (e.g.,

Table 9.1.   Risk factors for posttransplant cardiovascular disease

Risk Factor	Strength of Evidence
Pretransplant cardiovascular disease	++++
Diabetes (including posttransplant diabetes)	++++
Cigarette smoking	+++
Hyperlipidemia	+++
Hypertension	++
Platelet and coagulation abnormalities	++
Allograft dysfunction/rejection	++
Hypoalbuminemia	++
Erythrocytosis	+
Oxygen free radicals	+
Infections	+
Increased homocysteine	+

ischemic strokes) are at increased risk for ischemic heart disease. Although pretransplant CVD greatly increases the risk for posttransplant CVD complications, much of the risk for CVD in the late posttransplant period is acquired after transplantation. Identifying and aggressively managing high-risk patients is important.

Diabetes is the most common cause of ESRD leading to transplantation, and diabetes is the most important risk factor for posttransplant CVD. Both type 1 and type 2 diabetes greatly increase the risk for ischemic heart disease, cerebral vascular disease, and peripheral vascular disease. Diabetic control may become difficult after transplantation and patients with type 2 diabetes often become insulin dependent.

Approximately 20% of nondiabetic patients develop hyperglycemia after transplantation, and 5% to 10% require therapy with oral hypoglycemic agents or insulin. Older patients, obese patients, blacks, and patients with a strong family history of diabetes are at higher risk for posttransplant diabetes. The effect of diabetes developed after transplantation on morbidity and graft survival is similar to that of pretransplant diabetes. Corticosteroids and the calcineurin inhibitors (tacrolimus more so than cyclosporine) all contribute in varying degrees to glucose intolerance (see Chapter 4).

Numerous epidemiologic studies of the general population show that cigarette smoking is an important modifiable risk factor for CVD. Studies report that smoking is as prevalent in renal transplant recipients as it is in the general population. These same studies show that cigarette smoking is linked to CVD in the late posttransplant period.

Countless epidemiologic studies and numerous large, randomized, controlled trials in the general population show that hyperlipidemia causes CVD. The evidence is strongest that elevations in low-density lipoprotein (LDL) cholesterol contribute to the pathogenesis of atherosclerosis; however, evidence is also very strong that low levels of high-density lipoprotein (HDL) cholesterol also contribute to CVD risk. In addition, there is growing evidence that hypertriglyceridemia is an independent risk factor for CVD in the general population. Several studies have found the same associations between lipoprotein elevations and CVD in renal transplant patients. The most important cause of hyperlipidemia after renal transplantation is immunosuppressive medication. Sirolimus, cyclosporine, tacrolimus (in order of severity) all cause elevations in lipid levels to varying degrees (see Chapter 4). Other causes include corticosteroid dose, diet, genetic predisposition, proteinuria, and possibly decreased renal function.

Data from several epidemiologic and interventional studies show that hypertension contributes to CVD in the general population, although it has proved difficult to demonstrate that hypertension specifically causes CVD in renal transplant recipients. This may be because most transplant physicians treat blood pressure aggressively. Corticosteroids and the calcineurin inhibitors (cyclosporine more so than tacrolimus) can elevate blood pressure after renal transplantation. Graft dysfunction also contributes to hypertension. Several studies also found that the presence of the native kidneys is associated with increased blood pressure after renal transplantation.

Observational studies found that allograft dysfunction is also associated with subsequent CVD complications. Decreased renal function and proteinuria can contribute to other risk factors, such as hyperlipidemia, hypertension, and hyperhomocysteinemia. Allograft dysfunction is also more common in patients who have had acute rejection and have been treated with higher doses of immunosuppressive medications known to affect several CVD risk factors adversely. In some studies, however, allograft dysfunction was an independent risk factor for CVD. It is speculated that allograft rejection may be associated with a systemic, inflammatory response that may contribute to the pathogenesis of CVD; at least one study shows that hypoalbuminemia is an independent risk factor for posttransplant CVD, and that chronic inflammation may reduce serum albumin levels. Atherosclerosis could be both a cause and an effect of chronic inflammation.

Although epidemiologic studies have often reported an association between antioxidant vitamin usage and CVD, more convincing clinical data supporting a role for oxygen free radicals in the pathogenesis of CVD has been elusive. In particular, most large, randomized, controlled trials in the general population have failed to show that antioxidant vitamins protect against CVD events. Some evidence suggests that oxygen free radicals may be more prevalent and that antioxidant defenses may be more compromised in renal transplant recipients than in the general population.

A number of epidemiologic studies implicate various infections, including cytomegalovirus (CMV) infection, in the pathogenesis of CVD. In addition, some studies have found evidence for the presence of infectious agents in atherosclerotic lesions. It is certainly plausible, however, that individuals with CVD may be more susceptible to infection and that infectious agents may play an innocent-bystander role in systemic atherosclerosis. One study found that heart transplant recipients treated with CMV prophylaxis had less coronary artery disease (CAD). On the other hand, few studies have found an association between CMV or other infections and CVD in renal transplant recipients, despite the fact that the prevalence of such infections is very high. Thus, this interesting hypothesis remains unproved.

A number of observational studies found a strong association between increased levels of plasma homocysteine and CVD in the general population. It has been suggested that homocysteine may cause vascular endothelial damage and thereby lead to atherosclerosis. A large, multicenter, randomized trial is being conducted in the United States to determine whether lowering homocysteine with a fortified multivitamin preparation will reduce the incidence of CVD events in the transplant population [the FAVORIT study (Folic Acid for Vascular Outcome in Transplantation)]. The result of this trial will be particularly important because elevated levels of homocysteine are more common in transplant patients than in the general population. This is no doubt largely a result of the fact that renal dysfunction itself, which is common in allograft recipients, elevates plasma homocysteine levels.

Infection

Specific posttransplant infections are discussed in Chapter 10. Infection is an inevitable consequence of immunosuppression. Whereas CVD is linked to immunosuppressive medications through their adverse (nonimmunosuppressive) effects, posttransplant infection is attributable to the overall level of immunosuppression. Certain infections occur more frequently at certain time frames from the transplant (see Chapter 10, Fig. 10.1). CMV is arguably the most common infection after renal transplantation. Infection occurs most often in the early posttransplant period when patients are most immunosuppressed. Fortunately, the availability of effective antiviral therapy has greatly reduced its lethal potential. Occasionally, patients will develop chronic retinitis from CMV infection, but this is rarely life-threatening. BK virus is a human polyomavirus that has emerged as a serious infection that can cause graft dysfunction and, ultimately, graft failure (see Chapters 10 and 13). It is critical to identify BK virus because its morphologic characteristics can be confused with acute rejection and the therapeutic response is based on minimization of immunosuppression. Chronic liver disease, usually caused by viral hepatitis, is an important cause of posttransplant mortality (see Chapter 11). The hepatitis C virus is the most common cause of hepatitis after renal transplantation. Influenza is an important cause of preventable morbidity and mortality after transplantation. Viral infections are associated with malignancy in the late posttransplant period.

Bacterial infections are common in the late posttransplant period because of underlying risk factors and immunosuppression. As previously discussed, the high prevalence of peripheral vascular disease among diabetic patients and other transplant recipients greatly increases the risk for cellulitis and life-threatening bacterial sepsis. Ischemic bowel disease can also lead to septic shock and death. Bladder dysfunction, caused by diabetes and other anatomic urologic abnormalities, combine with immunosuppression to increase the risk for urinary tract infections and gram-negative bacterial sepsis. Tuberculosis is common in the late posttransplant period, especially among high-risk populations.

Several other, potentially life-threatening, opportunistic infections occur sporadically, but are nevertheless relatively common in the late posttransplant period. Examples include infection with *Pneumocystis carinii, Toxoplasma gondii, Nocardia* species, *Aspergillus* species, *Listeria monocytogenes, Candida* species, *Cryptococcus neoformans, Histoplasma capsulatum, Coccidioides immitis,* and *Blastomyces dermatitidis.* Infection with opportunistic organisms can present as pneumonia, meningitis, cellulitis, osteomyelitis, or generalized sepsis. Diagnosis requires a high index of suspicion and an aggressive diagnostic approach.

Malignancy

Malignancies are common after renal transplantation; they are also more common in chronic dialysis patients. Much of our knowledge of the malignancy–transplantation association comes from large registries, such as the Israel Penn Transplant Tumor Registry and the Australia-New Zealand Dialysis and Transplant Registry. Readers are also referred to Feng et al., *Tumors in Transplantation: The 2003 Third Annual State ASTS State of the Art Winter Symposium* (see Part I of the "Selected Readings," below). These data indicate that the incidence of non-skin malignancies in renal transplant recipients is up to 3.5-fold higher than that of age-matched controls. This increase can be attributed to an increased incidence of most tumors. However, the observed-to-expected incidence (the standardized incidence ration) is not uniform among different types of tumors. Some tumors, such as lung cancer, breast cancer in women, and prostate cancer in men, do not appear to be more common among renal transplant recipients than among the general population. Colon cancer and renal cell carcinoma are more common than in the general population, although renal cell carcinoma may be no more common than in the dialysis population. The differences in the observed-to-expected incidence of different malignancies are consistent with the notion that more than one mechanism may explain the increased incidence of cancer after renal transplantation.

Some malignancies are undoubtedly caused by viral infections. Viruses that may otherwise reside in the host without untoward complications may cause potentially lethal malignant transformations in immunocompromised renal transplant recipients. Some of the tumors that occur with the highest incidence, as compared with the general population, have possible viral causes. For example, the posttransplant lymphoproliferative disorders (PTLDs) have been linked to infection caused by the Epstein-Barr virus. The human herpesvirus-8 has been implicated in the high incidence of Kaposi sarcoma after renal transplantation. Human papillomaviruses have been implicated in the pathogenesis of squamous cell cancer of the skin, vulva, vagina, and possibly uterine cervix. Liver cancer may be caused by chronic infection with hepatitis B and C viruses.

Urinary malignancies may occur more frequently among renal transplant recipients because renal disease may sometimes be associated with malignant and premalignant conditions such as acquired cystic disease of the native kidneys. Similarly, an increased risk for the rarely occurring parathyroid cancer may be attributable to long-standing renal disease and events occurring before transplantation.

Other mechanisms are undoubtedly at play. Immunosuppressive agents may damage deoxyribonucleic acid (DNA) and lead to malignant transformation of cells and may also inhibit normal immune surveillance and thereby allow cells that have undergone malignant transformation to grow and divide unchecked. In an animal model, cyclosporine has been shown to promote cancer progression by a direct transforming growth factor (TGF)-β–related cellular effect that is independent of the host's immune cells. The antiproliferative effect of sirolimus may theoretically protect against tumor development and progression, although the clinical significance of this observation has yet to be confirmed (see Chapter 4, Part I).

Malignancies may occur at any time after transplantation. However, some are more likely than others to occur early after transplantation. These include PTLD (relatively common) and Kaposi sarcoma (relatively rare). Most other tumors tend to occur later. In the Australia-New Zealand Dialysis and Transplantation Registry, the mean time to the diagnosis of non-Hodgkin lymphoma (PTLD) was 8 to 10 years after transplantation. Moreover the incidence of malignant tumors continues to increase throughout the late posttransplant period. The cumulative incidence of nonskin malignancies is approximately 33% by 30 years after transplantation. The cumulative incidence of skin cancer is much higher, but few patients die of skin cancer after renal transplantation.

Few studies have systematically examined risk factors for posttransplant malignancies. Most investigators believe that the cumulative effects of immunosuppression per se, rather than any particular agent or agents, is principally responsible for the increased incidence of nonskin malignancies after renal transplantation. Age increases the risk for posttransplant tumors, and it may be wise to minimize the amount of immunosuppression used in transplant recipients older than 60 or 65 years of age. Cigarette smoking is also associated with a higher risk for posttransplant malignancies.

Tumor markers, carcinoembryonic antigen (CEA), cancer antigen 125 (CA125), and CA15-3 have a low specificity and sensitivity as screeners for malignancies in renal transplant recipients. The value of routine screening of the transplant population for common cancers (breast, colorectal, prostate) has been questioned because the risk-to-benefit ratio of such screening may be less favorable in the transplant population than in the general population because the life expectancy of transplant patients is intrinsically limited. Decisions regarding cancer screening should be made on an individual basis.

CHRONIC ALLOGRAFT NEPHROPATHY

Chronic allograft nephropathy is second only to death with a functioning allograft function as the most common cause of late allograft failure. The term chronic allograft nephropathy is preferred to the frequently used chronic rejection because the etiology includes factors that can be considered both immune, or alloantigen dependent, and nonimmune, or alloantigen independent (Table 9.2). The distinction between alloantigen dependent and alloantigen independent is a convenient one, but multiple factors often coexist, and early events may program later events. For example, ischemic injury may make the graft more susceptible to acute rejection and graft survival is impaired in the presence of hypertension.

In 1953, in one of the first reports of successful human deceased donor renal transplantation, the transplant pioneer David Humes and coworkers described pathologic findings from a patient who died almost 6 months after cadaveric renal transplantation.

The tubular degeneration, casts, focal cellular infiltration, and interstitial edema were felt to be consistent with the picture of ischemic nephritis. There were striking changes in the intrinsic blood vessels. A severe degree of arteriosclerosis had developed. There was marked thickening of the intima with narrowing of the lumen, in some vessels almost to the point of occlusion. The inner portion of the intima showed dense sclerosis, and the outer portion, just within the inner elastic lamina, contained numerous lipid-laden macrophages.

Table 9.2.   Putative risk factors for chronic allograft nephropathy

Alloantigen-Dependent Risk Factors

Acute rejection
Histocompatibility mismatch
Prior sensitization
Suboptimal immunosuppression
Medication noncompliance
Ongoing humoral injury

Alloantigen-Independent Risk Factors

Ischemic injury and delayed graft function
Older donor age
Donor and recipient size mismatching
Calcineurin-inhibitor nephrotoxicity
Hyperlipidemia
Hypertension
Cigarette smoking
Hyperhomocysteinemia
Oxygen free radicals
Infection (e.g., cytomegalovirus)
Proteinuria

This description fits well with what we now call chronic allograft nephropathy, the histologic features of which are described in Chapter 13. Clinically, chronic allograft nephropathy presents in one of three ways:

1. As a finding in patients undergoing biopsy for an acute increase in serum creatinine or proteinuria.
2. As a finding in patients undergoing biopsy for gradually declining allograft function or proteinuria.
3. As a finding on a protocol biopsy obtained in patients with no clinical or laboratory abnormality.

The biopsy findings of chronic allograft nephropathy are often poor predictors of the subsequent clinical course, particularly if the histologic findings are mild. Functional studies tend to underestimate the extent of morphologic injury. Patients with transplant glomerulopathy or severe arterial lesions on biopsy often have progressive declines in renal function. The chronic allograft disease index (CADI) described in Chapter 13 is an attempt to improve the prognostic value of the biopsy findings of chronic allograft nephropathy. Although chronic allograft nephropathy is a useful term, it should not be used as a wastebasket and every attempt should be made by the pathologist to identify the predominant lesion. Chronic allograft nephropathy can be considered to represent the "cumulative and incremental damage from time-dependent immunologic and nonimmunologic cause" (see Nankivell et al. in Part I of the "Selected Readings," below).

Alloantigen-Dependent Risk Factors

The most convincing evidence that alloantigen-dependent factors are important in the pathogenesis of chronic allograft nephropathy comes from several epidemiologic studies demonstrating an association between acute and chronic rejection. There is now little doubt that patients who have acute rejection episodes are more likely than patients with no acute rejection to develop chronic allograft nephropathy; an episode of acute rejection in the first 6 months after transplantation increases the risk for late graft loss by up to 50%. Not all acute rejection episodes, however, lead to chronic allograft nephropathy, and it is difficult in individual patients with acute rejection to predict the likelihood of developing chronic allograft nephropathy. Acute rejections that occur late (after the first 3 months) appear to be more predictive of chronic allograft nephropathy than those that occur during the first 3 months. It is unclear, however, whether acute rejection episodes that occur late because of attempts to withdraw immunosuppressive agents are as predictive of chronic allograft nephropathy as those that occur late on full doses of immunosuppression. It is clear that acute rejections that are more severe, either by histology or by increase in serum creatinine, are also more likely than less-acute severe rejections to herald chronic allograft nephropathy. Finally, multiple acute rejections also appear to be more predictive of chronic allograft nephropathy.

The number of major histocompatibility complex (MHC) antigens that are mismatched between the recipient and donor is associated with chronic allograft nephropathy and late allograft failure (see Chapter 3, Fig 3.3). Clearly, deceased donor kidney transplants that have zero MHC mismatches have the best long-term allograft survival. Less marked, but nevertheless statistically significant, are differences in late allograft survival between kidneys that have one through six MHC mismatches. The effect of MHC mismatches on graft half-life is further evidence that alloantigen-dependent factors are important in the pathogenesis of chronic allograft nephropathy.

Studies have also found an association between detection of preformed antibodies (see Chapter 3) at the time of transplantation and subsequent chronic allograft nephropathy. In some studies, the absence of preformed antibodies has correlated with long-term allograft survival. Anti-HLA antibodies are consistently detectable in the months prior to recognition of chronic rejection, although their finding does not accurately predict its development. This observation, together with the widespread application of the C4d stain (see Chapter 13) in the evaluation of renal transplant biopsy specimens, has enhanced the emphasis of the role of ongoing humoral injury in chronic allograft nephropathy. In some studies, up to 60% of patients with chronic allograft nephropathy show evidence of antibody mediated injury. The therapeutic implications of this finding are discussed in Chapter 4, Part V.

If it could be shown that higher doses of immunosuppression prevented chronic allograft nephropathy, this would be further evidence that alloantigen-dependent factors are important. Data showing that higher doses or more potent immunosuppression reduces the incidence of chronic allograft nephropathy, however, are equivocal. It is noteworthy that the introduction of cyclosporine in the 1980s led to dramatic (25% to 30%) reductions in the rate of acute rejection early after transplantation and greatly improved 1-year graft survival in most programs. During this era, however, there was minimal improvement in graft half-life, suggesting that cyclosporine had little effect on chronic allograft nephropathy. The nephrotoxicity of the calcineurin inhibitors may have canceled the benefit that a reduced incidence of acute rejection from the use of calcineurin inhibitors may have had on chronic allograft nephropathy. In the 1990s, this trend may have abated with the more judicious use of the calcineurin inhibitors and the availability of nonnephrotoxic immunosuppressive agents. The use of mycophenolate mofetil for at least 1 year posttransplant reduces the incidence of chronic allograft nephropathy.

Several studies show that poor adherence to medications increases the likelihood of late graft failure, presumably from chronic allograft nephropathy. This, too, has been cited as evidence supporting the hypothesis that chronic allograft nephropathy is caused by alloantigen-dependent factors. These same patients are likely to be noncompliant with followup visits, limiting the ability to detect treatable acute rejection and increasing the risk for chronic allograft nephropathy. Patients who are noncompliant with immunosuppression, however, may also be noncompliant with antihypertensive agents, as well as other medications, which could increase the risk for chronic allograft nephropathy. Thus, it is difficult to attribute the adverse consequences of noncompliance entirely to alloantigen-dependent mechanisms causing chronic allograft nephropathy.

Alloantigen-Independent Risk Factors

Patients with delayed, or "slow," graft function have a higher rate of late allograft failure. The serum creatinine level at the time of discharge from hospital is a predictor of late graft loss (see Chapter 8). One theory holds that ischemic injury and delayed graft function result in a reduced number of functioning nephrons and that inadequate "nephron dosing" causes chronic allograft nephropathy and late allograft failure. However, delayed graft function is also associated with an increased incidence of acute rejection that could also explain its adverse effects on late graft survival. If true, this might suggest that close surveillance of patients for acute rejection during and after periods of delayed graft function could reduce the rate of late allograft failure.

Donor age is clearly associated with a higher rate of late allograft failure. Expanded criteria donor kidneys are defined by their higher incidence of late graft loss (see Chapter 5). Many of the histologic characteristics of chronic allograft nephropathy are similar to those seen in normal aging. It is unclear exactly how age of the kidney increases the risk for late allograft failure. The inadequate number of nephrons may create a physiologic response that sets in motion mechanisms ultimately leading to graft failure. The accelerated senescence theory proposes that the intrinsic age of the kidney (genetically determined in every cell and expressed in telomere length) limits its longevity in the recipient; the aging process is further accelerated by the repeated injury and stress represented by the alloantigen-dependent and alloantigen-independent factors discussed previously. By whatever mechanisms, the use of older kidneys appears to be a major cause of chronic allograft nephropathy.

A test of the hypothesis that inadequate nephron dosing may lead to chronic allograft nephropathy is to determine whether the size of the kidney affects long-term outcomes. Clearly, larger kidneys have a proportionally greater filtration capacity (although not necessarily a greater number of nephrons) than smaller kidneys. It has been theorized that placing a small kidney into a large recipient may create a situation of inadequate nephron dosing for that recipient and thereby precipitate chronic allograft nephropathy. A number of studies, however, have failed to demonstrate that this donor–recipient size mismatching increases the risk for chronic allograft nephropathy or late allograft failure.

The calcineurin inhibitors are nephrotoxic. The histologic changes of chronic calcineurin inhibitor toxicity are nonspecific and can resemble those of chronic allograft nephropathy. The extent of interstitial fibrosis that is a feature of chronic allograft nephropathy and calcineurin inhibitor toxicity has been correlated to the expression of TGF-β messenger ribonucleic acid (mRNA), which, in turn, may be stimulated by cyclosporine. Therefore, chronic calcineurin inhibitor toxicity could be yet another alloantigen-independent mechanism contributing to the pathogenesis of chronic allograft nephropathy. Morphologic lesions attributable to chronic calcineurin inhibitor toxicity are near universal in long-functioning grafts. The fact that graft survival has not been reduced by the increased incidence of acute rejections after cyclosporine withdrawal in randomized, controlled trials may be a result of the offsetting effects of nephrotoxicity in the controls continuing to take cyclosporine in these studies. Withdrawing cyclosporine may produce a trade-off between the adverse effects of acute rejection and the beneficial effects of reduced nephrotoxicity, the net result being no difference in allograft survival. Additional studies with long-term followup are needed to confirm this hypothesis.

The most distinctive histologic characteristic of chronic allograft nephropathy is the fibrointimal proliferation seen in arteries. In some ways, this vasculopathy resembles accelerated atherosclerosis, prompting investigators to consider whether alloantigen-independent risk factors for atherosclerotic vascular disease may also be risk factors for chronic allograft nephropathy. In randomized controlled trials in heart transplant recipients, 3-hydroxy-3-methylglutaryl coenzyme A (HMG-CoA) reductase inhibitors reduced graft vasculopathy. As yet, there are no studies in renal transplant recipients demonstrating that lipid-lowering agents reduce chronic allograft nephropathy. Advanced glycation end products and oxidative stress, which have been implicated in the pathogenesis of atherosclerosis and the progression of renal disease, are increased in chronic allograft nephropathy to a degree that cannot be explained by renal dysfunction alone.

Registry data show that elevated blood pressure is also associated with graft failure. Of course, it is plausible that graft dysfunction causes hypertension, rather than hypertension causing graft dysfunction and chronic allograft nephropathy. Unfortunately, there are no randomized trial results to determine whether aggressive blood pressure lowering will reduce the rate of late graft failure. Cigarette smoking is another risk factor that could have a negative effect on graft vasculopathy and contribute to chronic allograft nephropathy. Homocysteine may be injurious to vascular endothelial cells, and transplant recipients have increased levels of plasma homocysteine compared with controls. Reduced renal function itself, however, is known to cause higher levels of homocysteine, and there are no data suggesting that reducing homocysteine improves graft survival. Similarly, oxygen free radicals are of theoretical importance in the pathogenesis of systemic atherosclerosis and could also play a role in endothelial injury and the vasculopathy of chronic allograft nephropathy. Finally, infections have long been considered a possible mechanism in the pathogenesis of systemic atherosclerosis. If true, the increased incidence of CMV and other infections could also contribute to the vasculopathy of chronic allograft nephropathy. To date, the evidence that infections contribute to chronic allograft nephropathy is largely circumstantial.

Most epidemiologic studies suggest that the incidence of persistent proteinuria after transplantation (more than 1 to 2 g per 24 hours for longer than 6 months) is approximately 20%. Of course, the incidence of proteinuria in these studies is greater with longer duration of followup. Cross-sectional studies suggest that about two-thirds of patients with persistent proteinuria have chronic allograft nephropathy on biopsy. Chronic allograft nephropathy is also the most common cause of posttransplant nephrotic syndrome. Although it is clear that chronic allograft nephropathy can cause proteinuria, proteinuria may also have toxic effects on the allograft that contribute to chronic allograft nephropathy. Indeed, a number of studies have identified proteinuria as an important risk factor for graft loss to chronic allograft nephropathy. Proteinuria causes interstitial nephritis in experimental animals. In addition, studies in humans with renal disease have consistently reported that the amount of urine protein excretion predicts renal disease progression. Thus, it is possible that proteinuria could cause tubulointerstitial damage and contribute to renal injury in chronic allograft nephropathy.

Renal Function Predicts Renal Function

Whatever the mechanism of chronic allograft failure, the bottom line remains the same: the better and more stable the graft function, the better is the long-term outcome. The serum creatinine measured at varying stages posttransplant (at discharge from hospital; 6 months; 1 year) is a valuable predictor of long-term outcome and events occurring in the first year are critical for long-term survival. Renal function is a better predictor of graft survival than the incidence of acute rejection, delayed graft function, HLA mismatch, and other risk factors. The utility of renal function as a reliable predictive tool for graft loss, however, has been questioned (see Chapter 4, Part III).There has been a trend to improved renal function in the U.S. transplant population. Patients with a 1-year creatinine of less than 1.5 mg/dL and a change of creatinine of less than 0.3 mg/dL can look forward to excellent long-term graft outcome. Higher values are accompanied by a steadily increasing risk of graft loss (Fig. 9.2).

ACUTE REJECTION IN THE LATE POSTTRANSPLANT PERIOD

A small proportion of renal allografts are lost to acute rejection in the late posttransplant period. Noncompliance with immunosuppressive medications may play an important role in some, if not most, late acute rejections, and should always be considered when they occur. Because most patients do not admit to missing doses of medications, it is difficult to know how often noncompliance causes acute rejection and graft failure. Transplant centers frequently attempt to reduce doses of immunosuppression, replace drugs with less-toxic or less-expensive alternatives, or withdraw an agent to convert stable patients from triple to double immunosuppressive therapy. Such changes in immunosuppression are always associated with some risk for acute rejection. If patients are monitored closely, acute rejection can be detected early and can usually be treated successfully. On the other hand, if acute rejection goes undetected, as is often the case with noncompliant patients, it can cause or accelerate graft failure.

RECURRENT AND DE NOVO RENAL DISEASE

Recurrence of glomerulonephritis is the third most common cause of graft loss after chronic allograft nephropathy and death with a functioning graft. The reported incidence of recurrence of the original renal disease in the allograft is variable, as is the resultant risk of graft failure. This variable incidence is reflected

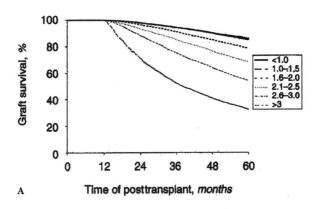

A   Time of posttransplant, *months*

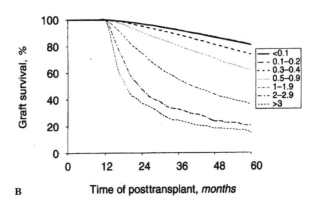

B   Time of posttransplant, *months*

Fig. 9.2.   Relationship of serum creatinine (mg/dl) (A) and change of serum creatinine (mg/dl) (B) at 1-year posttransplant to long-term graft function. (From Hariharan S, McBride M, Cherikh W, et al. Post-transplant renal function in the first year predicts long-term kidney transplant survival. *Kidney Int* 2002;62:311–318, with permission.)

in the wide ranges noted in Table 6.4 (see Chapter 6). Much of the variation is because of differences in the duration of followup, and because of differences in the frequency with which patients undergo biopsies. It is probable that as graft failures from death and rejection decline, the apparent incidence of graft failure from recurrent disease will increase. It is also frequently difficult to establish whether some diseases represent recurrences or *de novo* glomerular disease. For patients who did not have a specific biopsy diagnosis made for the cause of their native kidney disease, the diagnosis may become evident in the pathology of their transplant biopsy.

The incidence of recurrent and *de novo* disease among a large cohort (4,913 subjects, with 22% receiving living-related donor transplants) in the Renal Allograft Disease Registry was 3.4% over a mean followup period of 5.4 years. Diagnoses were focal segmental glomerulosclerosis (FSGS) (34.1% of the total), immunoglobulin (Ig) A nephropathy (13.2%), diabetes (11.4%), membranoproliferative glomerulonephritis (MPGN) (10.8%), membranous nephropathy (9.6%), hemolytic uremic syndrome (HUS) or thrombotic thrombocytopenic purpura (TTP) (4.8%), and other (16.1%). There was a significant increase in graft failures among the recurrent and *de novo* disease groups (55%) when compared with the others (25%; p<0.001). In contrast, in a small cohort of two-haplotype-matched living-related donor transplants followed for a mean of 8.3 years, the incidence of recurrent disease was 15%, and was 27% in patients with glomerulonephritis as the original kidney disease. The higher incidence of disease recurrence in the latter study may reflect the lack of competing graft loss to rejection in well-matched recipients exposed to relatively long followup.

In data from large registries, it may be more difficult to discern the incidence of disease recurrence than to define the outcome of patients after recurrent disease has been diagnosed. However, in a group of more than 1,500 Australian patients with biopsy-proven glomerulonephritis that were followed for 10 years, the incidence of graft loss as a consequence of any kind of glomerulonephritis was 8.4%. FSGS is clearly the form of glomerular disease most commonly associated with recurrence and graft loss, and patients who have lost a prior transplant because of recurrent FSGS are at much higher risk. Early recognition of recurrent FSGS is particularly important because it may respond to plasmapheresis. The prevention and management of recurrent FSGS, which is most common in children, is discussed in detail in Chapter 15. MPGN type 2 (dense-deposit disease) recurs in almost 100% of patients and often leads to graft failure. MPGN type 1 recurs in approximately 20% to 30% of patients and leads to graft failure in approximately 50%. Membranous glomerulonephritis can present as *de novo* disease but probably recurs in 5% to 10% of patients. Approximately 25% of patients may ultimately lose their grafts from recurrent membranous nephropathy. Histologic recurrence of IgA nephropathy is common. Allograft failure to IgA nephropathy is higher than once reported and may be as high as 25%. Henoch-Schönlein purpura recurs in a high proportion of patients and leads to graft failure in approximately 25%. Antiglomerular basement membrane disease recurs in 10% to 25% of patients, but rarely causes graft failure. Diabetes recurs histologically in 100% of patients after a few years. Graft failure as a consequence of diabetes occurs in approximately 5% to 10% patients, but this percentage may increase as graft failure caused by rejection declines.

ROLE OF NONCOMPLIANCE IN LATE ALLOGRAFT FAILURE

The frequency of noncompliance with immunosuppressive medications is difficult to measure, but it is probably more frequent than reported. As a group, transplant recipients may be especially reluctant to admit to noncompliance if they believe that doing so might jeopardize their chances of ever receiving another transplant. Some patients may admit to noncompliance and seek financial assistance in obtaining their medications (see Chapter 19). Noncompliance may also manifest as a failure to keep scheduled appointments or as inconsistent immunosuppressant drug levels. Patients who fail to have their serum creatinine measurements performed regularly are more likely to have late graft failure.

Patients may become noncompliant with medications for a number or reasons (see Chapter 19, Table 19.2). They may harbor the false belief that taking medication regularly is unnecessary. This belief may be reinforced by several years of an uneventful posttransplant course. Many patients believe that the effects of immunosuppression continue indefinitely, even when doses of medications are missed. Such patients are more likely to be noncompliant than are patients who have a better understanding of the duration of the action of immunosuppressive medications. Some patients may become noncompliant because they fear the adverse effects of medication more than they fear graft rejection. This is particularly true of adolescents, who abhor the social stigma of the body habitus changes caused by corticosteroids and, to a lesser extent, cyclosporine.

Patients may simply forget to take doses of medication. In a survey of 100 members of the Transplant Recipient International Organization (TRIO), less than 30% were taking fewer than 5 medications, and 35% reported taking 10 to 20 different medications each day. Only 2% of the medications required a single daily dose. (In general, studies show that the number of times a day that patients must take medications is a stronger predictor of noncompliance than is the total number of medications.) Of those surveyed, 25% admitted missing doses of medications, and 55% of these gave forgetfulness as the reason. It is likely that the members of the TRIO represent a highly motivated population of transplant recipients. Only 35% of the participants were kidney transplant recipients, and recipients of other, nonrenal organs may suffer lethal consequences if their grafts fail.

Noncompliance increases the risk of late graft loss three- to fivefold and may be the most common cause of late graft loss. Noncompliance can lead to graft failure through several different mechanisms. Patients who receive inadequate immunosuppression because of noncompliance may develop acute or chronic rejection that leads to graft failure. Noncompliance with clinic visits and laboratory followups can also contribute to late graft failure. Acute rejection in the late posttransplant period rarely presents with signs and symptoms until it is far advanced. Thus to be successfully treated, acute rejection must be detected early, which can only be done by detecting increases in serum creatinine levels soon after they occur. It follows that patients who do not see physicians and who do not have frequent measurements of serum creatinine levels are less likely to have rejection detected at an early stage, when it is treatable. It also follows that it is the responsibility of transplant physicians and transplant team members to constantly reinforce to the patients the importance of compliance and to make every effort to facilitate compliant behavior by minimizing the complexity of the medication protocol and other aspects of long-term posttransplant followup.

Caregivers often feel impatient when it comes to treating and preventing diseases that cause morbidity and mortality. Although convincing knowledge about the treatment of chronic allograft nephropathy is limited and we might not fully understand its etiology in an individual patient, we do know that it is a major cause of graft failure in the late posttransplant period. The dilemma is similar to that which caregivers face when they have patients suffering from inoperable, three-vessel coronary artery disease, inoperable cancer that responds poorly to chemotherapy, or other diseases and complications for which there may not be effective therapies.

On the other hand, there is a substantial amount of evidence to suggest ways to prevent at least some major disease complications that are common after renal transplantation. Studies show, however, that despite good evidence that a particular therapy or preventive strategy is beneficial, that therapy or preventive strategy may not be applied. Hypertension, for example, is a known risk factor for stroke and ischemic heart disease, and numerous studies document the safety and efficiency of antihypertensive medications. Nevertheless, many studies also show that hypertension is poorly controlled, even among patients who are seen regularly in hospitals and clinics. Attention to atherosclerotic risk factors may be the most important way to improve the longevity of transplant recipients and their grafts, yet these risk factors are often not addressed nor adequately emphasized. Part of the responsibility no doubt falls on the patients themselves; much also falls on physicians and other caregivers.

In the past, it has been common for patients to receive repeat transplants as each organ fails. Every transplant clinic follows patients who have had multiple transplants. In the current environment of an increasing shortage of deceased donor organs and waiting lists lasting years, repeat deceased donor transplants may become an infrequent luxury. Appreciation of the difficulty in attaining a second transplant makes it all the more critical to do all we know to protect the function of the first.

Resources are limited; there is only so much that can be done. It seems prudent, therefore, to adopt a priority system for delivering health care. Such a system should emphasize measures that are known to be effective, that is, strategies that are evidence based. In the case of renal transplantations, we know the major causes of morbidity and mortality in the late posttransplant period. In many cases, we have a substantial amount of evidence to suggest effective measures to prevent many common posttransplant complications. This evidence, if not available from studies in renal transplant recipients, can often be extrapolated from studies in the general population. The challenge is to make the most of what we have. This section outlines strategies for the management of renal recipients in the late posttransplant period. The emphasis is on specific complications for which we have

**Table 9.3.   The most important things to
do in the late posttransplant period**

Minimize immunosuppression whenever possible.
Adopt a strategy to prevent noncompliance.
Monitor renal function closely.
Make an accurate pathologic diagnosis of the cause of allograft
    dysfunction.
Aggressively treat hyperlipidemia.
Aggressively treat hypertension.
Encourage a healthy lifestyle.
Screen for cancer.
Prevent infection.
Protect the bones.
Regard impaired allograft function as a form of chronic kidney
    disease.

evidence that the problem is common and intervention is likely
to be effective (Table 9.3).

The intensity of followup that the following strategies require
will, of course, vary according to individual patient needs. As a
general rule, monthly followup is advised between 3 months posttransplant and the end of the first posttransplant year for stable
patients. In the second posttransplant year, patients should be
monitored every 1 to 2 months and thereafter every 3 to 6 months
in perpetuity. Followup can occur at the office of the transplant
program of origin, in the office of a nephrologist, or with an in-
ternist or family practitioner with experience in posttransplant
management. Patients and caregivers should always have free access to the expertise provided by transplant programs and transplant physicians and surgeons.

Strategy 1: Reduce Immunosuppression Whenever Possible

Death is a common cause of renal allograft failure in the late
posttransplant period. The ultimate goal is to have all our patients die with a functioning graft, but not prematurely, as is now
too often the case. Cardiovascular disease, cancer, and infection
are the leading causes of death in the late posttransplant period,
and immunosuppression plays a major role in the pathogenesis
of each of these complications. Each immunosuppressive agent
has both immune and nonimmune toxicity. Immune toxicity is
usually nonspecific; that is, immune toxicity is the result of the
total amount of all immunosuppression over a given period of
time. Immune toxicity can only be avoided if patients became tolerant to their transplanted kidney. Unfortunately, most patients
will reject their kidney if immunosuppression is completely withdrawn, and the best we can do is select the minimal amount immunosuppression that prevents rejection. This minimal amount
should ideally be tailored to the needs of specific patients, but we
are able to do that only in a crude way.

The principal obstacle to reducing the overall amount of immunosuppression is acute rejection. A number of risk factors for

Table 9.4. Tailoring the *amount* of immunosuppression to the individual

Risk Factor	Patients Who May Need More Immunosuppression	Patients Who May Need Less Immunosuppression
Donor source	Deceased	Living
Major histocompatibility	>0 Mismatches	0 Mismatches
Prior transplant experience	>1, Rejected quickly	0 or 1, Prolonged survival
Age	<18 years old	>60 years old
Race	African American	White
Timing of acute rejection	Late	Early
Severity of acute rejection	Severe, vascular	Mild, cellular
Number of acute rejections	>1	0 or 1

acute rejection have been identified (Table 9.4). These risk factors can be taken into account when determining the amount of immunosuppression that may be appropriate for individual patients in the late posttransplant period. In general, outcomes are better for living donor kidneys. This is especially true for living donor kidneys. This is especially true for 2-haplotype-identical, living-related transplants. For deceased donor kidney recipients, the number of major histocompatibility mismatches is associated with the rate of late allograft failure (see Chapter 3, Fig. 3.3). In particular, patients with zero mismatches are at significantly lower risk for late graft failure when compared with patients with as few as one mismatch, and at least one study has shown that the number of HLA-DR mismatches predicts acute rejections after elective withdrawal of cyclosporine. Patients who have had more than one previous transplant have a higher risk for graft failure. In addition, the chances of such a patient receiving yet another kidney are reduced, making the risk association with reducing immunosuppression higher. Patients younger than 18 years of age have a higher incidence of acute rejection and need more immunosuppression than do patients 30 to 50 years of age. On the other hand, elderly patients are more likely to die of complications of immunosuppression than to lose their kidneys to acute rejection, and many transplantation centers attempt to use less immunosuppression in elderly transplant recipients.

African American patients are at increased risk for late allograft failure. The reasons for this are probably multiple, but include possible differences in immunoreactivity to the graft and poor bioavailability of calcineurin inhibitors. Acute rejection is a strong predictor of outcome, particularly from chronic allograft nephropathy. However, not all acute rejections lead to graft failure. Characteristics of acute rejection that correlate to increased risk for graft failure and, by interference, an increased need for

**Table 9.5. Tailoring the *type*
of immunosuppression to the individual**

Risk Factor or Complication	Agents to Reduce or Withdraw
Severe hyperlipidemia	Cyclosporine, prednisone, sirolimus
Severe hypertension	Cyclosporine, prednisone
Severe tremor	Tacrolimus, cyclosporine
Difficult to control diabetes	Prednisone
New-onset diabetes	Tacrolimus, prednisone
Anemia, neutropenia, thrombocytopenia	Azathioprine, mycophenolate mofetil, sirolimus
Severely impaired renal function	Cyclosporine, tacrolimus
Gout requiring allopurinol	Azathioprine
Cosmetic changes	Switch calcineurin inhibitors
Inability to pay for medications	Simplify regimen, use inexpensive agents

long-term immunosuppression include late rejections, severe rejections, and multiple acute rejections. All of the above factors can be used to judge the amount of immunosuppression that may be best for individual patients in the late posttransplant period.

A number of randomized controlled trials have studied the feasibility of electively withdrawing immunosuppressive agents in the late posttransplant period. Withdrawal of both prednisone and cyclosporine has been studied extensively, yet withdrawal of these agents remains controversial (see Chapter 4, Part IV). Elective cyclosporine withdrawal is associated with approximately a 10% risk for acute rejection in the months following withdrawal. Most of these rejection episodes can be successfully treated and reversed. Despite this increased risk for rejection, controlled trials with long-term followup have been unable to demonstrate an increased risk for graft failure after cyclosporine withdrawal. In contrast, acute rejection after prednisone withdrawal appears to increase the risk for late allograft failure in randomized controlled trials. Additional studies are warranted to define better circumstances under which immunosuppression withdrawal is advisable.

In addition to deciding on the minimum amount of immunosuppression needed to prevent acute rejection, physicians and patients must also choose among the most effective, but least toxic, of several different agents. In general, it is prudent to tailor the choice of agents to the risk profile or adverse effects that are most troubling to the individual (Table 9.5). For patients who have severe hyperlipidemia, especially those who are at high risk for cardiovascular disease, it may be wise to minimize the use of cyclosporine, prednisone, and sirolimus. Each of these drugs causes hyperlipidemia. Switching a patient from cyclosporine to tacrolimus, for example, may reduce low-density lipoprotein cholesterol by the same amount as therapy with an HMG-CoA reductase inhibitor. Similarly, reducing cyclosporine or prednisone may help to control blood pressure. Patients with severe tremor will be especially eager to reduce or withdraw tacrolimus or cyclosporine in the late posttransplant period if this is possible. Similarly, patients with difficult-to-control diabetes may be good candidates for minimizing doses of prednisone. New-onset diabetes in a patient receiving tacrolimus may respond to switching to cyclosporine. Bone marrow suppression may be an indication for reducing doses of azathioprine, mycophenolate mofetil, or sirolimus. Patients with marginal renal function may sometimes delay starting dialysis by decreasing or stopping calcineurin inhibitors. Patients with severe liver disease may benefit from lowering or discontinuing azathioprine. Patients with cosmetic complications may choose to switch calcineurin inhibitors. Allopurinol can dramatically increase blood levels of azathioprine; hence, azathioprine may need to be reduced or discontinued for patients with gout and switched to mycophenolate mofetil. Tacrolimus may be the calcineurin inhibitor better for patients with gout. Finally, many patients cannot afford to pay the high cost of immunosuppression. The use of expensive medications for patients who cannot afford them increases the risk for noncompliance and graft failure. Prednisone and azathioprine are a fraction of the cost of newer immunosuppressive agents and yet may provide adequate immunosuppression for many patients.

Strategy 2: Adopt Strategies to Prevent Noncompliance

There are few randomized, controlled trials to suggest how to prevent noncompliance with immunosuppressive medications. On the other hand, a number of observational studies have demonstrated that noncompliance is an important, preventable cause of allograft failure. These same studies have provided clues to preventive measures that are most likely to be effective.

- Minimize the number of daily doses of medication. Whenever possible, use medications that can be dosed once daily.
- Educate patients. In particular, dispel the common misconception that the immunosuppressive effects of medications extend beyond the dosing interval. Patients need to be constantly reminded that failure to take medications regularly will eventually result in graft failure.
- Help patients to establish a system to remind them to take their medications. Enlist the help of friends, family, and public health aides. Use egg-carton-style pull containers or other mnemonic devices.
- Maintain close contact with patients throughout the late posttransplant period. Insist that patients have frequent followup with the transplant center, and make every effort to locate patients who are lost to followup. Clinic visits and laboratory checks are a valuable reminder to patients of the importance of taking medications. When negotiating contracts with providers, insist that patients be allowed to followup with the transplant center at regular intervals.

- Know whether your patients have trouble paying for their medications. If this is the case, assign someone to help them. Most transplant programs have found that it is often necessary to have a dedicated social worker or pharmacist available to help patients find ways to cover the cost of their immunosuppressive medications.
- Identify patients who are at high risk for noncompliance. Adolescent patients are at increased risk, often because they are fearful of cosmetic effects of prednisone and cyclosporine. Patients who are poorly educated are also at increased risk for noncompliance. Similarly, low family income is associated with noncompliance. Socioeconomic factors place members of racial minorities at increased risk for noncompliance. Studies show that patients who were noncompliant with medication, diet, and dialysis therapy before transplantation are more likely to be noncompliant after renal transplantation.
- Patients who are at high risk for noncompliance should be targeted with risk factor intervention in much the same way that we target patients who are at high risk for cardiovascular disease with intensive risk factor management. In both instances, the benefit is likely to be the greatest risk when the risk is the highest.

Strategy 3: Monitor Renal Function Closely

Frequent monitoring of renal function in the late posttransplant period helps to enforce noncompliance with immunosuppressive medications and provides the only reliable means to detect acute rejection when it may still respond to treatment. A program requiring patients to make certain that serum creatinine is measured regularly and reported to the transplant center also provides an indirect means for the center to monitor compliance. Patients should also keep a record of their own creatinine values and thereby learn to self-monitor for significant change. Patients who fail to have their serum creatinine level checked regularly should be contacted and reminded of the importance of close, ongoing followup to prevent graft failure. Patients and caregivers should be constantly reminded that acute rejection rarely presents with signs and symptoms in the late posttransplant period. Although immune monitoring holds promise as a more sophisticated way of recognizing acute rejection before it manifests clinically, the serum creatinine level is currently the only practical tool that can be used to screen for acute rejection in the late posttransplant period. It is not too much to ask patients to have their serum creatinine level measured regularly in the late posttransplant period.

At least once a year, and preferably more often, urine should be checked for protein excretion. Persistent proteinuria (i.e., more than 1 g in 24 hours for at least 6 months) is associated with an increased risk for graft failure. Proteinuria can be most reliably detected by either a timed urine collection (which is cumbersome) or a protein:creatinine ratio measured in a random "spot" urine sample (which is convenient). Dipstick screening is less reliable because the protein concentration is also dependent on the state of diuresis. There are two reasons why it is important to detect proteinuria.

1. Reducing high levels of proteinuria with angiotensin-converting enzyme (ACE) inhibitors or receptor antagonists may help to reduce levels of serum cholesterol and alleviate coagulation and other metabolic abnormalities associated with nephrotic-range proteinuria.
2. There is growing circumstantial evidence that proteinuria may itself be injurious to the kidney and may contribute to the pathogenesis of chronic allograft nephropathy.

Strategy 4: Make an Accurate Pathologic Diagnosis of the Cause of Graft Dysfunction

It is important to establish an accurate pathologic diagnosis in patients with deteriorating graft function. There is evidence to suggest that even low-grade tubulitis, or so-called borderline acute rejection, may increase the risk for chronic allograft nephropathy (see Chapter 13). A small, randomized, controlled trial demonstrated that treating acute rejection on protocol biopsies during the first few months after transplantation resulted in a lower serum creatinine level at 2 years, as compared with control patients who underwent less-frequent biopsies and who relied, instead, on increased serum creatinine levels to prompt biopsy and treatment (see Chapter 8). Few centers perform protocol biopsies—that is, biopsies on all patients at predetermined intervals—in the late posttransplant period. However, the message is clear. It is important to have a high level of suspicion for acute rejection and a low threshold for obtaining a renal allograft biopsy. An acute, sustained rise in serum creatinine should prompt immediate evaluation. The strategy of routinely monitoring serum creatinine levels will only be successful if biopsies are obtained quickly and acute rejection is treated. Such a strategy will also avoid unnecessary intensification of immunosuppression when rejection is not present. Unexpected diagnoses, such as recurrent disease, calcineurin inhibitor toxicity, polyomavirus infection, and posttransplant lymphoma may require radically different therapeutic approaches. If a diagnosis of chronic allograft nephropathy is established, repeated biopsies may be unnecessary because repeated treatment may be unwise (see Chapter 4).

Strategy 5: Treat Hyperlipidemia Aggressively

Hyperlipidemia is common after renal transplantation. Elevations in total cholesterol are almost invariably accompanied by elevations in LDL cholesterol. Triglycerides are also frequently elevated. Several studies have found correlations between hyperlipidemia and cardiovascular disease after renal transplantation. Studies in the general population provide incontrovertible evidence that treatment of elevated LDL reduces the risk for ischemic heart disease events and decreases mortality. A National Kidney Foundation task force on CVD concluded that transplant recipients with LDL cholesterol levels of greater than 130 mg/dL should be considered for pharmacologic treatment, especially if they have preexisting CVD, diabetes, or other risk factors. Tables 9.6 and 9.7 list recommendations for the primary and secondary prevention of CHD. Recognition of patients with the metabolic syndrome is important early posttransplant so that patients can

Table 9.6.   American Heart Association/American College of Cardiology primary prevention of coronary heart disease

Risk Intervention and Goals	Recommendations
Smoking cessation	• Query at each visit • Advise to quit • Help with counseling and pharmacotherapy • "Ask, advise, assess, assist and arrange"
Blood pressure control	Lifestyle modification (restrict salt intake, moderate ethyl alcohol use, and physical activity)
Dietary intake	Modify food choices to reduce saturated fats and transfat
Aspirin	Low-dose aspirin
Dyslipidemia	Treat appropriately; see below
Physical activity	At least 30 minutes of moderate-intensity physical activity on most days (and preferably all) days of the week
Weight management	10% weight reduction in the first year of therapy
Diabetes	Maintain hemoglobin A_{1c} <7%

be targeted for lifestyle modifications and drug therapy (Tables 9.8, 9.9, and 9.10).

Reduction of the urine protein excretion with an ACE inhibitor or receptor antagonist may help to reduce lipid levels for patients with nephrotic-range proteinuria. Reduction or discontinuation of cyclosporine, sirolimus, or prednisone may also help lower lipid levels. Diet is effective in reducing cholesterol and LDL, but the effect is usually modest. A number of studies have shown that HMG-CoA reductase inhibitors are safe and effective in lowering LDL cholesterol after renal transplantation. In the ALERT (Assessment of Lescol in Renal Transplantation) trial, fluvastatin lowered LDL by 32%, and although there was no significant reduction in the rate of coronary intervention or mortality, the incidence of cardiac deaths and nonfatal myocardial infarction seemed to be reduced. Approximately half of all kidney transplant patients receive these drugs. Plasma levels of HMG-CoA reductase inhibitors are increased in cyclosporine-treated renal transplant recipients, and it is generally prudent to use about half the usually prescribed dose. Patients who still have high LDL cholesterol levels may be candidates for combination therapy. Low-dose bile acid sequestrants can be combined with an HMG-CoA reductase inhibitor. Bile acid sequestrants should probably not be taken at the same time as cyclosporine and should not be used in patients with very high triglyceride levels. Fibric acid analogues, such as gemfibrozil, can also be used

Table 9.7. American Heart Association/American College of Cardiology secondary prevention for patients with coronary artery disease

Goals	Intervention
Smoking: *goal is complete cessation*	Ask, advise, assess, and arrange
Blood pressure control: *goal is maintain blood pressure <130/80*	See Table 9.10
Lipid management: *primary goal: LDL-C <100 mg/dL; secondary goal: If TG ≥200 mg/dL HDL ≤40 mg/dL*	See Table 9.9
Physical activity: *minimum goal: 30 min, 3–4 d/wk; optimum daily*	Assess risk
Weight management: *goal is BMI 18.5–24.9 kg/m²*	Calculate BMI and measure waist circumference Follow weight Waist circumference <88 cm (<35 inches) in women Waist circumference <102 cm (<40 inches) in men
Diabetes management: *goal HbA$_{1C}$ <7%*	Appropriate therapy to maintain HbA$_{1C}$ <7%
Antiplatelet agents/anticoagulants	Indefinitely on aspirin (75–325 mg)
ACE-I	Indefinitely for all post-MI patients unless contraindicated
Beta blockers	Indefinitely in all post-MI patients

ACE-I, angiotensin-converting enzyme inhibitor; BMI, body mass index; HbA$_{1C}$, glycosylated hemoglobin; HDL, high-density lipoprotein; LDL-C, low-density lipoprotein cholesterol; MI, myocardial infarction; TG, triglycerides.

in combination with HMG-CoA reductase inhibitors. Some fibric acid analogues (but not gemfibrozil), however, are reported to increase the serum creatinine level. Combination therapy should be used with caution because it increases the risk for myositis and rhabdomyolysis.

Strategy 6: Treat Hypertension Aggressively

Hypertension occurs in 60% to 80% of renal transplant recipients. It is associated with an increased risk for graft failure. Studies in the general population show that treatment with antihypertensive agents reduces the risk for cardiovascular disease. There is no reason to believe that treating blood pressure elevations would not be beneficial in renal transplant recipients.

Table 9.8.   National Cholesterol Educational Program Adult Treatment Panel III: metabolic syndrome

Diagnosis is established when ≥3 of these risk factors are present

Risk Factor	Defining Level
Abdominal obesity[a]	Waist circumference[b]
Men	>102 cm (>40 inches)
Women	>88 cm (>35 inches)
Triglycerides	>150 mg/dL
High-density lipoprotein cholesterol	
Men	<40 mg/dL
Women	<50 mg/dL
Blood pressure	>130/85 mm Hg
Fasting glucose	≥110 mg/dL

[a] Abdominal obesity is more highly correlated with metabolic risk factors than is increased body mass index.
[b] Some men develop metabolic risk factors when waist circumference is only marginally increased.
From *Third report of the expert panel on detection, evaluation, and treatment of high blood cholesterol in adults (Adult Treatment Panel III)*. Bethesda, MD: National Institutes of Health, National Heart, Lung, and Blood Institute, 2001, with permission.

All classes of antihypertensive agents can be used to lower blood pressure in renal transplant recipients, and each has its advantages and disadvantages (Table 9-10). Although there are limited data on the effects of reduced dietary sodium chloride intake on blood pressure in renal transplant recipients, this is a reasonable first step. A low dose of thiazide diuretic is also reasonable for patients with creatinine clearance estimated to be greater than 25 to 30 mL per minute. Low doses of thiazides (e.g., 12.5 to 25 mg per day) are effective and do not generally perturb lipid or glucose metabolism. Both a low-salt diet and thiazide diuretics may help with edema, which is a common problem after transplantation. A thiazide diuretic may also help in the management of the hyperkalemia that is common in calcineurin inhibitor-treated transplant recipients. Transplant recipients may be sensitive to volume contraction; therefore diuretics may cause a reversible increase in serum creatinine levels. Thiazides often potentiate the antihypertensive effects of other agents, especially ACE inhibitors. Thiazides are inexpensive. Beta blockers are also relatively inexpensive and are especially attractive for patients with ischemic heart disease, which is common after renal transplantation. Relative contraindications to beta-blocker therapy (e.g., peripheral vascular disease, reactive airways disease, and hypoglycemic reactions) are rarely a reason to forego the use of this important class of medication.

Physicians are sometimes reluctant to use ACE inhibitors and angiotensin II antagonists in transplant patients for fear of inducing hemodynamic impairment of allograft function. Several studies, however, show that these drugs are generally safe, effective, and well tolerated. They may reduce proteinuria and stabilize the deterioration in renal function in chronic allograft failure, possibly reducing the production of TGF-β. They may also have additional benefit in reducing the incidence of cardiovascular events in high-risk patients. Occasionally, ACE inhibitors may increase serum creatinine, but this is usually a transient and reversible effect. Hyperkalemia can often be managed by adding a thiazide diuretic or a loop diuretic to the treatment regimen. ACE inhibitors may cause anemia in transplant recipients; this side effect can be exploited for the treatment of posttransplant erythrocytosis. Cough occurs in approximately 15% of patients on ACE inhibitors, but is much less frequent with angiotensin II receptor antagonists. Otherwise, angiotensin II receptor antagonists appear to have all of the advantages and disadvantages of ACE inhibitors.

Calcium antagonists are also effective in renal transplant recipients. They can contribute to edema, which is already prevalent among transplant patients. Calcium antagonists appear to improve the preglomerular, arterial vasoconstriction that mediates cyclosporine-induced declines in renal blood flow. They may help to alleviate the propensity of the calcineurin inhibitors to exacerbate delayed graft function immediately after deceased donor transplantation. Nondihydropyridine calcium antagonists, for example, diltiazem and verapamil, increase calcineurin inhibitor blood levels and can be used to help reduce the immunosuppressive drug cost. Dihydropyridine calcium antagonists have less effect on blood levels (see Chapter 4, Part I). Vasodilators and alpha blockers are also effective in treating hypertension, although they can cause reflex tachycardia and may need to be used in combination with beta blockers. Excess hair growth with minoxidil, the most potent vasodilator, limits its long-term usefulness in women. Other agents that are useful include sympatholytics, central and peripheral alpha antagonists, and combined alpha/beta blockers. Table 9.11 lists the compelling indication for specific classes of antihypertensive drugs.

Most patients require combination therapy. Some require several agents. Useful combinations include the following:

- Diuretics with an ACE inhibitor or receptor antagonist. A calcium antagonist can also be added.
- Calcium antagonists, beta blockers, and diuretics.
- A vasodilator, a beta blocker, and a diuretic.

When hypertension cannot be controlled, particularly if attempts to reduce blood result in decreased graft function, the possibility of renal allograft artery stenosis should be considered (see Chapter 7). In addition, the presence of diuretic-resistant peripheral edema, a loud allograft bruit, renal dysfunction after administration of ACE inhibitors or angiotensin receptor blockers (ARBs), and polycythemia, should engender consideration of this diagnosis. Color-flow Doppler examination of the renal artery may aid the diagnosis, but interpretation of this test is difficult, and false-positive results are common. Radionuclide scanning is usually not helpful. Magnetic resonance angiography or renal arteriography should be used for diagnosis when suspicion of renal allograft artery stenosis is high (see Chapter 12). Percutaneous transluminal angioplasty may improve renal function and reduce

Table 9.9.   Drugs affecting lipoprotein metabolism

Drug Class, Agents, and Daily Doses	Lipid/Lipoprotein Effects	Side Effects	Contraindications	Clinical Trial Results
HMG-CoA reductase inhibitors (statins)[a]	LDL ↓ 18%–50% HDL ↑ 5%–15% TG ↓ 7%–30%	Myopathy Increased liver enzymes	Absolute: • Active or chronic liver disease Relative: • Concomitant use of certain drugs[b]	Reduce major coronary events, CHD deaths, need for coronary procedures, stroke and total mortality
Bile acid sequestrants[c]	LDL ↓ 15%–30% HDL ↑ 3%–5% TG No change or increase	Gastrointestinal distress; decreased absorption of other drugs	Absolute: • Dysbeta-lipoproteinemia • TG >400 mg/dL Relative: • TG >200 mg/dL	Reduced major coronary events and CHD deaths
Nicotinic acid[d]	LDL ↓ 5%–25% HDL ↑ 15%–35% TG ↓ 20%–50%	Flushing Hyperglycemia Hyperuricemia (or gout) Upper GI distress Hepatotoxicity	Absolute: • Chronic liver disease • Severe gout Relative: • Diabetes • Hyperuricemia • Peptic ulcer disease	Reduced major coronary events and possibly total mortality

Fibric acids[e]	LDL ↓ 5%–20% HDL ↑ 10%–20% TG ↓ 20%–50%	Dyspepsia Gallstones Myopathy	Absolute: • Severe renal disease • Severe hepatic disease	Reduced major coronary events
Intestinal cholesterol inhibitor[f]	LDL ↓ 18% TG ↓ 8% ApoB ↓ 16%	Well tolerated with few adverse reactions; similar to placebo in clinical trials	Absolute: • Active or chronic liver disease • Do not use in combination with resins or fibrates	No long-term clinical trial data

ApoB, apolipoprotein B; CHD, coronary heart disease; GI, gastrointestinal; HDL, high-density lipoprotein; HDL, high-density lipoprotein; LDL, low-density lipoprotein; TG, triglyceride.
[a]Lovastatin (20–80 mg), simvastatin (20–80 mg), fluvastatin (20–80 mg), atorvastatin (10–80 mg).
[b]Cyclosporine, macrolide antibiotics, various antifungal agents, and cytochrome P450 inhibitors (fibrates and niacin should be used with appropriate caution).
[c]Cholestyramine (4–16 g), colestipol (5–20 g), colesevelam (2.6–3.8 g).
[d]Immediate-release (crystalline) nicotinic acid (1.5–3 g), extended-release nicotinic acid (Niaspan) (1–2 g), sustained-release nicotinic acid (1–2 g).
[e]Gemfibrozil (600 mg b.i.d.), fenofibrate (54 mg + 160 mg), clofibrate (1,000 mg b.i.d.).
[f] Ezetimibe (10 mg).
From *Third report of the expert panel on detection, evaluation, and treatment of high blood cholesterol in adults (Adult Treatment Panel III)*. Bethesda, MD: National Institutes of Health, National Heart, Lung, and Blood Institute, 2001.

Table 9.10.   Some advantages and disadvantages
of antihypertensive agent classes

Class	Advantages	Disadvantages
Low-dose thiazide	↓Cost, ↓edema, ↓hyperkalemia	↑Creatinine
Beta blocker	↓Cost, ↑survival in IHD	↑Lipids
CEI	↓Proteinuria, ↓erythrocytosis, ↑cough	↓Creatinine, anemia, ↑potassium
AII-RA	↓Proteinuria, ↓erythrocytosis, ↓CEI-cough, ↓CEI-hyperkalemia	↑Cost, ↑creatinine, anemia
Calcium blocker	↑CsA levels, ↑RBF	↑Edema
Vasodilators	↓Afterload in CHF	↑Heart rate

AII RA, angiotensin II receptor antagonists; CEI, converting enzyme inhibitors; CHF, congestive heart failure; CsA, cyclosporine; IHD, ischemic heart disease; RBF, renal blood flow.

the need for antihypertensive medications in 60% to 85% of cases. Restenosis may occur in up to 30%. Surgery should probably be reserved for critical stenosis that threaten the integrity of the graft.

The native kidneys often contribute to hypertension after renal transplantation. Studies to determine the role of the native kidneys in causing hypertension, however, are probably not useful. In particular, renal vein renins do not reliably predict blood pressure reduction after native kidney nephrectomy. Therefore, in difficult-to-control hypertension, consideration should be given to empirical removal of the native kidneys. Laparoscopic surgery may reduce the morbidity of posttransplant native kidney nephrectomy.

Strategy 7: Encourage a Healthy Lifestyle

Regular aerobic exercise should be part of the therapeutic regimen of all patients at high CVD risk and may be particularly beneficial in counteracting the effects of corticosteroids on muscle and bone. Near-normal levels of physical functioning are possible after transplantation, particularly for those patients who engage in regular physical activity. Exercise may help to minimize posttransplant weight gain and may be particularly important for patients with the metabolic syndrome. Readers are referred to Chapter 18 for detailed dietary recommendations for transplant patients.

Cigarette smoking appears to be just as prevalent among renal transplant recipients as it is in the general population. Cigarette smoking contributes to cardiovascular disease and increases the already high risk for cancer after renal transplantation. Studies in nontransplanted populations also show smoking to be detrimental to renal function. Thus, every effort should be made to

Table 9.11.   Joint National Committee 7 guideline basis for compelling indications for individual drug classes

Compelling Indication	Recommended Drugs					
	Diuretic	BB	ACE-I	ARB	CCB	ALDOST ANT
Heart failure	•		•	•		•
Postmyocardial infarction		•	•			•
High coronary disease risk	•	•	•		•	
Diabetes	•	•	•	•	•	
Chronic kidney disease			•	•		
Recurrent stroke prevention	•		•			

ACE-I, angiotensin-converting enzyme inhibitor; ALDOST ANT, aldosterone antagonist; ARB, angiotensin receptor blocker; BB, beta blocker; CCB, calcium channel blocker.
From *The seventh report of the Joint National Committee on prevention, detection, evaluation, and treatment of high blood pressure.* Bethesda, MD: National Institutes of Health, National Heart, Lung, and Blood Institute, 2003.

encourage transplant recipients to quit smoking. Smoking cessation programs that make use of nicotine-replacement therapies have been shown, in clinical trials, to be effective. The American and Psychiatric Society and the Agency for Health Care Policy and Research have developed guidelines for smoking cessation.

Aspirin prevents CVD events for patients with known CVD. The role of aspirin prophylaxis in primary prevention is clear. Aspirin should be considered for renal transplant recipients with CVD, and possibly for patients who are at high risk for CVD events.

Strategy 8: Screen for Cancer

Knowledge that many posttransplant cancers are caused by viruses has not yet produced effective prophylactic strategies. Successful treatment of cancer after renal transplantation relies on surveillance and early detection. Typically, guidelines for cancer screening developed for the general population are presumed to be relevant to renal transplant recipients. However, because the life expectancy of most transplant patients is less than that of the general population, the presumptions underlying recommendations for cancer screening may not be relevant to them. Decisions regarding routine screening for breast and colorectal cancers should be made on an individual basis, because their incidence does not differ in the transplant population from the general population. Some, but not all, studies report an increased incidence of prostate cancer posttransplant and annual prostate-specific antigen (PSA) testing has been suggested. Cervical carcinoma is more prevalent in transplant recipients, and women who are older than 18 years of age should have an annual pelvic examination and Papanicolaou (Pap) smear. Anogenital carcinoma is common after renal transplantation. Yearly physical examination and pelvic examination in women are useful for screening for anogenital lesions.

Skin cancers are common after renal transplantation. Annual self-examination and examination by a physician are warranted to screen for squamous cell carcinoma and malignant melanoma. Suspicious lesions should undergo biopsy. Patients should be instructed to avoid sun exposure and to use sunblock, although the effectiveness of this strategy in adults is uncertain. Patients with multiple lesions should undergo formal dermatologic surveillance on a regular basis. In addition to local measures, oral isotretinoin may be beneficial and appears to be safe in transplant recipients.

The management of immunosuppression in patients who have developed cancer is difficult, and each case should be considered individually. There is a clinical evidence that higher cyclosporine levels are associated with an increased incidence of cancer and experimental evidence that cyclosporine may accelerate the growth of metastatic cancer. It is unlikely that this finding is specific for cyclosporine; therefore, it is wise to minimize the immunosuppressive protocol, and in some cases, discontinuation of immunosuppression may be appropriate. The potential for graft loss needs to be weighed against the natural history and the staging of the malignancy. It is the patient who must ultimately decide on his or her priorities after receiving consultation from oncologic and transplant physicians. There are theoretical reasons for using sirolimus-based immunosuppression in patients with posttransplant malignancies (see Chapter 4, Part I). The practical benefit of this approach, however, is unproven. Posttransplant lymphoproliferative disease is discussed later.

Strategy 9: Prevent Infection

Infections are common in the late posttransplant period (see Chapter 10). These are sporadic, and few specific measures are effective in reducing the risk for infection. Routine prophylaxis for *Pneumocystis carinii* infections with trimethoprim-sulfamethoxazole is probably not warranted late after transplantation. The exception may be for patients who are receiving high doses of immunosuppression to treat rejection or for patients receiving sirolimus (see Chapter 4, Part I). The same is true for CMV infection prophylaxis. Although recurrent urinary tract infections are common, there is no evidence that routine prophylactic antibiotic therapy is effective.

Influenza types A and B are likely to be at least as common, and probably more severe, in renal transplant patients as in the general population. Therefore, transplant recipients should receive annual influenza vaccination. Although vaccines are safe, they may be somewhat less effective in transplant recipients than in the general population because of the limitation in antibody response by immunosuppressant drugs. Nevertheless, the response to vaccination is high enough (50% to 100%) to warrant their use. During the influenza season, chemoprophylaxis with amantadine or rimantadine (effective only against influenza A) or one of the newer neuraminidase inhibitors (effective against influenza A and B) should be considered for patients who have not yet been vaccinated. Consideration should also be given to the early diagnosis of influenza. If begun early, therapy can shorten the course of influenza infection and is probably warranted in immunosuppressed transplant recipients. Infections from *Streptococcus pneumoniae* are also common after renal transplantation and can cause considerable morbidity and mortality. The polyvalent pneumococcal vaccine should probably be administered every 2 years.

Strategy 10: Protect the Bones

Corticosteroid-induced osteopenia and its consequences are a common cause of posttransplant morbidity. Cross-sectional studies consistently show that bone mass is lower in transplant recipients than in age- and sex-matched controls. Vertebral bone loss is the highest in the first 6 to 12 months posttransplant (3% to 9%), but tends to stabilize thereafter. A fracture rate of 7% to 11% has been described in nondiabetic kidney transplant recipients; in diabetic recipients of kidney and pancreas transplants, the fracture incidence has been reported to be as high as 45%. It is reasonable to screen for decreased bone mineral density at baseline and 6 months after transplantation with dual-energy x-ray absorptiometry (DEXA) of the lumbar spine and hip. Patients with decreased bone mineral density may be candidates for oral calcium and vitamin D supplementation. Patients with abnormal bone mineral density 6 months after transplantation should be considered for additional followup examinations to measure the effectiveness of therapy. Bisphosphonates, which inhibit osteoclast activity, are effective in treating posttransplant osteopenia. Both bisphosphonates and calcitriol reverse bone loss and increase bone mass, although the resultant impact on the fracture rate is unproven. Bisphosphonates are somewhat more effective than vitamin D metabolites, although they may be contraindicated in the occasional patient with bone disease characterized by low turnover. Low bone turnover can be diagnosed only with a bone biopsy. It is difficult to prove a direct relationship between corticosteroid dose and bone loss, but it is reasonable to minimize steroid dose or consider discontinuation in the patients at high risk. Most of the impact of corticosteroids on bone comes from the high doses given in the early posttransplant period or for the treatment of acute rejection. Very-low-maintenance doses appear to have little effect on bone.

Corticosteroids can also cause avascular necrosis (AVN) or osteonecrosis. The site for posttransplant AVN is the femoral head in nearly 90% of cases. The incidence of AVN is difficult to assess but has been reported to be close to 1% per year in the second and third posttransplant years, and an overall incidence of 5.5% has been reported. The pathogenesis of AVN is poorly understood, and although corticosteroids can be implicated in most cases, it has proved difficult to establish a meaningful dose–response effect. AVN usually presents as hip or groin pain exacerbated by weight bearing. Pain may also be referred to the knee. Magnetic resonance imaging is the most sensitive method for diagnosis. Core decompression before the femoral head collapses may relieve pain, but approximately 60% of cases require total hip arthroplasty.

Hypophosphatemia is common early after transplantation but is less common in the late posttransplant period. When hypophosphatemia is encountered in the late posttransplant period, it is often caused by tertiary hyperparathyroidism, and serum parathyroid hormone levels should be measured in all patients with late posttransplant hypophosphatemia. On the other hand, hyperphosphatemia may also be encountered, usually in transplant recipients with renal insufficiency. Attempts should be made to suppress elevated parathyroid hormone levels by increasing serum calcium to high-normal levels. Calcium can usually be increased by reducing elevated serum phosphorous levels (with dietary phosphorous restriction and phosphorous binders) or by administrating oral calcium and vitamin D supplements. If increased parathyroid hormone levels cannot be suppressed, particularly if hypercalcemia becomes problematic, then parathyroidectomy may be required.

Hypomagnesemia is seen in approximately 10% of renal transplant recipients treated with calcineurin inhibitors. Hypomagnesemia may play a role in posttransplant hyperlipidemia and hypertension. Treatment is usually by oral magnesium replacement.

Strategy 11: Regard Impaired Posttransplant Function as a Form of Chronic Kidney Disease

Even well-functioning kidney transplants may have a glomerular filtration rate (GFR) that falls within the definition of chronic kidney disease (CKD) (see Chapter 1, Table 1.1). Chronic allograft nephropathy is a form of CKD that progresses to endstage renal disease and the need for dialysis and transplantation. Caregivers often give mixed signals to successful transplant recipients—on the one hand, patients are encouraged to "lead a normal life," while on the other hand, they are bombarded with precise instructions for health maintenance. Somehow a balance needs to be struck by patients and their doctors between these contrasting attitudes. It is clear, however, that patients with impaired baseline renal function are not normal and their care should encompass the same principles that have become standard of care for other causes of CKD. Control of hypertension, use of ACE inhibitors, control of mineral metabolism, treatment of anemia, preparation for end-stage renal disease options, and timely dialysis access placement, are all fundamental to optimal long-term posttransplant care. The immunosuppressive management of the failing graft is discussed in Chapter 4, Part V.

SPECIFIC MANAGEMENT ISSUES IN THE LATE POSTTRANSPLANT PERIOD

Posttransplant Lymphoproliferative Disease

The reported incidence of PTLD in the recipients of solid-organ transplants ranges from 0.8% to 15%, and varies with the type of transplantation, the patient's age, and the immunosuppressive regimen employed. The incidence is approximately 12-fold higher than in the nontransplant population. For kidney transplant recipients, the incidence is typically 1% to 2%. Despite the widespread use of potent immunosuppressive protocols, the incidence of PTLD in kidney transplant recipients does not appear to be increasing.

PTLDs have several unusual features that distinguish them from lymphomas found in the general population.

1. Most are non-Hodgkin lymphomas (Hodgkin disease is the most common lymphoma in age-matched controls) and are of B-cell origin and are CD20+.
2. PTLD often presents as dysfunction of the transplanted organ and may be confused histologically with severe rejection. Disease is often localized near the allograft.
3. There is a high rate of association with Epstein-Barr virus (EBV) and infection. Seronegative recipients of an organ from a seropositive donor are at highest risk for PTLD.
4. Extranodal involvement (central nervous system, liver, lungs, kidneys, intestines) is common, and multiple sites are often involved.
5. The mortality rate is much greater with PTLD than for lymphomas in the general population. The course may be extremely fulminant, with progression to death within a few months of transplantation.
6. The prolonged or repeated administration of lymphocytic-depleting antibody preparations is a significant risk factor for the development of PTLD.
7. PTLD may respond to withdrawal or drastic reduction of immunosuppressive therapy. Standard chemotherapy and irradiation are not generally helpful and may exaggerate the degree of immune compromise.
8. Viral infection, particularly with CMV infection (see Chapter 10), may serendipitously reduce EBV replication and the incidence of PTLD.

Role of Epstein-Barr Virus

EBV is a human DNA-transforming herpes virus that primarily targets B lymphocytes. It is associated with an array of disorders ranging from infectious mononucleosis to nasopharyngeal carcinoma, Burkitt lymphoma, and B-cell lymphomas in immunocompromised patients.

Transmission of EBV in transplant recipients is most commonly through the transplanted organ. EBV undergoes lytic replication because of inadequate EBV immune surveillance. The resultant increased burden of EBV in the naive recipient then infects the recipient's B cells. EBV has the innate capability of transforming and immortalizing host B lymphocytes, producing *lymphoblastoid cells*. An extrachromosomal particle of EBV genome can be found within the B-cell nucleus. In an immunocompetent host, a latent carrier state is established when the proliferation of the transformed B cells is contained by a normal immune response with intact cell-mediated immunity. Approximately 95% of adults have serologic evidence of previous EBV infection. The presence of reactive T lymphocytes inhibits infected cell proliferation in a process called regression. Immunosuppressive agents, particularly the antilymphocytic antibody preparations (see Chapter 4), prevent regression, and EBV-transformed cells may proliferate uncontrollably. The number of EBV DNA copies has a high, positive, predictive value for the diagnosis of PTLD; however, renal transplant patients can have a fluctuating serologic load without development of PTLD and there is a poor correlation between the serologic evidence of EBV reactivation and EBV viral load.

EBV-associated PTLD appears to progress through stages of transformation to a malignant state. The first stage resembles an infectious mononucleosis syndrome, with the development of polymorphic diffuse B-cell hyperplasias without cytogenic abnormalities or gene rearrangements. The second stage produces a subpopulation of cells with cellular and nuclear atypia and cytogenic abnormalities. In the third stage, a malignant monoclonal B-cell lymphoma develops. A form of fulminant PTLD has been described, often following multiple courses of OKT3. The disease may initially resemble a severe infectious mononucleosis-like illness, but may progress rapidly, with death occurring within a few months of transplantation. At a later stage, the patient may present with localized lymphoproliferative tumor masses in the brain, lung, or gastrointestinal tract. Predictors of poor survival from PTLD include increased age, elevated lactic acid dehydrogenase values, severe organ dysfunction, multiorgan involvement, and constitutional symptoms (fever, night sweats, weight loss).

Clonality

The issue of clonality of posttransplant lymphomas has been a source of dispute. It has been suggested that polyclonal B-cell lesions are likely to be benign and to respond to withdrawal of immunosuppression and acyclovir, whereas monoclonal lesions are believed to be frankly malignant. In fact, polyclonal lymphoproliferative disorders may represent an early stage in a spectrum that progresses from polyclonal activation of B cells by EBV to latently infected, malignantly transformed, monoclonal B cell lymphomas.

Treatment

Restoration of host immunity is probably the most important therapy for the control of lymphoid proliferation. Patients with evidence of polyclonality are most likely to respond to reduction of immunosuppression. Acyclovir, which acts by inhibiting the EBV-associated DNA polymerase, has been used but is not of proven benefit. For patients with monoclonal tumors, immunosuppression should be drastically reduced or discontinued altogether.

Results with conventional cytoxic therapy and radiotherapy have been disappointing, with mortality rates remaining at greater than 80%. Several small series and cases of PTLD have been reported where treatment with the anti-CD20 monoclonal antibody rituximab has been successful. B cells, together with their EBV viral load, disappear from the blood after its administration. The success rate of rituximab is estimated to be 65%. Rituximab and rapamycin combinations have also been reported. Most patients in whom immunosuppression is stopped lose their grafts to inexorable rejection. Occasionally, tumors regress and the patients and their grafts can be maintained on very-low-dose immunosuppression.

Hematologic Disorders

Anemia

Anemia is common after renal transplantation. The presumption that the newly transplanted kidney will produce enough erythropoietin to lead to resolution of pretransplant and early posttransplant anemia is incompletely realized in many patients. Using a cut-off of a hematocrit of 33%, it has been estimated that 30% of patients are anemic at some time during the late posttransplant period, and that 25% are anemic at 5 years posttransplant. In addition to its clinical symptoms, anemia may be a factor in the progression of chronic allograft failure and it may further exaggerate left ventricular hypertrophy. Unrecognized iron deficiency is a frequent cause, and gastrointestinal bleeding should be excluded. Anemia from folate or vitamin B_{12} deficiency is unusual. Hemolysis is rare. In the late posttransplant period, anemia is most commonly caused by immunosuppression or decreased renal function. Azathioprine, mycophenolate mofetil, and sirolimus can cause anemia, thrombocytopenia, and leukopenia, and the doses of these medications may need to be reduced. ACE inhibitors or receptor antagonists may also cause anemia. Parvovirus infection may be a cause of refractory anemia and treatment with intravenous immunoglobulin might be effective. When no underlying cause can be found, treatment with subcutaneous erythropoietin or Aranesp might be effective, particularly when renal function is impaired and iron stores are adequate. The efficacy of therapy can be monitored by observing changes in the reticulocyte count that precede an increase in the hemoglobin level. Anemia in patients with chronic allograft failure should be treated no less aggressively than the anemia accompanying other causes of chronic renal failure.

Erythrocytosis

Erythrocytosis is encountered in up to 20% of patients posttransplant, most commonly during the first 2 years. It rarely occurs in patients who have undergone native kidney nephrectomy, suggesting that it is the native kidneys, rather than the transplant, that is the source of the problem. The cause of erythrocytosis appears to be related to defective feedback regulation of erythropoietin metabolism. Although increased erythropoietin production has been reported posttransplant, erythrocytosis is not directly related to erythropoietin levels, which may be low or undetectable in some cases. Elevated levels of insulin-like growth factor (IGF)-1 have been found, which may increase the sensitivity of erythroid precursors to erythropoietin. Erythrocytosis may also be a manifestation of transplant renal artery stenosis and this diagnosis should be considered in any patient with the combination of hypertension, edema, allograft bruit, and erythrocytosis.

Hematocrit levels higher than 60% are associated with increased viscosity and thrombosis, and treatment should commence at a hematocrit level of greater than 55%. Low doses of

ACE inhibitors or receptor antagonists are generally effective in reducing elevated hematocrit levels. Their mechanism of action may be related to the induction of apoptosis in erythroid precursors and to reduction of IGF-1 levels. Renal dysfunction after introduction of ACE inhibitors should raise the possibility of transplant renal artery stenosis. Theophylline is a potential alternative to the use of ACE inhibitors or receptor blockers, although it is less-well tolerated. Phlebotomy may be required in resistant cases.

POSTTRANSPLANT REPRODUCTIVE FUNCTIONS

Men

After successful transplantation, about two-thirds of male patients observe improved libido and a return of sexual function to predialysis levels. In some patients, there is no improvement, and occasionally sexual function deteriorates. Fertility, as assessed by sperm counts, improves in half of patients. The sex hormone profile tends to normalize; plasma testosterone and follicle-stimulating hormone levels increase; and luteinizing hormone levels, which may be high in dialysis patients, decrease to normal or low levels. Cyclosporine may impair testosterone biosynthesis through direct damage to Leydig cells and germinal cells, and a direct impairment of the hypothalamic–pituitary–gonadal axis has been suggested. Sirolimus may also reduce testosterone levels. There is no increased incidence of neonatal malformations in pregnancies fathered by transplant recipients.

Additional factors may account for failure of male sexual function to improve after transplantation. Antihypertensive medications may be responsible in some patients, autonomic neuropathy may impair erectile function, and interruption of both hypogastric arteries may occasionally impair vascular supply. Male patients should be asked about their sexual function and referred for urologic evaluation when necessary. There is no specific contraindication to the use of sildenafil (Viagra) in transplant recipients so long as standard precautions are taken regarding concomitant coronary artery disease.

Women

Women with chronic renal failure demonstrate loss of libido, anovulatory vaginal bleeding or amenorrhea, and high prolactin levels. Maintenance dialysis therapy results in improvement in sexual function in only a small percentage of women, and pregnancy is rare. Within a year of successful transplantation, menstrual function and ovulation typically return, and prolactin levels fall to normal.

Family Planning

All women of childbearing age should be counseled concerning the possibility and risks of pregnancy after kidney transplantation. Psychosocial issues should be discussed, genetic counseling should be provided for those with hereditary kidney disease, and consideration should be given to the long-term prognosis of the patient and the graft. Patients can be assured that birth defects are not increased with the use of azathioprine, cyclosporine,

Table 9.12.   Criteria for the reduction of posttransplantation pregnancy risk

At least 1 year posttransplant
Serum creatinine <2.0 mg/dL, preferably <1.5 mg/dL
No recent episodes of acute rejection
Normotensive or minimal antihypertensive regimen
Minimal or no proteinuria
Normal allograft ultrasound
Pregnancy-safe drug regimen (see text)

and tacrolimus during pregnancy, although intrauterine growth retardation and prematurity are common. Data regarding the stability of graft function during and after pregnancy should be discussed. All pregnancies should be planned and prepared for. Conception should be delayed 18 to 24 months after kidney transplantation and contraception practiced until then.

Contraceptive counseling should begin immediately after transplantation because ovulatory cycles may begin within 1 to 2 months of transplantation in women with well-functioning grafts. Low-dose estrogen-progesterone oral contraceptive preparations are advised. They should be used with caution because they may cause or aggravate hypertension or precipitate thromboembolism, especially in the context of cyclosporine immunosuppression. Calcineurin inhibitor levels should also be monitored soon after the contraceptive is started. The long-acting, subcutaneously placed hormone preparations are highly effective and well-tolerated. They have not yet been formally tried in the transplant situation and should be used only under careful supervision. The risk for infection may be increased with the use of an intrauterine device in immunocompromised patients, and their efficacy may be compromised by the antiinflammatory properties of the immunosuppressive agents. Barrier contraception is the safest modality but depends on user compliance for efficacy.

PREGNANCY

Women with end-stage renal disease sometimes seek transplantation with the knowledge that a well-functioning graft will give them the only real chance for natural motherhood. It has been estimated that 2% of women of childbearing age conceive after transplantation. The incidence of spontaneous abortion is reported to be 13%, and that of ectopic pregnancy is reported to be 0.5%. These frequencies are not different from those seen in the normal population. About one-third of pregnant transplant recipients seek therapeutic abortion, a number that likely reflects inadequate family planning in women who have not previously considered themselves to be fertile. More than 90% of conceptions that continue beyond the first trimester end successfully.

Table 9.12 lists the criteria that should be ideally be met before conception. A 90% incidence of successful pregnancies has been reported for women with a baseline serum creatinine of 1.5 mg/dL or less. A higher serum creatinine level increase the risk of posttransplant graft loss, which consistently occurs within 2 years of pregnancy in women whose baseline creatinine is greater than 2.0 mg/dL. Failure to meet all the listed criteria places the patient in a higher risk category, but is not necessarily an absolute contraindication to pregnancy. The U.S. National Transplantation Pregnancy Registry has been developed to provide current information concerning transplant recipient pregnancy for the benefit of patients and their physicians.

Antenatal Care

Pregnancy in a patient with a kidney transplant should be considered a high-risk condition and should be monitored in a tertiary care center with consultation by a transplantation nephrologist, obstetrician, and pediatrician. The pregnancy should be diagnosed as early as possible and accurate dating obtained by fetal ultrasound. For patients with good allograft function before conception, the GFR remains stable or increases, as it does during a normal pregnancy. The GFR may decline to pregnancy values during the third trimester. Most studies suggest that pregnancy itself does not have an unfavorable effect on long-term graft function as long as baseline function is excellent. Proteinuria may increase to abnormal pregnancy in the third trimester, but usually resolves postpartum and is of no prognostic significance unless it is associated with hypertension. About 30% of pregnant patients with kidney transplants develop pregnancy-induced hypertension, a figure that is fourfold greater than in uncomplicated pregnancies. The use of cyclosporine in pregnancy tends to increase the incidence of hypertension. If complications (usually hypertension, renal deterioration, and/or rejection) occur before 28 weeks gestation, successful obstetric outcome is reduced by 20%. Prematurity (60%), growth restriction (52%) and the need for hospitalization in a neonatal intensive care unit (35%) are reported to be more common in transplant recipients than in patients with renal diseases who are not on immunosuppression.

Urinary tract infections are the most common bacterial infections and occur in up to 40% of pregnant transplant recipients. Pyelonephritis may develop despite adequate antibiotic treatment. Urinary tract infections are particularly common in patients who develop end-stage renal disease as a consequence of pyelonephritis.

Immunosuppression in Pregnancy

Prednisone

Prednisone crosses the placenta, but a large proportion is converted to prednisolone, which allegedly does not suppress fetal corticotropin. Adrenal insufficiency in the neonate has been reported with maternal prednisone ingestion. Very large doses of corticosteroids administered to animals have resulted in congenital anomalies (cleft lip and palate), but no consistent abnormalities have been noted in the offspring of women treated with corticosteroids during pregnancy for rheumatologic disease or kidney transplantation. Overall, prednisone is considered to be relatively safe for use in pregnancy.

Azathioprine

At doses of 2 mg/kg or less, no anomalies attributable to azathioprine have been noted in human offspring. There are minimal data, however, on the long-term effects of azathioprine on first- or second-generation offspring. Azathioprine can cause transient gaps or breaks in lymphocyte chromosomes. Germ cells and other tissues have not been studied. It is not known whether the eventual sequelae could be the development of malignancies in affected offspring or other abnormalities in the next generation.

Calcineurin Inhibitors

There are no animal or human data showing teratogenicity or mutagenicity of cyclosporine or tacrolimus, which appear to be safe during pregnancy. Intrauterine growth retardation and small-for-gestational-age neonates have been reported with cyclosporine use and may reflect chronic vasoconstriction. Cyclosporine is present in the fetal circulation at the same concentration found in the mother. The increased volume of distribution may produce low maternal blood levels and dose elevations may be required.

Other Immunosuppressions

The U.S. Food and Drug Administration (FDA) categorizes the potential fetal risks of drugs used in pregnancy. Most immunosuppressive drugs fall into category "C," which implies that "risks cannot be ruled out." Limited data are available concerning the safety of pregnancy for patients receiving the newer immunosuppressive agents (see Chapter 4); for the present they should be avoided during pregnancy. Mycophenolate mofetil and sirolimus should be discontinued 6 weeks before conception is attempted. At present, there is insufficient information about the biologic effect of even small amounts of immunosuppressive agents on the neonate, and breastfeeding should be discouraged.

Hypertension Control

Many transplant patients require antihypertensive drugs in pregnancy. Drugs that have been consistently shown to be safe should be used, these include methyldopa, hydralazine, and labetalol. ACE inhibitors and receptor blockers are generally contraindicated in pregnancy but it is probably safe to continue a pregnancy if their administration is discontinued as soon as pregnancy is diagnosed.

Labor and Delivery

Vaginal delivery is recommended because the transplanted kidney is placed in the false pelvis and there is little risk for obstruction of the birth canal or mechanical injury to the allograft. Cesarean section is usually performed only for standard obstetric reasons. Great care should be taken to identify and protect the transplanted ureter. Preterm delivery occurs in about half of pregnancies in transplant recipients because of the frequent occurrence of declining kidney function, pregnancy-induced hypertension, fetal distress, premature rupture of membranes, and premature labor. The incidence of small-for-gestational-age neonates is 20%. There is no increase in fetal abnormalities.

In the perinatal period, the steroid dose should be augmented to cover the stress of labor and to prevent postpartum rejection. Hydrocortisone, 100 mg every 6 hours, should be given during labor and delivery. Maternal hypertension and fluid balance should be monitored carefully. Graft function and the immunosuppressive regimen should be monitored with particular care in the first 3 months postpartum. Occasional cases of postpartum acute renal failure resembling hemolytic uremic syndrome have been described.

SELECTED READINGS

Part I

Abbott K, Yuan M, Taylor A, et al. Early renal insufficiency and hospitalized heart disease after renal transplantation in the era of modern immunosuppression. *J Am Soc Nephrol* 2003;14:235–239

Briganti E, Russ G, McNeil J, et al. Risk of renal allograft loss from recurrent glomerulonephritis. *N Engl J Med* 2002;347:103–107.

Chkhotua A, Gabusi E, Altimari A, et al. Increased expression of p16(INK4a) and p27(Kip1) cyclin-dependent kinase inhibitor genes in aging human kidney and chronic allograft nephropathy. *Transplantation* 2003;41:1303–1307.

Collins AJ, Kasiske B, Herzog C, et al. Excerpts from the USRDS 2003 annual data report: atlas of end-stage renal disease in the United States. *Am J Kidney Dis* 2003;42[6 Suppl 5]:A5–A7.

Colvin RB. Chronic allograft nephropathy. *N Engl J Med* 2003;349:2287–2291.

Cosio F, Pesavento T, Kim S, et al. Patient survival after renal transplantation: IV. Impact of post-transplant diabetes. *Kidney Int* 2002;62:1440.

Feng S, Buell JF, Chari R, et al. Tumors and transplantation: the 2003 third annual ASTS state of the art winter symposium. *Am J Transplant* 2003;3:1481–1487.

Gourishankar S, Hunsicker L, Jhangri G, et al. The stability of the glomerular filtration rate after renal transplantation is improving. *J Am Soc Nephrol* 2003;14:2387.

Halloran P. Call for revolution: a new approach to describing allograft deterioration. *Am J Transplant* 2002;2:195.

Hariharan S, McBride M, Cherikh W, et al. Post-transplant renal function in the first year predicts long-term kidney transplant survival. *Kidney Int* 2002;62:311–318.

Heidenhain C, Reutzel-Selke A, Bachmann U, et al. The impact of immune-activating processes following transplantation on chronic allograft nephropathy. *Kidney Int* 2003;64:1125.

Karthikeyan V, Karpinski J, Nair R, et al. The burden of chronic kidney disease in renal transplant recipients. *Am J Transplant* 2003;4:262–269.

Lee P, Terasaki P, Takemoto S, et al. All chronic rejection failures of kidney transplants were preceded by the development of HLA antibodies. *Transplantation* 2002;74:1192–1195.

Matas A, Humar A, Gillingham K, et al. Five preventable causes of kidney graft loss in the 1990s: a single-center analysis. *Kidney Int* 2002;62:704–708.

Nankivell BJ, Borrows R, Fung C, et al. The natural history of chronic allograft nephropathy. *N Engl J Med* 2003,349:2326–2332.

Pascual M, Theruvath T, Kawai T, et al. Strategies to improve long-term outcomes after renal transplantation. *N Engl J Med* 2002; 346:580–590.

Ponticelli C, Villa M, Cesana B, et al. Risk factors for late kidney allograft failure. *Kidney Int* 2002;62:1848–1853.

Raj DS, Lim G, Levi M, et al. Advanced glycation products and oxidative stress are increased in chronic allograft nephropathy. *Am J Kidney Dis* 2004;43:154–160.

Part II

Abbott K, Oglesby R, Agodoa L. Hospitalized avascular necrosis after renal transplantation in the United States. *Kidney Int* 2002;62:2250–2255.

Brandenburg V, Ketteler M, Fassbender J, et al. Development of lumbar bone mineral density in the late course after kidney transplantation. *Transplantation* 2002;40:1066–1070.

Bruno S, Remuzzi G, Ruggeneti P. Transplant renal artery stenosis. *J Am Soc Nephrol* 2004;15:134–141.

Bustami R, Ojo AO, Wolfe R, et al. Immunosuppression and the risk of posttransplant malignancy among cadaveric first kidney transplant recipients. *Am J Transplant* 2004;4:87–92.

Carroll R, Ramsay H, Fryer A, et al. Incidence and prediction of nonmelanoma skin cancer post-renal transplantation: a prospective study in Queensland, Australia. *Transplantation* 2003;41:676–681.

Cohen D, Galbraith C. General health management and long-term care of the renal transplant recipient. *Am J Kidney Dis* 2001;38: S10–S24.

Cruz D, Brickel H, Wysolmerski J, et al. Treatment of osteoporosis and osteopenia in long-term renal transplant patients with alendronate. *Am J Transplant* 2002;2:62–67.

Danovitch G. Guidelines on the firing-line. *Am J Transplant* 2003;3:514–515.

Fernandez-Fresnedo G, Escallada R, Rodrigo E, et al. The risk of cardiovascular disease associated with proteinuria in renal transplant patients. *Transplantation* 2002;74:1345–1349.

Ferreira S, Moises V, Tavares A, et al. Cardiovascular effects of successful renal transplantation: a 1-year sequential study of left ventricular morphology and function, and 24-hour blood pressure profile. *Transplantation* 2002;74:1580–1585.

First R, Gerber D, Hariharan S, et al. Posttransplant diabetes mellitus in kidney allograft recipients: incidence, risk factors, and management. *Transplantation* 2002;73:379–385.

Howard A. Long-term management of the renal transplant recipient: optimizing the relationship between the transplant center and the community nephrologist. *Am J Kidney Dis* 2001;38[6 Suppl 6]:S51–S57.

Holdaas H, Fellström B, Jardine A, et al. Effect of fluvastatin on cardiac outcomes in renal transplant recipients: a multicenter, randomised, placebo-controlled trial. *Lancet* 2003;361:2024–2031.

Kasiske B, Cosio FG, Beto J, et al. Clinical practice guidelines for managing dyslipidemias in kidney transplant patients: a report of the Managing Dyslipedemias in Chronic Kidney Disease Work Group of the National Kidney Foundation Kidney Disease Outcomes Quality Initiative. *Am J Transplant* 2004;4(Suppl 7):13–53.

Kasiske B, Vazquez MA, Harmon WE, et al. Recommendations for the outpatient surveillance of renal allograft recipients. *J Am Soc Nephrol* 2000;11[Suppl 15]:1.

Morales J. Influence of the new immunosuppressive combinations on arterial hypertension after renal transplantation. *Kidney Int* 2002;62:S81–S87.

Opelz G, Dohler B. Lymphomas after solid organ transplantation: a collaborative study report. *Am J Transplant* 2003;4:222–230.

Paya C, Fung J, Nalesnik M, et al. Epstein-Barr virus-induced posttransplant lymphoproliferative disorders. *Transplantation* 1999;68:1517–1526.

Ramesh Prasad G, Ahmed A, Nash M, et al. Blood pressure reduction with HMG-CoA reductase inhibitors in renal transplant recipients. *Kidney Int* 2003;63:360–364.

Verschuuren E, Stevens S, van Imhoff G, et al. Treatment of posttransplant lymphoproliferative disease with rituximab: the remission, the relapse, and the complication. *Transplantation* 2002;73:100–104.

Wilkinson A. Use of angiotensin-converting enzyme inhibitors and angiotensin II antagonists in renal transplantation: delaying the progression of chronic allograft nephropathy? *Transplantation Rev* 2000;14:138–143.

Yorgin P, Scandling J, Belson A, et al. Late post-transplant anemia in adult renal transplant recipients. An under-recognized problem? *Am J Transplant* 2002;2:429–433.

10

Infections in Kidney Transplantation

Bernard M. Kubak, Cynthia L. Maree, David A. Pegues, and Andy Hwang

Among solid-organ transplants, kidney transplantation is associated with the lowest rates of infections, in part because of the elective or semielective nature of kidney transplantation. In contrast, liver, heart, or lung allograft recipients often have poor clinical and nutritional status before transplant that contributes to increased infection risk. Despite ongoing refinements in immunosuppressive agents, graft preservation, and surgical techniques, infection remains a significant cause of morbidity and mortality in renal transplant recipients. Infections related to transplant surgical complications or to postoperative nosocomial, opportunistic, or latent pathogens can affect graft function and transplant outcome. Graft dysfunction or chronic rejection leads to augmented immunosuppression, increasing the risk of infection with immunomodulating viruses. Infectious syndromes encountered in the kidney transplant recipient include device-associated infections; genitourinary infections, including infections associated with antimicrobial-resistant organisms; bacterial, mycobacterial, and fungal pneumonia, including pulmonary and disseminated infections with *Nocardia* bacteria, *Mycobacterium tuberculosis* on nontuberculous mycobacteria, and *Candida*, *Aspergillus*, *Cryptococcus*, and *Pneumocystis* fungi; reactivation mycoses such as histoplasmosis and coccidioidomycosis; and disseminated or organ-specific viral diseases [cytomegalovirus (CMV), human herpesvirus (HHV), varicella-zoster virus (VZV), Epstein-Barr virus (EBV), polyomavirus, adenovirus, and respiratory viruses including influenza A and B, respiratory syncytial virus (RSV), and parainfluenza viruses.]

This chapter highlights the infectious disease issues in kidney transplant recipients, posttransplant infection prophylaxis, and the recognition and treatment of common and emerging infectious syndromes with appropriate antimicrobial therapy to minimize allograft toxicity.

GENERAL GUIDELINES FOR INFECTION RECOGNITION

Table 10.1 summarizes the clinical risk factors for infection in the pretransplant and posttransplant settings. Recognition of the following factors may assist in the identification of the causative pathogen and the initiation of appropriate empiric antimicrobial therapy before laboratory confirmation:

1. The timing of an infectious episode following transplantation is critical (Fig. 10.1). The majority of infections occur in the first posttransplant month, and typically develop from new or preexisting or genitourinary infection in the recipient or donor.

Table 10.1. Risk factors for infection in renal transplant recipients

Pretransplantation (recipient)

- Medical conditions (renal failure, diabetes, malnutrition, disorders of immune function)
- Iatrogenic immunosuppression for chronic conditions (corticosteroids, cyclophosphamide)
- Unrecognized or inadequately treated infection in the recipient
- Colonization with unusual or resistant organisms (e.g., VRE in stool, MRSA in nares or on skin, drug-resistant Enterobacteriaceae or *Pseudomonas* in genitourinary tract, gastrointestinal tract, and upper respiratory tract; acquisition of yeasts on mucocutaneous and other mucosal surfaces; yeasts or molds on skin, mucosal surfaces)
- Preoperative antibiotic exposures
- Duration and frequency of hospitalizations

Perioperative

- Complexity of surgery and requirement for reexploration(s)
- Prolonged operative time
- Graft injury or prolonged ischemia; acute graft failure
- Bleeding or multiple blood transfusions
- Graft infection (donor) and/or unrecognized infection in the donor
- Perioperative bacteremia or sepsis
- Microbial contamination of preservation fluid or graft
- Retained foreign bodies

Posttransplantation

- Acute graft failure or dysfunction; requirements for augmented immunosuppression and prolonged cytolytic therapies
- Early reexploration or retransplantation
- Complicated postoperative management; development or worsening of comorbid medical conditions (hyperglycemia, hepatic disease, respiratory insufficiency, altered sensorium)
- Infection with immunomodulating viruses (CMV, HHV, respiratory viruses)
- Prolonged catheters, genitourinary stents, or mechanical ventilation
- Bladder-drained procedure; enteric-drained procedure (pancreas, kidney–pancreas transplant), pancreas transplant after kidney transplant
- Anastomotic breakdown or leaks; development of fluid collections, devitalized tissues, hematomas
- Leukopenia, thrombocytopenia, acquired hypogammaglobulinemia
- Prolonged antibiotic therapy; acquisition of antibiotic-resistant nosocomial pathogens
- Corticosteroids: maintenance dose and pulses
- Hospital exposures: construction, ventilation, and water supply
- Selected occupational, gardening, and recreational activities: composting, exposure to decaying vegetation, hunting
- Lack of appropriate hand hygiene by caregivers
- Marijuana use

CMV, cytomegalovirus; HHV, human herpesvirus; MRSA, methicillin-resistant *Staphylococcus aureus;* VRE, vancomycin-resistant *Enterococcus.*

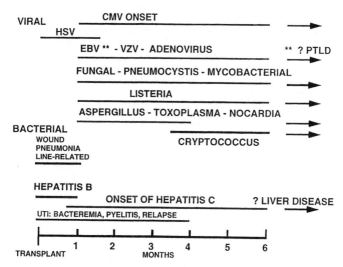

Fig. 10.1. Timetable for occurrence of infection after transplantation. Arrows indicate infections or other manifestations that may present more than 6 months to years after transplantation. **, indicates possible relationship of EBV to PTLD; CMV, cytomegalovirus; EBV, Epstein-Barr virus; HSV, herpes simplex virus; PTLD, posttransplantation lymphoproliferative disease; UTI, urinary tract infection; VZV, varicella-zoster virus; (Modified from Rubin RH. Infection in the organ transplant patient. In: Rubin RH, Young LS, eds. *Clinical approach to infection in the compromised host.* New York: Plenum, 1994, pp 629–669, with permission.)

Table 10.1 lists the host, surgical, and medical factors that are associated with an increased risk of infection.

During months 1 to 6, infections associated with postoperative complications or with enhanced immunosuppression can develop, persist, or recur. Augmented immunosuppression is associated with an increased risk of infection with immunomodulating viruses such as CMV, HHV, hepatitis B virus (HBV), hepatitis C virus (HCV), and EBV that enhance susceptibility to infection with opportunistic pathogens by altering the expression of inflammatory mediators and cytokines by a complex interrelated cascade. This leads to a permissive environment for opportunistic pathogens such as *Pneumocystis, Aspergillus,* and other molds and *Listeria monocytogenes, Nocardia, Cryptococcus, Toxoplasma,* and other viruses. CMV and other human herpesviruses also exert an immunomodulating effect that has been implicated in allograft rejection, obliterative transplant arteriopathy, and posttransplantation lymphoproliferative disorder (PTLD).

After posttransplant month 6, patients generally can be categorized as those with successful graft outcome and minimal long-term maintenance immunosuppression, those with poor graft function because of chronic rejection who require intensified immunosuppression, or those chronically infected with immunomodulating viruses such as CMV. Infections in patients with long-term successful allografts are typically similar to those that develop in persons in the community, while the latter two patient groups are at ongoing risk of opportunistic infections.

2. The *net state of immunosuppression.* This is a semiquantitative assessment that reflects the complex interaction of the following factors:

A. The dose, duration, and temporal sequence of immunosuppressive therapy, including augmented immunosuppression for episodes of rejection;

B. Quantitative immunodeficiency, including leukopenia, thrombocytopenia, and low immunoglobulin levels;

C. Breach of tissue barriers by foreign bodies (e.g., urinary and venous catheters; stents), open wounds, fluid collections, and devitalized tissues;

D. Metabolic abnormalities such as hyperglycemia, liver failure, malnutrition, uremia;

E. Infection with immunomodulatory viruses.

3. The infectious history of the donor, specifically any infectious syndromes and pathogen that can be directly transmitted with the allograft.

4. Preoperative recipient history of infections and exposures, such as tuberculosis, hepatitis viruses, HIV, VZV, CMV, or EBV. Immune-altering conditions, such as surgery or functional asplenia; pretransplant medical conditions including rheumatologic disorders such as systemic lupus erythematosus that require immunosuppressive therapy, diabetes mellitus, substance or injection drug use, liver dysfunction, malnutrition, and potential geographic exposures to endemic mycoses, toxoplasmosis, tuberculosis and *Strongyloides* species.

5. The acquisition of community and healthcare-associated pathogens, such as *Streptococcus pneumoniae,* Enterobacteriaceae, and *Pseudomonas* species, methicillin-resistant *Staphylococcus aureus* (MRSA), and vancomycin-resistant *Enterococcus* (VRE). Pretransplant dialysis patients and kidney recipients especially may harbor bacteria and yeasts on their skin, mucosal surfaces, and sinopulmonary and gastrointestinal tracts. Many candidates may have been hospitalized or treated for recent infections. Consequently, these patients may be colonized with healthcare-associated bacteria and fungi, some of which have intrinsic or acquired antimicrobial resistance. The clinical consequences this colonization after kidney transplant must be carefully considered, because in the setting of graft dysfunction, postoperative surgical complications, or rejection, these colonizing organisms have the potential to gain access to blood, urine, respiratory tracts, and fluid collections. Determining the species and antimicrobial susceptibility of these colonizing organisms may assist in directing empiric antimicrobial therapy if clinical infection develops.

6. Factors that confound the diagnosis of infection in the recipient include: an impaired host inflammatory response; the delay in clinical diagnosis because of the lack of "classic" clinical and radiologic signs associated with infection and inflammation

compared to the nonimmunocompromised host; the rapid progression of infections in this context, particularly with altered transplant anatomy; the failure to recognize "high-risk" patient characteristics (e.g., diabetes, enhanced and prolonged immunosuppression, multiple antibiotic courses, among others); and, the delays in laboratory diagnosis and paucity of reliable rapid diagnostic assays in cases of fungal, mycobacterial, and viral diseases.

7. Inherent diagnostic uncertainty: infection can occur during or following episodes of rejection or CMV infection, particularly with fungal pathogens, and can involve nonallograft sites. Infections can be well established and disseminated before cultures become positive or before histopathology confirms invasion and etiology. In addition, adverse effects of medications may mimic the signs and symptoms of infection.

PRETRANSPLANT SCREENING: RECIPIENT AND DONOR

Untreated or unrecognized infections in the recipient can become clinically apparent in the posttransplant period. These can include intravascular device infection, pneumonia, cellulitis, periodontal abscess, or smoldering intraabdominal, hepatobiliary, or genitourinary tract infection. Reactivation or exacerbation can occur postoperatively depending on the overall *net state of immunosuppression.* During pretransplant screening, the identification of latent infections or infectious exposures in the recipient can lead to a reappraisal of transplant candidacy or to alterations in standard posttransplant antimicrobial management. For the living-related donor, a careful history of prior infections and exposures and of any current signs or symptoms of infection should be obtained and active infections treated when appropriate. Donation should be deferred until the respective infection resolves (living-related donor and pretransplant evaluations are described elsewhere in this book).

Pretransplant Screening: Donor- and Allograft-Transmitted Infections

It may be difficult to differentiate between an infection acquired from the allograft, from an exogenous source, or from reactivation of latent disease in the recipient. The following agents have been implicated transmission from the donor allograft: aerobic gram-positive and gram-negative bacteria, anaerobic bacteria, *Mycobacteria* species, *Toxoplasma,* and *Strongyloides* species; HIV, CMV, HBV, HCV, herpes simplex virus HSV, VZV, EBV, and West Nile virus; and fungi including *Candida* species, *Histoplasma capsulatum, Coccidioides immitis, Cryptococcus neoformans, C. albicans, A. fumigatus,* and *Monosporium apiospermum.* Serious complications of donor allograft-transmitted infections include disruption of the vascular anastomoses, formation of "mycotic" (microbial) aneurysms, infective endocarditis, and sepsis. The risk of donor-transmitted infection can be reduced by scrupulous screening and epidemiologic evaluation (see Chapter 5).

Evaluation of the patient for infection risk should include a history of antibiotic allergies, assessment for endovascular infection,

Table 10.2.   Pretransplant screening

Underlying medical conditions (see Chapter 6)

Antibiotic and medication allergies and adverse reactions

Chest radiograph (e.g., any evidence of active infiltrates; prior granulomatous lesions; scarring)

Dental assessment

History of sexually transmitted diseases, high-risk behaviors, injection drug usage

PPD skin test with anergy panel; history of tuberculosis risk factors and exposure(s)

Urine culture

Endovascular repair or placement (e.g., valve, vascular graft)

Serologies:

    CMV IgG antibody

    Epstein-Barr Virus (EBV) antibody panel

    Herpes simplex virus (HSV), HHV-8 (HHV-6 in pediatric candidates) and varicella-zoster virus (VZV) IgG antibodies

    Hepatitis B virus (HBV) surface antigen (HBsAg), core antibody (HBcAb IgM and IgG), surface antibody (HBsAb)

    Hepatitis C virus (HCV) IgG antibody

    HIV 1 and 2 antibody

    Human T-cell lymphotropic virus (HTLV-I/II) antibody in patients from endemic regions

    West Nile virus (determine geographic and seasonal risk)

    SARS-CoV (no routine viral testing at present; check CDC guidelines)

    Rapid plasma reagin (RPR)

    Coccidioides IgM and IgG antibody by EIA (in patient from endemic areas)

    Trypanosoma cruzi serology (in patients from endemic areas)

CDC, Centers for Disease Control and Prevention; CMV, cytomegalovirus; EIA, electroimmunoassay; HHV, human herpesvirus; HIV, human immunodeficiency virus; Ig, immunoglobulin; PPD, purified protein derivative; SARS-CoV, severe acute respiratory syndrome-associated coronavirus.

a dental assessment, a preoperative urine culture, and a chest radiograph to exclude active pneumonic processes or evidence of prior granulomatous disease (Table 10.2). A chest radiographic suggestive of infectious granulomatous disease and a history of exposure to *Mycobacterium* or endemic mycosis should prompt an investigation of prior skin laboratory testing for infectious agents and a history of documented infection and treatment. Risk of infection with an endemic mycosis should be assessed, including history of travel to or residency in an at-risk area. Old "healed" granulomatous lesions may harbor latent organisms that can reactivate in the posttransplant setting during routine immunosuppression, especially after treatments for rejection. The risk of active or latent tuberculosis infection in the recipient or donor should be reviewed. Recipients should have a purified protein derivative (PPD) skin test performed with appropriate controls (e.g., mumps, *Candida*, tetanus). The higher incidence of cutaneous anergy in renal-failure patients will lead to false-negative PPD results, so clinical and radiographic history compatible with prior tuberculosis (TB) disease is critical. Living donors should undergo tuberculosis screening, and urine acid-fast bacillus (AFB) cultures should be performed if there is a history compatible with disseminated tuberculosis. While deceased donor history of prior tuberculosis often is difficult to ascertain, active infection in the donor should be avoided. Isoniazid prophylaxis in the recipient may be indicated despite a negative PPD skin test if the chest radiograph and history suggests a risk of latent tuberculosis. The American Thoracic Society recommendations for prophylaxis for latent tuberculosis should be followed.

Patients who previously completed a full-treatment course for active tuberculosis usually do not require additional antituberculous therapy after transplantation. Patients with polycystic kidney disease who have been treated for infected polycystic kidneys should have repeatedly negative urine cultures. Pretransplant polycystic nephrectomy is occasionally required (see Chapter 6).

Donor Screening

Postoperative infections can arise from inadequate donor screening. The donor's medical history and social history should include information on high-risk behaviors such as injection drug usage, prior hospitalizations and blood transfusions, incarceration histories, and tuberculosis exposures. These exposures may be associated with an increased risk of acute HIV, hepatitis B, and hepatitis C infection where serologies may be negative. The organ procurement agency should provide results of donor microbiology cultures, serum serologies, and history of infections, including bacteremias that may not be confirmed by the laboratory until after transplantation in some cases. Because many deceased donor kidneys may be recovered from patients in intensive care units, occult bacteremias or genitourinary tract infection should be excluded by appropriate cultures. In the case of donor-associated bacteremia, pathogen-directed antimicrobial therapy should be administered to the recipient and continued for a period based upon the virulence of the organisms, followup blood cultures, and careful clinical assessment. Infections of the vascular anastomosis, although rare, are associated with donor-derived bacteremia with *S. aureus, P. aeruginosa,* gram-negative bacilli, and *Candida* and *Aspergillus* species. In addition, donor history of any potential upper and lower urinary tract infections should ascertained. Deceased donor kidneys have been transplanted successfully from donors with localized, nongenitourinary infections, including pneumonia and meningitis. History of bacteremia should be ruled out and antimicrobial therapy administered to the recipient as clinically indicated. Syphilis has been transmitted in solid-organ transplants, but it is not a contraindication to organ donation. The recipient should receive treatment appropriate to the presumed stage of donor syphilis infection. During the allograft harvesting and transplant, contamination of the preservation media has been observed. If present, pathogen-directed antimicrobial therapy should be administered to the recipient and continued for approximately 2 weeks. Donors infected by fungal pathogens, particularly fungemia or genitourinary fungal infection should be avoided. Unspecified, ambiguous, or inadequate donor infectious or high-risk behavior history should preclude use of such donor organs. Donors with unspecified viral infections, or suspicion of encephalitis, or ambiguous causes of infectious death should also be avoided.

Serologic Testing

Preoperative antibody testing, where appropriate, should include CMV, VZV, EBV, HSV-1 and -2, human herpesviruses 6, 7, and 8, HIV, antihepatitis B virus surface antibody (anti-HBsAb), surface antigen (HBsAg), and core antibody [HBc immunoglobulin IgG and IgM]; and HCV antibody (see Chapter 11); and specific testing for endemic mycoses when appropriate (e.g., coccidioidal antibody detection in any patient with any exposure to an endemic area).

Cytomegalovirus

CMV is the most common viral infection after kidney transplantation, and the severity of infections ranges from asymptomatic to target-organ infection (central nervous system, lungs, intestine, allograft), dissemination, and death. The clinical implications of the CMV infection are discussed in Viral Infections and summarized in Table 10.3. The seroprevalence of CMV ranges from 40% to 97%, depending on the population screened. The incidence of CMV seropositivity increases with age, and most adult dialysis patients have detectable IgG antibody to CMV. The CMV antibody status of the donor and recipient should be ascertained before transplant. A CMV-seronegative recipient (R–) of a CMV-seropositive donor (D+) is at the highest risk of developing subsequent CMV infection and disease. After transplant, these recipients require preemptive antiviral therapy strategies for a period after transplantation, careful close vigilance for the signs and symptoms of CMV disease, and laboratory monitoring for CMV replication. While CMV seropositive recipients (D+/R+, D–/R+) have a lower risk of CMV disease, a similar prevention strategy should be employed, based on the individual patient risk factors and net state of immunosuppression.

Epstein-Barr Virus

Both EBV-seronegative recipients of grafts from EBV-seropositive donors and EBV-seropositive recipients may be at increased risk for PTLD, particularly if they receive prolonged or repeated courses of antilymphocytic therapy (see Chapter 9). EBV mismatch may occur more commonly in pediatric kidney recipients. In high-risk patients, the quantitative EBV viral load can be assayed by polymerase chain reaction (PCR) after augmenting immunosuppression or when clinically indicated, and can be used to prompt preemptive therapies.

Other Human Herpesviruses

Other human herpesviruses of significance to organ transplant recipients include HSV-1 and -2, VZV, and HHV-6, -7, and -8. While pretransplant screening for HSV may be performed, antiviral prophylaxis is routinely administered during the first posttransplant month. Awareness of VZV status is important as varicella infection may cause a spectrum of disease posttransplant. Before transplantation, VZV-seronegative recipients should receive varicella vaccine unless there are contraindications.

Table 10.3. Relationship between pretransplant CMV serostatus of donor and recipient and risk of CMV infection and disease

Donor	Recipient	Terminology	Cytomegalovirus Antibody Status		
			Infection (%)	Disease (%)	Pneumonitis (%)
+	−	Primary infection	70–88	56–80	30
−	+	Reactivation	0–20	0–27	Rare
+	+[a]	Reinfection or superinfection	70	27–39	3–14
−	+		Zero[b]		
+ or −	+	With antirejection ALA plus conventional immunosuppression[c]	—	65	—

[a]The source of infection and disease may be a new virus strain from the donor or latent virus in the recipient.
[b]Inadequate or incorrect donor/recipient screening, or viral acquisition during recent peritransplant periods may result in false-negative serologies; in this case, recent serologies are recommended.
[c]Results with conventional immunosuppression: Cyclosporine or tacrolimus, azathioprine (or mycophenolate mofetil), prednisone, and ALA (antilymphocyte antibody).
Data from Davis CL. The prevention of cytomegalovirus disease in renal transplantation. *Am J Kidney Dis* 1990;16:175–188; Rubin RH. Cytomegalovirus in solid organ transplantation. *Transplant Infect Dis* 2001;3:1–5.

Following transplantation, VZV immunoglobulin should be administered if the recipient is exposed to a person with varicella infection (chickenpox or zoster). Generally, screening for the human herpesviruses 6, 7, and 8 is not performed pretransplant because of the high rate of seropositivity in adults. HHV-6 has been implicated as a cofactor for CMV and other infections; no treatments are available. HHV-8 has also been implicated in the development of transplant-associated Kaposi sarcoma and EBV-negative lymphoproliferative diseases.

Hepatitis B and C

The detection of HBV and HCV in both transplant donors and recipients has improved with newer laboratory methods to detect viral-specific antibodies, antigens, and nucleic acids. The impact of latent or active HBV and HCV infection on transplant candidacy and kidney donation is discussed in Chapter 11.

Human Immunodeficiency Virus

All potential transplant donors should be tested for HIV-1 and HIV-2 antibody. A history of any high-risk behaviors must be obtained, because transplant-derived HIV infection has occurred associated with acute infection in the seronegative "window" or associated with massive blood transfusion and false-negative donor HIV antibody test results. Many centers reject kidneys from high-risk donors for fear of failure to detect antibody during the "window" during acute infection (see Chapter 5). Usually, HIV-seropositive donors have not been used. Although transmission of HIV by infected organs has been described, these precautions have reduced the risk for infection to an almost negligible degree. Recently, with the advent of highly active antiretroviral therapy (HAART), HIV-positive recipients meeting specific criteria requiring kidney transplant have been included in National Institutes of Health (NIH) protocols for transplantation (see Chapter 6). Further research is required.

Human T-Lymphotrophic Viruses I and II

Human T-lymphotrophic virus I (HTLV-1) is more common in individuals from the Caribbean and Japan than in persons from other geographic areas. Blood products, organ transplants, and intimate contact can transmit HTLV-1. Clinical syndromes include HTLV-1-associated myelopathy/tropical spastic paraparesis and progression and adult T-cell leukemia/lymphoma virus. HTLV-I myelopathy has been reported after transplant from an infected donor; recipient and donor deoxyribonucleic acid (DNA) homology was identical. HTLV-II is serologically similar to HTLV-I, but disease association is under investigation. Donors with HTLV-I seropositivity are generally not used.

West Nile Virus

West Nile virus (WNV) is a vector-borne flavivirus that was first recognized in the United States in 1999, and now has been reported in almost every continental state. Transmission is usually from the bite of an infected mosquito, but its transmission has been reported through blood and transplanted organs. In late 2002, the Centers for Disease Control and Prevention (CDC) confirmed the transmission of WNV to organ recipients from a single donor. First-generation serologic and PCR assays are available. The epidemiology of WNV has changed rapidly, so the extent of risk to the donor pool and recipients remains under investigation. During summer months, it appears prudent to avoid organs from donors from an area with active WNV infection who have symptoms of a viral illness, especially viral encephalitis or meningitis.

Severe Acute Respiratory Syndrome-Associated Coronavirus

First recognized in February 2003, a coronavirus called severe acute respiratory syndrome-associated coronavirus (SARS-CoV) has been implicated in the etiology and pathogenesis of severe acute respiratory syndrome (SARS). If SARS is present in the community, transmission is possible from a donor organ. Even with a rapid clinical test such as reverse transcriptase-PCR, a donor with incubating SARS or with early SARS may be missed. A donor SARS screening guideline tool has been proposed that includes donor hospital SARS exposure, clinical evaluation of donor for the signs and symptoms of a "viral-like" illness, and donor contact and travel history. Based on this donor screen tool, prospective donors can be risk stratified. Recipient history for possible incubating SARS also should be sought and screening with the proposed guidelines applied.

Coccidioidomycosis and Histoplasmosis

The detection of *C. immitis* antibody by complement fixation or immunodiffusion, or of *H. capsulatum* antibody by immunodiffusion during transplant evaluation, should alert the clinician to the possibility of disease reactivation after transplantation. Reactivation can occur during routine immunosuppression or after augmented immunosuppression for rejection. Patients who have resided in geographic areas at risk for coccidioidomycosis or histoplasmosis should be tested for antibody before transplantation and, if antibody-positive, they should receive prophylactic azole antifungal therapy following renal transplantation for an indefinite period.

Immunizations

The initial visit for transplant evaluation is the time to review prior immunization status. Up-to-date information on recommended adult and pediatric immunizations is available at www.cdc.gov/nip/rec/adult-schedule.pdf. Although the immune response to vaccination is often suboptimal among patients with end-stage renal disease, transplant candidates, especially those with functional or surgical splenectomy, should have their immunizations reviewed and updated early in the pretransplant evaluation process. Live-attenuated vaccines, such as measles-mumps-rubella (MMR) and varicella, should be administered no later than 4 to 6 weeks before transplantation to minimize the possibility of vaccine-derived infection in the posttransplant period. Ideally, household contacts of transplant recipients should be fully immunized to protect the transplant recipient. Live vaccines should be avoided before transplantation in immunocompromised candidates who require immunosuppressive medications and following solid-organ transplantation in all recipients. Other live-attenuated vaccines, including Bacille Calmette-Guérin, oral polio, and intranasal influenza vaccine, also should be avoided.

Inactivated vaccines that are safe to administer to transplant recipients, when appropriate, include hepatitis A and hepatitis B, intramuscular influenza A and B, pneumococcal, *Haemophilus influenza* B, inactivated-polio vaccine, diphtheria-pertussis-tetanus (DPT), and *Neisseria meningitidis.* Annual influenza vaccination is recommended. Although an increased risk of rejection with influenza immunization has been reported, a causal relationship remains undetermined. Immunization with *N. meningitidis,* inactivated polio, and smallpox vaccinations may be appropriate for special risk situations, including travel or occupational risk. An accelerated schedule for hepatitis B immunization has been used before and following transplant, especially if the organ is from an HBsAb-positive donor or the recipient has advanced HBV infection. The immunogenicity of HBV vaccination must be assessed following the vaccine series, and recipients may remain capable of transmitting HBV infection. Successful vaccination against CMV has not been achieved.

PATHOGENESIS OF INFECTION IN KIDNEY ALLOGRAFT RECIPIENTS

Approximately 80% of infections in kidney transplant recipients are bacterial. Tables 10.4 and 10.5 summarize the syndromes and microbial pathogens commonly encountered in kidney transplant recipients. Most bacterial infectious syndromes occurring in the first month after solid-organ transplantation are similar to those occurring after genitourinary surgery in immunocompetent patients, and the risk for infection increases with the complexity of the transplant surgery. Common infectious syndromes in kidney recipients include genitourinary tract infection, especially catheter-associated urinary tract infection (UTI), pneumonia, primary bacteremia that is often associated with vascular catheters, intraabdominal infections, and superficial or deep surgical site infections that are often associated with fluid collections or devitalized tissues.

Pulmonary bacterial infections are the most common life-threatening infections in kidney transplant recipients. The risk of pneumonia is increased among patients who require prolonged intubation, those with structural lung disease, and those with diminished gag reflex, prolonged nasogastric tube use, or impaired diaphragmatic function that increase the risk of aspiration. Hospital environmental exposure to certain species from contaminated water or aerosols, including *Legionella* and *Pseudomonas,* also increase the risk of pneumonia.

Among renal transplant recipients, the urinary tract is the most common primary site of infection associated with secondary bacteremia. Among patients with sepsis, poor outcome is associated with gram-negative species, multidrug-resistant organisms, and *Candida* species, especially when the empiric antimicrobial therapy is ineffective or delayed. Some studies suggest that bacterial sepsis increases the risk of CMV infection because of high levels of tumor necrosis factor-α or dysregulated immune response to CMV in the context of serious bacterial infections.

Table 10.4. Commonly encountered bacterial pathogens in renal transplant recipients listed by site of infection

Intraabdominal	Septicemia	Urinary Tract	Pneumonia	Wound	Dermatologic (Cellulitis)
Enterobacteriaceae	Enterobacteriaceae	Enterobacteriaceae	Enterobacteriaceae, P. aeruginosa	Mixed infection Enterobacteriaceae	Staphylococcus sp. Streptococcus sp.
Enterococcus sp.	Pseudomonas aeruginosa	P. aeruginosa	S. pneumoniae S. aureus (methicillin-sensitive and -resistant strains) Mixed flora from aspiration	P. aeruginosa	Enterobacteriaceae
Anaerobes (Bacteroides sp.)	S. aureus (methicillin-sensitive and -resistant strains)	Enterococcus sp.	Nocardia	Enterococcus sp.	P. aeruginosa (ecthyma)
S. aureus	Enterococcus sp. (vancomycin-sensitive and -resistant strains)		Legionella	S. aureus	Atypical Mycobacterium sp. (nodules)
Mixed infection	Rare: anaerobes (Bacteroides sp.)		M. tuberculosis, atypical Mycobacteria sp. Rhodococcus (rare)	Anaerobes (Bacteroides sp.)	
	Rhodococcus				

Table 10.5. Commonly encountered nonbacterial pathogens in renal transplant recipients listed by site of infection

Sinopulmonary	Genitourinary Tract	Gastrointestinal	Central Nervous System	Dermatologic
Aspergillus, Candida, Cryptococcus, Less common: *Zygomycoses, Coccidioides, Histoplasma, Pseudallescheria (Scedosporium)*	*Candida, Aspergillus* (rare)	CMV, HHV, adenovirus, EBV	*Cryptococcus neoformans, Aspergillus,* Less common: *Coccidioides, Pseudallescheria*	*Candida,* dermatophytes *(Microsporum, Trichophyton Epidermophyton), Malassezia* Less common: *Cryptococcus, Aspergillus, Coccidioides, Histoplasma,* phaeohyphomycosis
Pneumocystis CMV, HHV, respiratory viruses Less common: SARS-CoV, EBV	CMV, adenovirus, polyomavirus, papillomavirus	*Candida, Aspergillus,* zygomycoses	CMV, HHV, VZV, West Nile Virus, (rare: EBV, polyomavirus)	HHV, VZV

CMV, cytomegalovirus; EBV, Epstein-Barr virus; HHV, human herpes virus; SARS-CoV, SARS-associated coronavirus; VZV, varicella-zoster virus.

Historically, UTIs were the most common infectious complication of renal transplantation. Fortunately, antimicrobial prophylaxis with trimethoprim-sulfamethoxazole (TMP-SMX) or ciprofloxacin decreases the frequency of UTIs to less than 10% and essentially eliminates urosepsis unless urine flow is obstructed. Because of its broad-spectrum antimicrobial activity, TMP-SMX also reduces the incidence of infection with *N. asteroides, L. monocytogenes,* toxoplasmosis, *P. carinii, S. pneumoniae,* and bacterial gastroenteritis. The risk of genitourinary infection is directly related to complications of the surgical procedure, such as the urine leaks, wound hematomas, and lymphoceles, which can result in bacterial suprainfection. Genitourinary tract manipulation during transplantation, urinary catheters, anatomic abnormalities (e.g., ureterovesicular stenosis, ureteral stricture, vesicoureteric reflux), and neurogenic bladder also predispose to posttransplant UTI. Early catheter removal decreased the incidence of UTI in renal allograft recipients. Perinephric abscesses are uncommon after transplantation, but lymphoceles can promote abscess formation, often because of the need for repeated percutaneous drainage. Fever, graft tenderness, and a characteristic ultrasound appearance assist in diagnosis. Common organisms include staphylococci, enteric gram-negative bacteria, enterococci, and, rarely, anaerobic bacteria or *Candida* species.

The incidence of surgical wound infections following kidney transplantation ranges from 2% to 25%. Wound infections typically occur within 3 weeks after transplantation and are usually related to technical complications and recipient factors, such as obesity and diabetes. The process can involve the perinephric space or cause mycotic aneurysms at the site of the vascular anastomosis. Rarely, allograft nephrectomy is required; in pancreas–kidney transplant recipients, pancreatic abscess with gram-negative organisms or fungi may require surgical drainage or graft removal.

Preexisting medical conditions unrelated to end-stage renal disease, such as diverticulosis or biliary disease, can become apparent in the posttransplant period. Immunosuppression, including corticosteroids, increases the risk of diverticulitis and colonic perforation and gastric perforation by diminishing mucosal immune surveillance, mucosal integrity, and fibroblastic activity. Hypoperfusion of the gastrointestinal mucosa, from hypotension or use of vasopressor agents, also enhances the risk of mucosal perforation and secondary sepsis. Thrombocytopenia and acquired hypogammaglobulinemia have been implicated as risks factors for bacterial and fungal infections in some transplant patients.

Less-common bacterial infections in kidney transplant recipients include sinusitis associated with nasogastric or nasotracheal tubes, cannulation site abscess, tracheostomy site cellulitis, meningitis after a primary bacteremia, and prostatitis and prostatic abscess associated with urinary catheters. Catheters disrupt physical barriers and produce portals of entry for endogenous and nosocomial flora. The transplanted organ also may become a focus of infection as a result of ischemia and acute rejection after transplantation. Transfusion-associated infections (CMV, and much less commonly, hepatitis viruses and HIV) can occur among patients receiving large amounts of blood products.

Infections in kidney transplant recipients can be difficult to diagnose because concomitant immunosuppression and alterations in the immune response attenuate the usual clinical signs and symptoms of infection. In addition, infection may be difficult to differentiate from other causes of graft dysfunction, and diagnosis can be delayed. Rapid clinical discrimination of infection and early institution of antimicrobial therapy are essential for effective treatment and prevention of complications. Resistant infections or coinfection with more than one pathogen should be considered in an immunocompromised patient, especially when failing to respond to targeted antimicrobial therapy. For example, the immunomodulating effect of CMV infection can facilitate concurrent or subsequent infection with bacterial or fungal pathogens, such as *Pseudomonas* or *Aspergillus*.

Bacteremia and Fungemia

For the detection of bacterial or fungal septicemia, blood cultures ideally should be drawn before initiation of antimicrobial therapy. Specimens should be collected using both blood cultures and fungal isolator tubes. Fungal cultures are especially important if the patient has received corticosteroids for rejection; has a vascular, urinary, or drainage catheter; has been receiving total parenteral nutrition; has a suspicion of gastrointestinal inflammation or perforation; or has diabetes mellitus. Renal transplant recipients may *not* have systemic signs such as fever or leukocytosis with sepsis; consequently, a lower clinical threshold for bacteremia and sepsis is warranted in these patients.

Pneumonia

Diagnostic specimens for posttransplant pneumonia include blood, expectorated sputum, tracheal suction, bronchoalveolar lavage (BAL) fluid, transthoracic fine-needle aspirate, and, occasionally, lung biopsy. Blood cultures may assist in the etiologic diagnosis of pneumonia because 10% to 15% of patients with pneumonia have secondary bacteremia. Fiberoptic bronchoscopy with BAL and transbronchial biopsy is valuable in the diagnosis of severe pneumonia, especially when the episode is associated with an accessible pulmonary lesion. *Legionella* species can be cultured using charcoal media or detected using *Legionella*-specific nucleic acid probes or direct fluorescent antibody testing of respiratory specimens; additionally, *Legionella pneumophila* group 1 antigen can be detected in urine specimens. Specimens of respiratory secretions, pleural fluid, fine-needle aspirates, and biopsy specimens should be obtained for fungal culture and should be stained for fungal elements by sensitive methods, such as calcofluor staining. Fluorescein-labeled monoclonal antibody staining of BAL or sputum specimens increases the sensitivity for detection of *P. carinii. Nocardia* species can be identified presumptively when a modified acid-fast staining reveals delicately branching filamentous, beaded gram-positive rods. Acid-fast staining of respiratory specimens, biopsy specimens, nodules, and lymph nodes may reveal mycobacterial forms.

However, growth on culture is required for definitive identification. Specific DNA probes for *M. tuberculosis* and *M. avium* complex can decrease the time to diagnosis of infections associated with these species.

Chest computed tomography (CT) scanning is valuable in the diagnosis of infectious pneumonia and can be used to guide percutaneous or thoracoscopic biopsy of suspicious lesions. Concurrent immunosuppression and attenuated inflammatory response can modify the radiographic appearance and progression of pneumonia in transplant recipients. Noninfectious etiologies of pulmonary infiltrates are frequent in transplant recipients and include atelectasis, aspiration, contusion, hemorrhage, infarction or emboli, capillary leak, and pulmonary edema.

Although more common in the later posttransplant period, CMV infection also should be considered. Diagnosis is established by shell-vial culture with early antigen detection or by direct detection using PCR and DNA-hybridization from blood, respiratory specimens, or other sites.

Urinary Tract Infection

A clean-catch midstream urine specimen should be submitted for quantitative bacterial and fungal culture. In renal transplant recipients, lower levels of bacteriuria may be associated with a significant risk of systemic infection. The tips of genitourinary stents should be cultured for bacterial and fungal pathogens. If ureteral stents are required, infections may be more difficult to eradicate without removal of the foreign body. Antimicrobial agents achieve inadequate antimicrobial concentrations to eradicate biofilm-associated organisms and there is impaired immune and phagocytic function around the foreign body. Infected perigraft fluid collections or devitalized tissues will often require percutaneous or open incision, in addition to directed antimicrobial therapy, to resolve the infection.

Wound and Other Tissue Infections

Diagnosis of infection associated with surgical wounds, skin nodules, or necrotic ulcers should include aspiration of any drainable material, a deep swab specimen from the site, and a biopsy specimen, when appropriate. Gram stain, aerobic and anaerobic bacterial culture, and fungal and acid-fast stains and cultures should be performed. Percutaneous or open drainage may be necessary in case of infected perigraft collections, hematomas, or urinomas. Culture of fluid collections should be performed in patients with unexplained fever or other signs and symptoms of infection in the early postoperative period. Ultrasound or CT guidance can assist in localization and drainage catheter placement. In most circumstances, percutaneous or open drainage of infected fluid collections or hematomas is necessary for resolving the infection. If catheter-associated bacteremia is suspected, the intravascular device should be removed and the catheter tips should be cultured. Patient with diarrhea, colitis, or abdominal symptoms who have received antibiotic therapy should have stool specimens collected for *Clostridium difficile* toxin detection. Failure to remove the infected device or to drain the infected fluid collections may lead to prolonged antimicrobial therapy and an increased risk of resistance, treatment failure, drug toxicities, and graft dysfunction.

Approach to the Kidney Transplant Recipient with Fever

The differential diagnosis of fever in the kidney transplant recipient is broad and includes infection (i.e., bacterial, viral, fungal, parasitic), graft rejection, medication-associated adverse effect, noninfectious systemic inflammatory response (e.g., pancreatitis, pulmonary embolism, or cytokine release syndrome from murine-monoclonal antibody preparations), and combinations of infection and rejection. Although fever may accompany episodes of acute rejection, with current immunosuppressive drugs, patients with rejection are often afebrile. Temperature elevations may occur during treatment of rejection with both OKT3 and the polyclonal antibodies as a result of cytokine release (see Chapter 4). Other reported adverse effects of antibody treatment that can be confused with infectious symptoms include cephalalgia, photophobia, aseptic meningitis, and pulmonary infiltrates (edema).

MICROBIAL ETIOLOGY, TREATMENT PRINCIPLES, AND SPECIFIC THERAPY

Bacterial Infections

The bacterial pathogens in the early posttransplant period are similar to those causing nosocomial infections in a nontransplant surgical population (Tables 10.4 and 10.5). The antibiotic sensitivity patterns and prevalence of pathogens reflect hospital-specific antimicrobial usage and epidemiology. In the early posttransplant period, Enterobacteriaceae, *Staphylococcus,* and *Pseudomonas* species are the most commonly isolated nosocomial pathogens. Aerobic gram-negative bacilli constitute nearly half of all pathogens detected by blood culture, and infection is associated with a 2-week mortality rate of 11%. Secondary bacteremia most commonly arises from the lung, abdomen, surgical wound, and urinary tract, and can be associated with multidrug-resistant strains, including VRE and MRSA (Fig. 10.2). Although uncommon, infective endocarditis in the early posttransplant period has been associated with *S. aureus,* coagulase-negative staphylococci, *Escherichia coli, Acinetobacter* species, *Enterococcus* species including VRE, *Pseudomonas* species, and *Candida* species. Most of these episodes are associated primary intravascular device or surgical site infection.

Aerobic gram-negative bacilli (Enterobacteriaceae, *E. coli, P. aeruginosa*) are the most common organisms causing pneumonia and UTIs in kidney transplant recipients. Additional pathogens include *S. aureus* and enterococci (pneumonia and UTI), *S. pneumoniae,* and *Legionella* species, including as *L. pneumophila, L. bozemanii, L. micdadei*(pneumonia), and *Candida* species (UTI). Increasingly, *Klebsiella pneumoniae* and *E. coli* strains with chromosomal or plasmid-encoded resistance to extended-spectrum cephalosporins are associated with nosocomial urinary tract infections.

Bacterial organisms causing surgical site infection after solid-organ transplantation vary depending on the surgical

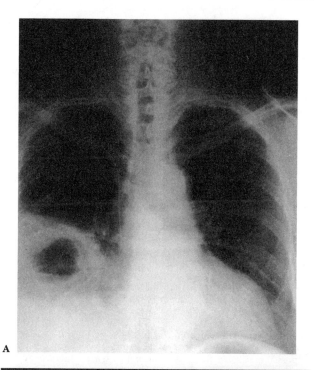

A

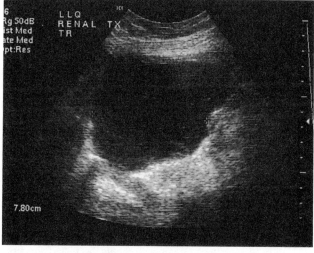

B

Fig. 10.2.   **Disseminated infection with methicillin-resistant** *Staphylococcus aureus* **(MRSA). A: Cavitary pneumonia on chest radiograph after bacteremic disease. B: Perigraft collection with MRSA in same patient.**

complications at the operative site. The most commonly isolated organisms are gram-positive species, such as *Staphylococcus* and *Streptococcus,* aerobic gram-negative bacteria, especially
E. coli, Enterobacter species, and *Pseudomonas* species, and enterococci, polymicrobial species, and anaerobes such as *Bacteroides
fragilis.* Other infrequently encountered bacterial pathogens reported in the early posttransplant period include *Nocardia, Mycobacterium, Salmonella, Mycoplasma hominis, Ureaplasma ure-
alyticum,* and *Rhodococcus equi.*

Vancomycin-Resistant Enterococcus

VRE colonization rates following solid-organ transplant have
ranged between 11% and 63% with infections occurring in 1%
to 16% of patients. The majority of VRE infections occur within
the first month following transplantation. Most commonly, infections include bacteremia, intraabdominal and biliary tract
sites, wounds, and urinary tract; also, endocarditis, mediastini-
tis, and intrathoracic infections have been reported. Although
enterococci are not typically virulent, VRE infections have been
associated with increased mortality. Retrospective reviews have
implicated certain risk factors for VRE acquisition, including prolonged hospitalization and intensive care unit stays; exposure to
other patients with VRE; broad-spectrum antibiotics; immunosuppression; renal insufficiency and hemodialysis; receiving a
CMV-seropositive donor organ; prolonged operative time; and reoperation. It is uncertain if VRE infections are a marker for de-
bilitated immunocompromised patients or an independent risk
factor for mortality. VRE should be suspected in any patient with
a positive culture for *Enterococcus* with risk factors. A single,
positive blood culture is significant if associated with a positive
culture from a normally sterile site or infected wound. Multiple positive blood cultures indicate significant bacteremia and
should be evaluated. A single, positive blood culture may indicate contamination and should be evaluated in the context of
the patient's clinical symptoms. VRE colonization can be seen in
open wounds, urine, and stool, and should be interpreted accordingly. VRE colonization may persist for months to years in kidney
transplant patients. Current recommendations to decrease the
risk of VRE infection and colonization include limiting the use
of vancomycin and broad-spectrum antibiotics, especially those
with anaerobic-directed activity; further, active surveillance for
VRE colonization; and use of contact precautions, including use of
gowns, gloves, and meticulous hand hygiene. Vancomycin should
not be used for the primary treatment of *C. difficile* colitis, routine surgical prophylaxis, selective bowel decontamination, or
for convenience of dosing regimens. VRE colonization may be
missed from a single stool or perirectal culture and three samples should be done at weekly intervals prior to discontinuing
isolation procedures. Treatment of VRE includes removal of infected medical devices, drainage of fluid collections, and relief
of biliary obstruction. Organisms should be tested for susceptibility to ampicillin, linezolid, quinupristin-dalfopristin, daptomycin, chloramphenicol, doxycycline, and gentamicin. Ampicillin
or one of the aminopenicillin or ureidopenicillin derivatives are
the agents of choice for treatment of infection associated with

ampicillin-susceptible enterococci. For serious infections, amino-glycosides should be used for synergistic bacterial activity; how-ever, kidney function must be closely monitored. Linezolid, quinupristin-dalfopristin (for *Enterococcus faecium* only), and daptomycin are agents available for treatment of VRE that are not susceptible to ampicillin or for patients with a penicillin and vancomycin allergy. Linezolid is associated with cytopenias and requires close monitoring. Second-line antibacterial agents that may have *in vitro* activity against VRE include chloramphenicol, doxycycline, and TMP-SMX.

Clostridium difficile

Diarrhea occurs in approximately 13% of kidney transplant recip-ients, usually in the first 2 years following transplantation. The etiology is most commonly infectious (41%) or medication associ-ated (34%). Of infectious etiologies, *C. difficile* is the most common agent. It occurs in 16% of pediatric kidney transplant popula-tion and is the most common bacterial infection during the first 2 weeks after transplantation. *C. difficile*-associated syndromes include asymptomatic carriage, diarrhea, pseudomembranous colitis, intestinal obstruction, and rare cases of intraabdomi-nal abscesses; bacteremia also has been reported. Occasionally, colectomy may be required for severe toxic megacolon. Most *C. difficile* infections are acquired nosocomially via either the hands of healthcare workers or from fomites. Risk factors include administration of broad-spectrum antianaerobic antimicrobial therapy; length of hospitalization; younger age; female gender; treatment for rejection with monoclonal antibodies; and intraab-dominal graft placement. *C. difficile* infection may result in fluid and electrolyte abnormalities, and can lead to malabsorption of medications, including immunosuppressive agents. Oral metron-idazole is the preferred first-line treatment for *C. difficile* infec-tion; if treatment failure occurs, oral vancomycin should be ad-ministered. In patients with severe gastrointestinal dysmotility or ileus, oral agents may not reach the colonic mucosa and intra-venous metronidazole should be administered.

Listeriosis

In renal transplant recipients, infection with *L. monocytogenes* most commonly presents as meningoencephalitis or septicemia but may also cause febrile gastroenteritis. Infection typically oc-curs 6 or more months after transplantation. Intravenous ampi-cillin (200 mg/kg in divided doses every 4 hours for 2 weeks) should be used to treat bacteremia. Meningitis should be treated with high-dose ampicillin and gentamicin for 3 weeks; repeat lumbar puncture should be performed to document cure. Many sporadic cases of listeriosis are associated with ingestion of pro-cessed meats. Patients should be instructed to eat only properly cooked meats and pasteurized dairy products.

Nocardiosis

The frequency of nocardia infections varies between 0.7% and 3% in solid-organ transplant recipients. Although the prophylactic use of TMP-SMX has decreased the incidence of nocardia infec-tion, *Nocardia* species should be considered in the differential diagnosis of infection occurring in the setting of early rejection, enhanced immunosuppression, neutropenia, and uremia. There are at least 12 species within the genus of *Nocardia*, with *N. asteroids* complex, *N. brasiliensis, N. otitidiscaviarum,* and *N. transvalensis* most commonly associated with infection among transplant recipients. Nocardia infection most commonly presents 1 to 6 months after transplantation with acute or subacute pneumonia, but hematogenous spread to the brain, skin and subcutaneous tissues, bone, and eye has been reported. Once pulmonary disease is established, dissemination to the brain is common, and cerebral CT or magnetic resonance imaging (MRI) should be performed. High-dose TMP-SMX (e.g., 10 to 15 mg/kg of trimethoprim in two to four divided doses, depending on the severity of illness) is the treatment of choice for most *Nocardia* species infections. However, resistance has been reported and antimicrobial susceptibility testing is recommended. Other agents, including imipenem, amikacin, second- and third-generation cephalosporins (cefuroxime, ceftriaxone, cefotaxime), minocycline, and quinolones, may be used with TMP-SMX or in combination in place of TMP-SMX when treating serious nocardia infection. Amikacin should be used with caution in the renal transplant patient because of the risk of nephrotoxicity. Surgical debridement and drainage may be required to manage brain abscesses or empyema. Because of the substantial risk for relapse in the setting of ongoing immunosuppression, treatment should be for at least 12 months and radiographic monitoring of the site(s) of infection should be performed at regular intervals.

Legionellosis

Legionella species infections have been reported in kidney transplant recipients. Risk factors include multiple corticosteroid boluses, prolonged mechanical ventilation, and exposure to *Legionella*-contaminated hospital water supplies. *L. micdadei* and *L. pneumophila* commonly cause pneumonia, but extrapulmonary involvement, including culture-negative endocarditis, and renal, hepatic, and central nervous system infection, have been reported. Signs and symptoms of *L. pneumophila* infection include a nonproductive cough, a temperature–pulse dissociation, elevated hepatic enzymes, diarrhea, hyponatremia, myalgias, and altered mental status. Radiographic findings include alveolar or interstitial infiltrates, cavities, pleural effusions, or lobar consolidation. Diagnosis can be confirmed by culture on special media or direct-fluorescent antibody testing of sputum, tissue, or bronchoalveolar fluid. In addition, a urinary antigen test should be performed; this test has a reported 70% sensitivity and 100% specificity for *L. pneumophila* serogroup 1. Delayed treatment is associated with increased mortality, and empiric treatment should be administered in suspected cases. Macrolides, quinolones, tetracyclines, rifampin and TMP-SMX have *in vitro* activity against *Legionella* species. In organ transplants, optimal treatment should include azithromycin and a quinolone. Erythromycin will increase and rifampin will decrease blood levels of the calcineurin inhibitors and should be avoided, if possible (see Chapter 4). Duration of treatment ranges from 14 to 21 days, depending on severity of illness.

Rhodococcus

Rhodococcus equi is an aerobic gram-positive coccobacillus that can cause infection in animals and in immunocompromised hosts, including renal transplant recipients. *Rhodococcus* most commonly causes pulmonary infection months to years after transplantation. Presentations include nodular or cavitary necrotizing pneumonia and empyema that may be confused with pulmonary tuberculosis. Aspiration of pulmonary nodules may reveal granulomatous inflammation with foamy macrophages with intracellular coccobacilli. Other clinical syndromes include sepsis, osteomyelitis, dermatologic disease, pericarditis, and lymphadenitis. Effective agents include quinolones, vancomycin, carbapenems, doxycycline, erythromycin, and TMP-SMX; β-lactams may be ineffective. Recurrences can occur, and surgical drainage may be required.

Mycobacterial Infection

Tuberculosis (TB) and nontuberculous mycobacteria (NTM) are potential causes of serious infection in renal allograft recipients that may present as early as the first posttransplant month. The incidence of active tuberculosis is estimated to be 1% to 4% following renal transplant, and is higher in those who resided in or traveled to a country with a high prevalence of TB infection. Radiographic presentations of pulmonary infection with *M. tuberculosis* and NTM include multilobar disease, focal infiltrates and nodules, empyema, pleuritis, or a combination of findings.

In the transplant population, atypical presentations of *M. tuberculosis* and NTM disease may delay diagnosis and contribute to morbidity. Special vigilance for reactivation tuberculosis is warranted, especially among transplant recipients with a prior history of mycobacterial infection, old granulomatous disease on chest radiograph, or from countries with high TB prevalence. Up to 40% of renal transplant recipients with reactivation tuberculosis will present with disseminated infection, with involvement of the skin, skeleton (bone and joint), or central nervous system. Finding granuloma in biopsy specimens from extrapulmonary sites should suggest disseminated disease. Because of the increase in multidrug-resistant (MDR) strains, appropriate therapy should include four agents: isoniazid (INH), rifampin (RIF), pyrazinamide (PZA), and ethambutol (EMB) or intramuscular streptomycin (SM) until susceptibility tests results are available. Although there are no controlled clinical trials in kidney transplant recipients, patients with TB infections associated with susceptible strains should receive INH and RIF for 6 additional months (12 total months). Adverse effects associated with antituberculous agents include hepatitis (INH > PZA > RIF), peripheral neuritis and optic neuropathy (INH, EMB), hearing loss and azotemia (SM), and gastrointestinal intolerance (INH, RIF, EMB, PZA). Both INH and RIF affect the cytochrome P450 enzyme system. INH increases cyclosporine and tacrolimus levels, and RIF decreases these drug levels, increasing the risk of rejection. These interactions are usually predictable and may occur within 1 to 3 days of initiating antituberculous therapy. Appropriate dosage adjustments and monitoring are required.

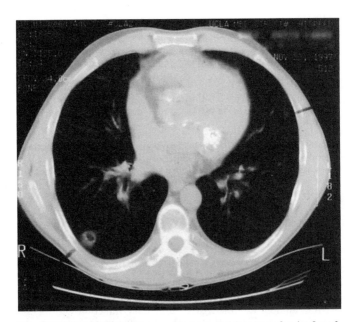

Fig. 10.3.   Chest CT scan from patient treated for several episodes of rejection; both nodular and cavitary infiltrates are observed. Bronchoalveolar lavage from this patient revealed *Aspergillus fumigatus*, cytomegalovirus, and *Mycobacterium fortuitum*. Combination therapies with amphotericin B lipid complex (ABLC), ganciclovir, and antimycobacterial agents were required for resolution.

Infection with NTM, including *M. kansasii, M. fortuitum, M. chelonei, M. xenopi, M. marinum, M. haemophilum,* and *M. abscessus,* have been reported in renal transplant recipients. These pathogens can be cultured from sputum, lung tissue, skin, bone, and other disseminated sites (Fig. 10.3). Many of the NTM are intrinsically resistant to standard antituberculous agents, and susceptibility testing should be performed against standard tuberculous agents, quinolones, macrolides, cephalosporins, and linezolid. Treatment typically includes combinations of agents for prolonged durations (e.g., longer than 12 months). Patients with osteomyelitis and extensive soft-tissue disease may require surgical intervention. *M. fortuitum* may cause bloodstream infection associated with intravascular devices and prompt device removal is critical.

Mixed Infections

Concurrent bacterial, fungal, and viral infections most often occurs in association with the following factors: repeated episodes of rejection and resultant enhanced immunosuppression from corticosteroids and anti-T-lymphocyte antibody preparations;

postoperative nosocomial infections (e.g., pneumonia or intraabdominal abscess); or immunomodulation from CMV or other virus infection, particularly respiratory viruses and hepatitis C. Figure 10.3 illustrates a case of pneumonia caused by multiple pathogens in a kidney transplant recipient. The presence of CMV in bronchoalveolar specimens or blood should always be investigated in fungal pulmonary infections or mixed infections.

ANTIMICROBIAL THERAPY

Antimicrobial therapy is given for the following indications:

- *Prophylaxis:* Antimicrobial agents are used to prevent a commonly encountered infection in the immediate postoperative period (e.g., surgical prophylaxis).
- *Empiric therapy:* Antimicrobials are administered without identification of the infecting pathogen.
- *Specific therapy:* Antimicrobials are administered to treat an infection with a diagnosed pathogen.

Surgical Prophylaxis

Perioperative antimicrobial prophylaxis reduces the frequency of surgical site infection. The agent should have activity against skin pathogens (e.g., staphylococci, streptococci) and urinary tract pathogens (*E. coli* and *Klebsiella* and *Proteus* species). Cefazolin (1 to 2 g) is generally preferred and should be administered within 1 hour of the surgical incision. The choice of antimicrobial agent for renal transplant prophylaxis should be based on institution-specific susceptibility patterns and a careful review of the patient's history of drug allergies. Surgical prophylaxis should given as a single dose or discontinued after no more than 24 hours to minimize the risk of toxicity and superinfection, and limit cost.

Empiric Therapy

For patients with suspected sepsis, the choice of empiric therapy should be guided by the potential site(s) of infection and bacterial or fungal pathogens; institution-specific susceptibility patterns; prior antimicrobial therapy; the time since transplantation; the severity of renal and hepatic dysfunction; and the net state of immunosuppression. Initial empiric therapy should use broad-spectrum agents. After a specific pathogen is isolated and sensitivities are available, a targeted, narrow-spectrum agent with appropriate antibacterial activity should be substituted to limit the risk for suprainfection and toxicity. Commonly used agents for empiric therapy include broad-spectrum penicillins (piperacillin), third-generation cephalosporins (ceftizoxime), β-lactam plus β-lactamase inhibitor combinations (ampicillin/sulbactam, ticarcillin/clavulanate, or piperacillin/tazobactam), carbapenems, or vancomycin, if line-associated infection is suspected.

Specific Therapy

With the isolation of a specific organism, therapy is focused on the specific pathogen to minimize the risk for suprainfection, toxicity, and cost of therapy. Table 10.6 lists specific treatment options for infectious pneumonia. Potential interactions between antimicrobials and immunosuppressive agents are discussed in

Table 10.6.   Pneumonia in the kidney transplant recipient

Pathogens	Suggested Therapy
Bacteria	
Staphylococcus aureus, methicillin susceptible	Oxacillin, nafcillin, first-generation cephalosporin, vancomycin (if penicillin allergic)
S. aureus, methicillin resistant	Vancomycin, quinupristin/ dalfopristin, linezolid, daptomycin
Enteric gram-negative bacilli	Third-generation cephalosporin, antipseudomonal penicillin ± aminoglycoside, quinolones (ciprofloxacin, levofloxacin), carbapenem, TMP-SMX
Streptococcus pneumoniae, penicillin susceptible	Penicillin G, ampicillin, second- or third-generation cephalosporin
S. pneumoniae, high-level penicillin resistant	Levofloxacin, gatifloxacin, moxifloxacin, vancomycin
Legionella pneumophila	Erythromycin (± rifampin), clarithromycin, azithromycin, quinolone
Mycobacteria tuberculosis	Isoniazid, rifampin, pyrazinamide and ethambutol; alternative agent directed by sensitivities and/or intolerance (e.g., quinolone, streptomycin)
Atypical mycobacteria	Determined by sensitivities of individual species (extended susceptibility testing recommended)
Nocardia asteroides	TMP-SMX, sulfisoxazole, minocycline, amikacin, imipenem, ceftriaxone, cefuroxime
Fungi	
Cryptococcus neoformans	Fluconazole, itraconazole, AmB ± flucytosine, LFAB
Aspergillus species	AmBd, LFAB, voriconazole, itraconazole, caspofungin
Coccidioides immitis	AmBd, fluconazole, itraconazole, LFAB
Histoplasma capsulatum	AmBd, itraconazole, LFAB
Candida albicans	AmBd, fluconazole, voriconazole, itraconazole, LFAB, caspofungin
Non-*albicans Candida* sp.	AmBd, LFAB, caspofungin, voriconazole, fluconazole or itraconazole (susceptible *Candida* sp. only and higher doses may be necessary)
Pneumocystis carinii	TMP-SMX, pentamidine, dapsone + TMP, atovaquone

continued

Table 10.6. (*Continued*)

Pathogens	Suggested Therapy
Viruses	
Cytomegalovirus	Ganciclovir, valganciclovir, foscarnet, cidofovir or fomivirsen (retinitis); CMV-immunoglobulin
Herpes group (non-CMV)	Acyclovir, ganciclovir, famciclovir, valacyclovir, penciclovir (topical for orolabial herpes simplex virus)
Varicella zoster	Acyclovir, famciclovir, valacyclovir
Respiratory syncytial virus	Ribavirin (aerosolized), palivizumab[a]
Influenza A/B	Oseltamivir (A/B), zanamivir (A/B), amantadine (A), rimantidine (A)

AmBd, amphotericin B deoxycholate; CMV, cytomegalovirus; LFAB, lipid-formulation of AmB; TMP-SMX, trimethoprim-sulfamethoxazole.
[a]Palivizumab is a humanized monoclonal antibody targeted to the F protein of respiratory syncytial virus (RSV).

Chapter 4 and are summarized in Table 10.7. Nosocomial gram-negative bacteria are associated with an increase in mortality in allograft recipients, and these pathogens warrant special attention. Organisms such as *Enterobacter cloacae* commonly may acquire resistance to β-lactam agents. In this case, effective therapies include carbapenems, fluoroquinolones, TMP-SMX, and cefepime. Aminoglycosides, although generally active against *E. cloacae* and most other gram-negative bacteria, should be used with caution in renal allograft recipients because of the increased risk of nephrotoxicity. When *P. aeruginosa* is suspected or documented, combination therapy with an antipseudomonal penicillin (piperacillin), carbapenem, ceftazidime, or cefepime, plus an aminoglycoside, or fluoroquinolone is recommended for synergistic bactericidal activity and to limit the emergence of resistance.

FUNGAL INFECTIONS

Despite ongoing refinements in immunosuppressive therapy, graft preservation, and surgical techniques, fungal infections remain a significant cause of morbidity and mortality in renal transplant recipients (Table 10.8). Although the incidence of fungal infections in renal transplant recipients is less than that reported for other solid-organ transplant recipients, the mortality from fungal infections remains high and is related to the pathogenicity of the organisms, site of infection, impaired host inflammatory response, limited diagnostic tools, potential for rapid clinical progression, failure to recognize a "high-risk" patient, and comorbid diseases such as renal failure and diabetes mellitus.

Colonization with yeasts and molds occurs frequently in transplant candidates with end-stage renal disease and after transplantation because of ongoing immunosuppression, particularly corticosteroid therapy. Fungal colonization is associated with

Table 10.7.   Interactions between frequently used antiinfective agents and immunosuppressives

Antibiotic Drug	Immunosuppressive Drug[a]	Findings/Implications
Aminoglycosides		
Amikacin, gentamicin, kanamycin, neomycin, streptomycin, tobramycin	CsA, Tac	Increases nephrotoxicity
Carbapenems		
Imipenem	CsA	Increases CsA level
Ertapenem[b], meropenem[b]	CsA, Tac, Sir, Aza, Evr, Myc	No interactions found
Cephalosporin		
Ceftriaxone[c]	CsA	Increases CsA level
Macrolides		
Azithromycin[d]	CsA, Sir	Increases CsA/Sir level
Clarithromycin	CsA, Tac, Sir	Increases CsA/Tac/Sir level
Dirithromycin	CsA	Increases CsA level
Erythromycin	CsA, Tac, Sir	Increases CsA/Tac/Sir level
Penicillins		
Nafcillin, Oxacillin[b]	CsA	Decreases CsA level
	Sir	Increases incidence of nephrotoxicity
Ticarcillin, piperacillin[b]	CsA	Decreases Sir level; increases CsA level
Quinolones		
Ciprofloxacin	CsA	Increases CsA level and nephrotoxicity
Gatifloxacin[b], moxifloxacin[b]	CsA, Tac, Sir	No interactions found
Levofloxacin[b]	CsA	No interactions found
Norfloxacin	CsA	Increases CsA level and nephrotoxicity
Ofloxacin	CsA	Increases CsA level
Sparfloxacin	Tac	Possible prolongation of QTc interval
Sulfonamides[e]:		
Sulfadiazine	CsA	Decreases CsA level, increases incidence of nephrotoxicity

continued

Table 10.7.   *(Continued)*

Antibiotic Drug	Immunosuppressive Drug[a]	Findings/Implications
Sulfamethoxazole and trimethoprim	CsA	Decreases CsA level, increases incidence of nephrotoxicity
	Aza, Myc	Anemia, neutropenia
Doxycycline	CsA	Increases CsA level
Antifungals		
Amphotericin B	CsA, Tac	Increases incidence of nephrotoxicity
Amphotericin B lipid complex	CsA, Tac	Increases incidence of nephrotoxicity
Liposomal amphotericin	CsA, Tac	Increases incidence of nephrotoxicity
Caspofungin[f]	CsA	Increases ALT/AST/caspofungin level decreases Tac level
	Tac	Decreases Tac level
Fluconazole[g], itraconazole[g], ketoconazole[g]	CsA, Tac, Sir	Increases CsA/Tac/Sir level
Voriconazole[h]	CsA, Tac	Increases CsA/Tac/Sir level
	Sir	Contraindicated
Mycobacterial and malarial agents		
Isoniazid	Sir	Increases Sir level
Pyrazinamide	CsA	Decreases CsA level
Rifampin[i], rifabutin[i]	CsA, Tac, Sir	Decreases CsA/Tac/Sir level
Rifapentine[i]	CsA, Tac	Decreases CsA/Tac level
Chloroquine	CsA	Increases CsA level
Quinine	CsA	Decreases CsA level
Antiviral agents		
Acyclovir[j], valacyclovir[j]	CsA	Neurotoxicity
	Aza, Myc	Anemia, neutropenia
Cidofovir	CsA	Nephrotoxicity
Foscarnet[k]	CsA	Neurotoxicity, electrolyte abnormalities
Ganciclovir[l]	CsA, Tac	Increases nephrotoxicity, leukopenia,
	Aza, Myc	Anemia, neutropenia
Lamivudine[b], oseltamivir[b]	CsA, Tac, Sir, Aza, Evr, Myc	No interactions found

continued

Table 10.7.   (*Continued*)

Antibiotic Drug	Immunosuppressive Drug[a]	Findings/Implications
Miscellaneous		
Atovaquone	Aza, Myc	Increases bone marrow suppression
Chloramphenicol[m]	CsA, Tac	Increases CsA/Tac level
Clindamycin	CsA	Decreases CsA level
Dapsone	Tac	Increases Tac level
Daptomycin[b]	CsA, Tac, Sir, Aza, Evr, Myc	No interactions found
Linezolid[n]	Aza, Myc	Increases bone marrow suppression
Metronidazole	CsA, Tac, Sir	Increases CsA/Tac/Sir level
Quinupristin and dalfopristin[o]	CsA	Increases CsA level

ALT, alanine transaminase; AST, aspartate transaminase; Aza, azathioprine; CsA, cyclosporin; Evr, everolimus; Myc, mycophenolate; Tac, tacrolimus; Sir, sirolimus.

[a] Less clinical data is available for antiinfective interactions with Tac, Sir, Myc, Aza, and Evr than for CsA. Antiinfectives that have a significant effect on the metabolism of CsA by CYP3A4 show similar effects on Tac and Sir.

[b] Although no drug interactions have been documented, immunosuppressive drugs, such as CsA, Tac, Sir, and Evr are increasingly used; what little data on drug interactions are available warrants ongoing surveillance for drug antiinfective interaction.

[c] There are no reported drug interactions with other cephalosporins.

[d] Elevations of serum cyclosporine levels may occur with the concomitant use of azithromycin. The manufacturer advises careful monitoring of patients. Studies in rats show that azithromycin does not affect the cytochrome P450 enzyme system; consequently, it would not be expected to interact with CsA.

[e] Effects of drug interaction differ between family members and are dependent on sulfa dose. More occurrences are reported for sulfadimidine, and less for sulfisoxazole and others. Monitor levels of sulfa and immunosuppressive drugs, especially in high-dose sulfa therapy as used for *Pneumocystis carinii* and *Nocardia* spp. Low-sulfa dose in prophylactic therapy is not problematic.

[f] Subjects receiving caspofungin and CsA had an increase of AST and ALT to two to three times the upper limit of normal and an increase of 35% in caspofungin. Concomitant use of caspofungin with cyclosporine is not currently recommended unless potential benefit outweighs potential risk of hepatotoxicity (elevation in transaminases); further analysis is required.

[g] Drug interaction side effects are seen mostly in high doses of fluconazole. Combination of ketoconazole and Sir is contraindicated in all cases. Sir can have a greater than tenfold increase in area under the curve in this combination. A similar effect can also occur with itraconazole and Sir.

[h] Voriconazole is contraindicated with Sir. Readjust the dose of CsA by half and Tac by two-thirds when taken with voriconazole.

[i] Drug interactions likely to occur with rifabutin and rifapentine. Magnitude of side effect is lower with rifabutin. Onset of adverse effect is seen in 2 days to

continued

Table 10.7. (Continued)

1 week with rifampin. Usually requires a dose increase (twofold) in CsA to maintain therapeutic serum level.

[j]Significant risk of nephrotoxicity with concurrent use of acyclovir or valacyclovir with CsA. Monitor renal insufficiency and adjust the dose as needed. Bone marrow toxicity of acyclovir and mycophenolate mofetil (MMF) is mild compared to the ganciclovir and MMF toxicity.

[k]No published clinical trials in solid-organ transplant patient. Concurrent use of foscarnet and CsA may increase nephrotoxicity to some degree in most patients.

[l]Controlled clinical trials of solid-organ transplant patients showed no evidence of synergistic bone marrow toxicity. In clinical practice, when initiating ganciclovir treatment with a patient, the dose of azathioprine is often reduced or held to avoid significant neutropenia. In the same trials, patients on IV ganciclovir were observed to have a significant decline in renal function while no pharmacokinetic interaction with CsA was found.

[m]Concurrent use of CsA and chloramphenicol has resulted in a transient decrease of CsA followed by an increase of 50% in levels. Tac levels have increased to 200% from baseline in 5 to 6 days with use of chloramphenicol.

[n]Additive risk of myelosuppression when initiated with Aza, MMF, or other myelo-depleting drugs.

[o]Manufacturer data have shown an increase of 63% in area under the curve, 30% in maximal drug concentration, and 77% in half-life, and a decrease of 34% in clearance of CsA.

use of broad-spectrum antibacterial agents, domiciliary exposures, pretransplant and posttransplant immunosuppressive therapy, and the presence of urinary catheters and endotracheal tubes. Fungal colonization may herald invasive fungal infection, particularly with certain *Candida* species such as *C. tropicalis*. Also, many solid-organ *donors* have been hospitalized in an intensive care unit setting and have received mechanical ventilation, broad-spectrum antibiotics, or corticosteroids, and have had urinary bladder and vascular catheters. Such conditions favor fungal growth on skin, mucosal surfaces, and within the gastrointestinal tract. Transplant *candidates* may also harbor fungal organisms as a consequence of these same risk factors.

In the posttransplant period, differentiating between fungal colonization and infection is often difficult and remains imprecise. Fungal colonization, defined as the isolation of yeast or mold from a nonsterile body site without local or systemic evidence of infection, occurs commonly in organ transplant recipients, especially from the oropharynx, upper respiratory tract and gastrointestinal (GI) tract. However, isolation of yeast or mold should be interpreted in the context of the patient's clinical status and net state of immunosuppression.

Candida spp., *Aspergillus* spp., and *C. neoformans* are the most common fungal pathogens reported in renal transplant recipients. *P. carinii*, Zygomycetes (*Mucor, Rhizopus*), hyalohyphomycoses, phaeohyphomycosis, and the geographically restricted mycoses (*Histoplasma, Coccidioides, Blastomyces*) are more commonly encountered under special clinical circumstances, such as immunomodulating viral infection, reactivation or residual

Table 10.8. Incidence of major invasive fungal infections (IFI) among kidney transplant recipients and proportion of those infections that are caused by *Aspergillus, Candida, Cryptococcus*, and other fungi

Organ Transplant	Incidence of IFI (%)	Proportion of IFI (%)				Mortality (%)			
		Aspergillus	*Candida*	*Cryptococcus*	*Other fungi*	*Aspergillus*	*Candida*	*Cryptococcus*	*Other fungi*
Renal	0–20	0–26	76–95	0–39	0–39	20–100	23–71	0–60	55
Pancreas and pancreas-kidney	6–38	0–3	97–100	—	—	100	20–27	—	—

Data derived from several series using varying definitions of fungal infection between 1980 and 1999.

disease for the endemic mycoses, chronic graft dysfunction, or during the treatment of posttransplant malignancies.

Donor-transmitted fungal infection is uncommon among kidney transplant recipients, but cases of *Candida, Aspergillus, Histoplasma, Coccidioides, Cryptococcus,* and *Monosporium (Scedosporium)* have been reported. Usually, these infections are associated with unrecognized infection within the donor allograft or in the blood compartment. All donors should be evaluated for evidence of active or occult fungal infection, particularly of the blood and urine. All fungal culture results and any history of exposure or infection with geographically restricted fungi should be ascertained.

Candida infections occur most commonly during the first month following transplant and are usually associated with technical complexities and complications of the renal transplant surgery or with early rejection and enhanced immunosuppression. *Candida* infection is most commonly associated with an endogenous source of colonization, but lack of handwashing of healthcare workers may contribute to acquisition from an exogenous source. *C. albicans* is the most commonly isolated species; other species include *C. glabrata, C. tropicalis, C. parapsilosis, C. krusei, C. lusitaniae, C. rugosa, C. kefyr,* and *C. guilliermondii.* Speciation is clinically useful because non-albicans *Candida* vary in *in vitro* susceptibility to azoles and newer antifungal agents. The spectrum of *Candida* infections includes mucocutaneous candidiasis and esophagitis; wound infections; cystitis, pyelonephritis, and ureteral obstruction (by *Candida* elements or "fungal ball"); intraabdominal infections, including infected perigraft fluid collections or peritonitis; and intravascular device-associated fungemia. Uncommon sites of infection include pneumonia, allograft vascular endocarditis, and hematogenous dissemination, including endophthalmitis. Renal parenchymal involvement with *Candida* is most often the result of hematogenous infection, although an ascending route from the bladder can occur. Candiduria may be asymptomatic but may associated with cystitis or upper tract infection. Recurrent candiduria should be treated with an antifungal agent to avoid these complications.

The risk of fungal infection after simultaneous pancreas-kidney (SPK) and pancreas after kidney (PAK) transplants is comparable to liver transplant recipients. More that 45% of these infections are caused by *Candida* species. Risk factors for fungal infection in SPK and PAK recipients include older donor or recipient age, enteric versus bladder drainage (SPK recipients), retransplant versus primary transplant (PAK recipients), and vascular graft thrombosis. In SPK transplant recipients, bladder drainage of pancreatic secretions may favor urinary tract colonization with *Candida* species. Alternative surgical drainage procedures where exocrine secretions are drained into the peritoneal cavity or via a pancreaticocystostomy may also predispose to fungal infections. Consequences of these infections include multiple exploratory laparotomies and a high risk of graft loss. Mortality was as high as 20% in one series of recipients with fungal or combined fungal and bacterial infections.

The period of 1 to 6 months after kidney transplant is marked by opportunistic, relapsed, residual, and viral-associated (e.g.,

CMV, hepatitis C) fungal infection. The type, dose, time, duration, and intensification of immunosuppression are important determinants of ongoing risk. *Pneumocystis* occurs most commonly during this period, especially among patients receiving increased doses of corticosteroids or inadequate prophylaxis. *Cryptococcus,* endemic mycoses, hyalohyphomycosis, phaeohyphomycosis, zygomycosis, and dermatophytes most commonly occur 6 or more months after transplantation. Conditions that alter the net state of immunosuppression may shift the timeline for fungal infection forward. Other fungal infections in renal transplant recipients include cryptococcal meningitis and space-occupying brain lesions—pulmonary, dermatologic, skeletal, organ-specific disease; aspergillosis—pneumonia and other tissue-invasive forms, including genitourinary, central nervous system, rhinocerebral, gastrointestinal, skin, wound, and musculoskeletal disease; zygomycosis with *Rhizopus* and *Mucor* species—pulmonary, rhinocerebral, cutaneous disease; coccidioidomycosis—pneumonia, meningitis, musculoskeletal, and skin involvement; histoplasmosis: pneumonia, mediastinal, disseminated disease, cutaneous disease; pneumocystosis—pneumonia and, rarely, extrapulmonary infection; *Penicillium marneffei*—pneumonia; and scedosporiosis—pneumonia and disseminated disease.

Additional fungal pathogens observed in renal transplant recipients include the dermatophytes (*Trichophyton, Microsporum,* and *Epidermophyton* species), hyalohyphomycosis (*Fusarium* and *Alternaria* species), and phaeohyphomycosis. These may present locally as cutaneous lesions or, rarely, with disseminated disease. The prevalence of dermatophytic infection is increased with enhanced immunosuppression, diabetes, and environmental exposures.

The diagnosis of fungal infection remains problematic and frequently leads to delays in clinical recognition.

Table 10.9 summarizes laboratory and radiologic methods for the diagnosis of *Candida, Aspergillus, Cryptococcus,* and other fungal infections. Isolation of yeast (e.g., *Candida* species) from cultures of stool, respiratory, and urine samples occurs commonly in kidney transplant recipients receiving corticosteroids and broad-spectrum antimicrobials, and does not necessarily imply infection. However, repeatedly positive fungal cultures from single sites or from multiple sites may be herald invasive candidiasis in the appropriate clinical setting. Patients with genitourinary tract stents and recurrent urinary fungal isolates often require removal of foreign body to eradicate fungal infection. The isolation of *Aspergillus* from respiratory cultures (particularly *A. fumigatus* and *A. terreus*) should prompt a search for invasive disease, including by high-resolution chest CT with biopsy of suspected pulmonary lesions. Patients at risk of aspergillosis include those receiving repeated courses of enhanced immunosuppression for rejection, or with chronic graft dysfunction, diabetes, comorbid medical illnesses, and CMV infection. Diagnosis of aspergillus infection depends upon a high clinical suspicion, isolation of *Aspergillus* from a sterile body site or repeated isolation from the respiratory tract, and typical radiographic findings. Radiologic appearances of pulmonary aspergillosis in kidney transplant recipients include nodules, diffuse or wedge-shaped opacities,

Table 10.9.   Laboratory and radiologic approaches in the diagnosis of *Aspergillus, Candida, Cryptococcus,* and select fungal pathogens

Agent	Method	Description and Comments
Aspergillus	Culture	• Respiratory or sterile site specimen. • Specificity of culture from nonsterile site limited
	Antigen detection	• Detection of galactomannan in serum, urine, BAL, or CSF by EIA • Platelia *Aspergillus* EIA (Bio-Rad Laboratories) or latex agglutination (LA test Pastorex *Aspergillus*); depending on index cut-off points, sensitivity 81% (45%–92%) and specificity 89% (81%–93%) • GM may be detected in serum at an early stage of infection • GM detected in BAL fluid specimens in patients with IA with good correlation between serum and BAL fluid • May be useful for monitoring response to therapy and detecting relapse
	Nucleic acid detection	• PCR detection of *Aspergillus* DNA (standardization lacking) • Specimens include BAL, serum/plasma/whole blood, or CSF • May not discriminate between invasive infection and colonization in BAL specimens • Potential use in monitoring response to antifungal therapy • Risk of contamination of PCR buffers by spores and other molds • Lacking multicenter trials in organ transplant recipients
	Antibody detection	• Clinical value unclear; sources include serum or CSF IgG/IgM • Antibody often absent in immunocompromised patients
	Histopathology	• Direct visualization permits assessment of tissue invasiveness

continued

Table 10.9. (*Continued*)

Agent	Method	Description and Comments
		• Stains include H and E, calcofluor white, GMS, PAS, Masson-Fontana • Pathologist must be experienced with fungal morphology to differentiate between similar-appearing fungal organisms (e.g., *Aspergillus, Scedosporium, Fusarium,* and filamentous fungi)
	Radiology	Chest • Plain radiograph; CT preferred • Linear and single or multiple nodular or patchy opacities (parenchymal or pleural based) • Wedge-shaped or diffuse infiltrates • Cavitary lesions with early "halo" sign progressing to air crescent sign • Halo sign may accompany pulmonary infection with mycobacteria, nocardia, and zygomycoces, and collagen vascular diseases • Bronchial wall thickening (tracheobronchial disease) • Pleural effusion and adenopathy are rare Brain • CT with contrast; MRI with gadolinium preferred • Single or multiple lesions with ring enhancement and surrounding edema • Scedosporium and phaeohyphomycoses may have a similar MRI appearance.
Candida	Smear and culture	• Blood or other sterile site specimen preferred • Limited specificity of isolation from nonsterile site • Identify to species level to guide antifungal therapy

continued

Table 10.9. (*Continued*)

Agent	Method	Description and Comments
	Nucleic acid detection	• PCR detection of *Candida* DNA from BAL, serum, or CSF • Direct detection by DNA probe • PCR contamination problematic because of the ubiquity of *Candida* • Species-specific DNA probes in development
	Antigen detection	• Detection of mannan or other protein in serum by latex agglutination, EIA, RIA or other method • Sensitivity improved by serial measurement
	Antibody detection	• Serum or CSF IgG, IgM, or total antibody • Limited usefulness as most patients have antibody
	Histopathology	• Direct visualization stains in order of utility calcofluor white, GMS, PAS, KOH wet preparation, Giemsa/Wright • Useful for detection of tissue infection, must demonstrate tissue-invasive organisms
	Radiology	Chest • Diffuse airspace consolidation • Pleural effusions, rare cavitation, adenopathy Organ space • CT or MRI of liver, spleen, kidney, bone or other tissues • Nodules, diffuse contrast enhancement
Cryptococcus	Cultures	• CSF India ink stain • Evaluate for disseminated disease: blood, respiratory, urine, skin may be involved • Large volume of CSF may be required • Positive smear must be confirmed by culture
	Nucleic acid detection	• PCR detection • DNA from BAL, serum, or CSF • Methods not standardized

continued

Table 10.9.   (*Continued*)

Agent	Method	Description and Comments
	Antigen detection	• Detection of capsular polysaccharide in serum, urine, or CSF by latex agglutination, coagglutination, EIA, or other method • May be useful for detecting invasive disease, monitoring response to therapy and detecting relapse • False negatives caused by prozone phenomena, immune complex formation, or noncapsular strains • False positives caused by other fungi (e.g., *Trichosporon*)
	Antibody detection	• Serum or CSF IgG, IgM, or total antibody • Not clinically useful because antibody often absent in immunocompromised patients and those with meningitis
	Histopathology	• Direct visualization in tissue with methenamine silver, PAS, GMS, mucicarmine • Permits assessment of tissue invasiveness
	Radiology	Chest • Single or multiple nodules or masses • Diffuse reticular or reticulonodular, segmental or lobar consolidation • Pleural effusion septal thickening paratracheal, hilar, and mediastinal adenopathy sometimes seen Brain • CT or MRI with contrast • Solitary lesions with ring enhancement and surrounding edema • Cerebral edema
Zygomycosis	Smear and culture	• Direct visualization of sparsely septate broad hyphae in tissue • Culture yield may be low

continued

Table 10.9. (*Continued*)

Agent	Method	Description and Comments
		• Identification to genus and species level may assist in determining prognosis and targeting therapy with newer antifungal agents
	Radiology	Chest • CT imaging useful for diagnosis • Consolidation, pleural effusion, and focal cavitation • Cavitation common but air crescent sign less frequently observed
		Rhinocerebral • MRI with gadolinium or CT with contrast of brain, sinuses, and orbits • Very useful to determine extent of infection, guide surgical resection, assess prognosis and risk of visual loss
Coccidioido-mycosis	Culture	• Cultures of BAL, CSF, skin, bone, joint/synovium, or other tissue • Blood culture rarely positive
	Histopathology	• Spherules detected by hemotoxylin and eosin stain, Papanicolaou smear, PAS stain
	Serology	• EIA, latex agglutinin, tube precipitin (IgM-early) • False positives of LA occur in CSF • Complement fixation (CF) IgG in serum or CSF: serum CF parallels disease severity low titers (1:2–1:8 found in pulmonary coccidioidomycosis, with >1:16 indicative of dissemination); may cross react with other mycosis; >1:2 CF in CSF indicates meningitis. • Immunodiffusion complement fixation: qualitative or semiquantitative confirmation of CF results

continued

Table 10.9.   (*Continued*)

Agent	Method	Description and Comments
	Radiology	Chest • Diffuse reticulonodular infiltrates, focal infiltrate, nodules • Apical cavitation common • Mediastinal adenopathy • Pleural-based lesions and pleural effusions Brain • CT to assess for hydrocephalus • MRI to visualize patency of aqueduct
Histoplas-mosis	Culture	• Cultures of BAL, blood, urine, bone marrow, skin, or other tissue • Blood culture rarely positive
	Histopathology	• Calcofluor white, KOH preparation, Giemsa, hemotoxylin and eosin stain, GMS, Papanicolaou smear, PAS
	Antigen detection	• EIA can detect urine *Histoplasma capsulatum* carbohydrate antigen • Cross-reactions can occur with other fungi
	Radiology	Chest • Patchy pneumonitis • Numerous small nodules (progressive disseminated forms of histoplasmosis) • Hilar and mediastinal lymphadenopathy.

BAL, bronchoalveolar lavage; CSF, cerebrospinal fluid; CT, computed tomography; DNA, deoxyribonucleic acid; EIA, electroimmunoassay; GM, granulocyte macrophage; GMS, Gomori methenamine silver; IA, invasive; Ig, imunoglobulin; KOH, potassium hydroxide; MRI, magnetic resonance imaging; PAS, periodic-acid Schiff; aspergillosis; PCR, polymerase chain reaction; RIA, radioimmunoassay;

empyema, cavitary forms, tracheobronchitis, or a combination of parenchymal lesions. Galactomannan assays may aid in the early diagnosis of invasive aspergillosis in the high risk setting.

Prophylaxis

During induction or periods of enhanced immunosuppression oral nonabsorbable or topical antifungal agents, such as clotrimazole or nystatin, are typically administered to prevent mucocutaneous *Candida* infection. These agents are ineffective in preventing systemic fungal infection. Although prophylaxis with a systemic antifungal agent is not recommended routinely after uncomplicated renal transplantation, it may be indicated in patients receiving prolonged broad-spectrum antibacterial therapy or enhanced immunosuppression, or with persistent candiduria. In such cases, an azole, echinocandin, or a lipid-based formulation of amphotericin B can be administered for a duration proportional to the risk for fungal infection. No randomized trails have been undertaken in kidney transplant recipients among these agents. Antifungal prophylaxis using agents with more limited spectrum of activity (e.g., fluconazole) may potentially increase the risk of colonization and infection with non-albicans *Candida* or *Aspergillus* species.

Renal transplant recipients with a history of prior treatment of an endemic mycosis or radiographic evidence of old "healed" granulomatous disease associated with coccidioidomycosis or histoplasmosis benefit from long-term (lifelong) azole prophylaxis with fluconazole or itraconazole. The cyclosporine and tacrolimus dosages should be adjusted with these agents.

Treatment

Historically, invasive candidiasis, cryptococcosis, coccidioidomycosis, histoplasmosis, and aspergillosis were treated with amphotericin B deoxycholate (AmB). Because of inherent toxicities and intolerance, especially at the high doses required for invasive aspergillosis, central nervous system disease, or invasive organ diseases (e.g., 1 to 1.5 mg/kg per day), newer agents have increasingly been use in renal transplant recipients. The lipid-formulations of amphotericin B (LFAB) are associated with lower risks for nephrotoxicity, metabolic derangements, and infusion-associated side effects than is AmBd. These agents include amphotericin B (AmB) lipid complex (Abelcet, ABLC), liposomal AmB (AmBisome), and AmB colloidal dispersion (Amphotec, ABCD). These agents originally were approved for the treatment of fungal infections in patients refractory to or intolerant of conventional AmB. Higher therapeutic dosages can be administered, and broad-spectrum antifungal activity is generally maintained. Figure 10.4 demonstrates the utility of a lipid-based AmB formulation (ABLC) in the treatment of pulmonary aspergillosis in a kidney transplant recipient.

Voriconazole appears to be superior to conventional AmB for the treatment of invasive aspergillosis and also has *in vitro* activity against *Fusarium* and *Scedosporium*. Available in both IV and oral formulations, the drug is generally well tolerated, but some patients experience visual hallucinations or severe photosensitivity. Although itraconazole has good *in vitro* activity

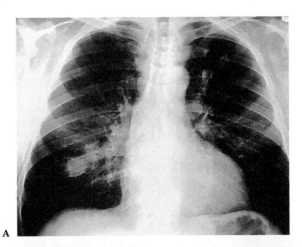

A

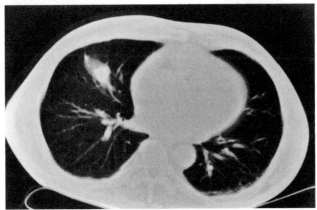

B

Fig. 10.4.   Pulmonary aspergillosis after kidney transplantation.
A: Multiple pulmonary nodules with hilar adenopathy are seen on
chest radiograph. B: Thoracic CT showing nodules some with central
cavitation. C: Chest radiograph showing resolution of pulmonary
nodules after AmB lipid complex (ABLC) and subsequent
itraconazole therapy.

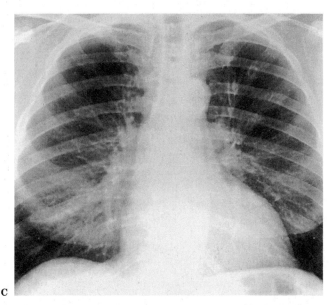

C

Fig. 10.4. *Continued*

against *Aspergillus* species, its use is generally reserved for treatment of less-severe aspergillosis or maintenance therapy following initial response to AmB, LFAB, or voriconazole, and for treatment of endemic mycoses, including of histoplasmosis, blastomycosis, sporotrichosis, and paracoccidioidomycosis. Itraconazole oral solution is more bioavailable than the capsule formulation and should be taken with meals, whereas the capsule requires an acid gastric pH for optimal absorption and should be taken on an empty stomach. Fluconazole is the first-line agent of the treatment or prevention of reactivation coccidioidomycosis in renal transplant recipients. The use of fluconazole at standard doses may be associated with the development of fungal resistance or tolerance, as well as with the risk for fungal superinfection with *C. glabrata, C. krusei,* or *C. tropicalis.* Ketoconazole, fluconazole, and itraconazole are useful for treating mucocutaneous fungal infection and infection of the genitourinary tract, gastrointestinal system, lungs, and, under specific conditions, central nervous system. Fluconazole and 5-flucytosine can be used for cryptococcal disease. All of the azole antifungals impair calcineurin inhibitor metabolism to some degree and increase blood levels (see Chapter 4). This effect is most consistent with ketoconazole, and its use may permit a reduction in cyclosporine or tacrolimus dose of up to 80%.

The echinocandins, including caspofungin and the investigational agents anidulafungin and micafungin, inhibit synthesis of fungal cell wall protein beta-1-3 glucan and are fungicidal for *Candida* species, including fluconazole-resistant species.

Available only as an IV infusion, caspofungin is well tolerated and increasingly is being used to treat serious infections associated with non-albicans *Candida* species in transplant recipients. Coadministration of caspofungin with tacrolimus results in modest (approximately 20%) reduction in tacrolimus levels, and an increased incidence of abnormal liver function tests with cyclosporin; combined usage in this latter case is a relative contraindication.

The development of any serious fungal infection in a transplant recipient mandates a critical evaluation of the immunosuppressive regimen. The corticosteroid dose should be minimized, the blood levels of cyclosporine and tacrolimus should be kept in the low therapeutic range, and adjunctive agents can often be temporarily discontinued. Failure of clinical response to an antifungal regimen may require discontinuation of immunosuppression, even at the cost of abandoning the graft.

Pneumocystosis

Pneumocystis carinii pneumonia most often occurs 1 to 6 months after transplantation. It typically presents with fever, nonproductive cough, arterial–alveolar mismatching, and diffuse interstitial infiltration or focal air-space consolidation on chest radiograph. BAL with transbronchial biopsy and staining is a highly sensitive method of identifying pulmonary disease. First-line treatment is with TMP-SMX for 14 to 21 days. Second-line agents include intravenous pentamidine (3 to 4 mg/kg per day) or dapsone-trimethoprim (100 mg dapsone daily with trimethoprim 15 mg/kg per day). Adverse effects of trimethoprim include nephrotoxicity, pancreatitis, and bone marrow suppression. Dapsone is associated with hemolytic anemia in patients with glucose-6-phosphate dehydrogenase deficiency. Mild to moderate *P. carinii* pneumonia can be treated with atovaquone (750 mg orally thrice daily for 21 days) in patients intolerant to TMP-SMX. Prophylactic agents, in order of efficacy, include TMP-SMX, bimonthly intravenous or aerosolized pentamidine, dapsone, and atovaquone.

VIRAL INFECTIONS

Viral infections are a major problem in allograft recipients, most commonly 1 to 6 months after transplantation. Clinical disease can occur later, especially after intensification of immunosuppression or physiologic insults that increase the net state of immunosuppression. EBV-related lymphoproliferative disorder is discussed in Chapter 9.

Cytomegalovirus

CMV infection occurs primarily after the first month of transplantation with an estimated incidence of 30% to 78% if prophylaxis is not administered, depending on the serologic status of the donor and recipient (Table 10.3). CMV can be transmitted by the allograft, via blood products, or by sexual contact. CMV establishes lifelong latency after primary infection. Among all organ transplants, renal transplant recipients have the lowest risk of CMV disease in the absence of antiviral prophylaxis. Pancreas transplant recipients are among the highest risk, with kidney–pancreas recipients also displaying increased risk. In general, the dose, duration, agents, and intensity of immunosuppression determine the risk of CMV among transplant recipients. Specific risk factors include CMV donor–recipient mismatching, and the use of lymphocyte-depleting preparations induction and for rejection therapy (see Chapter 4). Other risk factors include comorbid illnesses, neutropenia, and, potentially, coinfection with HHV-6 and -7.

Active CMV infection may be symptomatic or asymptomatic, and is characterized by viral replication and shedding with a specific immune response to CMV. *Primary CMV infection* represents infection in the previously uninfected seronegative host. *Secondary CMV infection* represents infection in a previously infected seropositive host caused by either reactivation of latent endogenous virus, reinfection or suprainfection with new virus strain. *CMV disease* refers to symptomatic acute CMV infection and can be further divided into the *CMV syndrome* (fever, fatigue, leukopenia and/or thrombocytopenia, and an increased CMV titer from a specific diagnostic assay) and *invasive CMV disease* (e.g., pneumonitis, hepatitis, or gastrointestinal involvement such as colitis or enteritis, or involvement of the allograft itself). *Latent CMV infection* represents lifelong persistence of virus without replication in healthy seropositive host. *Recurrent CMV disease* is defined as clinical manifestations of CMV disease arising after cessation of anti-CMV therapy. *Refractory CMV disease* may reflect viral resistance resulting from mutations in CMV strains or disease in a profoundly immunosuppressed host.

CMV infection is associated with immune modulation and dysregulation, especially of helper/suppressor T cells, and can culminate in opportunistic infection, allograft injury or rejection, and the development of PTLD. Host mediators implicated in reactivation of CMV include tumor necrosis factor (TNF), catecholamines, and proinflammatory prostaglandins. Tumor necrosis factor binds to the TNF receptor of cells latently infected with CMV and generates nuclear transcription factors protein kinase C and nuclear factor kappa B (NF-κB) that act as promoters of the immediate-early (IE) gene of CMV initiating replication. CMV infection induces antiendothelial cell antibodies that contribute to both acute and chronic rejection.

CMV disease most commonly presents as a viremic syndrome, manifest by fever, malaise, leukopenia, and transaminitis. Pneumonitis is the most serious CMV infection, characterized by dyspnea, hypoxemia, interstitial infiltrates, and the detection of CMV antigens, nucleic acids, or inclusion bodies on bronchoalveolar lavage. CMV upper and lower gastrointestinal disease includes esophagitis, cholecystitis, duodenitis, hepatitis, and colitis. Diagnostic endoscopy can reveal solitary or multiple mucosal ulcerations with hemorrhage. Tissue specimens should be stained for CMV using immunofluorescent anti-CMV antibody and examined for inclusion bodies. CMV retinitis is uncommon in transplant recipients and can be diagnosed by direct funduscopy. Central nervous system CMV disease (e.g., meningitis, encephalitis, myelitis) may be more difficult to diagnose. Neurologic disease caused by other neurotropic opportunistic pathogens, and drug toxicities, should be simultaneously investigated. Multiorgan involvement can be observed in disseminated CMV disease.

Diagnosis

Table 10.10 summarizes methods for the diagnosis of CMV infection and disease.

Historically, tissue-invasive CMV disease was diagnosed by histopathology, but this approach can be associated with diagnostic delays or inadequate specimen collection. Detection of serum CMV IgM or IgG antibody by electroimmunoassay (EIA) is useful for pretransplant screening and for documenting seroconversion, but is less useful for the diagnosis of CMV disease. Culture-based methods include conventional tissue culture and shell vial centrifugation and can be performed on blood, buffy coat blood fraction, urine, cerebrospinal fluid (CSF), respiratory secretions or other tissue specimens. Tissue culture is most commonly employed for antiviral-resistance testing. Staining conventional cell culture or shell vial culture with monoclonal antibody against early CMV viral antigens at 48 hours can decrease the time to diagnosis but is not as sensitive as traditional viral culture. Detection of CMV pp65 antigen in peripheral blood lymphocytes by a semiquantitative fluorescent assay also is more rapid than traditional culture methods. CMV DNA can be detected directly from blood, CSF or tissue specimens by PCR or other nucleic acid amplification method. CMV DNA hybridization uses signal-amplified detection and quantitation of CMV DNA in peripheral white blood cells, and increasingly is used to diagnose CMV disease associated with viremia. Delays in processing blood for CMV DNA hybridization may decrease the sensitivity of the test. Qualitative CMV DNA detection by PCR is extremely sensitive but cannot differentiate active disease from treated disease or latent infection.

Treatment

Effective antiviral agents for CMV prophylaxis and treatment have substantially decreased the morbidity and mortality associated with CMV disease. Most commonly, active CMV disease is treated with intravenous ganciclovir, usually for 14 to 21 days, with a reduction in the immunosuppression if the disease is severe. Oral valganciclovir also may be effective for treatment of mild to moderate CMV disease. After a course of treatment, low-risk patients should be monitored frequently for signs and symptoms of CMV disease; renal transplant recipients with ongoing risk factors for CMV should receive maintenance therapy with oral ganciclovir or valganciclovir. Adverse effects of ganciclovir include reversible, dose-related granulocytopenia and thrombocytopenia, fever, rash, seizures, nausea, myalgias, abnormalities in liver enzyme determinations, and, rarely, pancreatitis. Drug interactions include an increased seizure risk when used in combination with acyclovir and imipenem, and additive marrow suppression with azathioprine, mycophenolate, and TMP-SMX.

Experience in treating refractory CMV disease suggests that the addition of CMV hyperimmune globulin or intravenous pooled

Table 10.10. Current diagnosis of cytomegalovirus infection

Method	Description	Comments
Viral culture	• Cell culture and shell vial centrifugation techniques • Early antigen detection by staining cell culture or shell vial culture with labeled monoclonal anti-CMV antibody	• Cultivate virus from blood, buffy coat fraction, or other tissue • Detection by typical cytopathic effect, nuclear inclusions and direct staining for CMV antigen • Detection of CMV from throat swabs, urine, or saliva may not support the presence of CMV disease
Nucleic acid detection, antigen detection	• Qualitative PCR • Quantitative DNA hybridization • Antigenemia	• Qualitative PCR is sensitive but not specific for CMV disease • Specialized equipment and labor required for PCR, hybridization, antigenemia
Serology	Acute, convalescent CMV IgG or single CMV IgM titer	• Serologic response may be delayed or absent in primary infection • False-positive reactions or interference may occur • Potential variability in kit standardization
Histopathology, immunopathology	• Microscopic examination of tissue for inclusion bodies • Immunohistochemical staining with labeled monoclonal anti-CMV antibody • Electron microscopic examination of biopsy specimens for CMV	• Insensitive; inclusion bodies may be present only in advanced infection • Specialized equipment required

CMV, cytomegalovirus; Ig, immunoglobulin; PCR, polymerase chain reaction.

gammaglobulin (IVIG) to ganciclovir may improve the clinical response. Cidofovir and foscarnet can be used to treat disease associated with ganciclovir-resistant CMV strains. However, the risk for additive nephrotoxicity with calcineurin blockers has limited their usage.

Prevention

To minimize severe CMV infection, some transplantation centers avoid transplanting CMV-positive kidneys into CMV-negative recipients. However, this approach is limited by the competing needs for human leukocyte antigen (HLA) matching and the shortage of donor kidneys. Regimens to limit the risk of CMV disease and to improve patient and allograft survival vary from center to center and are based upon the CMV serostatus of the donor and recipient and an assessment of the net state of immunosuppression. Large, multicenter, randomized trials with strict enrollment criteria and consistent immunosuppressive regimens are lacking. In practice, two strategies are used for CMV prevention: universal prophylaxis and preemptive therapy. Universal prophylaxis involves giving antiviral therapy to all at-risk patients immediately after transplant for a defined duration. The duration of prophylaxis is dependent on the perceived duration of risk and net state of immunosuppression. Preemptive therapy, sometimes referred to as "targeted or guided prophylaxis," involves monitoring patients at regular intervals for early evidence of CMV replication by use of a laboratory assay such as p65 antigenemia or CMV DNA hybridization. Patients with laboratory evidence of early CMV replication are treated with antiviral therapy to prevent symptomatic disease. The approach of universal prophylaxis may be more useful for patients at high risk of CMV disease, while preemptive therapy may be more useful for those patients at low or intermediate risk of CMV disease.

Antiviral agents used for universal prophylaxis include acyclovir, valacyclovir, intravenous or oral ganciclovir, valganciclovir, CMV immune globulin (CMVIG), and a combination of antiviral agents and CMVIG (Table 10.11). Although oral acyclovir is effective in lower-risk recipients [e.g., donor (D) CMV-negative/recipient (R) CMV-negative or -positive], it is considered ineffective in high-risk patients. Oral valacyclovir administered for 3 months after transplant reduced the incidence of CMV disease in seropositive and seronegative kidney transplant recipients in some clinical trials. Oral and intravenous ganciclovir and oral valganciclovir are more active *in vitro* against CMV than acyclovir and are more effective than acyclovir in preventing CMV disease in both R+ and D+/R− patients. Compared to the IV formulation, oral ganciclovir is substantially less bioavailable (4% to 6%) and achieves significantly lower serum levels, but is more convenient to administer. Valganciclovir is the L-valine ester of ganciclovir and is administered 900 mg per day by mouth for CMV prophylaxis. This dose produces similar area under the curve (AUC) values to IV ganciclovir (5 mg/kg per day) and much higher values than oral ganciclovir (3 g per day). A clinical trial compared once-daily valganciclovir to thrice-daily oral ganciclovir given for approximately 90 to 100 days for the prevention

Table 10.11. Potential strategies for cytomegalovirus (CMV) prophylaxis

Prophylactic Regimens[a]	CMV Serologies		
	D +, R−	R +	D−, R−
Oral acyclovir	0	0	+
Ganciclovir or valganciclovir	+	+	0
IV ganciclovir followed by oral ganciclovir or valganciclovir	+	+	0
IV or oral ganciclovir and CMVIG[b]	+	+	0
Oral valacyclovir	+	+	0

CMVIG, cytomegalovirus immune globulin; D, donor; IV, intravenous; R, recipient.

[a]In D+/R− kidneys, oral ganciclovir (3 g/d), valganciclovir (900 mg/d) or IV ganciclovir (5 mg/kg/d) prophylaxis is effective for prevention of CMV disease. All doses are adjusted for renal function. Prophylaxis is initiated shortly after kidney transplant and continued for approximately 3 months. In R+ kidney, oral ganciclovir (3 g/d) for 3 months decreases the rate of CMV disease compared with placebo or acyclovir. In R+ kidneys, oral valganciclovir (900 mg/d) is an alternative; oral valacyclovir (8 g/d) has also been used in R+ and D+/R− recipients. All of the above regimens have been generally used for 90 to 100 days after transplant but may be continued for up to 180 days for patients who received antilymphocytic induction therapy.

[b]CMVIG can be considered as adjunctive prophylaxis in high-risk recipients. Doses range from 200 mg/kg on day 0, followed by 150 mg/kg/d at weeks 2, 4, 6, 8, 10, and 100 mg/kg/d at weeks 12 to 16.

of CMV disease in high-risk D+/R− solid-organ transplant recipients. Overall, the two agents were similarly effective. However, in a subanalysis, valganciclovir was more effective than ganciclovir in preventing CMV disease at 6 months among kidney transplant recipients. Oral valganciclovir and ganciclovir are appropriate agents for prevention of CMV disease in D+/R− or R+ pancreas-kidney recipients. In nonblinded, nonrandomized trials, CMVIG reduced the incidence of virologically confirmed CMV-associated syndromes and secondary opportunistic infections in D+/R− renal transplant. Further research is required.

CMV-positive transplant patients who are treated with OKT3, or who require multiple treatments for rejection, have a high incidence of symptomatic CMV disease. Although controlled trials are lacking, IV ganciclovir therapy (2.5 to 5 mg/kg per day) administered during antibody treatment or intensified immunosuppression courses followed by a period of oral ganciclovir or valganciclovir may reduce this risk. Ganciclovir treatment presumably inactivates latent virus that has the potential for reactivation when immunosuppression is intensified. Ganciclovir and valganciclovir require dosage adjustment for decreased creatinine clearance.

Herpes Simplex Virus and Varicella-Zoster Virus

HSV infection typically develops within the first 6 weeks after transplantation and most commonly involves mucosal surfaces. Infection occasionally can disseminate to visceral organs and cause esophagitis, hepatitis, and pneumonitis. The majority of infections are caused by reactivation of endogenous latent virus, although primary infection transmitted from the allografts has been described. Both acyclovir and ganciclovir are active against herpesviruses *in vitro,* and both are useful in the treatment or prophylaxis of HSV. Alternative agents include valacyclovir and famciclovir. Acyclovir can be given intravenously or orally for mucocutaneous infections. For treatment of HSV encephalitis, a higher dosage is given by slow infusion to prevent crystallization within the renal tubules.

Herpes zoster ("shingles") develops in approximately 10% of adult renal transplant recipients and may involve two or three adjoining dermatomes. Infection is usually caused by reactivation of latent disease. The 10% of transplant candidates who are VZV seronegative should receive varicella vaccine before undergoing transplant. Acyclovir, famciclovir, and valacyclovir can be used for treatment of herpes zoster and primary varicella infection. While uncommon, disseminated VZV is usually associated with primary VZV infection and can cause pneumonia, encephalitis, disseminated intravascular coagulation, and graft dysfunction. Susceptible individuals should be given VZV immunoglobulin as soon as possible for maximal effectiveness but no later than 96 hours following an exposure. Intravenous acyclovir (10 to 15 mg/kg every 8 hours as a slow infusion) should be given for the treatment of primary varicella and disseminated zoster. Oral acyclovir, valacyclovir, famciclovir, or ganciclovir may be appropriate for treatment of mild dermatomal zoster.

Other Human Herpesviruses

HHV types 6, 7, and 8 may reactivate following renal transplant. While more than 90% of adults are seropositive of HHV-6 and HHV-7, only 0% to 5% are seropositive for HHV-8. HHV-6 reactivates in 31% to 55% of organ transplant recipients, most commonly occurring during episodes of acute rejection, associated with calcineurin inhibitor toxicity, and the first 4 weeks posttransplant. Reactivation of HHV-6 is associated with CMV disease and an increased risk of invasive fungal infection, and can cause hepatitis, pneumonitis, and encephalitis. The manifestations of HHV-7 infection are poorly characterized. Neither serology nor PCR of peripheral blood lymphocytes can reliably distinguish active from latent infection with these viruses, and routine monitoring in asymptomatic individuals is not recommended. Prevention strategies are unclear. Ganciclovir, foscarnet, and cidofovir have activity *in vitro* against HHV-6. Symptomatic HHV-6 infection should be treated with antiviral therapy and reduction of immunosuppression. The role for treatment of asymptomatic patients is undefined. HHV-8 seroconversion occurs in up to 12% of seronegative kidney transplants, usually within 3 months of transplantation. Posttransplant infection can be primary or transmitted from the donor kidney and is associated with

Kaposi sarcoma occurring a median of 30 months posttransplant. Diagnosis is supported by pathology and by the presence of HHV-8 DNA sequences in involved tissue. Treatment consists of radiation and chemotherapy. Pretransplant donor and recipient serologic screening may be helpful for risk stratification.

Adenovirus

Adenovirus can cause hemorrhagic cystitis, fever, renal dysfunction, and, rarely, dissemination with pneumonia, hepatitis, and death. Following transplantation, infection may result from reactivation of latent adenovirus or primary infection from an exogenous source or from the renal allograft. Disseminated disease is more common following primary infection. Definite diagnosis is by kidney biopsy that typically reveals granulomatous interstitial nephritis, tubular necrosis, and ground glass-like intranuclear viral inclusion bodies in tubular cells. Intravenous ribavirin either alone or in combination with intravenous immunoglobulin has been used with some success and reduction in immunosuppression may be of benefit.

BK Virus

Polyomaviruses associated with human disease include BK virus and JC virus. BK virus causes latent infection of the kidney; with reactivation during immune suppression, it may cause tubulointerstitial nephritis and ureteral stenosis or stricture. The peak incidence of primary BK infection occurs in children 2 to 5 years of age, and 60% to 80% of adults are seropositive. Rates of infection in renal transplant recipients' range between 10% and 60%, with a bimodal distribution of disease between 10 days and 6 weeks posttransplantation for primary infection and 5 weeks and 17 months for reinfection or reactivation. Risk factors for infection and disease include donor seropositivity, degree of immune suppression, use of tacrolimus and mycophenolate mofetil, and allograft rejection. Definitive diagnosis requires a renal biopsy. BK virus DNA PCR of urine and serum, and the identification of decoy cells in the urine, may assist in establishing the diagnosis. Management involves reduction of immunosuppression with close monitoring for rejection. Leflunomide, cidofovir, IVIG, and corticosteroids may be of clinical benefit. Leflunomide is the drug of first choice because of its combined antiviral and immunosuppressive properties and its lack of nephrotoxicity (see Chapter 4). A maintenance dose of 20–40 mg daily is usually adequate.

Influenza Types A and B, Parainfluenza Virus, and Respiratory Syncytial Virus

Community respiratory viruses may cause significant morbidity and mortality in renal transplant recipients. These seasonal viruses can be transmitted by virus-laden respiratory droplets and aerosols by direct person-to-person contact or by contact with fomites, and can occur in healthcare settings. Renal transplant recipients may be the "sentinel" cases for a community influenza outbreak. Community respiratory virus disease usually presents with upper respiratory tract symptoms and high fever, myalgias, arthralgias, anorexia, and mucosal inflammation. Illness ranges from mild upper respiratory illness, to bronchiolitis, progressive viral pneumonia with respiratory failure, and suprainfection with fungal or bacterial pathogens, such as *S. aureus, Streptococcus* species, and gram-negative bacilli. Simultaneous CMV reactivation may occur as a result of immunomodulation.

Rapid detection of virus-infected upper respiratory cells (e.g., nasopharyngeal washing, respiratory secretions) using virus-specific fluorescent-labeled antibody probes can facilitate the diagnosis, appropriate isolation, and treatment of patients with viral respiratory infections. Annual influenza immunization should be considered in all renal transplant recipients. Influenza immunization is less effective in inducing viral-neutralizing antibody titers and in preventing disease in immunocompromised patients than in healthy persons, but results in a substantially decreased risk of hospitalization and mortality. Live, intranasal influenza vaccine should not be administered to renal transplant recipients or their household contacts. Treatment of influenza A includes early administration of amantadine or rimantadine, but neither agent is effective against influenza B. The neuraminidase inhibitors oseltamivir and zanamivir are active against both influenza A and B and are effective if started within 36 to 48 hours after onset of symptoms. They result in a modest decrease in the duration of illness and significantly decrease the risk of secondary bacterial complications. During community or institutional outbreaks of influenza, susceptible persons should be vaccinated and antiviral prophylaxis administered for 2 weeks until antibodies develop. RSV pneumonitis may respond to aerosolized ribavirin delivered in a controlled contained administration system given over 24 hours. RSV monoclonal antibody (palivizumab) may be combined with aerosolized ribavirin before respiratory failure develops, although their use has not been studied in renal transplant recipients. Parainfluenza virus (types 1–4) is a paramyxovirus; it can occur during fall and winter months, or sporadically. Disease spectrum in renal transplants can mimic influenza and can include mild upper respiratory disease to frank pneumonia and death. Transmission occurs by infected respiratory droplets and fomites. Handwashing is essential in hospitalized patients to reduce transmission. Coinfection with bacterial and fungal pathogens should be ruled out. Diagnosis of parainfluenza includes viral isolation, shell vial assays, and rapid antigen detection kits on cultured material or direct clinical specimens; variation in commercial kits has been noted and should be properly standardized. Treatment options are poor for parainfluenza infections. With all viral infections, immunomodulation can occur; associated effects may include systemic suprainfection and allograft rejection.

Parvovirus

In transplant recipients, parvovirus B19 infection is a cause of refractory severe anemia, pancytopenia, thrombotic microangiopathy, fibrosing cholestatic hepatitis, and graft dysfunction. Parvovirus occurs in up to 23% of renal transplant recipients with severe anemia, and 80% of infections occur within the first 3 months of transplantation. Donor transmission has been reported. Examination of bone marrow reveals typical giant proerythroblasts, and the diagnosis should be confirmed by detection of B19 virus DNA in serum by PCR assay. Some patients may have concurrent CMV disease. Treatment consists of high-dose IVIG (0.5 mg/kg per day for 5 to 10 days), reduction of immunosuppression, and, if possible, discontinuation of tacrolimus therapy.

West Nile Virus

The clinical manifestation of WNV in the immunocompetent host typically consists of 3 to 6 days of malaise, anorexia, arthralgia, vomiting, nausea, rash, and lymphadenopathy. In elderly or immunocompromised individuals, more severe neurologic manifestations can occur, including encephalitis or meningitis, mental status changes, seizures, optic neuritis, muscle weakness, flaccid paralysis, and movement disorders. Symptoms that begin in the first 2 weeks posttransplantation suggest transmission via the allograft, whereas symptoms that begin later suggest community acquisition. Diagnosis is confirmed by detection of West Nile virus IgM antibody in the CSF. Treatment includes reduction of immunosuppression and supportive care. IVIG anecdotally has been associated with improvement in some severely ill transplant patients. Interferon alpha-2b and ribavirin have activity *in vitro* against WNV. All transplant recipients from at-risk areas should limit the risk of mosquito exposure by using insect repellents and wearing long-sleeve clothing and long pants while outdoors during summer months.

Severe Acute Respiratory Syndrome-Associated Coronavirus

In 2002, cases of SARS were reported associated with a new viral pathogen, SARS-CoV. The spectrum of disease ranges from asymptomatic or mild respiratory illness to rapidly fatal respiratory failure. Mortality rates ranged from 3% to 12% and were higher among the elderly (age greater than 60 years) and immunocompromised, including transplant recipients. Symptoms include fever [greater than 38°C (100.4°F)], chills, headache, myalgias, cough, shortness of breath, difficulty breathing, or hypoxia, and radiographic evidence of pneumonia or adult respiratory distress syndrome (ARDS). Laboratory findings include lymphopenia, thrombocytopenia, and mild increases in transaminases. Diagnostic assays include detection of viral ribonucleic acid (RNA) by real-time reverse transcription PCR and acute and convalescent antibodies to SARS-CoV by enzyme immunoassay. Therapy includes supportive care, empiric antimicrobial treatment active against both typical and atypical respiratory pathogens associated with community-acquired pneumonia, and the investigational use of intravenous ribavirin and corticosteroids. Standard precautions (hand hygiene), airborne precautions (N-95 respirator and placement in a negative-pressure isolation room) and contact precautions (gowns, gloves, and eye protection) are recommended when caring for patients hospitalized with suspected SARS.

Human Papillomavirus

Human papillomavirus causes cutaneous and anogenital warts and is associated with cervical intraepithelial neoplasia, squamous cell carcinoma, and anogenital carcinoma. Premalignant skin and cervical lesions are more common and progress more rapidly to cancer among organ transplant recipients. Cutaneous warts, keratotic skin lesions, and anogenital warts should be monitored and referred for early dermatologic or colorectal evaluation, biopsy, and treatment. Treatments include topical keratolytic and caustic agents, topical and oral retinoids, podophyllin, 5-fluorouracil, bleomycin, physical ablation, and investigational immunotherapies.

SELECTED READINGS

Centers for Disease Control and Prevention. Severe acute respiratory syndrome (SARS). Available at www.cdc.gov/ncidod/sars.

de Jong-Tieben LM, Berkhout RJ, ter Schegget J, et al. The prevalence of human papillomavirus DNA in benign keratotic skin lesions of renal transplant recipients with and without a history of skin cancer is equally high: a clinical study to assess risk factors for keratotic skin lesions and skin cancer. *Transplantation* 2000;69:44–49.

Delmonico FL, Snydman DR. Organ donor screening for infectious diseases. *Transplantation* 1998;65:603–610.

Fishman JA. BK nephropathy: what is the role of antiviral therapy? *Am J Transplant* 2003;3:99–100.

Fishman JA, Rubin RH. Infections in organ-transplant recipients. *N Engl J Med* 1998;338:1741–1751.

Hart GD, Paya CV. Prophylaxis for CMV should now replace preemptive therapy in solid organ transplantation. *Rev Med Virol* 2001;11:73–81.

Herbrecht R, Denning DW, Patterson TF, et al. Voriconazole versus amphotericin B for primary therapy of invasive aspergillosis. *N Engl J Med* 2002;347:408–415.

Ho M. Human herpesvirus 8: let the transplant physician beware. *N Engl J Med* 1998;339:1391–1392.

Humar A, Kumar D, Boivin G, et al. Cytomegalovirus (CMV) virus load kinetics to predict recurrent disease in solid-organ transplant patients with CMV disease. *J Infect Dis* 2002;186:829–833.

Imirizaldu JJ, Esteban JC, Axpe IR, et al. Post-transplantation HTLV-1 myelopathy in three recipients from a single donor. *J Neurol Neurosurg Psychiatry* 2003;74:1080–1084.

Jassal SV, Roscoe JM, Zaltzman JS, et al. Clinical practice guidelines: prevention of cytomegalovirus disease after renal transplantation. *J Am Soc Nephrol* 1998;9:1696–1708.

Jha V, Sakhuja V, Gupta D, et al. Successful management of pulmonary tuberculosis in renal allograft recipients in a single center. *Kidney Int* 1999;56:1944–1950.

Kumar D, Tellier R, Draker R, et al. Severe acute respiratory syndrome (SARS) in a liver transplant recipient and guidelines for donor SARS screening. *Am J Transplant* 2003;3:977–981.

Meier-Kriesche HU, Friedman G, Jacobs M, et al. Infectious complications in geriatric renal transplant patients: comparison of two immunosuppressive protocols. *Transplantation* 1999;68:1496–1502.

Mora-Duarte J, Betts R, Rotstein C, et al. Comparison of caspofungin and amphotericin B for invasive candidiasis. *N Engl J Med* 2002;347:2020–2029.

Murer L, Zacchello G, Bianchi D. Thrombotic microangiopathy associated with parvovirus B19 infection after renal transplantation. *J Am Soc Nephrol* 2000;11:1132–1137.

Nickeleit V, Hirsch HH, Binet IF, et al. Polyomavirus infection in renal allograft recipients: from latent infection to manifest disease. *J Am Soc Nephrol* 1999;10:1080–1089.

Patterson JE. Epidemiology of fungal infection in solid organ transplant recipients. *Transpl Infect Dis* 1999;1:229–236.

Paya C. Prevention of cytomegalovirus disease in recipients of solid-organ transplants. *Clin Infect Dis* 2001;32:596–603.

Rubin RH. Cytomegalovirus in solid organ transplantation. *Transpl Infect Dis* 2001;3:1–5.

Walsh TJ, Finberg RW, Arndt C, et al. Liposomal amphotericin B for empirical therapy in patients with persistent fever and neutropenia. *N Engl J Med* 1999;340:764–771.

Kidney Transplantation and Liver Disease

Fabrizio Fabrizi, Suphamai Bunnapradist, and Paul Martin

Liver disease, most notably caused by hepatitis B virus (HBV) and hepatitis C virus (HCV), remains a major cause of morbidity and mortality in long-term survivors of renal transplantation. Appropriate evaluation of the renal transplant candidate with chronic viral hepatitis includes assessment of viral replication, liver histology, and consideration of antiviral therapy. HCV infection is also implicated in posttransplant graft dysfunction.

RENAL TRANSPLANT RECIPIENTS WITH VIRAL HEPATITIS

Hepatitis B

Diagnostic Tests and Their Interpretation

Table 11.1 describes diagnostic tests for hepatitis B virus and their interpretation.

Serum hepatitis B surface antigen (HBsAg) is the first detectable viral marker in acute HBV infection. After an incubation period of up to 140 days, the patient may develop symptoms such as malaise and anorexia, or become frankly icteric. By this time, other serum markers of HBV infection also appear, including antibody to the hepatitis B core antigen (anti-HBc). Hepatitis B core antigen (HBcAg) is present exclusively in nuclei of infected hepatocytes, but the corresponding antibody circulates in blood. During acute HBV infection, anti-HBc is predominantly immunoglobulin (Ig) M. Over the subsequent 6 months IgM levels decline while IgG anti-HBc levels persist. Although anti-HBc is not a neutralizing antibody, it is the most durable marker of prior HBV infection. With successful resolution of acute HBV, protective antibody against HBsAg (anti-HBs) appears, signifying immunity against HBV. Anti-HBs antibody tends to decline and even disappear over time, leaving an "isolated" core antibody (IgG anti-HBc) as the only marker of prior HBV infection. If HBsAg persists for more than 3 months, HBV deoxyribonucleic acid (DNA) and hepatitis B e antigen (HBeAg) levels should be checked to assess level of active viral replication.

Natural History

Only approximately 5% of infected immunocompetent adults fail to recover from acute hepatitis B infection and develop chronic hepatitis B. In these individuals, HBsAg persists in serum and anti-HBs fails to appear. Chronicity is more likely in individuals with impaired immune response such as uremic patients, the elderly or children. Symptomatic acute HBV with jaundice is more likely to lead to successful clearance of HBV infection than a

Table 11.1.   Tests for hepatitis B virus (HBV)

Tests		Interpretation
HBsAg	Hepatitis B surface antigen	HBV infection
IgM Anti-HBc	Antibody to hepatitis B core antigen	Acute or recent HBV infection
IgG Anti-HBc	Antibody to hepatitis B core antigen	Chronic or remote HBV infection
HBsAb	Antibody to hepatitis B surface antigen	Immunity to HBV (vaccine induced or a result of prior infection)
HBe	Hepatitis B e antigen	Active replication
HBV DNA	HBV viremia	Active replication

subclinical acute HBV. This apparent paradox is explained by the prominent role the host immunity plays in the expression of the clinical course of HBV. The original immune response during acute HBV infection results in more liver injury with more symptoms, but also a greater likelihood of recovery. Two phases of chronic HBV infection can be identified. In the early months and years of chronic HBV infection, the "replicative" phase occurs, which is often accompanied by necroinflammatory changes in the liver and elevated aminotransferase levels in serum. The "replicative phase" is characterized by active viral replication: HBeAg and high titers of HBV DNA are detectable in serum. The second phase of chronic HBV infection is the "nonreplicative" phase, which is often heralded by a transient increase in aminotransferase levels. The "nonreplicative" phase follows HBeAg clearance. With HBeAg loss, antibodies to HBeAg appear in serum, HBV DNA levels decrease, and, generally, liver disease activity subsides both biochemically and histologically. After HBeAg clearance, infectivity is much reduced, but low levels of HBV DNA may persist for variable periods of time. Patients with persistent HBsAg positivity and normal aminotransferase activity were previously defined as "healthy carriers" of HBV, but are now referred to as "inactive" carriers. These patients, however, still are at risk for developing progressive liver disease triggered by immunosuppression after renal transplant. The HBV genome shows significant heterogeneity and various mutant forms of HBV have been identified in which amino acid substitutions at crucial sites in the viral genome occur. An important subset of patients clear HBeAg and develop the corresponding anti-HBe antibody, but continue to have active replication with strongly positive serum HBV DNA with elevated transaminases. This HBeAg-negative form of chronic HBV is characterized clinically by a more poorly sustained response to antiviral therapy than is found in chronically infected patients who remain HBeAg-positive. The HBeAg-negative form of chronic HBV is becoming more prevalent worldwide.

HBV infection is a major cause of morbidity, with as many as 350 million people infected worldwide, resulting in an estimated 2 million deaths per year. Despite the availability of a vaccine since the early 1980s, HBV remains a major cause of chronic hepatitis, cirrhosis, and hepatocellular carcinoma. Mutants with "YMDD" motif variants in the polymerase gene have been discovered as a result of lamivudine resistance. Six genotypic groups of HBV have been identified (A to F). Although their clinical significance is yet to be fully defined, studies suggest that specific HBV genotypes may be associated with more severe liver disease and lower response rates to therapy.

Prevention of HBV acquisition in dialysis centers has been an important aspect of its management in end-stage renal disease (ESRD) patients. The incidence and prevalence of HBV infection in dialysis patients in developed countries has fallen over the past three decades as a result of strict attention to relatively simple precautions. Outbreaks of HBV infection in dialysis units are usually a result of nonadherence to these precautions, including serologic surveillance, isolation of HBV-infected patients, use of dedicated dialysis machines, and rigorous disinfection. HBsAg rates remain higher in patients on dialysis in less-developed countries where HBV remains prevalent in the population as a whole. Despite availability of HBV vaccination for more than two decades, recent surveys in the United States reveal that fewer than 50% of patients on chronic dialysis have been vaccinated. Although response with development of protective levels of anti-HBs is not universal in this population, at least 60% of chronic dialysis patients do respond adequately.

Disease Progression After Renal Transplantation

The prevalence of HBV infection among renal transplant recipients has decreased overall because of less HBV infection in the dialysis population. Because of concern about posttransplant progression of liver disease, HBV infection has been regarded as a relative contraindication to transplantation. HBV infection in transplant recipients may be associated with only minor elevations of aminotransferase levels despite histologic progression. Progression of HBV-related liver disease may be promoted by several factors, most notably immunosuppression, HCV coinfection, and alcohol abuse. Immunosuppression may increase HBV replication by various mechanisms, including diminished activity of cytotoxic T lymphocytes. In addition, the HBV genome contains a glucocorticoid-responsive element that augments HBV replication. Azathioprine and the calcineurin inhibitors may also enhance HBV replication.

The adverse effect of immunosuppressive therapy on HBV infection has been recognized in several clinical settings. Severe, even fatal, HBV reactivation was noted in patients who had received systemic chemotherapy. Reactivation of HBV has been observed in renal transplant recipients whose prior markers of HBV infection had resolved with reappearance of HBsAg in serum despite its absence pretransplant. Liver transplantation in HBV-infected patients is associated with frequent graft reinfection followed by progressive liver disease if immunoprophylaxis is not given.

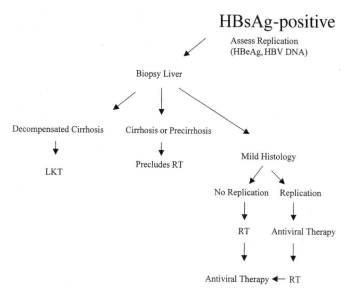

Fig. 11.1. **Approach to the workup of the kidney transplant candidate with viral hepatitis B. HBV, hepatitis B virus; LKT, combined liver and kidney transplant; RT, renal transplant.**

The adverse effect of HBsAg positivity on patient survival in renal transplant recipients is well established. The effect of HBsAg status on graft survival is less clear, although there are reports that suggest that graft survival might be enhanced in HBV infected recipients as a result of a diminished immune response resulting from chronic viral infection.

Role of Pretransplant Liver Biopsy

Figure 11.1 illustrates an approach to the kidney transplant candidate with a diagnosis of HBV. Liver biopsy should be incorporated in the evaluation of renal transplant candidates with HBsAg because it is difficult, on clinical grounds alone, to estimate the severity of liver disease in uremic patients. Aminotransferase levels may be depressed despite active histologic changes on biopsy. Administration of desmopressin acetate (DDAVP) at the time of biopsy should be considered to lessen the risk of bleeding caused by platelet dysfunction. A decision concerning transplant candidacy in HBsAg-positive patients should be based on both liver histology and evaluation of HBV replication by serum markers (i.e., HBeAg and HBV DNA). The absence of serum marker of replication, that is, HBV DNA or HBeAg positivity, before transplantation, however, does not preclude reactivation of HBV infection posttransplant. Patients with established cirrhosis (stage IV) on liver biopsy are at risk for frank hepatic decompensation after transplantation, and kidney transplantation alone is contraindicated. In patients with normal renal function, antiviral therapy has been reported to lead to regression of advanced histologic lesions. In transplant candidates with active HBV replication, pretransplant antiviral therapy should be attempted to arrest the course of liver disease and to suppress HBV replication. In patients with histologically mild liver disease, renal transplant is not precluded. However, all patients infected with HBV must be cautioned that even histologically mild disease can progress when immunosuppression is introduced. The advent of effective antiviral therapies now offers the opportunity to prevent posttransplant progression of HBV. If active replication is present (i.e., positive HBeAg or HBV DNA), antiviral therapy should be started pretransplant to slow the progression of liver disease. If the initial histology shows more advanced changes, liver biopsy should be repeated. All patients with HBV should be placed on posttransplant antiviral therapy. Better patient outcomes can be achieved if antiviral therapy is used posttransplant to prevent progressive liver disease.

Current Status of Antiviral Therapy

The options for antiviral therapy have expanded over the last several years from the initial introduction of interferon (IFN) to the more recent use of lamivudine and now adefovir. Although IFN may be efficacious in the treatment of chronic HBV, its use is contraindicated in renal transplant recipients. The immunomodulatory actions of IFN may lead to the precipitation of severe and often irreversible graft dysfunction.

The introduction of lamivudine has been a major advance in the management of posttransplant HBV-related liver disease. Lamivudine is a nucleoside analogue that suppresses HBV replication by interfering with the reverse transcriptase activity of HBV, causing termination of the proviral DNA chain. Lamivudine suppresses HBV replication and improves aminotransferase levels in renal transplant recipients. Lamivudine is well tolerated, is administered orally, and has no adverse immunomodulatory activity. Because lamivudine is metabolized by the kidney, its dose should be reduced in patients with impaired renal function. The standard dose is 100 mg once daily, which is reduced to 50 mg daily for a creatinine clearance of 30 to 49 mL per minute. Prolonged use of lamivudine is associated with the development of drug resistance, as a consequence of the induction and selection of HBV mutants at the YMDD motif of DNA polymerase, which may cause clinical worsening of liver disease. Adefovir has been approved for treatment of chronic HBV and is efficacious in the presence of lamivudine resistance. Resistance to adefovir is substantially less frequent than with lamivudine. A reduced adefovir dose is also necessary in the presence of renal dysfunction. No information is available yet about its use in renal transplant recipients, but it is well tolerated in liver transplant recipients and does not affect immunosuppressant drug levels.

Hepatitis C

Interpretation of Diagnostic Tests

Table 11.2 describes diagnostic tests for hepatitis C virus and their interpretation.

Table 11.2.   Tests for hepatitis C virus (HCV)

Tests	Uses	Comments
Anti-HCV ELISA 3.0	Initial diagnosis	Excellent sensitivity
HCV PCR qualitative	Confirmation of HCV infection	Helpful in dialysis of seronegative patients
HCV PCR quantitative	Assessment of viral load	Less sensitive than qualitative tests; more reproducible than qualitative tests; useful for monitoring response to IFN
HCV genotyping	Treatment decision	Role in predicting responsiveness to IFN

ELISA, enzyme-linked immunoabsorbent assay; IFN, interferon; PCR, polymerase chain reaction.

Serologic testing is the initial mode of diagnosis of HCV infection. Third-generation enzyme-linked immunoabsorbent assays (ELISAs) have been introduced and have further enhanced specificity and sensitivity of serologic testing, including in patients with ESRD. The gold standard for the diagnosis of HCV remains the detection of HCV viremia [HCV ribonucleic acid (RNA)] in serum by reverse-transcriptase polymerase chain reaction (PCR) and has effectively replaced the recombinant immunoblot assay. PCR-based tests may be either quantitative or qualitative with the latter having a lower limit of detection of viremia. Laboratory standardization varies and it may be difficult to compare results from one laboratory to another. Reliability may be further reduced by imperfect handling or storage of blood samples. Because of the occurrence of HCV viremia in a small minority of patients with ESRD who are negative by serologic testing, a PCR test should be performed if there is unexplained transaminitis or if a clinical concern about HCV infection remains despite negative serologic tests.

Natural History

Chronic HCV infection remains highly prevalent in the hemodialysis population despite elimination of HCV from the blood supply, reflecting, in part, nosocomial spread in hemodialysis units. HCV infection, and its potential for acceleration, is a frequent cause of concern in potential renal transplant recipients.

Because the natural history of HCV extends over decades rather than years, adverse consequences of chronic HCV infection in patients followed for a short period of time may not be apparent. ESRD patients have higher morbidity and mortality rates than does the general population because of comorbidities and thus the long-term consequences of HCV infection are difficult to assess in this population. Evaluation of HCV infection in renal transplant candidates is further complicated by the observation that aminotransferase levels in the dialysis population and patients with predialysis chronic renal failure are usually lower than the nonuremic population. Dialysis patients who are HCV viremic have aminotransferase levels greater than those who are not HCV viremic, although typically, the values are still within the "normal" range.

Six major HCV genotypes have been described; they differ little in clinical expression but vary in their responsiveness to IFN therapy. Response rates among patients with genotype 1 are much lower than patients with HCV genotypes 2 and 3.

Disease Progression After Renal Transplantation

The frequency of HCV infection among renal transplant recipients is influenced by various factors, including prior blood transfusion, history of previous transplant, type and duration of pretransplant renal replacement therapy, and the geographic origin of the recipient. The majority of anti-HCV seropositive renal transplant recipients have persistent HCV viremia. HCV RNA titers may increase markedly as a result of posttransplant immunosuppression.

A particular concern is that studies with serial liver biopsies have shown that posttransplant HCV-related liver disease is progressive. Factors implicated in the more rapid posttransplant progression include alcohol abuse and HBV coinfection. Liver disease is more aggressive in recipients who acquire HCV at the time of transplant because they develop an acute hepatitis at a time of maximum immunosuppression. Azathioprine and antilymphocyte agents have been implicated in more severe liver disease. Administration of high-dose steroids and antilymphocytic antibodies should be avoided and only used after a critical evaluation of potential risk and benefit, especially the risk of accelerating the course of liver disease.

Detailed studies with adequate followup have documented adverse effects of HCV infection on patient survival after kidney transplantation alone, as well as for combined kidney–pancreas transplantation. However, the outcome of HCV-infected hemodialysis patients is worse than for matched patients who undergo transplantation. Recipients of a first deceased donor transplant have an initially greater perioperative risk for death than those who remain on dialysis therapy, but a subsequent long-term benefit. Glomerulonephritis and mixed cryoglobulinemia, well described in the nontransplant setting, has been described in renal grafts either recurrent or *de novo*.

HCV infection in the general population is associated with an increased risk of type 2 diabetes mellitus. In HCV-positive renal transplant recipients, an overall incidence of type 2 diabetes of close to 40% has been described. The incidence is even higher if tacrolimus is used for immunosuppression and if other risk factors are present (see Chapter 9). HCV-positive transplant candidates should be warned of this increased risk.

Role of Pretransplant Liver Biopsy

Figure 11.2 illustrates an approach to the evaluation of renal transplant candidates with HCV. Liver biopsy is essential in the

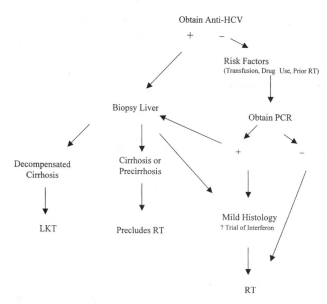

**Fig. 11.2.   Approach to the workup of the kidney transplant
candidate with viral hepatitis C. HCV, hepatitis C virus; LKT,
combined kidney and liver transplant; RT, renal transplant.**

evaluation of liver disease in renal transplant candidates because
reliance on clinical and biochemical findings may underestimate
its severity. Pretransplant liver biopsy provides useful prognostic information. Patients with minimal to mild chronic hepatitis
(stages I and II) can be safely transplanted, and a pretransplant
trial of antiviral therapy should be considered. Patients with cirrhosis on biopsy should not be transplanted because of the risk
for posttransplant hepatocellular failure. If there is a sustained
virologic response to antiviral therapy, and if repeat liver biopsy
shows improvement, transplant candidacy can be reconsidered.
For cirrhotic patients, combined liver–kidney transplant may be
a consideration if they subsequently develop hepatocellular failure (see Kidney and Liver Transplantation). For patients whose
histology precludes renal transplantation yet whose hepatic function is too well compensated to require liver transplantation, it
may be safer to remain on dialysis. In the event that decompen-
sated cirrhosis develops, combined orthotopic liver and kidney
transplantation may be indicated (Table 11.3)

Current Status of Antiviral Therapy
The major concern limiting the posttransplant use of IFN is the
risk, noted earlier, of precipitating graft loss. However successful pretransplant antiviral therapy for HCV has been followed
by a durable absence posttransplant of HCV RNA viremia. No

**Table 11.3.   Indications for combined
kidney and liver transplant**

Orthotopic liver transplant (OLT) candidate with severe irreversible
renal dysfunction caused by

1. Polycystic kidneys with massive hepatomegaly
2. Primary oxalosis
3. Prolonged pre-OLT dialysis dependence
4. Glomerulonephritis (especially as a consequence of IgA, HBV,
    and HCV)
5. Repeat OLT with calcineurin inhibitor toxicity
6. Diabetic nephropathy

effective noninterferon-based therapy is currently available for
HCV.

OTHER CAUSES OF LIVER DISEASE IN RENAL TRANSPLANT RECIPIENTS

Viral infections, such as herpes simplex (HSV) and cytomegalovirus (CMV), and drugs used in the posttransplant period should
be considered in the differential diagnosis of posttransplant hepatic dysfunction. Patients with elevated levels of serum aminotransferases and/or gamma-glutamyl transpeptidase, should be
questioned about ingestion of alcohol and hepatotoxic drugs. Specific inquiry should be made about use of herbal and health food
store products. Serum aminotransferase and gamma-glutamyl
transpeptidase levels should be rechecked after the patient has
abstained from potential toxic substances. A low grade, transient
elevation of serum aminotransferases is commonly seen in patients receiving calcineurin inhibitors. If these elevations persist or are severe, a thorough workup including liver biopsy is
indicated.

In the 1970s and 1980s, hemosiderosis was common in patients
with ESRD. The widespread use of erythropoietin and the lowered requirement for blood transfusion have made hepatic iron
overload less common in both dialysis patients and transplant recipients. Quantitative iron determined on liver biopsy and genetic
testing for hemochromatosis may be necessary to confidently distinguish primary hemochromatosis from secondary ion overload.
Another form of liver disease receiving increased attention is
nonalcoholic fatty liver disease. Important predisposing factors
include obesity, hyperlipidemia, and diabetes mellitus. Diagnosis is by liver biopsy, and management involves correcting the
precipitating factor. An important consideration in a transplant
recipient with unexplained hepatic dysfunction is viral hepatitis acquired from the donor graft. This should be excluded by
appropriate serologic workup. Intermittent hepatic dysfunction
may result from biliary colic, and pain might not be prominent in
older patients. Ultrasound is the initial investigation.

THE KIDNEY DONOR WITH POSITIVE HEPATITIS SEROLOGIES

Effects on Recipient

Donor HBsAg positivity precludes kidney donation. The use of organs from HBsAg-negative/anti-HBc antibody-positive deceased donors has the potential to transmit HBV infection because of amplification of minute quantities of residual HBV DNA by immunosuppression. The rate of transmission is significantly higher in hepatic recipients than in other solid-organ recipients. In contrast, use of a renal graft from an IgG anti-HBc antibody-positive donor is associated with a very small risk of infection transmission, and these kidneys can be safely considered for donation, especially for recipients who have been successfully immunized with HBV vaccine. If the potential donor is IgM anti-HBc-positive, recent acute HBV is likely even in the absence of HBsAg, and there is a greater risk of HBV transmission; thus, the graft should be declined.

Transmission of HCV by renal transplantation has been unequivocally demonstrated with occasionally severe acute, even fatal, hepatitis. There are wide variations in the rate of transmission of HCV from anti-HCV-positive donors, which may be a result of several factors, including donor HCV viral load and the technique used for preservation of donor grafts. The rate of transmission of HCV from HCV-infected donors appears to be much higher if flush preservation instead of pulsatile perfusion is used. Transplantation of kidneys from anti-HCV-positive donors into anti-HCV-positive recipients is safe in the short-term. However, among anti-HCV-positive recipients, those who received anti-HCV-positive kidneys may have a somewhat worse survival rate than did recipients of anti-HCV-negative kidneys.

HCV infection is more common in deceased donor donors than in the general population. For an HCV-positive transplant candidate, the waiting time for a kidney may be greatly foreshortened by the acceptance of a kidney from a HCV-positive donor. Because survival following renal transplant is enhanced when compared to survival on chronic dialysis, it may be advantageous for an HCV-positive transplant candidate to accept an HCV-positive graft after a short wait than to accept an HCV-negative kidney after a protracted wait. The benefits and risks of accepting an HCV-positive graft must be carefully discussed with HCV-positive transplant candidates.

KIDNEY AND LIVER TRANSPLANTATION

Combined Liver and Kidney Transplant

Approximately 20% of patients undergoing orthotopic liver transplantation (OLT) have clinically significant preoperative renal insufficiency, and approximately 2% of patients undergo a combined liver and kidney transplant (LKT). Most patients with pre-OLT renal dysfunction do not require concomitant kidney transplantation because their renal dysfunction is potentially reversible. A diagnosis of the hepatorenal syndrome or acute tubular necrosis is not an indication for LKT, although patients with pre-OLT dialysis dependence for more than several weeks may develop irreversible parenchymal changes that might limit their capacity for recovery. Table 11.3 lists the common indications for LKT. Graft and patient survival rates are lower in patients requiring LKT than in patients receiving a kidney transplant alone, primarily because of the high mortality rate during the first 3 posttransplant months as a consequence of increased surgical risk and other comorbid conditions. However, if survival data are censored for patients who died during the first 3 months, long-term graft and patient survival rates of LKT and kidney transplant alone are similar. The kidney transplant adds little to the morbidity of the concomitant OLT.

Liver transplantation appears to provide a form of immunologic "protection" to concomitantly transplanted organs. This allograft-enhancing effect of the liver on other transplanted organs from the same donor can be demonstrated even for patients with a positive pretransplant cross-match. Several immunologic mechanisms for this phenomenon have been proposed, including the development of antiidiotypic antibodies to major histocompatibility complex (MHC) class I and class II antibodies, the absorption of lymphocytotoxic antibodies onto reticuloendothelial cells of the liver allograft, and a soluble MHC class I molecule, which is principally made in the liver, that may inhibit cytotoxic T-lymphocyte activity. Another important mechanism may be the development of hematopoietic chimerism occurring after liver transplantation, resulting in tolerance.

There are practical implications to the protective effect of the concomitant liver transplant. It is not necessary to routinely cross-match unsensitized patients prior to LKT. If the cross-match is positive in a sensitized patients, the LKT may not necessarily be contraindicated and some programs progress with transplantation with addition of a perioperative infusion of intravenous immune globulin (see Chapter 4, Part II). The aggressiveness of immunosuppression after liver transplantation alone is generally less than that after other organ transplants, and fear of recurrent disease is greater than the fear of rejection. The immunosuppressive protocol after LKT is generally less intense than that after kidney transplant alone. Calcineurin inhibitor dosage and blood levels are kept lower and antibody-depleting agents are avoided for fear of an increased risk of infection and recurrence of hepatitis. The incidence of acute rejection after LKT is low.

Allocation of Liver Transplants

Kidney transplants are allocated based on waiting time and human leukocyte antigen matching (see Chapter 3), but not on disease severity or patient prognosis. To the contrary, liver transplants are allocated based on disease severity. The Model of End-Stage Liver Disease (MELD) score is a formula that give points to objective laboratory parameters (serum bilirubin, international normalized ratio, serum creatinine) that have been shown to predict survival. The higher the MELD score the greater the chances of liver allocation. The inclusion of the creatinine in the MELD score means that liver transplant candidates with pretransplant renal impairment are more likely to be allocated a liver. For LKT recipients, it is the MELD score that determines allocation and not the kidney allocation algorithm. Thus, paradoxically, candidates for a double-transplant LKT are likely to wait much less time for their kidney than will candidates "only" waiting for a kidney.

Kidney After Liver Transplant

Chronic renal failure develops in up to 18% of OLT recipients at 5-year followup and is associated with an increased risk of death after transplantation. The etiology of renal failure is likely multifactorial, including preexisting renal disease, perioperative renal damage, calcineurin inhibitor therapy, nephrotoxic effects of other drugs, hypertension, HCV with associated glomerulonephritis, and diabetes mellitus. Renal transplantation may be a consideration in otherwise robust OLT recipients who develop end-stage renal disease.

SELECTED READINGS

Bloom RD, Rao V, Weng F, et al. Association of hepatitis C with posttransplant diabetes in renal transplant recipients on tacrolimus. *J Am Soc Nephrol* 2002;13:1374–1380.

Bucci JR, Matsumoto CS, Swanson SJ, et al. Donor hepatitis C seropositivity: clinical correlates and effect on early graft and patient survival in adult cadaveric kidney transplantation. *J Am Soc Nephrol* 2002;13:2974–2982.

Davis CL, Gonwa TA, Wilkinson AH. Identification of patients best suited for combined liver-kidney transplantation: part II. *Liver Transpl* 2002;8:193–211.

Fabrizi F, Poordad FF, Martin P. Hepatitis C infection and the patient with end-stage renal disease. *Hepatology* 2002;36:3–10.

Fabrizi F, Bunnapradist S, Martin P. Transplanting kidneys from donors with prior hepatitis B infection: one response to the organ shortage. *J Nephrol* 2002;15:605–613.

Fabrizi F, Dulai G, Dixit V, et al. Lamivudine for the treatment of hepatitis B virus-related liver disease after renal transplantation: Meta analysis of clinical trials. *Transplantation* 2004;77:859–864.

Fong TL, Bunnapradist S, Jordan SC, et al. Analysis of the United Network for Organ Sharing database comparing renal allografts and patient survival in combined liver–kidney transplantation with the contralateral allografts in kidney alone or kidney–pancreas transplantation. *Transplantation* 2003;76:348–353.

Fong TL, Bunnapradist S, Jordan SC, et al. Impact of hepatitis B core antibody status on outcomes of cadaveric renal transplantation: analysis of United Network for Organ Sharing database between 1994 and 1999. *Transplantation* 2002;73:85–89.

Fornairon S, Pol S, Legendre C, et al. The long-term virologic and pathologic impact of renal transplantation on chronic hepatitis B virus infection. *Transplantation* 1996;62:297–299.

Ganem D, Prince AM. Hepatitis B infection—natural history and clinical consequences. *N Engl J Med* 2004;350:1118–1129.

Lee WC, Wu MJ, Cheng CH, et al. Lamivudine is effective for the treatment of reactivation of hepatitis B virus and the fulminant hepatic failure in renal transplant recipients. *Am J Kidney Dis* 2001;38:1074–1081.

Mahmoud I, Elnabashi A, Elsawy E, et al. The impact of hepatitis C viremia on renal graft and patient survival: A 9-year perspective. *Amer J Kidney Dis* 2004;43:131–139.

Martin P, Carter D, Fabrizi F, et al. Histopathological features of hepatitis C in renal transplant candidates. *Transplantation* 2000;69:1479–1484.

Natov SN, Pereira BJ. Management of hepatitis C infection in renal transplant recipients. *Am J Transplant* 2002;2:483–490.

Ojo AO, Held PJ, Port FK, et al. Chronic renal failure after transplantation of a nonrenal organ. *N Engl J Med* 2003;349:931–940.

Diagnostic Imaging in Kidney Transplantation

Peter Zimmerman, Nagesh Ragavendra,
and Christiaan Schiepers

The clinician evaluating a patient with renal transplant dysfunction has the choice of a variety of imaging procedures, including ultrasound (US), nuclear medicine (NM) or molecular imaging, computed tomography (CT), magnetic resonance imaging (MRI), and excretory urography. Imaging evaluation is usually initiated either with duplex US, which provides cross-sectional imaging and physiologic information quickly, noninvasively, and portably, or with NM studies, which provide physiologic information and some morphologic information. CT provides superb anatomic information but involves the use of iodinated contrast medium and lacks portability. MRI provides superb anatomic information, can noninvasively image large vessels, and can evaluate function using relatively nonnephrotoxic contrast medium (gadolinium). MRI, however, is not portable, is expensive, and requires special equipment for guided interventions. This chapter emphasizes the use of US and NM techniques in renal transplantation, although CT, MRI, and urography may, on occasion, be the optimal imaging modalities for certain clinical problems encountered in renal transplant recipients.

RADIOLOGIC EVALUATION OF THE LIVING DONOR

The process of evaluating a potential living donor is discussed in Chapter 5, Part II. The radiologic studies used to screen potential living donors are done to ensure that after nephrectomy, the donor is left with an anatomically and functionally normal kidney. They also permit the surgeon to decide which kidney is to be removed and to determine the suitability for laparoscopic or open nephrectomy (see Chapter 5). The traditional donor radiologic workup typically consisted of an intravenous urogram followed by angiography. With advances in CT and MRI technology, angiographic-type images can be obtained with these modalities, with peripheral intravenous access, often obviating the need for catheter angiography.

Computed Tomographic Angiography, and Urography

The helical, or spiral, CT scan, followed in the same session by several postcontrast radiographs, produces a modified intravenous urogram, usually called a *computed tomographic urogram* (CTU). Helical (also called spiral) CT allows very rapid acquisition of a volume of data, and the advent of multidetector helical CT has further improved this technique. *Computed tomographic angiography* (CTA) differs from usual CT in that intravenous contrast is injected rapidly (4 to 5 mL per second), imaging begins at peak contrast concentration in the aorta (20 seconds after injection), and very-thin-beam collimation (0.5 to 3 mm) is employed, yielding high-resolution images of vessels. The resulting volume of data can be computer rendered and displayed in a variety of ways, and made to look like a projectional radiographic angiogram. This technique can reliably delineate relevant vascular anatomy for surgical planning, such as number of renal arteries and veins and other variants (Plate 2). This method has replaced catheter angiography in most centers.

The urographic images of the CTU permit an evaluation of the intrarenal collecting system, ureters, and bladder. This allows detection of anatomic variants and pathology, such as supernumerary ureters, ureteropelvic junction obstruction, papillary necrosis, calyceal diverticula, extrarenal pelves, ureteroceles, and urolithiasis.

Magnetic Resonance Angiography and Urography

MRI and MR angiography and venography can provide similar information to CT and CT angiography. Relative drawbacks include less optimal evaluation of collecting systems and insensitivity for stone detection.

RADIOLOGIC TECHNIQUES IN THE EARLY POSTTRANSPLANT PERIOD

The indications for radiologic investigations in the early posttransplant period are discussed in Chapter 8.

Allograft Size

Renal transplant size increases in most acute processes and is thus a nonspecific indicator of renal dysfunction. Some studies show that an increase in graft cross-sectional area of more than 10% (measured by US) is suggestive of acute rejection, but the finding is too nonspecific to be clinically reliable. Practical use of allograft size is also limited by the fact that a normally functioning graft may be increased in size by up to 30% at 2 months after transplantation. The volume of a normal renal transplant usually stabilizes by 6 months.

Collecting System Dilation

Collecting system dilation may be obstructive or nonobstructive. The degree of dilation is often expressed using a grading system (grades I to IV) for US or excretory urography, or as mild, moderate, or severe; however, both of these systems are subjective. Obstruction of the transplant collecting system may occur secondary to extrinsic processes (e.g., peritransplant fluid collection), ureteral stricture (as a consequence of vascular insufficiency or rejection), or intraluminal lesions, such as kidney stone, blood clot, or sloughed papilla (Fig. 12.1). A mild, self-limited obstruction may result from early postoperative edema at the ureteroneocystostomy site, and minimal dilation may persist despite resolution of obstruction. Other causes of nonobstructive collecting system dilation include a full bladder, rejection, infection, and resolved, prior obstruction. This latter cause of nonobstructive dilation is particularly relevant in the transplanted kidney, because the collecting system is denervated and has no tone.

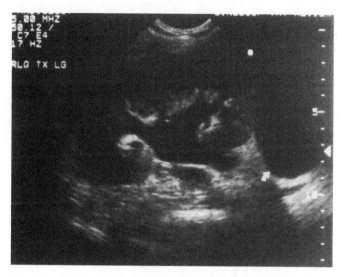

Fig. 12.1. Sonogram demonstrating hydronephrosis secondary to peritransplant fluid collection *(arrow).*

Use of the resistive index (RI; see "Acute Rejection," below) to distinguish obstructive from nonobstructive pyelocaliectasis has been proposed, but data regarding its reliability are inconclusive. The absence of collecting system dilation does not entirely exclude the possibility of obstruction. The most reliable noninvasive method to diagnose obstruction is progressive collecting system dilation on serial sonograms. Antegrade pyelography, a mini-nephrostomy, or a Whitaker pressure-flow study may be necessary to determine whether collecting system dilation has an obstructive or nonobstructive cause.

NM imaging of ureteral obstruction, typically shows normal perfusion and parenchymal uptake of tracer by the transplant, but pooling of tracer in the renal pelvis and prolonged pelvic retention. An obstructed system does not respond to the administration of diuretics such as intravenous (IV) furosemide. A system with an emptying half-time of more than 20 minutes is considered obstructed (normal emptying half-time is less than 15 minutes). Table 12.1 gives an overview of radiopharmaceuticals currently in use.

Peritransplant Fluid Collections

Peritransplant fluid collections may be produced by lymphoceles, urinomas, hematomas, and abscesses; all of these may compress the ureter and iliac veins, resulting in hydronephrosis and lower extremity edema. They all manifest as fluid collections on cross-sectional imaging studies (US, MRI, CT) or as photopenic regions on NM scans or scintigrams. Although there are imaging features suggestive of the nature of the fluid collection, their appearance

Table 12.1.   Radiopharmaceuticals for use in the quantification and evaluation of renal transplant function or morphology

Radionuclide		Biologic Compound	Physiologic/Biochemical Mechanism	Imaging	Application	Comment
^{51}Cr	EDTA	ethylenediaminetetraacetic acid	glomerular filtration	>95%	No	GFR	Not available in the USA
^{111}In	DTPA	diethylenetriamine pentaacetic acid	glomerular filtration, no resorption	>90%	No	GFR	2-sample method
^{131}I	OIH	orthoiodohippurate	glomerular filtration, 80% tubular secretion	20%	No	ERPF	1-sample method
^{99m}Tc	DTPA	diethylenetriamine pentaacetic acid	glomerular filtration, no resorption	>90%	Yes	Flow & Function	Plasma binding higher than MAG3
^{131}I or ^{123}I	OIH	orthoiodohippurate	glomerular filtration, 80% tubular secretion	20%	Yes	Flow & Function	High radiation dose of ^{131}I
^{99m}Tc	MAG3	mercaptoacetyltriglycine	tubular secretion	>95%	Yes	Flow & Function	Most commonly used
^{99m}Tc	EC	ethylenedicysteine	tubular secretion	>85%	Yes	Flow & Function	Not available in the USA

Isotope	Abbreviation	Agent	%	Mechanism		Application	Limitation
^{99m}Tc	DMSA	dimercaptosuccinic acid	7–14%	excreted into urine, binds to SH groups in cortical tubule cells	Yes	Parenchyma	Pyelonephritis, infarct, scar
^{99m}Tc	GHA	glucoheptonate	>50%	glomerular filtration, 10–15% bound to tubules	Yes	Parenchyma	Morphology kidney
^{67}Ga	Ga	citrate		Localizes in sites of inflammation, and certain neoplasms	Yes	Inflammation	Nonspecific
^{111}In or ^{99m}Tc	WBC	white blood cells		Localizes in inflammatory tissue	Yes	Infection	
^{111}In		lymphocytes		Localizes in inflammatory tissue	Yes	Rejection	Difficult to extract and label
^{111}In or ^{99m}Tc		platelets		Localizes in developing blood clots	Yes	Thrombosis	Difficult to label

Cr, chromium; ERPF, effective renal plasma flow; Ga, gallium; GFR, glomerular filtration rate; I, iodine; In, indium; Tc, technetium.

is usually not sufficiently specific; imaging-guided aspiration is often necessary.

Hematomas

Hematomas are common in the immediate postoperative period, they may be extrarenal or subcapsular in location, and usually resolve spontaneously. They may also occur after a biopsy or result from rupture of a graft pseudoaneurysm. On occasion, the hematoma may be large enough to obstruct the ureter. The US appearance of a hematoma varies with time, being echogenic in the acute phase and decreasing in echogenicity as clot lysis occurs. An acute hematoma is of high attenuation on CT and also decreases with time. The signal intensity of a hematoma on MRI is variable.

Urinomas

Urinomas resulting from extravasation of urine from the renal pelvis, ureter, or ureteroneocystostomy usually occur in the first 1 to 3 weeks after transplantation and may be caused by disruption of the ureterovesical anastomosis, incomplete bladder closure, ischemia of the collecting system, postbiopsy injury, or severe obstruction.

US reveals a nonspecific, usually nonseptated, fluid collection, often adjacent to the lower pole of the transplant. The CT appearance of a urinoma is a peritransplant fluid collection that may contain contrast-opacified fluid that is isodense to collecting system fluid if the leak is active at the time of the scan. MRI reveals a fluid collection that has identical signal characteristics to urine in the bladder. The leak may be extraperitoneal, intraperitoneal, or both, and in the latter circumstance, ascites may also be present. Characterization of the fluid can be achieved by obtaining a sample using US-guided aspiration and then determining the creatinine concentration (see Chapter 8).

Cystography is the examination of choice to confirm or exclude the bladder as the source of leak. If the bladder is not the source, the extravasation must be from above the ureterovesical anastomosis. If kidney function is adequate, a nuclear medicine study or a urogram may visualize the urinoma, although the precise location of the leak may be difficult to identify. NM imaging typically shows abnormal accumulations of activity outside the collection system (Fig. 12.2). Occasionally, this finding may be confused with ureteral stasis, in which case the abnormal accumulation will resolve when the patient voids or is given intravenous furosemide.

Lymphoceles

Lymphoceles are the most common type of peritransplant fluid collection and are the product of extraperitoneal or renal lymphatic disruption at surgery or during graft harvesting (see Chapter 7). They usually occur several weeks to months after surgery. The incidence of lymphoceles has been reported to be higher when rapamycin is used for early posttransplant immunosuppression. Small lymphoceles are common and are usually asymptomatic, but larger ones can cause obstruction.

The typical US appearance of a lymphocele is a fluid collection inferior and medial to the transplant that often contains

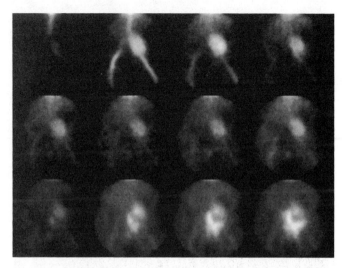

Fig. 12.2.   NM images of a left iliac transplant kidney
[radiopharmaceutical: ^{99m}Tc diethylenetriamine pentaacetic acid
(DTPA)]. The top left image shows activity in the abdominal aorta and
the beginning of the transplant. The next two images show prompt
visualization of the kidney, reflecting normal tracer concentration. In
the bottom row, enlarging irregular activity is seen between the
kidney and urinary bladder, indicative of urinary extravasation.

septations and low-level echoes (Fig. 12.3). The MRI signal characteristics of a lymphocele tend to be of low signal intensity on
T1-weighted images and of high signal intensity on T2-weighted
images.

Abscesses

A peritransplant abscess is usually secondary to infection of a
preexisting fluid collection and generally occurs 4 to 5 weeks after transplantation. The US appearance is a fluid collection that
contains debris, low-level echoes, and occasionally gas; the latter
manifests as mobile, nondependent, echogenic foci with "dirty"
shadowing or "ring-down" artifact.

The CT appearance is a heterogeneous fluid attenuation lesion (Fig. 12.4) that may contain gas. In the acute setting, cross-
sectional imaging techniques (US, CT) enable rapid diagnosis and
potential treatment of a suspected abscess by providing guidance
for aspiration and drainage. The absence of any imaging features suggestive of an abscess does not exclude the presence of
infection.

NM imaging employs different radiopharmaceutical agents for
infection surveys. Labeled white blood cells (WBCs), lymphocytes, antileukocyte antibodies, and gallium are available for this
purpose. These tracers localize in inflammatory tissue and may
be helpful in detecting a renal or perirenal abscess. A rejecting

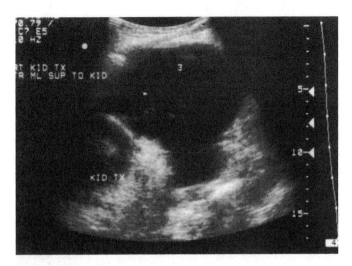

Fig. 12.3. Sonogram demonstrating lymphocele (*3*) with septations (*arrowhead*).

transplant, however, may also "light up," and interpretation of the results need to be approached cautiously. NM techniques are based on injection of the labeled compound, which travels through the body and accumulates at the site of infection or inflammation. The dose administered and half-life of the attached radionuclide determine the time of imaging after injection, from 2 to 24 hours for ^{99m}Tc, 1 to 2 days for ^{111}In, and 1 to 3 days for ^{67}Ga.

Acute Rejection

A variety of morphologic alterations may occur with acute rejection. All of these abnormalities may be seen with other medical complications of transplantation. Because many are subjective, these findings are insufficiently sensitive or specific to diagnose rejection definitively and to obviate the need for biopsy. These US abnormalities include graft enlargement, obscured corticomedullary definition, decreased echogenicity of the renal sinus, thickened urothelium, prominent hypoechoic medullary pyramids, increased or decreased cortical echogenicity, and scattered heterogeneous areas of increased echogenicity, the latter probably representing foci of hemorrhage (Fig. 12.5).

Resistive Index

With the advent of duplex US (combining grayscale imaging with Doppler capability), it was hoped that the physiologic parameters that could be measured with this technique would be diagnostic of rejection. The major parameter studied was vascular resistance (impedance), which is measured as the percentage reduction of the end-diastolic flow as compared with the systolic flow. The resistive index [RI = peak systolic velocity (PSV)

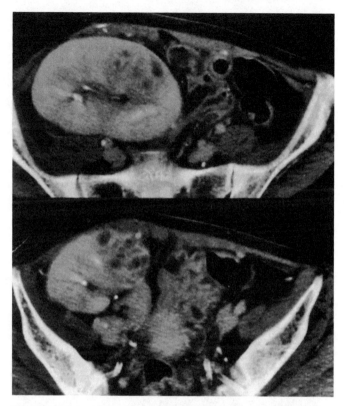

Fig. 12.4. Abscess in a renal allograft. There is a heterogeneous mass on contrast-enhanced computed tomography. Many small compartments preclude percutaneous drainage. Renal function was surprisingly well preserved. Abscess resolved after intensive antibiotic therapy.

minus end-diastolic velocity divided by PSV] or the pulsatility index (PI = PSV minus end-diastolic velocity divided by the mean velocity) are often elevated in rejection (Fig. 12.6), but because any cause of renal dysfunction may increase vascular resistance in the kidney, the finding of an elevated RI itself is nonspecific. Elevation of the RI (greater than 0.9) has been reported in rejection, severe acute tubular necrosis (ATN), renal vein obstruction, pyelonephritis, extrarenal compression, obstruction, and cyclosporine toxicity. The RI is also correlated with established cardiovascular risk factors.

Although the renal transplant RI is nonspecific, it is a valuable predictor of long-term allograft performance. An RI of 0.8 or greater, measured at 3 months posttransplant has been reported to be associated with poor subsequent graft function and death.

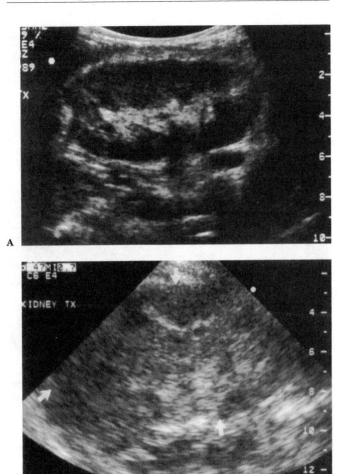

Fig. 12.5.   A: Sonogram of normal transplant kidney. **B:** Sonogram of transplant undergoing rejection reveals graft enlargement, decreased echogenicity of renal sinus (compare to echogenic sinus in A), and obscured corticomedullary delineations. Margins of graft marked by arrows.

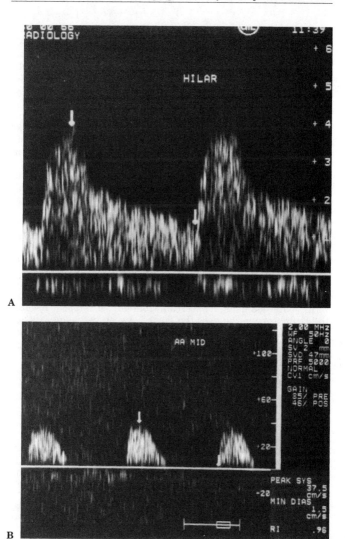

Fig. 12.6.   A: Normal pulsed-gate Doppler spectrum from kidney transplant with considerable flow throughout diastole and normal resistive index (RI = 0.65). B: Doppler spectrum of graft undergoing acute rejection with no diastolic flow (RI = 1). This is a nonspecific indicator of graft dysfunction.

Duplex Ultrasonography

Duplex US (or, more accurately, "triplex" if color, pulsed, and grayscale are employed simultaneously) combines a two-dimensional image with flow information, the latter being in the form of color, pulsed, and, most recently, power Doppler. These techniques employ the same sound waves as real-time imaging but measure the frequency and energy of the Doppler shift from the echoes interacting with flowing blood, allowing determination of flow presence, velocity, and direction (power Doppler does not assess the latter two). Color Doppler US provides an estimate of the mean velocity and direction of flow within a vessel by color-coding the information and displaying it superimposed on the gray-scale image. Power Doppler (also known as *amplitude* or *energy map*) measures the power of the Doppler signal and displays a greater range of signal strengths, thus allowing improved sensitivity to flow and visualization of smaller vessels. Power Doppler is displayed as a single color map of flow superimposed on a grayscale image but does not provide directional or velocity information as does color Doppler. Pulsed Doppler allows a sampling volume to be positioned in a vessel visualized on the grayscale image and provides a spectrum, or graph, of velocities of blood within the gate plotted as a function of time. A read-out of absolute velocities and calculation of the RI and PI are obtained using a spectrum from pulsed Doppler. Because the Doppler equation uses the angle between the beam axis and the vessel to calculate the velocity (performed by the machine software) and this angle is estimated by the ultrasonographer, incorrect angle correction may yield spurious velocities.

NUCLEAR MEDICINE IMAGING OF GRAFT FUNCTION AND DYSFUNCTION

NM imaging is noninvasive and does not jeopardize renal function. The widespread use of sophisticated US techniques, however, has reduced reliance on NM in the posttransplant period. Two types of radiopharmaceuticals are used for the evaluation of renal transplant function, based on their clearance from the plasma either by glomerular filtration or by tubular secretion. Table 12.1 provides an overview. Currently, the most frequently used radiopharmaceutical is ^{99m}Tc-mercaptotriglycine (MAG3). Of the older agents, ^{99m}Tc-DTPA is still a viable alternative. Iodine-labeled tracers are not ideal for imaging, because the ^{123}I-labeled tracers are not standard in the United States. ^{131}I as a label is not preferred, because the β emission causes a significant radiation dose, severely limiting the dose that can be administered. Evaluation of transplant flow and perfusion is not possible with ^{131}I radiopharmaceuticals.

The NM study most often applied is dynamic nephroscintigraphy (or NM-renography), in which three phases are distinguished. The first phase assesses the flow and perfusion of the transplant and is known as the *angiographic phase.* The second phase reflects the concentration of tracer in the renal cortex, the *parenchymal phase.* The third phase is the *excretory phase,* reflecting the clearance of tracer, which permits an assessment of the

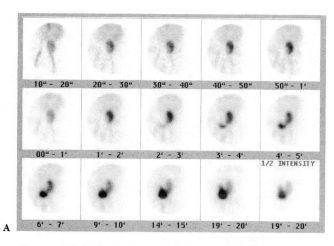

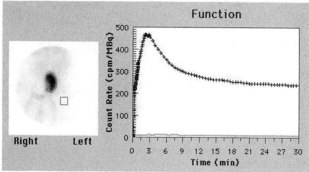

Fig. 12.7.   A: Dynamic images of a normal functioning transplant.
The top row shows flow/perfusion images, each of 10 seconds
duration. The middle and bottom rows are 1-minute images during
the subsequent 20 minutes. B: Regions of interest are drawn around
the kidney and background (*box*) and curves generated of the
activity within that region as function of time.

integrity of the ureteral system. A time-activity-curve is generated, depicting the activity in the transplant kidney in function
of time. Because dynamic NM renography is a planar imaging
technique, the measured counts from the kidney suffer from attenuation by tissues between kidney and camera, and from activity contributed by nonkidney tissue within the kidney region.
After proper correction, a curve is generated corresponding to the
renogram of the transplant. The NM images of a normal functioning transplant are shown in Fig. 12.7A and the corresponding
regions and curves in Fig. 12.7B.

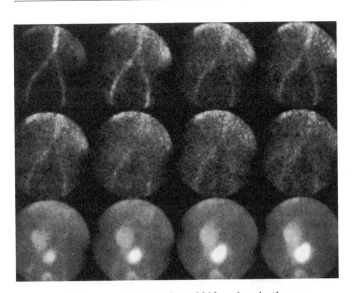

Fig. 12.8. NM images of a transplanted kidney in rejection [radiopharmaceutical: ^{99m}Tc MAG3 (mercaptotriglycine)]. Note the poor perfusion to the transplant, that is, delayed renal visualization in the initial images of the top two rows (5 seconds per image). The bottom row shows poor function (4 minutes per image). Overall, reduced function is represented by high surrounding background tissue activity, poor parenchymal washout of accumulated tracer, and reduced collecting system or urinary bladder activity.

Acute Rejection

Typically, acute transplant rejection appears on dynamic NM-renography as decreased perfusion, delayed transplant visualization, with poor parenchymal uptake and high background activity because of decreased clearance (Fig. 12.8). Transplant rejection may also be detected by static imaging techniques. Increased uptake can be seen with ^{67}Ga-citrate, ^{99m}Tc-sulfur colloid, or ^{111}In-labeled blood components. Unfortunately, the low specificity of uptake of these latter agents prevents them from being of much value in the differential diagnosis of graft dysfunction. These latter scans are considered obsolete for detecting rejection.

Despite the availability of various types of radiopharmaceuticals and the advancement of image technology, the differentiation between rejection and calcineurin inhibitor nephrotoxicity remains problematic. Attempts to use the renal cortical imaging tracer dimercaptosuccinic acid (DMSA) for this purpose have been unsuccessful.

Acute Tubular Necrosis

Acute tubular necrosis (ATN) typically shows good renal perfusion on the first-phase images, with preserved concentration during the second phase by the transplant. The third phase shows no excretion of tracer into the collecting system and bladder (Fig. 12.9). In addition, high surrounding tissue background activity is seen because of poor overall plasma clearance of the radiopharmaceutical. The renogram has the typical rising branch that reaches a plateau after 3 to 6 minutes. There is no descending branch, because there is no excretion. These findings are consistent with the pathophysiology of ATN, in which renal blood flow is preserved relative to glomerular filtration.

POSTTRANSPLANTATION VASCULAR COMPLICATIONS

Arterial Thrombosis

Renal arterial thrombosis is an uncommon complication of transplantation and usually occurs in the early postoperative period. The most common causes are faulty surgical anastomoses, a thrombogenic state, severe acute rejection, and progression of a stenosis to thrombosis. The findings in color and pulsed Doppler imaging consist of absent arterial and venous blood flow within the graft. There is some controversy regarding the necessity of further imaging to confirm this diagnosis because there are several reported cases in which no flow was demonstrated by Doppler, but digital subtraction angiography revealed patent vessels. Power Doppler should, in theory, reduce false-positive results, but this remains to be proven.

The dynamic NM images show lack of perfusion, absent visualization of the transplanted kidney, poor background clearance of activity, and sometimes a photopenic space in the transplant bed (Fig. 12.10). Renal vein thrombosis, acute cortical necrosis, and hyperacute rejection may all have similar scintigraphic findings.

Infarction

Acute segmental infarction may be diagnosed with Doppler US by demonstration of lack of flow to the infarcted region of parenchyma (Fig. 12.11). This diagnosis is facilitated by use of color and power Doppler, which both provide a global evaluation of flow to the organ, and help to identify segmental arteries, which can then be interrogated individually with pulsed Doppler.

Segmental renal infarction on NM scan (Table 12-1 lists the applicable radiopharmaceuticals) appears as a wedge-shaped, "cold" defect. DMSA is a radiopharmaceutical of the tubular secretion type, with a high uptake in the renal cortex (approximately 40%). This allows visualization of the mass of functioning renal tissue. Infarcts and scars appear as photopenic defects, demonstrating absence of functioning renal cells.

Renal Vein Thrombosis

Renal vein thrombosis is an uncommon complication that usually occurs in the first postoperative week. The US diagnosis is mainly dependent on the Doppler portion of the examination because the grayscale diagnosis is limited by the difficulty of direct visualization of the anechoic or hypoechoic acute thrombus and the nonspecificity of the frequently associated graft swelling

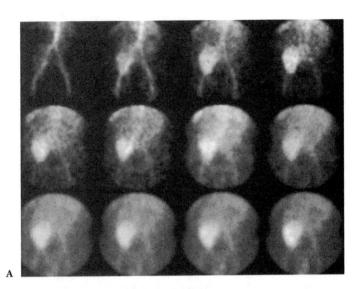

A

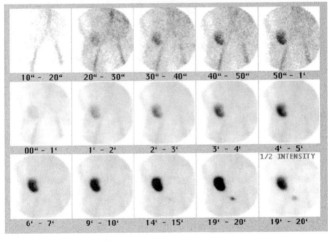

10" – 20"	20" – 30"	30" – 40"	40" – 50"	50" – 1'
00" – 1'	1' – 2'	2' – 3'	3' – 4'	4' – 5'
6' – 7'	9' – 10'	14' – 15'	19' – 20'	19' – 20'

4' – 5'
1/2 INTENSITY

B

Fig. 12.9.   A: NM images of acute tubular necrosis. Note the
well-preserved perfusion in the transplant, that is, prompt renal
visualization in the initial six images. Concentration of tracer by the
transplant is maintained, but there is no excretion and no collecting
system or urinary bladder activity. Radiopharmaceutical: 99mTc
DTPA (diethylenetriamine pentaacetic acid). B: Study performed
with 99mTc MAG3 (mercaptotriglycine) as radiopharmaceutical. Top
row is the flow/perfusion phase (10 seconds per image). Middle and
bottom rows show 1-minute images with normal renal concentration.
There is visualization of tracer in the bladder in the last two frames,
indicative of minimal function. Note the superior quality of 99mTc
MAG3 (mercaptotriglycine) over 99mTc DTPA in panel A.

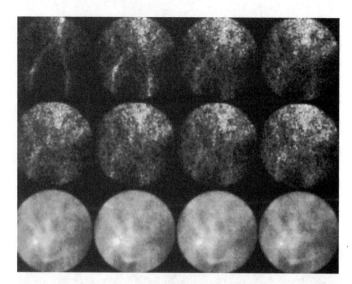

Fig. 12.10. **NM images of a transplanted kidney with renal artery thrombosis. Note the absence of renal perfusion, that is, nonvisualization of the transplant in the top two rows. In addition, there is no activity in the collecting system and bladder. Background tissue activity remains high, indicative of absent excretion. Radiopharmaceutical:** ^{99m}Tc **DTPA (diethylenetriamine pentaacetic acid).**

and hypoechogenicity. The combination of Doppler findings of high-impedance renal arterial waveforms with reversed, prolonged diastolic flow, a spike-like systolic component, and no detectable venous flow in the graft is highly suggestive of renal vein thrombosis (Fig. 12.12). Reversal of diastolic flow is a nonspecific finding that is reflective of increased arterial impedance in the graft. It may also be seen in ATN, acute rejection, and severe obstruction.

Chronic Rejection

In chronic rejection, there is gradual deterioration of kidney function, and the allograft is usually decreased in size. Angiographic findings include decreased blood flow and reduction of the number of arteries, which may be narrow and irregular. The nephrogram is patchy. US findings include decreased size of kidney, cortical thinning, and altered cortical echogenicity, often with increased echogenicity. Doppler US may show a nonspecific elevation in RI. NM images show reduced perfusion, shift of the renogram peak to the right, and decreased excretion.

Renal Artery Stenosis

Renal NM angiography may be useful in the diagnosis of renal artery stenosis (RAS) in a native kidney because the contralateral

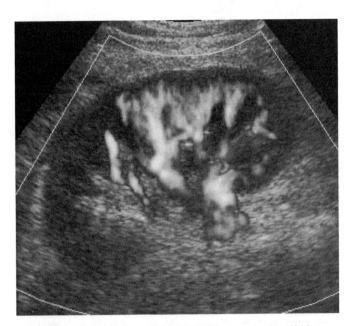

Fig. 12.11.   Color Doppler image reveals flow to majority of kidney, with absence of flow to area in upper pole, compatible with hypoperfusion/possible ischemia.

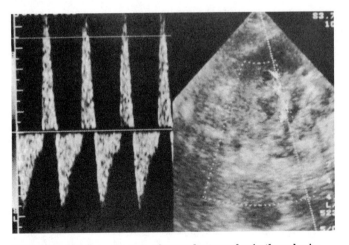

Fig. 12.12.   Duplex sonogram of transplant renal vein thrombosis demonstrates reversed flow in diastole and a spike-like systolic peak. No venous flow was detectable in the kidney, renal hilum, or location of the renal vein.

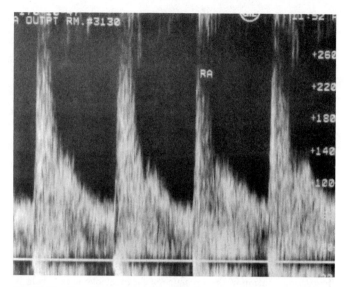

Fig. 12.13. Renal artery stenosis. Doppler spectrum demonstrates focal elevated peak systolic velocity (faster than 260 cm per second) with mild spectral broadening at the anastomosis.

kidney acts as a control for comparison. In the transplanted kidney with RAS, there may be a delayed blush on scanning, but in the absence of a paired kidney, this finding is too nonspecific to be diagnostically reliable.

The diagnosis of RAS by Doppler US is made by demonstration of a focal, segmental region of flow abnormality, characterized by elevated PSV and turbulent flow (Fig. 12.13). Various threshold values for PSV have been proposed for optimal detection of RAS, ranging from 100 to 300 cm per second; reported sensitivities and specificities range from fair to excellent. Because the normal range of PSV in the transplant renal artery may be variable, a ratio of PSV in the renal artery compared with the external iliac artery may be more useful. The accurate calculation of velocity by the machine's software, however, is highly dependent on the accuracy of the operator's estimate of the angle of insonation, and errors in this regard can yield spuriously elevated velocities. The accuracy of this estimate (*angle correction*) is dependent on the adequacy of delineation of the course of the renal artery, which is often small and tortuous. Color and power Doppler, by providing a map of the vascular anatomy, are helpful in tracing a vessel and therefore in determining the appropriate angle. A confident diagnosis of RAS using Doppler US can be made if the characteristic findings occur in a well-delineated vessel, allowing accurate angle correction. Conversely, high velocities without associated turbulence in a region where the accuracy of angle correction is equivocal must be viewed with skepticism.

Angiography remains the gold standard for diagnosis of RAS, and the threshold for performance of this study remains a matter of clinical judgment (see Chapters 7 and 9). CO_2 angiography provides a useful alternative to nephrotoxic iodinated contrast agents, but it may be less reliable than standard angiography.

Arteriovenous Fistulas

Postbiopsy arteriovenous fistulas most often resolve spontaneously but can produce persistent hematuria or hypertension. Grayscale US cannot identify these small vascular communications, but they are readily demonstrated on color Doppler as an area of artifactual color assignment in the renal parenchyma (Plate 3). This finding is believed to be caused by high-velocity flow in the fistula, which results in localized turbulence and vessel wall vibrations that are transmitted to the perivascular tissues. The vibrating interfaces in the perivascular tissue produce phase shifts in the reflected sound wave and result in random color assignment in this region. This phenomenon is essentially the Doppler equivalent of a bruit.

After an area of suspicion is identified, the fistulized vessels may be visualized on color Doppler by virtue of their high-velocity flow. Confirmation of the presence of an arteriovenous fistula is achieved by performing waveform analysis with pulsed Doppler and by demonstrating high-velocity, low-resistance flow in the supplying artery, and arterialization (highly pulsatile flow) of the waveform in the draining vein. A focal, intrarenal arterial stenosis can produce high-velocity flow and tissue vibration, thereby mimicking a fistula, but no changes in the venous waveform should occur.

Doppler US is readily able to demonstrate many fistulas and should be the initial, primary imaging modality. If no fistula can be demonstrated by US in a patient with persistent gross hematuria and hypertension, angiography may be necessary. Angiography is the examination of choice for defining the extent of the fistula and for treatment planning. Superselective occlusion of the segmental or interlobar branches is possible using a variety of occlusive devices, including steel coils and detachable balloons. CT and MR angiography could play a role in the diagnosis of a fistula, but may be limited by spatial resolution issues.

Pseudoaneurysms

Pseudoaneurysms in a renal transplant may be intrarenal, usually secondary to a biopsy, or, less commonly, extrarenal, usually as a consequence of faulty surgical anastomosis or perianastomotic infection. Extrarenal pseudoaneurysms have a much higher risk for spontaneous rupture and are therefore treated as a relative surgical emergency. Arteriovenous fistulas may be associated with pseudoaneurysms. The US findings are the same for intrarenal and extrarenal pseudoaneurysms and consist of a spherical fluid collection that may or may not contain thrombus. Color Doppler reveals swirling internal flow (Plate 4) and occasionally adjacent tissue vibrations.

Measurement of Glomerular Filtration Rate

Clinicians generally rely on the serum creatinine level as a marker of graft function, and although this simple test is indisputably invaluable in transplant management, its accuracy as a marker of glomerular filtration rate (GFR) is inconsistent. In chronic renal failure with proteinuria, tubular secretion of creatinine may form a significant percentage of total creatinine excretion and overestimation of GFR results. Radiolabeled diethylenetriamine pentaacetic acid (DTPA), ethylenediaminetetraacetic acid (EDTA), and iothalamate are all accurate filtration markers that, like inulin, reach the urine by filtration but without any element of tubular secretion or reabsorption. The clearances of these compounds are equivalent to the classic inulin clearance. They are more convenient to use than inulin because their plasma and urine levels can be measured with a scintillation counter.

Absolute renal function can be measured with true clearance techniques. After bladder emptying, the radiopharmaceutical is administered intravenously, and serial blood and urine samples are taken over several hours. From the obtained curve, the rate of tracer disappearance from blood and concentration in urine is determined, from which the GFR is calculated with the standard clearance formula. GFR can also be assessed with this plasma tracer disappearance curve, by measuring rate and extrapolating the volume of distribution, the so-called plasma clearance. One- and two-sample methods have been developed for routine clinical use (see Table 12.1).

SELECTED READINGS

Bruno S, Ferrari S, Remuzzi G. Doppler ultrasonography in post-transplant renal artery stenosis: a reliable tool for assessing effectiveness of revascularization? *Transplantation* 2003;76:147–153.

Budihna NV, Milcinski M, Kajtna-Koselj M, et al. Relevance of ^{99m}Tc DMSA scintigraphy in renal transplant parenchymal imaging. *Clin Nucl Med* 1994;19:782–784.

Cochran ST, Krasny RM, Danovitch GM, et al. Helical CT angiography for examination of liver renal donors. *Am J Roentgenol* 1997; 168:1569–1573.

Dubovski EV, Russell CD, Erbas B. Radionuclide evaluation of renal transplants. *Semin Nucl Med* 1995;25:49–59.

Grant EG, Perrella RR. Wishing won't make it so: duplex Doppler sonography in the evaluation of renal transplant dysfunction. *AJR Am J Roentgenol* 1990;153:538–539.

Kuo PC, Petersen J, Semba C, et al. CO_2 angiography—a technique for vascular imaging in renal allograft dysfunction. *Transplantation* 1996;61:652–654.

Loubeyre P, Abidi H, Cahen R, et al. Transplanted renal artery: detection of stenosis with color Doppler US. *Radiology* 1997;203:661–665.

Middleton WD, Kellman GM, Melson GL, et al. Postbiopsy renal transplant arteriovenous fistulas: color Doppler US characteristics. *Radiology* 1989;171:253–257.

Nankivell BJ, Cohn DA, Spicer ST et al. Diagnosis of kidney transplant obstruction using MAG3 diuretic renography. *Clin Transpl*
2001;15;11–18.

O'Neill WC. Sonographic evaluation of renal failure. *Am J Kidney Dis*
2000;35:1021–1038.

Phillips AO, Deane C, O'Donnell P, et al. Evaluation of Doppler ultrasound in primary non-function of renal transplants. *Clin Transpl*
1994;8:83–86.

Slakey DP, Florman S, Lovretich J, et al. Utility of CT angiography
for evaluation of living kidney donors. *Clin Transpl* 1999;13:104–
107.

Radermacher J, Mengel M, Ellis S, et al. The renal artery resistive
index and renal allograft survival. *N Engl J Med* 2003;349:115–
124.

Pathology of Kidney Transplantation

Cynthia C. Nast and Arthur H. Cohen

The gold standard for assessing structural abnormalities in the transplanted kidney is standard tissue histopathology of a biopsy or transplant nephrectomy. Immunofluorescence also is necessary for identification of certain types of acute rejection, and electron microscopy may be required to evaluate glomerular lesions. Fine-needle aspiration with cytologic evaluation of cells aspirated from the graft using a thin needle has been used in the past to determine the cause of acute allograft dysfunction. The advent of thinner core needles with relative safety of the core biopsy procedure has minimized the use of aspiration cytology in the clinical setting.

CORE-NEEDLE BIOPSY

Indications and Technique

Kidney transplant biopsies are most frequently performed at times of graft dysfunction when the etiology cannot be accurately elucidated by clinical or noninvasive means. Protocol biopsies are performed at predetermined intervals after transplantation at some centers in an attempt to recognize so-called subclinical rejection (see Chapter 8); they also may be required as part of clinical trials for the evaluation of new immunosuppressive drugs (see Chapter 4). More precise clinical indications for biopsy are reviewed in Chapters 8 and 9. Transplant programs vary in their reliance on biopsies and the clinical setting in which biopsies are performed.

Preparations for transplant biopsy are similar to those for biopsy of the native kidney. Informed consent is required from patients, who should be specifically warned of the risk for bleeding and occasional damage to the graft (see "Complications," below). Before biopsy, coagulation studies are usually performed, although in the absence of liver disease, use of anticoagulants, thrombocytopenia, or a clinical history of bleeding, these may not be necessary. The blood pressure should be controlled at a level of less than 160/100 mm Hg.

The locations of the graft and biopsy site can be determined by palpation or by ultrasound guidance. A small pillow or towel rolled in the small of the patient's back may facilitate palpation. Ultrasound offers the advantage of more precise localization of the graft and its depth, and may reduce the frequency of inadequate specimens. Ultrasound may detect perinephric fluid collections or hydronephrosis. It is unwise to perform biopsy through a fluid collection because of the inability to tamponade the biopsy site adequately. Significant hydronephrosis should be relieved before the biopsy is performed because it may be the cause of the graft dysfunction; a small blood clot after the biopsy may exaggerate the degree of obstruction. Generally, the upper or lower pole of the transplant is sought, depending on which is more easily palpated or near the surface. If the location of the biopsy site is difficult to ascertain or if the kidney is deep, it is wise to use real-time ultrasound with visual guidance or a fixed biopsy guide device (see Chapter 12).

Disposable automatic spring-loaded needles (18-gauge is usually adequate) have largely replaced the traditional modified 14-gauge Vim-Silverman needle and may be less traumatic to the kidney. The site chosen for the biopsy is locally anesthetized with 1% lidocaine, and a small stab wound in the skin is made to facilitate the passage of the needle. Precise instructions for use of the newer needles are provided in the package inserts. The needles are advanced up to the depth determined by ultrasound or until an increase in resistance is felt as the needle makes contact with the kidney. When the automatic needles are used, it may be advisable to withdraw the needle slightly before taking the sample to avoid excessive depth and ensure a cortical sample.

Two biopsy cores should be adequate. It is advisable to inspect the specimen immediately with a stereomicroscope to ensure adequacy. As soon as the needle is withdrawn, hemostasis should be augmented by manual compression or with a sandbag. Postbiopsy orders should include observation of the patient's vital signs every 15 minutes for at least 2 hours and then hourly for several hours. Patients initially should be immobile; in the absence of macroscopic hematuria, ambulation can begin after 6 to 8 hours. Many transplant centers permit outpatients to go home the same day the biopsy is performed.

Complications

Core needle biopsy is an invasive technique and is not risk free; these risks must be weighed against the benefit gained from the information obtained from the procedure. Careful assessment of potential risks and benefits must precede every decision to subject a patient to a biopsy.

All major complications after needle biopsy manifest as perinephric or urinary bleeding. Transient macroscopic hematuria is common and is of little clinical significance. Macroscopic hematuria follows about 3% of biopsies and may prolong hospitalization or lead to blood transfusion or placement of a bladder catheter for clot drainage. Ureteral obstruction occasionally occurs, requiring placement of a percutaneous nephrostomy; massive hemorrhage necessitating surgical exploration, graft nephrectomy, or angiographic embolization is rare. Postbiopsy arteriovenous fistulas sometimes may be detected by Doppler ultrasound and usually can be treated expectantly. Angiographic embolization may occasionally be required, and graft loss has been reported.

Specimen Handling

Detailed methods for handling tissue specimens are beyond the scope of this chapter. For all specimens, portions are obtained for each of the three traditional methods of evaluating renal parenchyma: light microscopy, electron microscopy, and immunofluorescence. For the initial biopsy, all methods should be used; for subsequent biopsies, electron microscopy is performed only if indicated. This approach allows the pathologist to obtain maximal diagnostic and prognostic information. In selected instances, rapid processing or frozen sections can be performed on the tissue placed in fixative for light microscopy when an immediate assessment of the changes in the graft is necessary for initiating or modifying therapy.

TRANSPLANT REJECTION

Traditionally, three major forms of rejection are recognized: hyperacute, acute, and chronic. Each has reasonably distinctive changes, although acute and chronic rejection may be present simultaneously, resulting in a mixture of histopathologic features. Table 13.1 lists the pathologic findings in the major lesions responsible for functional impairment of the graft.

Hyperacute Rejection

Hyperacute rejection is produced by preformed cytotoxic antibodies and is an infrequent event so long as the pretransplant cross-match is negative (see Chapters 3 and 5). It may manifest shortly after vascular anastomoses are established, or may be delayed up to 3 days. It is characterized by rapid and widespread vascular thrombosis, predominantly affecting arteries, arterioles, and glomeruli, often with polymorphonuclear leukocytes incorporated in the thrombi. The kidney is usually cyanotic, slightly edematous, and flaccid, and urine production suddenly ceases or does not begin at all. If the kidney is not removed immediately, extensive cellular necrosis ensues, followed after 24 hours by numerous cortical and medullary infarcts. Immunofluorescence may disclose capillary and arterial wall immunoglobulin (Ig) G or IgM, C3, and fibrin, with fibrin also in the thrombi. Electron microscopy in the early lesions indicates degeneration and early necrosis of vascular endothelium.

Hyperacute rejection needs to be differentiated from other circumstances in which extensive vascular thrombi occur. The differential diagnosis includes physical perfusion-related injury to vascular endothelium and injury caused by cold-reacting IgM antibodies against blood cells. Both of these conditions rarely may manifest in the immediate posttransplant period and may produce entrapment of leukocytes in thrombi. It is only in hyperacute rejection, however, that polymorphonuclear leukocytes are typically and regularly incorporated in the thrombi. Recurrent hemolytic uremic syndrome and a thrombotic microangiopathy associated with administration of the calcineurin inhibitors (discussed in Calcineurin Inhibitor Nephrotoxicity) are characterized by thrombi, usually without leukocytes, and are generally later-occurring lesions.

Acute Rejection

When the term "acute rejection" is used, it is typically acute *cell-mediated* rejection that is being referred to. However, two distinct immunopathologic mechanisms are responsible for acute rejection: cell-mediated immunity and antibody-mediated (humoral) immunity. It is critical to differentiate them.

Table 13.1. Histopathologic findings in the major causes of allograft dysfunction

Type	Interstitium	Tubules	Glomeruli Capillary lymphocytes	Arteries
Acute cellular rejection	Edema, lymphocytes	Lymphocytes, cell degeneration	Capillary lymphocytes	Swollen endothelium, lymphocytes, foam cells
Classic acute humoral rejection	Hemorrhage, zonal infarction, PTC C4d	Necrosis	Neutrophils, thrombosis	Necrosis, neutrophils, thrombosis
C4d+ acute humoral rejection	PTC C4d ± PTC neutrophils	± Necrosis	Neutrophils	Normal
Acute tubular necrosis	Edema	Cell degeneration, necrosis, mitoses	Normal	Normal
Acute cyclosporine toxicity	Edema	Isometric vacuoles, cell degeneration	Normal	Normal
Chronic rejection	Fibrosis, lymphocytes	Atrophy, dropout	Chronic transplant glomerulopathy	Fibrosis, lymphocytes narrowed lumina
Chronic cyclosporine toxicity	"Striped" fibrosis	Atrophy	Ischemic collapse	Arteriolopathy, hyalinization

PTC, peritubular capillary.

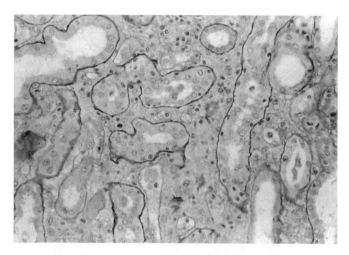

**Fig. 13.1.   Acute cell-mediated interstitial rejection. There is
interstitial edema with lymphocytes in both the interstitium and
tubular walls in association with tubular cell degeneration. (Periodic
acid-methenamine silver stain, ×200.)**

Cell-Mediated Acute Rejection

Cell-mediated acute rejection is the most common form of early
rejection, and has tubulointerstitial and vascular forms. Light microscopy and immunofluorescence microscopy with C4d immunostaining (see Antibody-Mediated Acute Rejection and the C4d
Stain) are the major procedures in diagnosing these lesions
and in all cases of graft dysfunction. At times, routine immunofluorescence and electron microscopic evaluation may be
helpful for the differential diagnosis. In *tubulointerstitial cell-
mediated acute rejection,* primary abnormalities are in the interstitium, which is diffusely edematous and infiltrated by numerous leukocytes, most of which are mature and transformed
lymphocytes (T4, T8) with fewer monocytes and plasma cells
(Fig. 13.1). Eosinophils are either absent or found focally in small
numbers; polymorphonuclear leukocytes are not a regular feature. Peritubular capillaries are dilated and filled with lymphocytes that may be seen migrating into the interstitium. A characteristic lesion, called *tubulitis,* occurs, whereby lymphocytes and
monocytes extend into the walls and lumina of tubules, with associated degenerative changes of epithelial cells. The cells and
basement membranes of tubular walls may be damaged and
discontinuous. When this lesion affects cast-containing distal
tubules, cast matrix (Tamm-Horsfall protein) may be found in
the interstitium, and occasionally in peritubular capillaries and
small veins. For tubulitis to have diagnostic significance, the
inflammation should be documented in normal (nonatrophied)
tubules. The significance of tubulitis solely in atrophied tubules
is not known.

Interstitial
inflammation
and edema

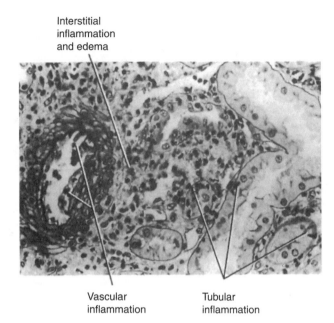

Vascular   Tubular
inflammation   inflammation

**Fig. 13.2. Acute cell-mediated vascular rejection. A small artery
contains lymphocytes in the lumen and in the intima beneath swollen
endothelial cells. Note the interstitial edema and infiltration by
lymphocytes, which are also in the walls of tubules. (Periodic
acid-Schiff stain, ×220.)**

In *cell-mediated vascular rejection*, lymphocytes, monocytes,
and foam cells may undermine arterial endothelium, but rarely
extend into the muscularis (Fig. 13.2). The endothelial cells
are swollen and often vacuolated, but arterial wall necrosis is
not a feature of this type of acute rejection. This form of vascular rejection often, but not always, occurs in concert with
tubulointerstitial rejection. *Acute transplant glomerulopathy* is a
form of glomerular cell-mediated rejection in which lymphocytes
and monocytes accumulate in glomerular capillary lumina and
mesangial regions (Fig. 13.3). Endothelial and mesangial cells
are swollen, and capillary walls display subendothelial lucencies,
with occasional segmental peripheral mesangial migration and
interposition on ultrastructural examination. In cellular rejection, immunofluorescence typically discloses fibrin in the interstitium; segmental linear or granular IgM, C3, and fibrin may be
found in glomerular capillary walls in acute transplant glomerulopathy. C4d staining is negative within peritubular capillaries.
Ultrastructural examination usually confirms the light microscopic findings and provides additional diagnostic information
only for the glomerular lesion. When acute cell-mediated rejection
is treated successfully, the interstitial inflammatory infiltrate

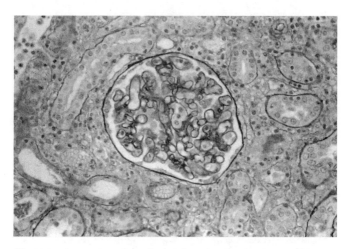

Fig. 13.3.   Acute transplant glomerulopathy. Glomerular capillary lumina contain monocytes and lymphocytes. There are also lymphocytes in tubular walls and interstitial rejection with interstitial edema and inflammation. (Periodic acid-methenamine silver stain, ×200.)

diminishes rapidly, whereas edema, tubular inflammation, and tubular cell damage may persist for some time.

Antibody-Mediated Acute Rejection and the C4d Stain

There are two types of antibody-mediated acute rejection: the classic vascular type and a more common type that is also C4d-positive but without vascular involvement. The vascular form is an uncommon type of rejection and is characterized primarily by necrotizing arteritis, with mural fibrinoid necrosis and variable inflammation, including a proliferation of lymphocytes, monocytes, and neutrophils (Fig. 13.4). Endothelial cells are severely damaged or absent, and luminal thrombosis is common. This lesion typically results in cortical infarction with focal interstitial hemorrhage. Although hyperacute rejection described above is also antibody mediated, it differs from antibody-mediated vascular rejection in that it does not have an inflammatory or fibrinoid component at its outset.

In antibody-mediated rejection, immunofluorescence discloses IgG and sometimes IgM accompanied by C3 in the walls of arteries. In these structures, fibrin may be intramural and intraluminal, and also may be in the interstitium when hemorrhage is present. Some investigators consider intimal arterial lymphocytic infiltration, described previously for cell-mediated rejection, to be a part of the vascular pathology of antibody-mediated rejection. However, the two forms of arterial inflammation are distinct and unrelated to one another. *Vascular rejection* is, therefore, an imprecise term that signifies merely inflammation of arteries, which can result from either cell-mediated or antibody-mediated

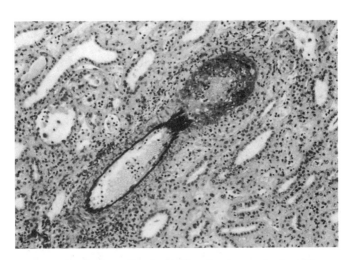

Fig. 13.4.   Antibody-mediated rejection, classic vascular type. The arterial wall is infiltrated by neutrophils and lymphocytes and has segmental fibrinoid necrosis. There are edema and inflammation in the adjacent interstitium. (Elastic-van Gieson stain, ×175.)

immunity. When arterial inflammation is present, it should be further categorized to indicate the etiologic mechanism. The antibody-mediated form is characterized by arterial mural necrosis, neutrophilic infiltrate, and luminal thrombosis, and represents a more severe lesion that is poorly responsive to therapy.

The more frequent form of antibody-mediated acute rejection is characterized by diffuse peritubular capillary staining for the complement component C4d. C4d was first associated with renal allograft rejection in the early 1990s and subsequently linked to the presence of donor-specific antibodies and humoral rejection. The recognition of the importance of the C4d stain has been a major step forward in the understanding of the role of antibodies in the rejection process. C4d has been described as a "footprint" for the presence of humoral rejection.

C4d is a split product of C4 involved in the classical complement cascade. Its formation is illustrated in Figure 13.5 and the accompanying legend. C4d is covalently bound to peritubular capillary endothelium or basement membrane collagen, and is a marker for the complement activation associated with humoral rejection (Fig. 13.6). The histologic appearance of this type of rejection is diverse, usually with scattered glomerular, peritubular capillary, and tubulointerstitial neutrophils. It also may appear only as acute tubular necrosis or accompany cell-mediated rejection. The only way to diagnose this antibody-mediated process is with immunostaining for C4d, which is most reliable in frozen-section specimens and should be performed on all biopsies obtained for renal transplant dysfunction. The treatment and prognosis for this type of rejection are different

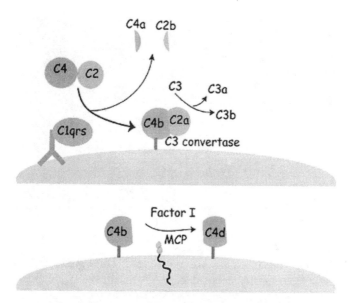

**Fig. 13.5.   Complement activation and formation of C4d. (Top)
Binding of complement fixing antibodies to a cell surface recruits
C1qrs complexes. C1qrs cleaves and activates C4 and C2. C4b formed
in this way may form covalent bonds with the cell surface and
associate with C2a to form C4b2a, the classical complement pathway
C3 convertase. C4b2a catalyzes cleavage of C3 and C5, amplifying
complement activation. (Bottom) C3 convertases are controlled by
various mechanisms. One mechanism involves cleavage of C4b by
factor I plus MCP or C4-binding proteins as cofactors to yield C4d,
which is catalytically inactive. Although C4d is catalytically inert, it
can interact with C4d receptors on B cells and follicular dendritic
cells. These interactions may help to regulate humoral immune
responses. (From Platt JL. C4d and the fate of organ allografts. *J Am
Soc Nephrol* 2002;13:2417–2419 with permission.)**

than for cell-mediated and classic vascular humoral rejection (see
Chapters 4 and 8).

Differential Diagnosis of Acute Cell-Mediated Rejection

Other forms of acute interstitial nephritis may have many of the
same structural lesions as acute rejection, including infectious interstitial nephritis (viral, bacterial) and drug-induced acute hypersensitivity interstitial nephritis. Certain viral and bacterial
interstitial nephritides may be characterized by a mononuclear,
rather than polymorphonuclear, infiltrate, thereby simulating
rejection. Glomerular inflammation and arterial inflammation,
when present, indicate rejection. Because of the negligible role
of polymorphonuclear leukocytes in acute cellular rejection, their
presence should be taken to signify acute infection or C4d humoral rejection, especially when fresh infarction is excluded.
Acute hypersensitivity lesions induced by drugs may have a
prominent component of eosinophils and sometimes granulomas.

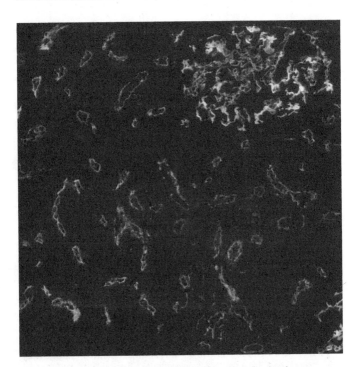

Fig. 13.6.   Acute microvascular antibody-mediated rejection. Peritubular capillaries stain diffusely for C4d. There is constitutive glomerular staining. (Immunofluorescence, ×200.)

Some biopsy specimens with calcineurin inhibitor toxicity may have focal interstitial lymphocytic perivenous infiltrates that do not extend into tubules. These infiltrates are not usually associated with diffuse edema.

Subclinical rejection describes a morphologic pattern of acute cell-mediated rejection that may occur in up to 30% of patients without clinical signs or symptoms of rejection or after apparently successful treatment of rejection. The significance of this asymptomatic inflammatory process relative to short-term or long-term renal function is discussed in Chapter 8.

Differential Diagnosis of Antibody-Mediated Rejection

The arterial inflammation in classic vascular antibody mediated rejection may be indistinguishable from a systemic necrotizing arteritis, but recurrence of vasculitic lesions in the transplant is rare. The effects of vascular occlusion, infarction, and parenchymal hemorrhage may be manifestations not only of arteritis but also of arterial occlusion from other causes, including surgical ligation of a large artery and emboli of any nature. C4d humoral rejection may appear to mimic other lesions in the renal allograft and requires immunostaining for accurate diagnosis.

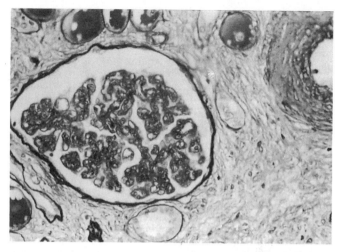

Fig. 13.7. **Chronic rejection with chronic transplant glomerulopathy. The arterial wall is thickened and the lumen narrowed a result of intimal fibrosis. Glomerular capillary walls often display "double contours," and monocytes are within widened mesangial regions and few capillary lumina. (Periodic acid-methenamine silver stain, ×200.)**

Chronic Allograft Nephropathy

Chronic allograft nephropathy (CAN) is the preferred term to the more loosely used "chronic rejection" (see Chapter 9). It is characterized by chronic changes in arteries, tubules, interstitium, and glomeruli. The pathogenesis is mixed; it may be the result of repeated episodes of overt or covert acute rejection (allogeneic factors) and exaggerated by nonimmunologic factors related to the kidney donor and recipient (nonallogeneic factors). From both the clinical and pathologic standpoints, the umbrella term CAN is a better term than chronic rejection because many of the chronic changes may result from different forms of immunologically and nonimmunologically mediated chronic injury to the transplant. These include chronic rejection, chronic calcineurin inhibitor toxicity, nephrosclerosis, partial obstruction, reflux, and chronic infection.

The pathologic changes of CAN are primarily cortical. There is patchy *interstitial fibrosis* with infiltrates of lymphocytes, plasma cells, and mast cells associated with *tubular atrophy*, or dropout. There may be neoexpression of the α_3 chain of type IV collagen and laminin B2 in the proximal tubular basement membrane, and significant increase in interstitial type I collagen. The walls of arteries are thickened with intimal fibrosis and sometimes with medial fibrosis, variable mononuclear leukocyte inflammation (including foam cells), with disruption and duplication of the internal elastic lamina, all resulting in luminal narrowing (Fig. 13.7). Immunofluorescence may document IgG, IgM, C3, and fibrin in the walls of arteries. In addition, juxtaglomerular apparatus hyperplasia may be present and is indicative of large artery involvement.

The glomeruli in CAN are often abnormal and exhibit a variety of changes, many of which constitute the lesion of *chronic transplant glomerulopathy,* which may occur as early as 4 months after transplantation (Fig. 13.7). This abnormality probably represents chronic glomerular rejection and most likely evolves from acute transplant glomerulopathy. Capillary walls are thickened with a double-contoured appearance; mesangial matrix, mesangial cells, or both are increased. The glomeruli may have a lobular appearance, and segmental sclerosis can occur. *Mesangiolysis,* or dissolution of mesangial matrix, is occasionally seen, with resulting capillary microaneurysms. Immunofluorescence often discloses mesangial and capillary wall granular deposits of IgM, C1q, and C3, with linear fibrin along capillary walls. When segmental sclerosis also is present, these same immune reactants are in a segmental distribution in a coarsely granular-to-amorphous pattern. Electron microscopy reveals a variety of abnormalities, including peripheral migration of mesangium, subendothelial new basement membrane formation, subendothelial flocculent material, and, infrequently, subendothelial and mesangial electron-dense deposits. The basement membranes of peritubular capillaries are often thickened and *multilayered*; this change has been correlated with the presence of chronic transplant glomerulopathy.

As with other forms of chronic renal parenchymal diseases, acquired cystic disease has been documented in the chronically rejected transplant. In an attempt to provide prognostic information and standardization of the pathologic changes of chronic allograft failure, a *chronic allograft disease index* (CADI) was developed. Its use may permit prognostication and evaluation of therapeutic interventions for chronic allograft failure, although its reliability has not yet been fully validated.

Differential Diagnosis

As noted previously, the parenchymal changes of CAN need to be differentiated from those of hypertension and chronic calcineurin inhibitor toxicity. The presence of transplant glomerulopathy, arterial fibrosis with or without inflammation and exaggerated interstitial type I collagen suggest CAN. In the absence of these findings, these lesions may be difficult to differentiate from one another.

Calcineurin Inhibitor Nephrotoxicity

Cyclosporine and tacrolimus produce similar renal structural and functional effects, and the pathologist cannot differentiate between the nephrotoxic affects of these two drugs. The pathogenesis of calcineurin inhibitor nephrotoxicity is discussed in Chapter 4.

Acute Toxicity

The structural abnormalities of acute calcineurin inhibitor toxicity are minimal; the dysfunction likely relates to calcineurin inhibitor-induced alterations in renal blood flow. There may be tubular dilation, tubular cell flattening, and occasional individual tubular cell necrosis, all with little or no interstitial edema or inflammation. Giant mitochondria and focal tubular calcification

Isometrically vacuolated
tubular cells

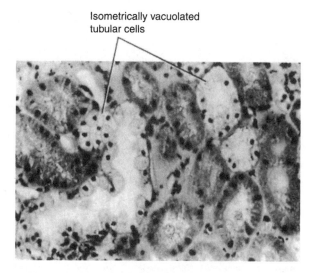

Fig. 13.8.   Cyclosporine toxicity with tubular cell isometric vacuoles. The cells of the lighter-staining tubules contain numerous closely packed uniform vacuoles. Note the lack of interstitial edema or inflammation. (Hematoxylin and eosin stain, ×200.)

also may be present. Unlike the lesions of acute rejection, lymphocytes, when present, are usually restricted to peritubular capillaries and small perivenous foci in the interstitium. They rarely are observed in tubules and are not in any other vascular location. Uniform, clear, small isometric vacuoles may be seen in a variable number of proximal tubular cells, often involving many cells of only few tubular profiles (Fig. 13.8).

Vascular Effects

A number of structural lesions of the vasculature are ascribed to the calcineurin inhibitors. *Arteriolopathy* consists of a variety of abnormalities that occur separately or together. There is necrosis of individual myocytes, often with large plasma protein precipitates; these insudates (hyalinization) are characteristically nodular, occurring on the adventitial aspect of arteriolar walls (Fig. 13.9). In contrast, in hypertension and diabetes mellitus, the insudative lesions are more typically subendothelial or within the muscularis. Cessation or reduction of the cyclosporine dose has resulted in amelioration or resolution of the arteriolopathy in some patients.

Thrombotic microangiopathy (TMA) is an uncommon but well-recognized complication of calcineurin inhibitor administration; its clinical diagnosis and manifestations are discussed in Chapters 4 and 8. In its mildest form, bland thrombi are present within lumina of arterioles and glomerular capillaries. These lesions are rarely widespread or associated with extensive tissue necrosis. If severe and prolonged, however, TMA may result in more

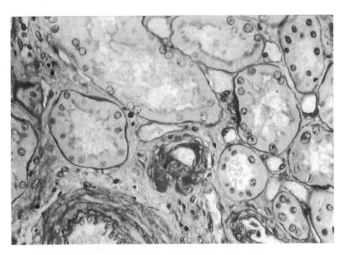

Fig. 13.9. Cyclosporine-associated arteriolopathy. The arteriole has plasma protein insudates ("hyalinization") along the outer aspect of the hypertrophied muscularis. There is no significant edema or inflammation in the interstitium. (Periodic acid-Schiff stain, ×285.)

severe arterial and arteriolar alterations with extensive cortical necrosis similar to that observed in the full-blown thrombotic thrombocytopenic purpura (TTP). In patients whose renal failure is caused by TTP, it may be impossible to differentiate recurrent disease from calcineurin inhibitor-induced TMA. However, the pronounced intimal changes ("onionskin" lesions) of interlobular arteries seen in TTP are not regular features of the calcineurin inhibitor-associated process. Hepatitis C virus infection has been linked to anticardiolipin antibodies, which may induce TMA in allograft recipients.

Chronic Toxicity

The changes of chronic calcineurin inhibitor toxicity are similar to chronic renal ischemia. In their purest form, they consist of focal fibrosis, or "striped" *interstitial fibrosis,* and tubular atrophy without inflammation. The interstitium may show a generalized increase of collagen types III and IV with lesser increases in type I. Glomerular ischemic collapse or complete sclerosis is also present. These features appear not to be a consequence of intrarenal arterial narrowing because the arteries are largely unremarkable; therefore, the combination of normal arteries with a vascular pattern of parenchymal fibrosis is highly suggestive of chronic calcineurin inhibitor nephrotoxicity. Juxtaglomerular apparatus hyperplasia may be pronounced.

Differential Diagnosis

Differentiation between CAN, nephrosclerosis, and chronic calcineurin inhibitor nephrotoxicity may be difficult. Perhaps the most salient feature permitting this distinction is the status of the interlobular and arcuate arteries which are often fortuitously included in the biopsy. Normal arteries usually indicate chronic calcineurin inhibitor nephrotoxicity. Intimal and medial fibrosis of arteries, often with lymphocytic infiltrates, are diagnostic of CAN. If the arteries disclose the usual features of hypertension, nephrosclerosis is likely. These three lesions may coexist and cloud the picture. In addition, characteristic findings may only be present in large arcuate and interlobar arteries and thus may not be included in a core biopsy specimen, further causing diagnostic difficulty.

OTHER PATHOLOGIC TRANSPLANT LESIONS

Acute Tubular Necrosis

Acute tubular necrosis in transplants is similar histologically to the lesion found in native kidneys, although there may be more overt necrosis of epithelial cells and sloughing of nonpyknotic epithelium into tubular lumina (Fig. 13.10). It is most often encountered in a biopsy performed within the first month or so after transplantation because of delayed graft function (see Chapter 8). In addition to the usual changes of tubular necrosis, focal interstitial lymphocytic infiltrates may be present without tubular inflammation.

Infections

Although the transplanted kidney may be the site of various infections, it may be difficult to diagnose them on the basis of tissue examination. This is not the case for usual forms of acute bacterial interstitial nephritis (acute pyelonephritis), in which the predominant interstitial and tubular infiltrating cells are polymorphonuclear leukocytes. Some uncommon nonsuppurative bacterial infections, however, are characterized by mononuclear leukocytic tubular and interstitial infiltrates. Viral infections typically produce a mononuclear tubulointerstitial nephritis, which may be morphologically similar to cell-mediated acute rejection. Specific agents, such as cytomegalovirus (CMV), may be difficult to diagnose because intranuclear or cytoplasmic inclusions are rare.

Human Polyomavirus Infection

Human polyomavirus BK infection has become a more frequently recognized infectious agent in immunosuppressed patients (see Chapter 10). Infection presents clinically as an elevated creatinine level with biopsy findings suggestive of severe acute rejection. If the diagnosis is unrecognized and immunosuppression is intensified, renal function will typically deteriorate further. Polyomavirus infection may also be associated with ureteric stenosis (see Chapter 7). In biopsy specimens with severe tubulointerstitial nephritis, infection is suggested by the finding of large basophilic intranuclear inclusions, occasionally with central clearing in enlarged tubular epithelial cells (Fig 13.11). The inflammatory infiltrate may be focal or mild, associated only with tubules containing infected cells. Special staining with polyomavirus monoclonal antibody confirms the diagnosis, which may have critical therapeutic repercussions.

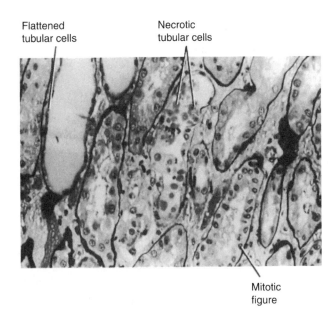

Fig. 13.10.   Acute tubular necrosis. The tubule in the center is incompletely lined by epithelial cells; sloughed cells and cellular debris are in the lumen. There is mild interstitial edema with few accompanying lymphocytes. (Periodic acid-methenamine silver stain, ×250.)

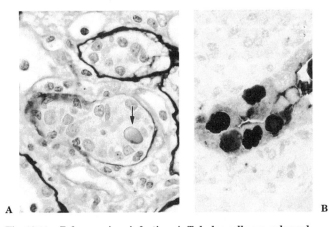

Fig. 13.11.   Polyoma virus infection. A. Tubular cells are enlarged with nuclear viral inclusions (*arrow*) and show necrosis. There is an adjacent lymphocytic inflammatory infiltrate (Jones methanamine silver, ×225). B. Immunoperoxidase stain for SV40 (polyoma virus) showing positive staining in infected tubular epithelial cells (×250).

De Novo Glomerulopathies

De novo membranous glomerulonephritis is found in up to 10% of kidneys in place for more than 1 year, and the capillary wall deposits are not infrequently combined with lesions of CAN. Membranous glomerulonephritis is often clinically silent or mild and is usually detected as an incidental finding. Focal and segmental glomerulosclerosis, including the usual and collapsing types, may occur as an independent lesion, although it often accompanies transplant glomerulopathy and may be associated with heavy proteinuria. Other forms of *de novo* glomerulonephritis are uncommon. The most reliable manner in which to diagnose these lesions is with immunofluorescence and electron microscopy, because the deposits and basement membrane changes often are not readily visible by light microscopy or are overshadowed by transplant glomerulopathy.

Recurrent Lesions

GLOMERULAR LESIONS

Although a variety of glomerulonephritides may recur in the posttransplant course, the recurrences are often of immunopathologic rather than clinical significance and do not necessarily affect graft survival or function (see Chapter 9). These lesions include IgA nephropathy, membranoproliferative glomerulonephritis type II (dense deposit disease), and, occasionally, membranous glomerulonephritis. Focal and segmental glomerulosclerosis may recur early after engraftment and is the recurrent lesion that is most likely to be responsible for graft loss. Antiglomerular basement membrane disease rarely recurs but can arise in a normal kidney transplanted into a patient with Alport syndrome (see Chapter 6). The vasculitides may recur after transplantation.

OTHER LESIONS

Amyloidosis, multiple myeloma, light-chain deposit disease, fibrillary nephropathy, and oxalosis can recur, often with significant graft dysfunction. The structural changes of diabetic nephropathy may recur in the transplanted kidney but are infrequently responsible for graft loss (see Chapter 14). Nodular glomerulosclerosis and arteriolar hyalinization are the usual morphologic manifestations of the recurrent lesion.

CLASSIFICATION SCHEMA

In an attempt to develop an organized and consistent approach to the classification and grading of the various structural lesions in the transplanted kidney, a series of workshop type conferences was held in Banff, Canada. The resulting schema, which came to be known as the *Banff classification,* was then combined with a separately developed classification resulting from a National Institutes of Health-sponsored study (Cooperative Clinical Trials in Transplantation). Although there remain some differences in the schemata, the combined approach, termed *Banff 97,* defines the abnormalities of rejection and assigns them a numeric score.

There are two parts to the schema: (a) the diagnostic classifications and (b) the grading of each pathologic component in the

Table 13.2.   Selected features of the
modified Banff 97 classification

Grade	Criteria
Acute humoral rejection	
I	C4d+, tubular necrosis
II	C4d+, capillary pmns and/or thrombosis
III	C4d+, transmural arteritis/fibrinoid necrosis
Acute cellular rejection	
I	Interstitial inflammation (>25% of parenchyma) Tubulitis (>4 lymphocytes per tubular cross-section)
II	Intimal arteritis (mild to severe)
III	Transmural arteritis and/or fibrinoid necrosis with lymphocytes
Chronic allograft nephropathy	
I	Mild interstitial fibrosis and tubular atrophy
II	Moderate interstitial fibrosis and tubular atrophy
III	Severe interstitial fibrosis and tubular atrophy or dropout

pmns, polymorphonuclear leukocytes.

tissue sample. The grading is somewhat cumbersome and involves assigning a degree of severity to changes affecting the tubules, interstitium, vessels, and glomeruli. The diagnostic categories include antibody-mediated hyperacute and accelerated acute rejection; a borderline lesion; acute rejection grade I (Fig. 13.1), grade II (Fig. 13.2), and grade III (Fig. 13.4) acute rejection; acute tubular necrosis; acute cyclosporine or FK506 toxicity; grade I (mild), grade II (moderate), and grade III (severe) chronic rejection (chronic nephropathy); and other lesions (e.g., infection, glomerulonephritides, posttransplant lymphoproliferative disorder). Table 13.2 summarizes the important aspects of the Banff 97 classification.

According to the Banff 97 classification, mild interstitial edema, patchy (10% to 25%) interstitial lymphocytic infiltration, and mild tubulitis (one to four lymphocytes per tubular cross-section) in the absence of arterial intimal inflammation are considered *borderline lesions,* suspicious for acute rejection. There remains some controversy regarding the clinical significance of borderline lesions; some, but not all, studies associate these lesions with treatment-responsive clinical acute rejection. The grade III rejection criteria do, however, appear to correlate with more severe clinical rejections, which may be unresponsive to treatment with high-dose steroids alone (see Chapter 4). Further work is required to clarify the clinical usefulness of the Banff 97 classification, and classification schemata with specific quantifiable criteria require further validation in clinical studies. There also remains concern regarding the consistency of grading between observers.

NEW TECHNIQUES IN EVALUATING TRANSPLANT DYSFUNCTION

The evaluation of acute and chronic renal allograft dysfunction is an area ripe for the application of new technologies including gene profiling with microarrays and proteomics. Several studies have examined gene expression of T lymphocyte activation markers using real-time polymerase chain reaction (PCR) of peripheral blood mononuclear cells, urine, and renal biopsy tissue for diagnosing acute rejection. These studies have identified upregulated T-cell factors such as granzyme B and perforin, often in combination with other rejection-associated factors, including human leukocyte antigen (HLA)-DR, as promising molecular means of rejection assessment. Noninvasive methods for identifying rejection are being explored, and have demonstrated donor-specific deoxyribonucleic acid (DNA) and proteomics of urine specimens as potential tools in this area. Gene microarray study biopsies of patients with acute and chronic rejection are identifying markers for diagnosis, therapeutic effectiveness, and prognosis. A defined collection of genes in renal biopsy specimens has been found to be predictive of chronic rejection prior to clinical or histologic features of chronic damage. Genomics and proteomics undoubtedly will continue to open new avenues of early diagnosis and treatment for rejection and other causes of declining allograft function.

KIDNEY DONOR HISTOPATHOLOGY

The ever-widening gap between the supply and demand for cadaveric kidneys has led to the increasing use of organs from "marginal" donors (see Chapters 3 and 5). Histopathology of these kidneys is often requested as a guide to the wisdom of transplanting them. The most common clinical situations in which donor pathology is requested are for older donors, donors with a history of hypertension or vascular disease, or donors with preharvesting evidence of renal dysfunction. Baseline histology may be required in the clinical trials evaluating new immunosuppressive drugs.

The time constraints imposed by the need for rapid decision making prevent routine histopathologic processing of biopsy material. Use of frozen tissue may impair diagnostic precision and rapid-processing techniques are preferred. A superficial wedge biopsy specimen may be provided; however, the subcapsular parenchyma often has chronic changes and is not representative of the whole organ. Additionally, arteries may be absent from superficial biopsy specimens, precluding adequate evaluation for nephrosclerosis. Therefore, such specimens should be interpreted with caution. The number and percentage of sclerosed glomeruli should be determined and an assessment made of the degree of tubulointerstitial and vascular disease. Transplant teams tend to give more prognostic credence to numeric values that may reflect the degree of nephrosclerosis, and kidneys with more than 20% sclerosed glomeruli often are discarded. Interstitial and vascular changes, however, which are more difficult to quantitate, may have more prognostic importance.

SELECTED READINGS

Ahsan N, Cheung JY. Pathogenesis and molecular mechanisms of chronic allograft nephropathy. *Contrib Nephrol* 2003:139:187–195.

Bhalla V, Nast C, Stollenwerk N, et al. Recurrent and *de novo* diabetic nephropathy in renal allografts. *Transplantation* 2003:75:66–69.

Bohmig GA, Exner M, Habicht A, et al. Capillary C4d deposition in kidney allografts: a specific marker of alloantibody-dependent graft injury. *J Am Soc Nephrol* 2002;13:1091–1099.

Bosmans JL, Woestenburg A, Yserbaert DK, et al. Fibrous intimal thickening at implantation as a risk factor for the outcome of cadaveric renal allografts. *Transplantation* 2000;69:2388–2393.

Briganti EM, Russ GR, McNeil JJ, et al. Risk of renal allograft loss from recurrent glomerulonephritis. *N Engl J Med* 2002:347:103–107.

Clark W, Silverman BC, Zhang Z, et al. Characterization of renal allograft rejection by urinary proteomic analysis. *Ann Surg* 2003;237:660–664.

Curtis JJ, Julian BA, Sanders CE. Dilemmas in renal transplantation: when the clinical course and histologic findings differ. *Am J Kidney Dis* 1996;27:435–440.

Furness PN, Taub N. International variation in the interpretation of renal transplant biopsies: Report of the CERTRAP project. *Kidney Int* 2001;60:1998–2006.

Gaber LW, Moore LW, Alloway RR, et al. Correlation between Banff classification, acute renal rejection scores and reversal of rejection. *Kidney Int* 1996;49:481–486.

Mauiyyedi S, Colvin RB. Humoral rejection in kidney transplantation: new concepts in diagnosis and treatment. *Curr Opin Nephrol Hypertens* 2002:11:609–618.

Muruve NA, Steinbecker KM, Luger AM. Are wedge biopsies of cadaveric kidneys obtained at procurement reliable? *Transplantation* 2000;69:2384–2388.

Nankivell BJ, Borrows RJ, Fung CL, et al. The natural history of chronic allograft nephropathy. *N Engl J Med* 2003;349:2326–2333.

Nickeleit V, Klimkait T, Binet IF, et al. Testing for polyomavirus type BK DNA in plasma to identify renal allograft recipients with viral nephropathy. *N Engl J Med* 2000;342:1309–1315.

Nickerson P, Jeffrey J, McKenna R, et al. Identification of clinical and histopathologic risk factors for diminished renal function 2 years post-transplant. *J Am Soc Nephrol* 1998;19:482–487.

Platt JL. C4d and the fate of organ allografts. *J Am Soc Nephrol* 2002;13:2417.

Racusen LC, Solez K, Colvin RB, et al. The Banff 97 working classification of renal allograft pathology. *Kidney Int* 1999;55:713–723.

Racusen LC, Solez K, Colvin R. Fibrosis and atrophy in the renal allograft: interim report and new directions. *Am J Transplant* 2002;2:203–207.

Randhawa PS, Finkelstein S, Scantlebury V, et al. Human polyoma virus-associated interstitial nephritis in the allograft kidney. *Transplantation* 1999:67:103–107.

Sabek O, Dorak MT, Kotb M, et al. Quantitative detection of T-cell activation markers by real-time PCR in renal transplant rejection and correlation with histopathologic evaluation. *Transplantation* 2002;74:701–705.

Sarwal M, Chua MS, Kambham N. Molecular heterogeneity in acute renal allograft rejection identified by DNA microarray profiling. *N Engl J Med* 2003;349:125–138.

Scherer A, Krause A, Walker JR, et al. Early prognosis of the development of renal chronic allograft rejection by gene expression profiling of human protocol biopsies. *Transplantation* 2003;75:1323–1328.

Yilmaz S, Tomlanovich S, Mathew T. Protocol core needle biopsy and histologic chronic allograft damage index (CADI) as surrogate end point for long-term graft survival in multicenter studies. *J Am Soc Nephrol* 2003;14:773–779.

Kidney and Pancreas Transplantation in Diabetic Patients

John D. Pirsch, Hans W. Sollinger, and Craig Smith

Diabetes mellitus is the leading cause of end-stage renal disease (ESRD), accounting for one-third of new ESRD patients each year. Approximately 40% of the ESRD population has diabetes; 12% of cases are classified as type 1 and 28% as type 2. The incidence of ESRD as a consequence of type 2 diabetes is increasing progressively in all countries with a Western lifestyle. Diabetes is second only to glomerular disease as an indication for transplantation, and it is the cause of ESRD in 20% of transplant recipients each year. Because of the growth in diabetes in the population, by 2006 the number of diabetics with new ESRD will equal the number of patients with ESRD from other primary diagnosis. The encouraging news is the incidence of diabetic nephropathy in insulin-dependent diabetes mellitus appears to be falling. However, most of the new cases of diabetic ESRD will occur in older patients with type 2 diabetes. This diagnosis remains the one that most commonly leads to kidney transplantation in adult whites, Asians, and Native Americans.

There is little question that kidney transplantation, alone or combined with pancreas transplantation, is the treatment of choice for end-stage diabetic nephropathy. Living donor kidney transplantation in diabetic recipients is associated with a survival advantage when compared with deceased donor transplantation; however, both forms of transplantation offer a pronounced survival advantage over chronic dialysis (see Chapter 1). Care must be taken in comparing transplant and dialysis patient groups because, as a whole, they are not strictly comparable. Patients with the least-severe morbid manifestations of diabetes are more likely to select, or be selected for, transplantation. When transplanted diabetic patients are compared with diabetics awaiting transplants, the transplanted group has a clear-cut survival advantage. Controlled studies evaluating the quality-of-life benefits of these treatment modalities clearly illustrate the benefits of transplantation over dialysis for patients with diabetes. Although all forms of kidney replacement therapy can stabilize or slow some of the secondary complications of diabetes, successful transplantation with correction of uremia and control of blood pressure can stabilize or improve complications, such as neuropathy, diabetic gastroparesis, and retinopathy.

This chapter considers the management issues associated with kidney and pancreas transplantation in diabetic patients and the pros and cons of the different forms of pancreas transplantation.

Figure 14.1 illustrates the options available for diabetic patients with advanced renal disease.

KIDNEY TRANSPLANTATION

Preoperative Assessment

The preoperative evaluation of potential kidney transplant recipients is discussed in Chapter 6. This section considers issues particularly relevant to diabetic patients. The propensity for the premature development of atherosclerosis in diabetic patients mandates careful screening for overt and covert vascular disease.

Coronary Artery Disease

About one-third of potential diabetic transplant recipients have significant coronary artery disease. Most of these patients do not suffer typical angina or other cardiac symptoms; hence, the possibility of covert coronary artery disease should be considered in every diabetic transplant candidate. In many transplantation programs, all diabetic patients undergo some form of stress test screening to help determine which patients should undergo further evaluation with cardiac catheterization. If exercise stress is used, it is usually supplemented with thallium or sestamibi scintigraphy or echocardiography to increase its specificity. Many diabetic patients with kidney failure, however, have poor functional capacity or are physically unable to exercise adequately to reach a target heart rate. These patients should undergo an oral or intravenous dipyridamole-thallium stress test or a dobutamine stress echocardiogram designed to simulate the effect of exercise on the heart. The sensitivity and specificity of noninvasive tests for detecting covert coronary artery disease varies from 50% to 75% so that excessive reliance on these tests can be misleading.

A meta-analysis of myocardial perfusion studies in patients with ESRD referred for kidney and kidney pancreas transplantation concluded that patients with evidence of an inducible perfusion abnormality or wall motion abnormality had a sixfold higher risk of myocardial infarction (MI) and fourfold higher risk of cardiac death. Patients with noninducible fixed defects also had a nearly fivefold increased risk of cardiac death, but not MI. In the diabetic subgroup, reversible defects were associated with a ninefold increase in MI. Fixed and reversible defects conferred a relative risk of 4.0 to 4.7 for cardiac death. These data would suggest that a negative nuclear scintigraphy or dobutamine stress test in this population is associated with a low event rate for MI and cardiac death following transplantation.

Because of the uncertainty of noninvasive testing, recipients with multiple risk factors or a positive or inadequate stress test should undergo cardiac catheterization before transplantation. Patients with coronary lesions amenable to bypass or angioplasty should be treated before transplantation. Patients with significant coronary artery disease who are not candidates for intervention may not be transplant candidates, although centers differ in their approach to such patients.

In an attempt to avoid an expensive and invasive workup in all diabetic patients, attempts have been made to determine which

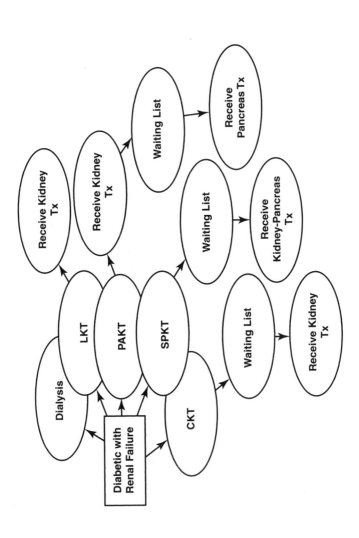

diabetic candidates are most unlikely to suffer covert coronary artery disease. Patients without cardiac symptoms who are younger than 45 years of age and have had diabetes for fewer than 25 years, who have not smoked for more than 5 pack-years, and who have a totally normal electrocardiogram have a low incidence of covert coronary artery disease; consequently, further workup may be unnecessary. Figure 14.2 shows an algorithm for screening diabetic transplant candidates for coronary artery disease.

Diabetic patients who wait for prolonged periods on the deceased donor transplant waiting list should have their cardiac status reassessed at intervals of 1 to 2 years, with repetition of noninvasive testing; coronary angiography should be repeated when indicated (see Chapter 6, Table 6.5). Known risk factors for coronary artery disease should be repeatedly reviewed and addressed.

Cerebrovascular and Peripheral Vascular Disease

The increased susceptibility of diabetic transplant recipients for cerebrovascular and peripheral vascular disease mandates particular attention to these issues in the pretransplantation evaluation. A history of cerebrovascular events or intermittent claudication and the finding of carotid bruits or poor peripheral pulses may require further assessment. Noninvasive studies should precede angiography, and consultation with a vascular surgeon may be warranted.

Infections

Patients should be free of significant infections, such as peritonitis, osteomyelitis, or unhealed foot ulcerations at the time of transplantation. If a patient develops these complications while awaiting a transplant, the patient's candidacy should be placed on hold until the problem is resolved.

Predialysis Transplantation

For patients with diabetic nephropathy, transplantation should be strongly considered before the initiation of dialysis (glomerular filtration rate of 20 mL per minute or less, or a serum creatinine level of 4 to 5 mg/dL). Early transplantation can obviate the need for dialysis access, can prevent episodes of congestive heart failure and volume overload, and can correct hypertension, which may contribute to loss of vision. Early transplantation may slow retinopathy and correct neuropathy secondary to uremia, which can exacerbate diabetic neuropathy. The development of diabetic

←

Fig. 14.1.   Options for diabetics with renal failure. A diabetic with renal failure can choose one of five treatment strategies: dialysis, living kidney transplantation (LKT), pancreas after living kidney transplantation (PAKT), simultaneous pancreas–kidney transplantation (SPKT), or deceased donor kidney transplantation (CKT). (From Knoll GA, Nichol G. Dialysis, kidney transplantation, or pancreas transplantation for patients with diabetes mellitus and renal failure: a decision analysis of treatment options. *J Am Soc Nephrol* 2003;14:500–515, with permission.)

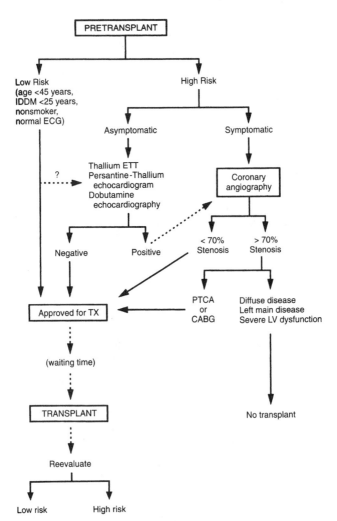

Fig. 14.2. Algorithm for screening of diabetic transplant candidates for coronary artery disease based on data that suggest that noninvasive evaluation of low-risk patients may be unnecessary. CABG, coronary artery bypass graft; EKG, electrocardiogram; ETT, exercise treadmill testing; IDDM, insulin-dependent diabetes mellitus; LV, left ventricle; PTCA, percutaneous transluminal coronary angioplasty; TX, transplantation. (From Williams ME. Management of the diabetic transplant recipient. *Kidney Int* **1995;48:1660–1674, reprinted with permission of Blackwell Science, Inc.)**

complications on dialysis may impair the rehabilitation potential of transplantation.

Predialysis diabetic transplant candidates who require coronary angiography risk precipitation of dialysis by contrast nephropathy. This risk needs to be carefully weighed against the risks associated with delaying transplantation or leaving coronary artery disease undiagnosed. Predialysis transplantation is also discussed in Chapter 6.

Insulin Requirements

By the time many diabetic patients develop advanced nephropathy or the need for dialysis, their insulin requirements have often diminished, or their diabetes may be controlled by oral agents or diet alone. After transplantation, improved appetite, carbohydrate intolerance induced by corticosteroids, and the use of calcineurin inhibitors, particularly tacrolimus (see Chapter 4) may lead to increased insulin requirements and cause non–insulin-dependent diabetic patients to require insulin. Patients should be forewarned.

Preoperative Preparation

For patients with severe gastroparesis, a nasogastric tube may need to be placed. Poor gastrointestinal function may compromise absorption of immunosuppressive therapies, and intravenous formulations of mycophenolate and corticosteroids should be considered in the early postoperative period. Most centers have abandoned the use of intravenous cyclosporine and tacrolimus, which are usually well absorbed, even from the malfunctioning gastrointestinal tract. Slow resumption of bowel function may follow transplantation, and, occasionally, nasogastric suction may be required in cases of prolonged ileus. In the immediate preoperative period when the patient is receiving nothing by mouth, half the normal dose of insulin should be given. Blood glucose levels should be monitored every 4 hours and a sliding scale used for dosing regular insulin. Patients should undergo dialysis if there is significant evidence of volume overload or congestive heart failure. The immunosuppressive protocol used does not differ in diabetic transplant recipients, although attempts may be made to lessen the reliance on corticosteroids.

Postoperative Complications

Several studies have shown no significant difference in major postoperative complications in diabetic versus nondiabetic patients, especially with regard to wound complications. Postoperative ileus, nausea, and vomiting are more common but are secondary to diabetic enteropathy. Because of the use of high-dose corticosteroids, frequent blood sugar monitoring is essential, and an insulin drip may be necessary in the first 24 to 48 hours after transplantation. All patients should receive instruction in blood sugar self-monitoring and in using sliding-scale administration of regular insulin for the control of episodes of hyperglycemia. Long-acting insulin, such as NPH or glargine insulin should be used. Occasionally, dividing the prednisone dose into a morning and afternoon dose helps to control postprednisone hyperglycemia.

Graft Dysfunction

REJECTION

The incidence of rejection and calcineurin inhibitor toxicity in diabetic patients is not different from that in nondiabetic patients. When possible, a kidney biopsy should be employed to determine the cause of graft dysfunction to prevent unnecessary immunosuppression in this high-risk population. Therapy with high-dose corticosteroids is frequently accompanied by poor blood sugar control and requires close monitoring.

PSEUDOREJECTION

In patients with poor blood sugar control, hypovolemia can cause elevations in the blood urea nitrogen and creatinine levels and mimic a rejection episode. Careful review of the previous blood sugar record and careful assessment of volume status are usually sufficient to make this diagnosis. Occasionally, functional obstruction secondary to neurogenic bladder also simulates rejection. This condition is usually diagnosed by ultrasound or renal scan, which shows a large distended bladder and a prominent renal pelvis. The volume of the postvoid residual may be more than 500 mL, and Foley catheter drainage with a fall in creatinine level confirms the diagnosis.

URINARY TRACT INFECTION

Urinary tract infections (UTIs) are more common in diabetic recipients because of the higher incidence of neurogenic bladder. Prophylaxis with daily double-strength trimethoprim-sulfamethoxazole is recommended.

Long-Term Complications

Peripheral Vascular Disease

Although successful kidney transplantation is a solution for the nephropathy associated with insulin-dependent diabetes mellitus, many other diabetic manifestations, including peripheral vascular disease, continue to progress. Up to 30% of patients are reported to have undergone at least one amputation within 3 years of transplantation. Meticulous foot care is essential to help prevent amputations. Although many ischemic ulcers are secondary to microvascular disease, macrovascular occlusion secondary to atherosclerotic plaquing is not uncommon. Angiography should be employed when indicated to identify patients with peripheral vascular lesions that are amenable to bypass grafting.

Retinopathy

Stabilization of retinopathy is common after transplantation, with most patients experiencing no change in visual acuity or showing some improvement. Recipients with severely impaired vision may note some improvement, although some patients progress to blindness.

Neuropathy

Neuropathy shows initial improvement with the correction of uremia; however, there is slow deterioration with the progression of the diabetes.

DIABETIC GASTROPATHY

Diabetic gastropathy is common, and gastroparesis is best treated with metoclopramide (10 mg four times daily before meals). Side effects associated with metoclopramide include mental confusion and a Parkinson-like syndrome with cogwheel rigidity, which is an indication to decrease the dose or discontinue the medication. Many patients who require metoclopramide before transplantation may discontinue it afterward. Diabetic diarrhea can be treated with oral or transdermal clonidine.

NEUROGENIC BLADDER

Neurogenic bladder is a frequent complicating factor after transplantation. Intermittent self-catheterization may be necessary in some patients.

ORTHOSTATIC HYPOTENSION

Orthostatic hypotension with supine hypertension is common secondary to autonomic neuropathy and may be transiently exacerbated after successful transplantation, particularly if the patient was in a fluid-positive state before transplantation. Treatment includes fludrocortisone acetate (Florinef), 0.1 to 0.3 mg daily; midodrine (an α-adrenoreceptor agonist) up to 10 mg three times a day; or sodium chloride tablets, if the patient is not edematous. Clonidine improves orthostatic hypotension, probably by a peripheral venoconstricting effect. Orthostatic hypotension typically resolves as the hematocrit rises; this process can be expedited with erythropoietin injections if necessary.

Hypertension

Hypertension is common after transplantation and may be caused by the effects of cyclosporine or tacrolimus, retained native kidneys, or, rarely, renal artery stenosis (see Chapter 9). Agents useful in treatment include the spectrum of antihypertensives; however, diuretics and beta blockers should be used with caution. Diuretics may impair glucose control or increase cholesterol levels; beta blockers may block the hypoglycemic response to norepinephrine and epinephrine and predispose the patient to severe hypoglycemic episodes. Calcium channel blockers are effective; however, verapamil and diltiazem increase cyclosporine levels. Close monitoring of cyclosporine or tacrolimus levels is necessary if these agents are used. The dihydropyridines do not interfere with cyclosporine metabolism and are effective in controlling posttransplantation hypertension. The long-acting preparation is preferred. Alpha blockers are also effective, but side effects at higher doses may limit their use. Angiotensin-converting enzyme inhibitors or receptor blockers are effective for blood pressure control, and these agents may have additional cardiac and renoprotective benefits. Kidney function may decline during their use, especially in undiagnosed renal artery stenosis or chronic rejection, and hyperkalemia and anemia may occur.

Hyperlipidemia

Hyperlipidemia should be treated aggressively in diabetic transplant recipients, particularly in the presence of coronary artery disease. Dietary treatment alone is usually ineffective; beta-hydroxy-β-methylglutaryl-coenzyme A (HMG-CoA) reductase inhibitors, starting at low doses with careful monitoring of muscle and liver enzymes, are the agents most likely to be effective (see Chapter 9).

Bone Disease

Diabetic transplant recipients are particularly susceptible to osteoporosis and its consequences (see Chapter 9), and a fracture rate of up to 40% has been described on long-term followup. Ideally, lumbar spine and hip bone mineral density should be measured by dual x-ray absorptiometry at the time of transplantation and at yearly intervals thereafter. The bisphosphonates represent the most effective means of prevention and treatment.

Recurrent Diabetic Nephropathy

Pathologic changes in the allograft consistent with diabetic nephropathy are common after transplantation; graft loss secondary to recurrent diabetic nephropathy, however, is unusual. In the future, with longer survival of transplant recipients, recurrent diabetic nephropathy may become a more significant problem.

Pregnancy

Pregnancy in transplant recipients is discussed in Chapter 9. Pregnant diabetic transplant recipients represent a particularly high-risk group; a limited number of successful pregnancies have been reported. Prematurity is universal, and deterioration of graft function is common. These factors, together with the potentially limited maternal life span, should be considered in the decision to proceed with the pregnancy.

KIDNEY–PANCREAS TRANSPLANTATION

Surgical Options

To provide the pancreatic islets needed to produce insulin and cure diabetes, it is necessary to transplant both the exocrine and endocrine pancreas. This situation will change if and when pancreatic islet transplantation becomes a readily available clinical reality (see the section on transplantation of pancreatic islets). Three patient groups can be considered for whole-organ pancreas transplantation: *pancreas transplantation alone* (PTA), for patients who have not yet developed advanced kidney disease; *simultaneous pancreas–kidney* (SPK) transplantation, for patients with renal failure; and *pancreas after kidney* (PAK) transplantation, for patients who have previously undergone successful kidney transplantation. Each of these approaches has advantages and disadvantages, which must be considered when determining the indications for pancreas transplantation (Table 14.1 and Fig. 14.3). In 1999, in the United States, Medicare approved reimbursement for pancreas transplantation for patients with ESRD (i.e., SPK and PAK but not PTA), making the procedure feasible for a much larger population of patients.

Much of the success of all types of cadaveric pancreas transplantation depends on meticulous attention to the technical aspects of donor selection, organ harvesting, and back-table preparation. Detailed discussion of these issues is beyond the scope of

Table 14.1. Pancreas transplantation options

	Pro	Con	1-Year Survival in 1999–2000
Preuremic pancreas alone	Good surgical risk; complications at early stage	Major surgical procedure; side effects of immunosuppressive therapy may outweigh potential benefits; relative risk (Fig. 14.3).	Patient 98%; pancreas 77%
Pancreas after kidney transplantation	Patient already immunosuppressed	Surgical procedure; advanced diabetic complications; relative risk (Fig. 14.3)	Patient 96%; pancreas 79%
Simultaneous kidney and pancreas transplantation	Only one surgical procedure; same immunosuppression; good results; relative benefit (Fig 14.3)	Advanced diabetic complications	Patient 95%; pancreas 85%; kidney 92%

this text; the reader is referred to the article by Frezza et al. (see "Selected Readings," below).

Preuremic Pancreas Transplantation

Some centers offer PTA transplantation as a therapeutic alternative for recurrently ketotic "brittle" patients and for patients with hypoglycemic unawareness. The number of patients receiving these transplants has increased over the past several years with improving immunosuppression. In 2002, 168 patients underwent PTA in the United States. The prolonged normoglycemia that follows the successful procedure may not lead to resolution of established nephropathy or retinopathy. For most diabetic patients, the risk:benefit ratio for PA transplantation is unfavorable because a pancreas transplant exposes them both to the risks of surgery and to the long-term side effects of immunosuppressive therapy. The procedure should be considered in diabetics with severe hypoglycemic unawareness or significant secondary complications of diabetes.

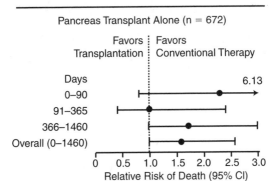

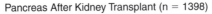

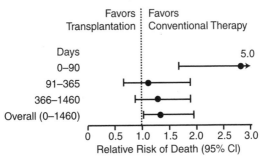

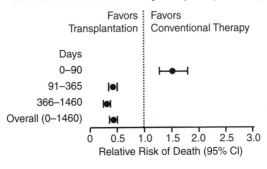

Transplantation of the Pancreas After the Kidney

PAK transplantation is the second most common pancreas transplant with 676 patients transplanted in 2002. In PAK transplantation, immunosuppressive therapy is not a major concern. In the long-term, the drug therapy the patients are already receiving for their kidney transplant is not significantly changed after the addition of a pancreas transplant. The significant risks for these patients are the risk of the surgical procedure itself and the short-term risk of a temporary postoperative boost in their immunosuppressive therapy. Unfortunately, these patients have already suffered significant secondary diabetic complications, and it is uncertain whether a well-functioning pancreas transplant will accomplish more than rendering these patients insulin independent. The results of PAK transplantation are worse than those of SPK transplantation, but have improved with the availability of the newer immunosuppressive agents (see Chapter 4). PAK transplantation may be a particularly relevant option for patients with a living donor, in which case the kidney is placed on the left side in anticipation of the pancreas transplantation several months later.

Simultaneous Kidney and Pancreas Transplantation

SPK transplantation is the preferred and most common type of pancreas transplantation. Since 1999, 1,800 SPK transplants have been performed per year in the United States. It has the advantage that only one surgical procedure is required and there is only one source of foreign histocompatibility antigens. Immunosuppressive therapy is similar to the therapy that these patients would receive with a kidney transplant alone. As in PAK transplantation, however, many patients have already suffered substantial secondary diabetic complications, and the extent to which these complications will reverse or stabilize is uncertain (see the section on the effect of pancreas transplantation on secondary diabetic complications). Nevertheless, SPK transplantation is established as a therapeutic and effective procedure; substantial improvement in the quality of life, as compared with kidney transplantation alone, has been documented by several centers (see the section on choice of procedure).

Outcome of Pancreas Transplantation

For SPK transplants since 1996, the 1-, 3-, and 5-year pancreas graft survival was 85%, 77%, and 70%, respectively. Pancreas transplantation does not adversely affect kidney graft survival.

←

Fig. 14.3. Relative risk of mortality, by transplant type. Days are posttransplant (recipients) or additional days waiting (patients not transplanted). Relative risk of 1.0 indicates that the risk of transplantation equals the risk for those not transplanted. CI, confidence interval. (From Venstrom JM, McBride MA, Rother KI, et al. Survival after pancreas transplantation in patients with diabetes and preserved kidney function. *JAMA* 2003;290:2817–2823, with permission.)

The 1-, 3-, and 5-year kidney graft survival was 92%, 84%, and 74%, respectively. Pancreas graft survival for PAK and PTA recipients was worse than for SPK recipients. The 1-, 3-, and 5-year pancreas graft survival for PAK was 77%, 65%, and 41%, respectively. For PTA, the corresponding pancreas graft survival was 79%, 67%, and 47%, respectively.

Accurate comparison of survival statistics for SPK versus kidney transplantation alone for diabetics is difficult because the SPK recipients tend to be younger, with less vascular disease. However, studies suggest a significant survival benefit for SPK recipients compared to diabetics receiving a kidney transplant alone. If survival after the different types of whole-organ pancreas transplant is compared to remaining on the waiting list for an organ there is a significant long-term survival advantage for SPK recipients but a survival disadvantage for PTA and PAK recipients (Fig. 14.3).

Surgical Techniques

Much of the controversy with respect to the optimal surgical technique for pancreas transplantation has been focused on the handling of the exocrine pancreatic secretions. The most commonly used techniques are enteric drainage and bladder drainage. Other management techniques (duct injection and obliteration) account for less than 1% of cases.

Enteric Drainage of Exocrine Secretions

Enteric drainage of exocrine pancreas secretions has become the most popular of the drainage options. In the past 3 years, nearly 80% of U.S. SPK transplants were performed with enteric drainage. Fifty-five percent of PAK and PTA transplants were performed with enteric drainage over the same time period. Some centers still prefer bladder drainage in PAK and PTA in order to monitor serial urine amylase determinations.

With enteric drainage, the whole pancreas, together with a segment of donor duodenum, is transplanted with side-to-side anastomosis into the recipient's small bowel (primary enteric drainage) (Fig. 14.4). Enteric drainage of the pancreas has several advantages over bladder drainage. It is associated with fewer urologic problems, fewer UTIs, a lower incidence of pancreatitis, and less-severe metabolic disturbance. The major problem with enteric drainage is an anastomotic leak, which may lead to early graft loss, intraabdominal sepsis, and the inability to monitor urine amylase for rejection.

Bladder Drainage

The number of centers choosing bladder drainage as their procedure of choice is decreasing. Whole pancreatic grafts are used with a side-to-side pancreatic duodenocystostomy (Fig. 14.5). The advantages of bladder drainage include a lower surgical complication rate and the use of urinary amylase for monitoring rejections (see the section on the diagnosis of rejection). The pancreas is placed contralateral to the simultaneously performed kidney transplantation. The disadvantages of bladder drainage are discussed later (see the section on complications) and are the primary reason for its decreasing popularity.

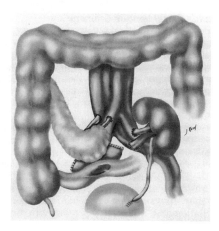

Fig. 14.4. Enteric drainage (ED) technique. The donor duodenal segment is anastomosed in a side-to-side fashion to the ileum or distal jejunum. (From Pirsch JD, Odorico JS, Sollinger HW. Kidney–pancreas transplantation. In: Schrier RW, Henrich WL, Bennett WM, eds. *Atlas of diseases of the kidney.* Vol. 5. Philadelphia: Current Medicine, 1999, with permission.)

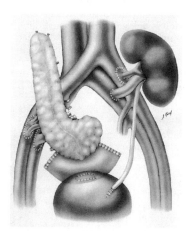

Fig. 14.5. Schematic diagram of the bladder drainage technique for simultaneous kidney and pancreas transplantation. Note side-to-side pancreaticoduodenocystostomy. (From Pirsch JD, Odorico JS, Sollinger HW. Kidney–pancreas transplantation. In: Schrier RW, Henrich WL, Bennett WM, eds. *Atlas of diseases of the kidney.* Vol. 5. Philadelphia: Current Medicine, 1999, with permission.)

Systemic Versus Portal Venous Drainage

Carbohydrate metabolism in successful pancreas transplant recipients is similar to that in immunosuppressed nondiabetic kidney transplant recipients. Most transplantation centers use systemic venous drainage of the transplanted pancreas (Figs. 14.4 and 14.5), but the number of portal-venous-drained pancreas transplants is increasing. With systemic venous drainage, basal and stimulated peripheral serum insulin levels are two to three times higher than normal because the insulin does not undergo first-pass hepatic uptake and degradation. Patients may be susceptible to postprandial hypoglycemia, and the high ambient insulin levels, insulin resistance, and abnormal lipoprotein metabolism may accelerate atherosclerosis. Portal venous drainage of the transplanted pancreas is preferred in some centers. Portal drainage reduces peripheral hyperinsulinemia and is theoretically more "physiologic." The technique is somewhat more technically challenging, and its relative benefits are not clearly established.

Complications

Significant surgical complications after pancreas transplantation with bladder drainage occur in about half of patients (Table 14.2), although most are manageable. Even at centers with the best results, the rate of early reoperation and the length of hospital stay are considerably greater for SPK transplantation than for kidney transplantation alone.

For bladder-drained pancreas transplants, urologic complications are common (Table 14.3). Approximately 35% of bladder-drained pancreas transplants eventually need enteric conversion by removing the pancreas with its duodenal segment from the bladder and reanastomosing it to a loop of small bowel. If possible, the conversion is delayed until at least 6 months after transplantation, at which time the risk for acute rejection is small and the doses of immunosuppressants are relatively low.

Table 14.2.   Technical complications in the first year after transplantation in 500 SPK transplants

Complication	Number of Patients[a] (%)
Enzymatic leak after bladder drainage	60/388 (15.5)
Enzymatic leak after primary enteric drainage	9/112 (8)
Pancreas thrombosis	5 (1)
Kidney thrombosis	4 (0.8)
Ureteral leak/stricture	7 (1.4)
Intraabdominal abscess	15 (3.0)
Peritonitis and fluid collections	58 (11.6)
Wound infection/dehiscence	60 (12.0)
Other	4 (0.8)

[a]Denominator of 500 transplants unless otherwise stated.
From Sollinger HW, Odorico JS, Knechtle SJ, et al. Experience with 500 simultaneous pancreas–kidney transplants. *Ann Surg* 1998;228:284–296, with permission.

Table 14.3.   Urologic complications in 388 bladder-drained SPK transplants

Complication	Number of Patients (%)
Urinary tract infection	242 (62.5)
Hematuria	69 (17.7)
Duodenal segment/bladder leak	60 (15.4)
Urethral stricture	11 (2.8)
Urethral disruption	10 (2.5)
Ureteral stricture	4 (1.03)
Ureteral leak	3 (0.77)

From Sollinger HW, Odorico JS, Knechtle SJ, et al. Experience with 500 simultaneous pancreas-kidney transplants. *Ann Surg* 1998;228:284–296, with permission.

Enzyme and Urine Leaks

A leakage from the duodenal segment is most often encountered within the first 3 months after transplantation and is the most frequent serious postoperative complication. For bladder-drained pancreas transplants, leaks occur in about 15% of patients. Enteric-drained pancreas transplants have a lower leak frequency (8%), but the complication more often leads to graft loss. Patients present with sudden onset of abdominal pain, which may be agonizing, and the serum amylase level is often elevated. For bladder-drained pancreas transplants, the diagnosis of urine leak is most often made with a cystogram or radionuclide scan (see Chapter 12). Reexploration is usually required, with closure of the leak or enteric conversion. In some patients with very small leaks, conservative therapy, consisting of placement of a Foley catheter for several weeks, is adequate. Small leaks may be difficult to detect radiologically and are suggested by recurrence of pain after removal of the Foley catheter.

Leaks from enteric-drained pancreas transplants are heralded by the sudden onset of severe abdominal pain, rising amylase and creatinine levels, and fever. They are particularly dangerous because of the intraperitoneal spillage of enteric succus. Diagnosis must not be delayed. Urgent operative intervention is usually required, although contained leaks can sometimes be managed successfully by percutaneous drainage.

Graft Pancreatitis

Pancreatitis of the allograft is a common postoperative complication and can occur in a variety of settings. In the immediate postoperative period, the effects of preservation and handling of the pancreas may induce a transient mild hyperamylasemia without significant clinical consequence. Pancreas rejection may also be heralded by an increase in serum amylase levels, which may be an important marker of rejection in PAK or PTA transplantation. Enzymatic leaks may also cause hyperamylasemia.

For bladder-drained pancreas transplants, reflux pancreatitis has been described and is believed to be caused by the irritant effects of refluxing urine on the pancreas. It is most common in patients with distended neurogenic bladders. It is managed by Foley drainage, often followed by self-catheterization to avoid high urinary residuals; α_1-adrenergic receptor blocking agents such as terazosin (Hytrin) may be useful. Enteric conversion may be required.

Vascular Thrombosis

Vascular thrombosis is a well-recognized complication after pancreas transplantation. Systemic anticoagulation with low-dose heparin or dextran infusions is routinely employed at many centers for several days after transplantation. Dextran infusion occasionally causes acute renal failure with tubular vacuolization—an occurrence that may cause diagnostic confusion. Vascular thrombosis of the pancreas can be caused by either arterial or venous thrombosis. In the case of arterial thrombosis, which is rare, the pancreas on reexploration appears soft and pale. In contrast, venous thrombosis is characterized by a large, engorged, dark-blue discolored pancreatic graft.

Pancreatic vascular thrombosis usually presents as abdominal pain with persistent elevation of blood sugar levels and hyperamylasemia. It may be difficult to differentiate from other causes of postoperative pain and graft dysfunction. Diagnosis is usually made radiologically with US or magnetic resonance angiography (MRA), but exploration is required if the results of diagnostic tests are equivocal or if the clinical situation deteriorates. The thrombosed pancreatic graft must be removed immediately because it constitutes a life-threatening focus of infection and toxemia.

Intraabdominal Abscess

Serious infections are more common after pancreas transplantation than after kidney transplantation alone, and in most series, they are the most common cause of death. The most feared complication is the formation of intraabdominal abscesses or infected peripancreatic fluid collections. In most instances, conservative therapy with antibiotics and percutaneously inserted drains is adequate; if the patient does not respond or infection persists, however, abdominal exploration and possible pancreatectomy should be considered early on. A late complication of peripancreatic infection is the development of a mycotic aneurysm at the site of the arterial anastomosis, resulting in life-threatening bleeding. If the diagnosis of a mycotic aneurysm is suspected, it must be confirmed by angiography, and the pancreas must be removed.

Complications Specific to Bladder-Drained Pancreas Transplants

Urinary Tract Infections

UTIs occur with a high frequency after pancreas transplantation with bladder drainage. In some cases, persistent UTIs are caused by sutures protruding from the anastomotic site; these sutures have to be removed through a cystoscope. In some cases, stone formation around retained sutures is noted. Use of absorbable sutures may prevent this problem.

Recurrent UTIs are a troublesome clinical problem. They are likely a result of the altered physiologic milieu of the bladder because of pancreatic exocrine secretions. Multiple recurrent UTIs are best treated by enteric conversion.

Hematuria

Hematuria after pancreas transplantation with bladder drainage may occur in the acute postoperative period or chronically. Whereas acute postoperative hematuria is usually caused by a bleeding vessel, either from the suture line or from the duodenal segment, chronic hematuria may be caused by an ulcer in the duodenal segment, granulation tissue at the suture line, or persistent cystitis. In acute cases, cystoscopy, clot evacuation, and cauterization of the bleeding point are usually sufficient. Chronic hematuria is usually treated by excision of the inflammatory focus, removal of sutures, or enteric conversion.

Urethritis

Sterile urethritis with dysuria and balanitis occurs after bladder-drained pancreas transplantation because of the irritant effect of pancreatic enzymes on the lower urinary tract mucosa; urethral strictures sometimes result. They can usually be treated conservatively by Foley drainage or suprapubic cystostomy; enteric conversion is sometimes required.

Metabolic Abnormalities

Complications can arise in bladder-drained pancreas transplantation as a consequence of the loss of large quantities of alkaline, enzyme-rich pancreatic fluid through the urinary tract. Metabolic acidosis, hyponatremia, and extracellular fluid volume depletion may develop, and oral, and sometimes intravenous, sodium chloride and bicarbonate supplementation are required. If patients are receiving tacrolimus, the bicarbonate should be administered at least 2 hours before or after the dose to avoid impaired tacrolimus absorption.

Immunosuppressive Therapy

Immunosuppressive therapy for all forms of whole-organ pancreas transplantation is the same in principle as for kidney transplantation alone and is discussed in detail in Chapter 4. Because of the frequency of acute rejection episodes in SPK transplantation, there is a tendency to use more aggressive immunosuppressive protocols with antibody induction and tacrolimus maintenance therapy often in combination with mycophenolate mofetil. It may be wise to maintain somewhat higher than usual cyclosporine or tacrolimus levels.

Diagnosis of Rejection

The diagnosis of rejection after pancreas transplantation may be extremely difficult and is best diagnosed with percutaneous biopsy. This difficulty can be explained by the histologic sequence of events, which is characterized by a cellular infiltrate first involving the exocrine pancreatic tissues. In the initial phases of the rejection process, the islets are spared, and serum glucose remains normal. Only at the later stages of rejection, when fibrosis, inflammation, and destruction of the islets occur, does the patient become hyperglycemic. At this stage, rejection is usually irreversible. Rejection must be recognized early, before the development of hyperglycemia, to prevent complete destruction of islet tissues.

In SPK transplantation, the kidney allograft is usually involved first in the rejection process, and a significant elevation of serum creatinine levels or a kidney biopsy permits the diagnosis of rejection to be made. Treating the kidney allograft rejection usually adequately treats the concomitant pancreas rejection.

The timely diagnosis of pancreas rejection in PAK and PTA transplantation is much more difficult, which may explain their inferior results. Markers of pancreas injury include levels of serum amylase, lipase, and human anodal trypsinogen. Timed urine collections for amylase (expressed as units per hour, typically in a 4-hour collection) are useful in bladder-drained pancreas transplants; the excretion decreases in the early phase of rejection when only the exocrine gland is involved. The definitive diagnosis of pancreas rejection requires invasive techniques, such as transcystoscopic biopsy of the head of the pancreas or percutaneous biopsy using an 18-gauge disposable automatic needle (see Chapter 13), both of which carry a small risk for bleeding and fistula formation. A classification system has been proposed for the pathologic diagnosis of rejection and as a guide to therapy (see Papadimitriou et al. in "Selected Readings," below).

Effect of Pancreas Transplantation on Secondary Diabetic Complications

The purpose of pancreas transplantation is to improve the quality of life of patients with end-stage diabetic nephropathy over and above that which can be achieved by kidney transplantation alone. This is achieved by normalization of carbohydrate metabolism, which frees the patients from years of insulin therapy and dietary constraint, and by arresting, preventing, and even reversing secondary diabetic complications. Although there is no question that a successful procedure makes the patient insulin independent, the effect on secondary manifestations of diabetes is less clear-cut and is the subject of ongoing research and controversy.

Nephropathy

When renal allografts from nondiabetic donors are placed into a diabetic recipient, morphologic signs of diabetic nephropathy in the form of thickening of the glomerular basement membrane appear as early as 2 years after transplantation. No microscopic evidence of diabetic nephropathy is seen up to 4 years after SPK transplantation. Mesangial and glomerular volume and basement membrane thickness are less after SPK transplantation than after kidney transplantation alone. Whereas changes of diabetic nephropathy can often be seen on biopsy specimens of kidneys transplanted alone into diabetic patients, loss of grafts to diabetic nephropathy is unusual, although renal function is better maintained in recipients of SPK transplants. Within the time frame of followup presently available, the benefit of SPK transplantation with respect to diabetic nephropathy is usually more evident histologically than clinically.

Neuropathy

Pancreas transplantation alone in preuremic patients results in significant improvement in motor and sensory nerve conduction velocity. Subjective and objective improvement of established neuropathy occurs after both SPK and kidney transplantation alone, although a variety of markers of autonomic function improve more after SPK transplantation. It is difficult to differentiate between improvement in the uremic and diabetic components of neuropathy, and the added benefit of SPK transplantation may take months or years to manifest clinically.

Retinopathy

Initial studies reported that neither PTA nor SPK transplantation produced a greater improvement in retinopathy than kidney transplantation alone. It is possible that this disappointing failure to show benefit related to the relatively short period of followup. Long-term studies have observed a trend in favor of pancreas transplantation during followup of at least 3 to 4 years.

Microcirculation

Using thermography, muscle oxygen tension measurements, and laser Doppler determination, SPK transplantation has been shown to have a beneficial effect on the microcirculation that is greater than with kidney transplantation alone. This objective determination is strengthened by the clinical observation that SPK transplant recipients suffer fewer amputations and diabetic ulcers of the lower extremities than do diabetic patients receiving kidney transplantation alone.

Coronary Artery Disease

Many centers apply more stringent criteria to exclude significant coronary artery disease in candidates for SPK transplantation than in candidates for kidney transplantation alone. Such a policy prevents comparative evaluation of the effect of the pancreas transplantation on the progress of the coronary artery disease. As greater confidence with SPK transplantation has developed, some centers are accepting patients at greater cardiac risk, and comparative groups have shown that the risk for early cardiac-related mortality is equal or greater in the SPK transplant recipients.

Quality of Life

After the first few months following a successful SPK transplantation, patients generally report a better quality of life than that of recipients of kidney transplants alone. SPK transplant recipients reportedly require less sickness pension, have more full-time employment, and have fewer lost workdays. It is difficult to quantitate the sense of liberation felt by lifetime diabetic patients who no longer must self-inject insulin and monitor every morsel they eat.

Patient Survival

Randomized, controlled trials comparing the survival benefit of kidney alone versus SPK transplantation for diabetics have not been performed. Uncontrolled data, however, suggest that SPK recipients have improved patient survival rates over diabetic patients transplanted with a kidney alone. The observed survival advantage may be a result of patient selection, but is reassuring in that the higher morbidity of pancreas transplantation does not appear to be reflected in a survival disadvantage.

Choice of Procedure

Patients and their physician advocates may be faced with a difficult dilemma when choosing between a kidney transplantation alone and an SPK transplantation. This dilemma is reflected in the ongoing discussions on this topic in the medical and transplantation literature. SPK transplantation is associated with increased early morbidity but may offer better long-term quality of life and the greater potential for stabilization or improvement of diabetic complications. Most centers recommend kidney transplantation alone when a living donor is available because this option offers the best long-term patient and graft survival; a PAK transplantation may follow. Patients choosing between SPK and deceased donor kidney transplantation must be thoroughly informed regarding the comparative risks and benefits of the two procedures and, in particular, must have realistic expectations regarding the effect of pancreas transplantation on secondary complications. Patients should also be aware that, in most regions of the United States, the waiting time for an SPK transplant is about one-third of that for a deceased donor transplant alone, and that a prolonged period of dialysis may expose them to additional risk. Patients seeking an isolated pancreas transplant in the presence of normal or near-normal renal function (PTA or PAK) should be made aware of the data suggesting a relative survival disadvantage of this procedure (Fig 14.3). This survival disadvantage is likely a reflection of the excellent survival of diabetics whose renal function is good. The rationale to proceed with an isolated pancreas transplant should be based on the judgment that quality of life will be so improved by the avoidance of the need for insulin that the survival disadvantage is outweighed.

TRANSPLANTATION OF PANCREATIC ISLETS

Transplantation of the islets of Langerhans is an appealing alternative to whole-organ pancreas transplantation, primarily because of the lowered risk of surgical complications. Recall that the pancreas is predominantly an exocrine gland and that clusters of endocrine cell, the islets, are scattered throughout the gland. These islets contain the glucose-responsive, insulin-secreting beta cells. The autoimmune destruction of these beta cells is the cause of type 1 diabetes mellitus. Replacement of the beta cell mass provides the freedom from insulin therapy enjoyed after successful pancreas transplantation, and the exocrine pancreas is unnecessary for insulin independence. Separation of the islets from the exocrine pancreas allows transplantation with minimally invasive techniques. More importantly, islet transplantation does not require vascular and allograft duodenal anastomoses, thus avoiding the major sources of surgical complications.

Until recently, success with islet transplantation has been poor when compared to whole-organ pancreas transplantation. The results of more than 400 islet transplants performed up to 1998 showed insulin independence in only 8% of recipients at 1 year, compared to 80% or more of pancreas transplant recipients. The so-called Edmonton protocol (see Shapiro et al. in "Selected Readings," below) generated new optimism for the success of islet transplantation. Using a steroid-free immunosuppression protocol (based on sirolimus, tacrolimus, and daclizumab), insulin independence was achieved in a small group of type 1 diabetic patients, without renal failure, receiving islet transplants alone. The recipients selected for this trial suffered hypoglycemic unawareness and/or "metabolic instability." The investigators transplanted the islets immediately after isolation, using a radiologically guided, transhepatic portal venous infusion technique. Besides the steroid-free immunosuppression, the success of the Edmonton protocol clearly depended on transplantation of an adequate islet mass, which often necessitated multiple transplants with islets isolated from two to four donors. Since the original publication of this protocol, several other programs have reported similar experience and approximately 80% of patients remain insulin-independent after 2 years.

Current Status

The knowledge, expertise, and expenses required to isolate a large number of quality human islets for transplantation are substantial. The U.S. Food and Drug Administration (FDA) deems isolated human islets for transplantation a biological product and currently requires an approved investigational new drug application and Institutional Review Board (IRB) approval for investigators conducting clinical islet transplantation research (see Chapter 4, Part III). The FDA also requires that investigators isolating human islets for transplantation use current "Good Manufacturing Processes (cGMP)," such as clean room facilities, careful record keeping, and quality controls. As of 2004, the National Center for Research Resources and the National Institute of Diabetes and Digestive and Kidney Diseases, components of the United States National Institutes of Health, support geographically dispersed Islet Resource Centers to provide pancreatic islets of cGMP-quality to eligible investigators for use in FDA-approved, IRB-approved transplantation protocols. Islet transplantation thus remains an experimental technique and is yet to become part of the routine diabetic care.

Islet Isolation

Fundamental steps in the process of islet isolation are procurement of the donor pancreas, transportation to the isolation laboratory, enzymatic digestion of the glandular tissue, separation, and purification of the islets. In most laboratories, it may take from one to four donor pancreases to yield enough islets for investigators to consider the mass adequate for a recipient. In the case of a patient who requires 3 transplants, for example, it may take as many 12 donor pancreases to provide persistent insulin independence. The preferential allocation of pancreases from the best donors to whole-organ transplantation may explain the multiple organs required to provide adequate islets.

Improved transplant success may result from postisolation culture of the islets for up to 72 hours prior to transplantation, and this may permit insulin independence with a single-donor transplant. The culture period may improve success by providing the time to measure the viability of the islets, time that is not available with immediate transplants. It is not clear whether the culture actually decreases the number of isolations required per recipient. Careful recipient and donor selection may also be a factor allowing single-donor success.

Recipient Selection

Like other allografts, islet transplant recipients require immunosuppression to prevent rejection. Therefore, patients are selected for clinical trials based on the risks of immunosuppression as compared to ongoing insulin therapy for diabetic control. Like whole-organ pancreas transplantation, the majority of recipients who received islets prior to the Edmonton protocol received a renal transplant either prior to or simultaneously with the islet transplant. For these patients there is a minimal additional risk of immunosuppression for the islet transplant, beyond that required for the renal transplant. For this reason, investigators continue to enroll type 1 diabetic patients with renal failure in clinical trials of islet after kidney and simultaneous islet kidney transplantation.

For islet transplantation alone in nonuremic patients, investigators look for life-threatening, or at least severe, problems with blood glucose control to balance the risks of immunosuppression. Hypoglycemic unawareness is a readily documented indication. "Metabolic instability" is a less-precise inclusion criterion for clinical trials, but a limited number of fully compliant patients working diligently with an attentive diabetologist, clearly manifest this severe problem.

Future Directions

For the near future, it is likely that islet transplantation will remain an investigational procedure, although efforts are underway to achieve FDA licensing for the biologic product of isolated human islets. Achieving insulin independence with one donor pancreas per recipient is one goal investigators look to meet through improving the isolation process, quality assessment, and, potentially, donor islet or recipient therapies. *In vitro* culture methods and cryopreservation of the islet product may allow precise timing of the islet transplant, perhaps in conjunction with recipient therapies designed to minimize immunosuppression or induce tolerance. Transplantation tolerance, eliminating the need for long-term immunosuppression, might allow patients to undergo islet transplantation earlier in the course of their disease, providing improved quality of life, and lowering the risk of long-term complications. Encapsulation of the islets within a device that bars the immune response, for example, by preventing recipient immune cells from contacting the islets, is an enticing means to achieve tolerance, but has met with limited success to date. At the time of this writing, information for professionals and patients about current clinical trials is available at http://www.isletservice.org.

SELECTED READINGS

Frezza EE, Corry RJ. Donor management and selection for pancreas transplantation. In: Hakim N, Stratta R, Gray D, eds. *Pancreas and islet transplantation.* Oxford: Oxford University Press, 2002:79–92.

Gruessner AC, Sutherland DER. Pancreas transplant outcomes for United States (US) and non-US cases as reported to the United Network for Organ Sharing (UNOS) and the International Pancreas Transplant Registry (IPTR) as of October 2002. In: Cecka JM, Terasaki PI, eds. *Clinical transplants 2002.* Los Angeles: UCLA Immunogenetics Center, 2003:41–46.

Hariharan S, Pirsch JD, Lu CY, et al. Pancreas after kidney transplantation. *J Am Soc Nephrol* 2002;13:1109–1118.

Herzog CA, Marwick TH, Pheley AM, et al. Dobutamine stress echocardiography for the detection of significant coronary artery disease in renal transplant candidates. *Am J Kidney Dis* 1999;33:1080–1090.

Joseph JT, Baines LS, Morris MC, et al. Quality of life after kidney and pancreas transplantation: a review. *Am J Kidney Dis* 2003;42:431–445.

Knoll GA, Nichol G. Dialysis, kidney transplantation, or pancreas transplantation for patients with diabetes mellitus and renal failure: a decision analysis of treatment options. *J Am Soc Nephrol* 2003;14:500–515.

Lederer E. Pancreas transplants for diabetic nephropathy: a time for reassessment. *Am J Kidney Dis* 2000;35:1238–1241.

Manske CL, Thomas W, Wang Y, et al. Screening diabetic transplant candidates for coronary artery disease: identification of a low risk subgroup. *Kidney Int* 1993;44:617–621.

Papadimitriou JC, Drachenberg CB, Wiland A, et al. Histologic grading of acute allograft rejection in pancreas needle biopsy: correlation to serum enzymes, glycemia, and response to immunosuppressive treatment. *Transplantation* 1998;66:1741–1745.

Pirsch JD. Medical evaluation for pancreas transplantation: evolving concepts. *Transplant Proc* 2001;33:3489–3491.

Rabbat CG, Treleaven DJ, Russell JD, et al. Prognostic value of myocardial perfusion studies in patients with end-stage renal disease assessed for kidney or kidney–pancreas transplantation: a meta-analysis. *J Am Soc Nephrol* 2003;14:431–439.

Reddy KS, Stablein D, Taranto S, et al. Long-term survival following simultaneous kidney–pancreas transplantation versus kidney transplantation alone in patients with type 1 diabetes mellitus and renal failure. *Am J Kidney Dis* 2003;41:464–470.

Robertson PR. Islet transplantation as a treatment for diabetes—a work in progress. *N Engl J Med* 2004;350:694–705.

Shapiro AM, Lakey JR, Ryan EA, et al. Islet transplantation in seven patients with type 1 diabetes mellitus using a glucocorticoid-free immunosuppressive regime. *N Engl J Med* 2000;243:230–238.

Troppman C, Gjertson DW, Cecka JM, et al. Impact of portal venous pancreas graft drainage on kidney graft outcomes in simultaneous pancreas-kidney recipients reported to UNOS. *Amer J Transplant* 2004;4:544–553.

Kidney Transplantation in Children

Samhar I. Al-Akash and Robert B. Ettenger

Kidney transplantation is universally accepted as the therapy of choice for children with end-stage renal disease (ESRD). Approximately two-thirds of pediatric patients with ESRD ultimately receive a kidney transplant. Successful transplantation in children and adolescents not only ameliorates uremic symptoms, but also allows for significant improvement of delayed skeletal growth, sexual maturation, cognitive performance, and psychosocial functioning. The child with a well-functioning kidney transplant can enjoy a quality of life that cannot be achieved by any form of dialysis therapy.

Current success in pediatric renal transplantation is attributed to improvements in transplantat technology, immunosuppressive therapy, and the provision of age-appropriate clinical care. For pediatric patients of all ages, transplantation results in better survival than dialysis. Five-year survival rates in transplant patients range from 94% to 97%, while in dialyzed patients the survival rate ranges from 75% to 87%. Nevertheless, success in pediatric kidney transplantation remains a challenging undertaking. Children and adolescents are constantly growing, developing, and changing. Each developmental stage produces a series of medical, biologic, and psychologic challenges that must be appropriately addressed if truly successful graft outcome and rehabilitation are to be realized.

Much of the statistical data reviewed in this chapter comes from databases that have provided an invaluable resource for the advancement of pediatric transplantation. These databases have enabled the evaluation and extrapolation of data from multiple pediatric renal transplant programs that tend to be small when compared with their adult counterparts. Major databases referred to are the *North America Pediatric Renal Transplant Cooperative Study* (NAPRTCS), the *Scientific Registry of Transplant Recipients* (SRTR), and the *United States Renal Data System* (USRDS) annual report (see Websites).

EPIDEMIOLOGY OF END-STAGE RENAL DISEASE IN CHILDREN

Incidence

The incidence and prevalence of treated pediatric ESRD have been increasing since 1989. As of 2000, the incidence rate of new cases of ESRD in children 0 to 19 years of age was 15 per million U.S. child population per year. The point prevalence of ESRD in this population is 70 per million U.S. child population. The incidence of ESRD increases with age, with the highest incidence observed in children between 15 and 19 years of age (28 per million).

Adolescents comprise approximately 50% of treated pediatric ESRD patients.

There is a wide variation by ethnic group in the incidence rates of treated ESRD. African American children have the highest incidence rate of 27 per million, as compared with 12 per million white children, 15 per million Asian and Pacific Islander children, and 17 per million Native American children. The incidence is higher in African Americans across all age groups, but is most prominent in the 15- to 19-year-old age group (60 per million African Americans compared with 20 per million whites). Over the past 20 years, incident rates for white pediatric patients have remained constant. For African American patients and other nonwhite ethnicities, however, the rates of ESRD have more than doubled. The incidence of glomerulonephritis as a cause of ESRD is up to three times higher in African American pediatric patients than in white pediatric patients; there is no racial predilection for other causes of pediatric renal disease. According to the NAPRTCS Dialysis Registry, patients with focal segmental glomerulosclerosis (FSGS) make up almost 24% of all pediatric African American dialysis patients, and more than 30% of adolescent African American dialysis patients. Boys have higher incidence of treated ESRD than girls in all age groups.

Etiology

Glomerular diseases account for about 30% and congenital, hereditary, and cystic diseases for 26% of cases of pediatric ESRD (Table 15.1). Although incidence rates for glomerular diseases have remained steady in the pediatric population, the incidence rates for patients with congenital, hereditary, and cystic diseases have trended upward over the past 20 years. In contrast to adults, ESRD caused by diabetes mellitus or hypertension is rare in children.

The etiology of ESRD varies significantly by age. Congenital, hereditary, and cystic diseases cause ESRD in more than 50% of children 0 to 4 years of age, whereas glomerulonephritis and FSGS account for nearly 40% of cases of ESRD for patients 10 to 19 years of age. The most common diagnosis in transplant children is structural disease (49%), followed by various forms of glomerulonephritis (14%) and focal segmental glomerulosclerosis (12%).

Access to Transplantation

As of 2003, the NAPRTCS registry reported that 7,651 children have received 8,399 transplants since 1987. At the time of transplantation, approximately 46% of pediatric recipients of kidney transplants are older than 12 years of age, 34% are 6 to 12 years of age, 15% are between the ages of 2 and 5 years, and approximately 5% are younger than 2 years of age. Approximately 60% are male, 62% are white, 16% are African American, and 16% are Hispanic.

Pediatric transplants constitute 4% to 6% of all kidney transplants in the United States. The number of pediatric kidney transplants has remained essentially constant during the last decade at approximately 700 each year. Over the same period the number

Table 15.1. Incidence of treated end-stage renal disease in pediatric patients[a] according to primary disease, 1993–1997

Primary Renal Disease	Incidence (%)
Glomerulonephritis (GN)	**29.8**
Focal segmental glomerulosclerosis	10.0
Membranoproliferative GN	2.5
Rapidly progressive GN	2.1
IgA nephropathy	1.6
Goodpasture syndrome	0.7
Membranous nephropathy	0.5
Other proliferative GN	1.5
Unspecified GN	10.3
Cystic, hereditary, and congenital disease	**26.0**
Renal hypoplasia, dysplasia	8.9
Congenital obstructive uropathy	6.7
Alport syndrome, other familial disease	2.7
Autosomal dominant polycystic disease	2.0
Autosomal recessive polycystic disease	1.0
Prune belly syndrome	1.1
Congenital nephrotic syndrome	1.2
Medullary cystic disease (nephronophthisis)	1.1
Cystinosis	0.7
Other	0.3
Interstitial nephritis, pyelonephritis	**9.1**
Nephrolithiasis, obstruction, gout	3.2
Chronic interstitial nephritis	2.0
Chronic pyelonephritis, reflux nephropathy	2.7
Nephropathy caused by other agents	0.9
Secondary GN, vasculitis	**8.9**
Systemic lupus erythematosus	4.6
Hemolytic uremic syndrome	1.9
Henoch-Schönlein purpura	0.9
Wegener granulomatosis	0.7
Hypertension	**4.8**
Hypertension, no primary renal disease	4.5
Renal artery stenosis or occlusion	0.3
Miscellaneous conditions	**3.8**
Diabetes mellitus	1.6
Neoplasms	0.6
Tubular necrosis (no recovery)	1.0
Uncertain etiology	**7.1**

[a] Patients younger than 20 years of age.
Modified from the USRDS 1999 annual report.

of adult kidney transplants has increased by nearly 50% (see Chapter 1, Fig 1.1). The rates for both living-related and deceased donor renal transplantation (measured as transplants per 100 dialysis patient years) are more than double in children than in adults, and are highest in the 5- to 9-year-old group. As of 2003, close to 60% of all pediatric kidney transplants came from living donors (compared to approximately 40% in adults) and there is a trend toward a decrease in the numbers of deceased donor transplants. This trend is undoubtedly a result of the awareness that early transplantation is the best therapeutic option for children with ESRD combined with the increased waiting times for deceased donor organs.

Children continue to represent an ever-decreasing percentage of the national waiting list for deceased donors. Over the last decade their number has increased by 11%, while the adult list has more than doubled in number. Median waiting times have remained roughly constant for pediatric patients. For the last year that these data could be calculated (2001), children 1 to 5 years of age waited a median time of 205 days for a kidney transplant; children 6 to 10 years waited a median of 338 days, and adolescents waited a median of 422 days. The median waiting time for all pediatric transplants is less than half of that for adults. This difference reflects kidney allocation rules (see Chapter 3, Table 3.4) that are specifically designed to favor children because of their unique needs for growth and development.

Timing of Transplantation

Renal transplantation should be considered when renal replacement therapy is indicated. In children, dialysis may be required before transplantation to optimize nutritional and metabolic conditions, to achieve an appropriate size in small children, or to keep a patient stable until a suitable donor is available. Many centers want a recipient to weigh at least 8 to 10 kg, both to minimize the risk for vascular thrombosis and to accommodate an adult-sized kidney. In infants with ESRD, a target weight of 10 kg may not be achieved until 12 to 24 months of age. At experienced centers, however, transplantation has been successful in children who weighed less than 10 kg or who were younger than 6 months of age.

Preemptive transplantation (i.e., transplantation without prior dialysis) accounts for 24% of all pediatric renal transplantations. The major reason cited by patients and families for the decision to undertake preemptive transplantation is the desire to avoid dialysis. Candidates for preemptive transplantation should have careful psychological assessment before transplantation because there may be a greater tendency for noncompliance in children who have not experienced dialysis. Nevertheless, there appears to be no impairment in graft outcome in pediatric recipients who have undergone preemptive transplantation when compared with those who have undergone dialysis before transplantation, and some data suggest a small improvement in allograft outcome. The reasons for the improved graft survival are unknown. Because of the prolonged waiting time for deceased donors, most preemptive kidney transplants are from living donors.

Patient and Graft Survival

Both patient and graft survival rates have improved steadily since systematic recording began in 1987. Patient survival after transplantation remains superior to that achieved by dialysis for all pediatric age groups. The overall 1- and 5-year patient survival rates are now 97% and 95%, respectively, for all primary transplants, and are marginally better for recipients of living donors than for deceased donors. Patients younger than 2 years of age have lower survival rates. The 3-year patient survival rate for deceased donor recipients is 90% and 94% for living donor recipients. Infection accounts for more than 30% of deaths. Other causes include cardiopulmonary disease (16%), malignancy (11%), cardiopulmonary (16%). Approximately 45% of patients who die do so with a functioning graft.

Graft survival rates for pediatric transplants are somewhat better than for adult transplants. One- and 5-year graft survivals are 95% and 83%, respectively, for living donor recipients and 91% and 73%, respectively, for deceased donor recipients. Of the more than 8,000 pediatric kidney transplantations reported to NAPRTCS since 1987, approximately 26% have failed. Chronic rejection accounts for 33% of graft failures, with acute rejection accounting for 16%. Other causes include vascular thrombosis (11%), recurrence of original disease (6.6%), and patient noncompliance (4.6%). Although some causes of graft failure, such as graft thrombosis and recurrence of the original disease, have remained constant during the past 10 years, loss from acute rejection has decreased dramatically. Technical issues remain a challenge and are a more common cause of graft loss in children than in adults.

PROGNOSTIC FACTORS INFLUENCING GRAFT SURVIVAL

The following factors are important determinants of the improving graft survival reported in pediatric patients. Long-term renal function is a particularly important consideration in pediatric renal transplantation because of its impact on posttransplant skeletal growth.

Donor Source

As noted above, short- and long-term graft and patient survival rates are better in recipients of living donor transplants in all pediatric age groups. Younger transplant recipients benefit the most from living donor transplantation and enjoy a 20% to 30% better graft survival rate 5 years after transplantation. Shorter cold ischemia time, better human leukocyte antigen (HLA) matches, lower acute rejection rates, and better preoperative preparation help to account for the better outcome in recipients of living donor kidneys.

Recipient Age

In the past, there has been a trend for younger children, especially those younger than 2 years of age, to have lower graft survival rates than older children, especially with deceased donor kidneys. Now that trend seems to be reversed. Some studies even suggest that infant recipients of adult kidneys with immediate function may have the longest half-lives of any type of kidney transplant.

Data from the SRTR published in 2003 documents that pediatric recipients younger than age 11 years who received living donor transplants had 5-year graft survival rates that were as good as, if not better than, recipients in older age groups. The rates were 92% for infants younger than 1 year, 81% for children 1 to 5 years old, and 80% for children 6 to 10 years old. The results for deceased donor recipients were also better in this age group than in adults generally. Recipients 1 to 5 years of age have a 5-year graft survival of 68% and recipients 6 to 10 years of age have a 5-year rate of 72%, the best of all age groups.

On the other hand, the long-term graft survival rates in adolescents are not as good as those seen in younger children, even though the short-term outcome is similar. The 1- and 5-year graft survival rates for adolescent recipients of living donor kidneys is 94% and 73%, respectively. For deceased donor kidneys, the graft outcomes were 91% and 54%, respectively. The results for 5 years are the poorest of all age groups. Higher rates of medication noncompliance, an unexplained high incidence of graft thrombosis, and a high recurrence rate of FSGS, which is the most common acquired cause of ESRD in this age group, have all been cited as potential causes for the reduced long-term outcome.

Donor Age

For all deceased donor recipients, kidneys from donors age 11 to 17 years provide optimal graft survival and function. This group is followed next by donors ages 18 to 34, 6 to 10, and then 35 to 49 years. Grafts from donors younger than 5 years old fare more poorly, and grafts from patients older than 50 years fare most poorly. Although transplanted kidneys grow in size with the growth of the recipient, transplantation with deceased donor kidneys from donors younger than age 6 years is associated with markedly decreased graft survival. The 5-year graft survival rate for recipients of deceased donor kidneys from donors younger than 1 year of age is only approximately 45%, compared with 58% and 64% for recipients of grafts from donors 2 to 5 years of age and older than 6 years of age, respectively. Kidneys from donors age 11 to 17 years have the best 5-year graft survival of approximately 72%. Children younger than 5 years old receiving a kidney from donors younger than 6 years old have the highest relative risk of graft failure.

Ethnicity

African American ethnicity is associated with a worse outcome. At 5 years posttransplant, African American children have graft outcomes of 53% and 69% for recipients of deceased donor and living-related kidneys, respectively. For white and Hispanic recipients, graft survival at 5 years is 70% and 64%, respectively, for recipients of deceased donor kidneys, and 82% for living donor grafts. African American children not only have poorer graft survival, but poorer renal function.

Human Leukocyte Antigen Matching in Children

In pediatric transplantation, most living donor transplants come from parents. Long-term graft survival is best when the donor is an HLA-identical sibling. When considering transplants from

HLA haplotype-identical sibling donors, studies suggest that there is improved outcome when donor and recipient share "noninherited maternal antigens," as distinct from "noninherited paternal antigens" (see Chapter 3). With regard to deceased donor transplantation, improved outcome has been reported with the sharing of both HLA-B and HLA-DR antigens.

Presensitization

Repeated blood transfusions expose the recipient to a wide range of HLA antigens and may result in sensitization to these antigens, leading to higher rates of rejection and graft failures. The graft failure rate increases by up to 40% for recipients with more than five blood transfusions before transplantation, as compared with those who had fewer transfusions. Blood transfusions have become less common since human recombinant erythropoietin became an integral part of ESRD therapy. It is surprising, however, that current USRDS data finds that hemoglobin levels in children on dialysis are lower than levels in their adult counterparts, and there is support for more aggressive management of anemia to forestall transfusions. Sensitization may also result from rejection of a previous transplant, and the 5-year graft survival for repeat deceased donor transplantations is approximately 20% lower.

Immunologic Factors

Immunologic parameters in younger children are different from those in adults and older children. Such differences include higher numbers of T and B cells, higher CD4+:CD8+ T-cell ratio, and increased blastogenic responses. These differences may account for increased immune responsiveness to HLA antigens and may be partly responsible for the higher rates of rejection that had been observed in children. With improved understanding and management of immunosuppression in pediatric patients, these higher rates of rejection have been significantly ameliorated.

Technical Factors and Delayed Graft Function

Surgical kidney transplant techniques for older children are similar to those in adults (see Chapter 7). Placement of the vascular anastomoses depends on the size of the child and the vessels. An extraperitoneal approach is usually accomplished with the venous anastomoses to the common or external iliac vein, and the arterial anastomoses to the common or external iliac artery. These vascular anastomoses tend to be more cephalad than for adult transplants.

Small children present difficult operative challenges. The relatively large size of the graft may result in longer anastomosis times, longer ischemia time, and subsequently higher rates of early graft dysfunction. When possible, the transplanted kidney is usually placed in an extraperitoneal location, although with very small children, the placement can be intraabdominal. The aorta and inferior vena cava are usually used for anastomoses to ensure adequate blood flow, but smaller vessels may be used. Vascular anastomosis may be problematic in a child with a previous hemodialysis access placed in the lower extremities or with a previous kidney transplant. Children should be evaluated thoroughly before transplantation to identify any potential anastomotic difficulties. Unidentified vascular anomalies may lead to prolonged anastomosis times and subsequently higher rates of delayed graft function (DGF) and graft thrombosis.

Occasionally, native kidney nephrectomy is necessary at the time of transplantation. While this can be done routinely in living donor transplantations where there is little cold ischemia time, it is preferable to avoid this, when possible, in recipients of deceased donor transplants. Native nephrectomy at the time of transplantation prolongs the surgical procedure and may predispose to "third spacing," which can complicate fluid management and contribute to an increase in DGF.

DGF is discussed in detail in Chapter 8. It occurs in approximately 5% of living donor and 18% of deceased donor transplants, and is associated with a reduced graft survival. In children with DGF, the 3-year graft survival rates are reduced by up 30%. Risk factors for DGF in children are more than five prior transfusions, prior transplantation, native nephrectomy, African American ethnicity, and a cold ischemia time of longer than 24 hours.

Antibody Induction

Antibody induction, with either polyclonal or monoclonal antibodies, is used either for prophylaxis against rejection or in a sequential manner to avoid nephrotoxicity resulting from early use of calcineurin inhibitors (see Chapter 4, Part IV). While the NAPRTCS database continues to show a nearly 14% reduction in the proportional hazard of graft loss with the use of antibody induction, this effect has decreased over time. In addition, the agents used for induction have changed markedly; nondepleting antibodies (see Chapter 4, Part II) are used in approximately 60% of all pediatric transplants done presently in the United States, whereas OKT3 is now rarely used for induction purposes.

Transplantation Center Volume

Transplant outcome in high-volume pediatric renal transplant centers has been reported to be superior to that found in lower-volume centers. High-volume centers (defined as the performance of more than 100 pediatric transplants between 1987 and 1995) reported a lower incidence of graft thrombosis and DGF, improved long-term graft survival, and more frequent use of antibody induction.

Cohort Year

The results of pediatric renal transplantation have been steadily improving. The current graft survival data at 1-year noted above represents an up to 15% improvement over the last 15 years. Five-year graft survival has improved by up to 5% over the same period. Graft outcome in transplants from deceased donors performed between 1995 and 2001 is now equivalent to the graft survival in living donor transplantation performed between 1987 and 1994.

RECURRENT RENAL DISEASE IN PEDIATRIC TRANSPLANTATION

Recurrent disease in the renal graft accounts for graft loss in almost 7% of primary transplantations and 10% in repeat transplantations. This is more than double that reported for adult transplantation (see Chapters 6 and 9, Part I). Both glomerular and metabolic diseases can recur with most recurrences caused by glomerular disease.

Glomerular Diseases

Focal and Segmental Glomerulosclerosis

FSGS is the most common cause of graft loss as a result of recurrent disease. For patients whose original disease was steroid-resistant nephrotic syndrome or confirmed FSGS, the disease recurs in 30% to 40% of patients undergoing primary transplantation. When the first transplant was lost to recurrence, FSGS recurs in 50% to 80% of those undergoing subsequent transplantation. The NAPRTCS database reports that grafts in approximately 20% to 30% of patients with the diagnosis of FSGS fail because of recurrence. The mean time to graft failure from recurrence is 17 months.

Recurrence is usually characterized by massive proteinuria, hypoalbuminemia, and nephrotic syndrome with edema or anasarca and hypercholesterolemia. It may present immediately or weeks to months after transplantation. Predictors of recurrence include rapid progression to ESRD from the time of initial diagnosis (less than 3 years), poor response to therapy, younger age at diagnosis (but older than 6 years of age), African American ethnicity, and the presence of mesangial proliferation in the native kidney. A protein permeability factor has been isolated from sera of patients with FSGS, and its concentration was found to correlate with recurrence and severity of disease in the transplanted kidney. The precise nature of this factor remains unclear, and there is no clinically approved assay to detect it.

Early posttransplant recognition of recurrent FSGS is important because plasmapheresis (which may lower the serum levels of protein permeability factor), and/or high-dose calcineurin-inhibitor may lead to significant reduction in graft losses because of recurrence. *In vitro* studies using rat glomeruli show that cyclosporine or tacrolimus, incubated with sera from FSGS patients, will inhibit the proteinuric effect of such sera. Thrice-daily cyclosporine may be used in doses that maintain whole-blood trough levels, as measured by fluorescent polarization immunoassay or enzyme-multiplied immunoassay technique, of between 200 and 400 ng/mL or higher, and is tapered slowly after achieving remission of the nephrotic syndrome and as cholesterol concentration decreases, or if significant toxicity develops. Some centers have used a high-dose continuous intravenous infusion of cyclosporine with similar improvement, or have used high dose or thrice-daily tacrolimus. Cyclophosphamide has also been reported to induce remission and sirolimus may prevent recurrence. Plasmapheresis is generally used with a frequency that matches disease severity and is occasionally required on a weekly basis for prolonged periods.

Some studies report that living-related donor transplant recipients suffer from a higher rate of recurrence. NAPRTCS data suggests that the graft outcome in recipients of living donor grafts with FSGS recurrence is no better than the outcome observed in recipients of deceased donor grafts that have not experienced recurrence. These data have led some pediatric transplant centers to reduce or discontinue the use of living-related donation for patients with FSGS. However, the controlled settings of living donor transplantation may allow certain benefits in the event that FSGS does recur. The lower incidence of DGF in living donation may permit augmentation of the calcineurin inhibitor dose. In addition, the preplanning implicit in living donation permits preoperative and early postoperative plasmapheresis, an approach that may potentially prevent or decrease the severity of recurrent disease.

Alport Syndrome

Alport syndrome, or hereditary glomerulonephritis, is a progressive disease often associated with neurosensory hearing loss and ocular abnormalities such as anterior lenticonus and cataracts. The inheritance pattern can be X-linked, autosomal recessive, and autosomal dominant. The abnormality in almost all patients stems from mutations in the α_3, α_4, or α_6 helices of type 4 collagen. In more than 80% of patients, Alport syndrome results from mutations in the COL4A5 gene on the X chromosome.

Strictly speaking, Alport syndrome itself does not recur; however, antiglomerular basement membrane (anti-GBM) glomerulonephritis may occur in approximately 3% to 4% of patients after transplantation and lead to graft loss. The antibodies causing the anti-GBM nephritis are usually directed against the α_5 chain of the noncollagenous portion of type IV collagen in the GBM, but antibodies against the α_3 chain have also been described. The risk appears to be greatest in patients with mutations of COL4A5 that prevent synthesis of the α_5 chain.

Anti-GBM glomerulonephritis presents as rapidly progressive crescentic glomerulonephritis with linear deposits of immunoglobulin (Ig) G along the basement membrane and commonly leads to graft loss. It usually occurs within the first posttransplant year. Asymptomatic cases with linear IgG deposits have also been reported. Treatment consists of plasmapheresis and cyclophosphamide, but such treatment is of only limited benefit. Retransplantation is associated with a high recurrence rate.

Membranoproliferative Glomerulonephritis

Histologic evidence of recurrence of membranoproliferative glomerulonephritis (MPGN) type I varies widely, with reported rates ranging from 20% to 70%. Graft loss occurs in up to 30% of cases. Histologic recurrence of type II disease occurs in virtually all cases, but graft loss is not inevitable and has been reported in up to 50% of patients (13% in the 2000 NAPRTCS database at a meantime posttransplant of 29 months). The presence of crescents in the native kidney biopsy may predict severe recurrence that often leads to graft loss. There is no proven treatment for recurrence of MPGN in children. Anecdotal case reports describe success with high dose corticosteroids, mycophenolate mofetil (MMF), or plasma exchange.

IgA Nephropathy and Henoch-Schönlein Purpura

Histological recurrence with mesangial IgA deposits is common and occurs in about half of patients with IgA nephropathy and in about 30% of patients with Henoch-Schönlein purpura (HSP). Most of the recurrences are asymptomatic, but graft loss may occur, often associated with crescent formation. Data from adult centers suggest that a fulminant presentation of IgA nephropathy as the original cause of ESRD predicts poor outcome in the transplanted kidney with disease recurrence. In the NAPRTCS database, only 5% to 8% of graft failures were because of recurrence in patients with IgA nephropathy or HSP.

Hemolytic Uremic Syndrome

Hemolytic uremic syndrome (HUS) accounts for up to 4.5% of primary renal disease in children leading to ESRD. In children, the most frequent form of HUS is diarrhea-associated (D+), or "typical," and is caused by verocytotoxin-producing *Escherichia coli* (VTEC). Although this is the most common form of HUS in childhood, it results in ESRD in only 10% of cases. "Atypical" HUS is far less frequent in children. It is characterized by a prodrome that lacks diarrheal association (i.e., "D–"), it has a relapsing course, and a very poor renal prognosis.

When considering transplantation in patients whose original cause of ESRD was HUS, care must be directed to the form of HUS that the patient suffered. The diarrhea-associated, or "typical," form does not usually recur after transplantation, while atypical HUS has a high propensity for recurrence. However, there are pitfalls in assessing recurrence of HUS. The D+/D– terminology can sometimes be misleading. Occasionally, patients with VTEC-associated HUS do not have diarrhea and therefore may be mistakenly labeled as D–. Similarly, diarrhea disease can trigger HUS in a patient who is genetically predisposed to HUS, and therefore erroneously be characterized as D+ HUS. In addition, it may be difficult to distinguish antibody-mediated vascular rejection from recurrent HUS, which presents histologically as thrombotic microangiopathy (TMA) (see Chapter 13). Finally, the calcineurin inhibitors may cause TMA in the transplanted kidney and produce a clinical picture that resembles HUS (see Chapters 4, Part I, and 8). With these reservations in mind, it is reasonable to conclude that D+ HUS has a minimal recurrence rate while the aggregate recurrence rate in D– HUS is 20–25%. The use of calcineurin inhibitors in both D– and D+ patients does not appear to trigger HUS recurrence and avoidance of calcineurin inhibitors does not appear to prevent recurrence.

Previously, it was recommended that at least 1 year of clinical quiescence occur before transplantation is attempted for patients with D– HUS, although this hiatus may not reduce the risk of recurrence. The patient and graft outcome in recurrent atypical HUS is poor. Ten percent of patients have died and 83% have lost the graft. For patients who have experienced recurrence, it is estimated that HUS will recur in approximately 50% of subsequent grafts.

A genetic defect of complement factor H production has been associated with a severe form of D– HUS. Factor H deficiency results in a state of continued complement activation with resulting low C3 and C4 levels. While there are only a few cases of this condition in pediatric renal transplantation, this form of D– HUS appears to have an associated rate of recurrence of greater than 50%. High-dose fresh-frozen plasma with plasma exchange have been advocated for this condition. Liver transplantation and combined liver–kidney transplantation have also been successful in a limited number of patients; the rationale for these approaches is that factor H is synthesized in the liver. The recurrence rate in the few reported patients with factor H gene mutations but normal factor H concentrations appears to be markedly less than for those with factor H deficiency.

Living donor transplantation is not contraindicated for patients whose original disease was D+ HUS. On the other hand, living donor transplantation is not advocated for patients with D– HUS. This is because of the high recurrence rate in such patients. In addition, it has been noted that some parental carriers of D– HUS might not manifest the disease until later in life, and organ donation would put such carriers at excessive risk.

Antiglomerular Basement Membrane Disease

Anti-GBM disease is rare in children. A high level of circulating anti-GBM antibody before transplantation is thought to be associated with higher rate of recurrence. Therefore, a waiting period of 6 to 12 months with an undetectable titer of anti-GBM antibody is recommended before transplantation to prevent recurrence. Reappearance of anti-GBM antibody in the serum may be associated with histologic recurrence. Histologic recurrence has been reported in up to half of cases, with clinical manifestations of nephritis in only 25% of these cases. Graft loss is rare, and spontaneous resolution may occur.

Congenital Nephrotic Syndrome

Congenital nephrotic syndrome occurs in the first 3 months of life. It can be classified as either congenital nephrotic syndrome of the Finnish type (CNSF) or diffuse mesangial sclerosis (DMS). CNSF is an autosomal recessive disease that occurs as a result of a mutation in the *NPHS 1* gene. While it is most commonly seen in Finnish patients, it is also found in other countries. The *NPHS 1* gene is located on chromosome 19 and has as its gene product the protein *nephrin*. Nephrin is a transmembrane protein, which is a member of the immunoglobulin family of cell-adhesion molecules. It is characteristically located at the slit diaphragms of the glomerular epithelial foot processes. More than 50 mutations of *NPHS 1* have been identified in CNSF, but more than 90% of all Finnish patients have one of two mutations—the so-called Fin major and Fin minor mutations.

Infants with CNSF are usually born prematurely and exhibit low birth weight and placentomegaly. CNSF manifests as heavy proteinuria, edema, and ascites, often in the first week of life and always by 3 months of age. Untreated, these children suffer from malnutrition, poor growth, frequent infections, and thromboembolic complications. ESRD occurs invariably by mid-childhood. Corticosteroids do not ameliorate CNSF, but in mild forms, angiotensin-converting enzyme inhibition, together with indomethacin, may be successful. The best therapeutic success has come from the approach of early dialysis, nephrectomy, and transplantation.

CNSF does not recur after transplantation. However, *de novo* nephrotic syndrome has been reported in approximately 25% of cases. It presents with proteinuria, hypoalbuminemia, and edema that may start immediately or as late as 3 years after transplantation. All of the patients with posttransplant nephrotic syndrome have been reported to have the homozygous Fin major genotype. Antibodies against fetal glomerular structures are found in the majority of patients with posttransplant nephrotic syndrome, and antibodies to nephrin are found in more than 50%. Approximately half of patients with this nephrotic syndrome respond to steroids and cyclophosphamide, but in those who do not respond, the graft is usually lost. Within the NAPRTCS database, vascular thrombosis and death with a functioning graft (mostly as a consequence of infectious complications) occur in 26% and 23% of cases, respectively, and account for higher rate of graft failure in this particular group.

DMS can be found in isolated form, or as part of Denys-Drash syndrome. The latter is a syndrome composed of progressive renal disease with nephrotic syndrome and DMS, Wilms tumor, and male pseudohermaphroditism. Most patients with DMS have mutations of the WT-1 gene located on chromosome 11p13. Patients with DMS who have received kidney transplants have not been reported as developing nephrotic syndrome.

Membranous Nephropathy

Membranous nephropathy is uncommon in children, so that posttransplant recurrence is rarely seen. *De novo* membranous nephropathy occurs more frequently and affects up to 10% of transplanted children. It usually presents later than the recurrent disease, which usually becomes apparent within the first 2 posttransplant years. The occurrence *de novo* membranous nephropathy does not appear to affect graft outcome in the absence of rejection.

Systemic Lupus Erythematosus and the Vasculitides

In the pediatric transplant literature, recurrence of systemic lupus erythematosus (SLE) is rarely seen. Recurrence in adults is more common and may not manifest till several years posttransplant. In pediatric nephrology, it is most common to observe lupus nephritis progress to ESRD in adolescence. Because it is standard practice to defer transplantation until SLE has become clinically quiescent for at least 6 to 12 months, it is likely that the pediatric patient with SLE who receives a kidney transplant may not suffer from recurrence until young adult life.

Antineutrophil cytoplasmic antibody (ANCA)-positive glomerulonephritides can recur in the transplanted kidney. Wegener granulomatosis and pauci-immune glomerulonephritis recurs in a small number of patients and can cause graft loss. Treatment with cyclophosphamide appears to be beneficial and patients must be monitored carefully for signs of recurrence.

Metabolic Diseases

Primary Hyperoxaluria Type I

Oxalosis results from deficiency of hepatic peroxisomal alanine glyoxylate aminotransferase (AGT). Deficiency of this enzyme leads to deposition of oxalate in all body tissues, including the kidneys, myocardium, and bone. Renal transplantation alone does not correct the enzymatic deficiency and graft loss is common because of oxalate mobilization from tissue deposits and subsequent deposition in the graft. Therapy with a combined liver and kidney transplantation has led to higher rates of success (see Chapter 11). The transplanted liver corrects the enzymatic deficiency and thus prevents further oxalate production. The well-functioning transplanted kidney excretes the mobilized plasma oxalate. Success of this approach is greatly facilitated by immediate graft function with a good diuresis. If possible, combined liver and kidney transplantation occurs early in the course of renal disease, preferably before the glomerular filtration rate (GFR) decreases below 20 to 25 mL per minute per 1.73 m^2. This serves to optimize outcome and prevent severe complications of the disease that may lead to irreversible morbidity.

Ideally, aggressive hemodialysis before transplantation is employed to decrease oxalate load to safe levels and minimize tissue oxalate deposition. The target plasma oxalate level is less than 50 mg/mL. At transplantation, a large donor kidney is used whenever possible to permit effective excretion of the oxalate burden. Early use of a calcineurin inhibitor may be deferred until the serum creatinine falls to the range of 1.0 to 2.0 mg/dL. Until this occurs, immunosuppression is accomplished with MMF, corticosteroids, and antibody induction. If early renal transplant dysfunction occurs, daily hemodialysis is continued. Once good renal function is established, calcineurin-inhibitor therapy is begun. In addition, posttransplant treatment includes pyridoxine, neutral phosphate, citrate, and noncalciuric diuretics.

Nephropathic Cystinosis

Transplantation in children with cystinosis corrects the transport defect in the kidney, but not in other organs affected by the disease. Hypothyroidism, visual abnormalities, and central nervous system manifestations are not corrected by transplantation and require ongoing therapy with cysteamine and thyroid hormone. Cystine crystals can be found in the renal graft interstitium within macrophages of host origin. This does not result in recurrence of Fanconi syndrome or graft dysfunction.

Sickle Cell Anemia

The graft survival rate for patients with sickle cell disease is low, with only about 25% of grafts functioning beyond 1 year after transplantation. The improvement in the hematocrit results in higher numbers of abnormal red blood cells, leading to sickling episodes in the renal graft.

PRETRANSPLANT EVALUATION

Evaluation of the Potential Living Donor

The evaluation and preparation of a living donor for a child is essentially the same as for an adult (see Chapter 5). As a general rule, it is possible to consider an adult donor of almost any size for a child, no matter how young. Living donation from siblings is usually restricted to donors older than age 18 years, although the courts have given permission for younger children to donate under extraordinary circumstances.

Histocompatibility matching considerations are not different for pediatric recipients of kidneys from living donors than for adult recipients. HLA-identical transplants are optimal and enable the lowest amount of immunosuppression to be used, thereby minimizing steroid and other side effects. The first living donor for a child is usually a one-haplotype-matched parent. Siblings may become donors as they reach the age of consent. When considering transplantation from siblings, data suggest that kidneys from haploidentical donors with noninherited maternal HLA antigens function better in the long-term than do those from donors with noninherited paternal HLA antigens (see Chapter 3). Second-degree relatives and zero-haplotype-matched siblings may also be considered as donors. The excellent results of nonbiologically related living donor transplants are not dependent on high degrees of HLA matching.

Evaluation of the Recipient

The evaluation of the potential pediatric transplant recipient is similar to that performed in adults (see Chapter 6), but because certain problems occur with more frequency in children, the emphasis may be different. It is important to establish the precise cause of ESRD in children whenever possible. Surgical correction may be required for certain structural abnormalities before transplantation. The precise cause of metabolic or glomerular disease should also be established if possible, because of the possibility of posttransplantation recurrence. Discussions of some common medical, surgical, and psychiatric issues in pediatric transplant candidates follow.

Neuropsychiatric Development

INFANTS

Infants with ESRD during the first year of life may suffer neurologic abnormalities. These include alterations in mental function, microcephaly, and involuntary motor phenomena, such as myoclonus, cerebellar ataxia, tremors, seizures, and hypotonia. The pathogenesis is unclear, although aluminum toxicity has been incriminated. Preemptive kidney transplantation or institution of dialysis at the earliest sign of head-circumference growth-rate reduction or developmental delay may ameliorate the problem. Some studies describe an improvement in psychomotor delay in some infants with successful transplantation, with a significant percentage of infants regaining normal developmental milestones. Tests of global intelligence show increased rates of improvement after successful transplantation.

OLDER CHILDREN

It is often difficult to assess to what extent uremia contributes to cognitive delay and impairment in older children. Uremia has an adverse, but often reversible, effect on a child's mental functioning, and it may often cause psychological depression. It may be necessary to institute dialysis and improve the uremic symptomatology before making a precise assessment of the child's mental function. Initiation of dialysis often clarifies the picture and permits progression to transplantation in situations in which it might otherwise have not seemed feasible. On the other hand, severely retarded children respond poorly to the constraints of ESRD care. A child with a very low IQ cannot comprehend the need for procedures that are often confusing and uncomfortable. In this situation, the family must be involved and supported in the decision to embark on a treatment course that does not include chronic dialysis or transplantation.

SEIZURES

Up to 10% of young pediatric transplant candidates have a seizure disorder requiring anticonvulsant treatment. Before transplantation, seizures should be controlled, whenever possible, with drugs that do not interfere with calcineurin inhibitor, sirolimus, or prednisone metabolism (see Chapter 4, Part I). Benzodiazepines are a good choice when circumstances permit. Carbamazepine does reduce calcineurin inhibitor and prednisone levels, but its effect is not as strong as that of phenytoin (Dilantin) or barbiturates. Should it prove necessary to use a drug that lowers immunosuppressive drug levels, a moderately augmented dose of prednisone may be given twice daily. The calcineurin inhibitor may need to be administered three times per day, or the dose adjusted upward, to achieve the desired trough levels, which should be monitored closely.

Psychoemotional Status

Psychiatric and emotional disorders are not, by themselves, contraindications to dialysis and transplantation; however, the involvement of healthcare professionals skilled in the care of affected children is mandatory. Primary psychiatric problems may be amenable to therapy and should not exclude children from consideration for transplantation. Experience with psychotropic drugs, such as selective serotonin reuptake inhibitors (SSRIs), has been very positive. As with antiseizure medications, it is important to recognize that certain drugs may interfere with the metabolism of some immunosuppressive medications. This has not been found to be a major issue with SSRIs such as citalopram, escitalopram, and sertraline (see Chapter 16).

Noncompliance is a particularly prevalent problem in adolescent transplant recipients. Patterns of medication and dialysis compliance should be established as part of the transplant evaluation. Psychiatric evaluation should be performed in high-risk cases. If noncompliance is identified or anticipated, interventions should be in place before transplantation. These should include both social and psychiatric interventions, where possible. Psychosocial support systems must be identified and nurtured. Frequent medical and social work monitoring is crucial if the patient is to be rehabilitated both medically and psychosocially to the point where the patient is a candidate for transplantation. The best outcomes will be achieved when there is close coordination between the medical and mental health providers. It is particularly important for the transplant and dialysis teams to stay in close communication as they prepare the patient for transplantation.

Cardiovascular Disease

Children and adolescents are unlikely to have overt cardiovascular disease that requires invasive diagnostic workup. Hypertension and chronic fluid overload during dialysis predisposes to left ventricular hypertrophy (LVH), hypertensive cardiomyopathy, and congestive heart failure. LVH may be present in up to 75% of pediatric transplant recipients and peripheral resistance is often elevated. In children, as in adults, transplantation may be beneficial to cardiac function. Occasionally, the degree of pretransplant cardiac compromise is so severe that heart transplant must accompany kidney transplantation.

The importance of hypertension control in children with ESRD cannot be overemphasized. In the pretransplant evaluation, blood pressure profiles and dialysis management must be carefully scrutinized. In the child who is hypertensive on dialysis, echocardiograms should be performed annually to assess ventricular hypertrophy and valve competence. In patients who require multiple antihypertensive drugs, bilateral nephrectomies may be required prior to transplant.

Premature cardiovascular disease is a common feature of adults who have suffered childhood ESRD, and attention to "adult" cardiovascular disease risk factors in childhood may serve to minimize long-term morbidity and mortality. The coronary vessels of young adult dialysis patients have significant premature calcification (see Chapter 1). This may be the harbinger of atherosclerotic lesions. Control of calcium/phosphorus metabolism in the pretransplant period is a potential way of ameliorating posttransplant coronary heart disease.

Infection

COMMON BACTERIAL PATHOGENS

Urinary tract infections and infections related to peritoneal dialysis are the most common sources of bacterial infection in children with ESRD. Aggressive antibiotic therapy and prophylaxis of urinary tract infections in children may effectively suppress infection, although pretransplant nephrectomy is occasionally required for recalcitrant infections in children with reflux. Peritonitis and related infections with peritoneal dialysis are discussed later (see Children Receiving Peritoneal Dialysis).

CYTOMEGALOVIRUS

The incidence of cytomegalovirus (CMV) infection increases with age, and young children are unlikely to have developed CMV seropositivity. CMV IgM and IgG levels should be obtained with the pretransplant evaluation, and these studies should be considered when planning posttransplantation CMV prophylaxis.

EPSTEIN-BARR VIRUS

It is important to establish the Epstein-Barr virus (EBV) antibody status of the child. As with CMV, EBV infections and resultant seropositivity increase with age. Primary EBV infection, in the context of potent immunosuppression, may predispose to a particularly aggressive form of posttransplantation lymphoproliferative disorder (PTLD).

IMMUNIZATION STATUS

Immunizations must be brought up to date whenever possible. Live viral vaccines are contraindicated in the immunosuppressed patient and every effort must be made to complete these vaccinations before transplantation. This includes varicella vaccination. Vaccination of the immunosuppressed host may fail to induce an adequate immune response, especially with the use of agents, such as MMF, that suppress antibody production.

Diphtheria and tetanus vaccine, as well as hepatitis B, can be given safely after transplantation, although pretransplantation administration is preferred. *Haemophilus influenzae*-type vaccine is also safe. Influenza and pneumococcal vaccines are recommended for the pediatric transplant recipient. Most of the available data on their effectiveness come from transplant recipients treated with cyclosporine or azathioprine. Studies are needed to address the immune responsiveness to vaccines under immunosuppression with newer agents.

Hemostasis

Up to 13% of graft loss in pediatric patients is caused by graft thrombosis. For this reason, it is particularly important to search for clues of a patient's tendency toward hypercoagulability, such as recurrent hemodialysis access clotting. If such a history is obtained, a full coagulation workup is indicated.

Patients with Glomerulonephritis of Unknown Etiology

Pediatric patients will often be referred for a pretransplant evaluation without having had the diagnosis of their ESRD established. As noted above, recurrence of glomerulonephritis or glomerulopathy is a significant concern in pediatric and adolescent recipients. For this reason, any patient with significant proteinuria or hypertension accompanying ESRD should have a serologic profile that can help classify the diagnosis of ESRD. This includes C3, C4, ANA, anti–single-stranded and –double-stranded deoxyribonucleic acid (DNA), and ANCA titers.

Urologic Problems

Obstructive uropathy is the cause of ESRD in approximately 16% of transplanted children. Other causes of ESRD that are commonly associated with abnormalities of the urinary tract, such as reflux nephropathy, neurogenic bladder, prune belly syndrome, and renal dysplasia, account for another 20% of transplanted children. Because of this high frequency, urologic abnormalities should always be considered as a cause of ESRD of uncertain etiology in children and young adults. A history of voiding abnormalities, enuresis, nocturia, or recurrent urinary tract infections may be the only clue to an underlying urologic defect.

The presence of an abnormal lower urinary tract is not a contraindication to transplantation. Urologic problems are best addressed before transplantation. Malformations and voiding abnormalities (e.g., neurogenic bladder, bladder dyssynergia, remnant posterior urethral valves, urethral strictures) should be identified and repaired if possible. Children with urologic disease and renal dysplasia often require multiple operations to optimize urinary tract anatomy and function. Such procedures include ureteric reimplantation to correct vesicoureteric reflux; bladder augmentation or reconstruction; Mitrofanoff procedure (creation of a vesicocutaneous fistula using the appendix to provide for continent and cosmetically acceptable intermittent catheterization); and excision of duplicated systems or ectopic ureteroceles that may cause recurrent infections.

BLADDER AUGMENTATION

Urodynamic studies can provide important information about bladder capacity and function, and help to define those situations that require bladder augmentation. Bladders that have high intravesical pressures are at risk to produce serious hydronephrosis in a transplanted kidney. Bladder augmentation is often required for patients with posterior urethral valve and some cases with small bladder capacity. Augmentation can be done using dilated ureter tissue, small intestine, or large intestine. Ureteric augmentation provides the best results because the ureteric mucosa is identical to the urinary bladder mucosa. Intestinal or colonic augmentation often requires frequent bladder irrigation, and is often complicated by significant mucus secretion that can cause intermittent obstruction of the bladder stoma, and lead to frequent urinary tract infections. Augmentation using gastric tissue causes severe dysuria because of the acidity of gastric secretions, and has been abandoned in most centers. Following bladder augmentation, most children will require chronic intermittent catheterization. Forceful hydrodilation as a substitute to bladder augmentation is used at some centers, but most physicians agree that it is very painful and futile, especially in children awaiting deceased donor transplantation.

If a child has a neurogenic bladder, a bladder augmentation, or other voiding abnormality, it is usually possible to teach a parent or the patient clean, intermittent self-catheterization. This can be done in transplant recipients safely and successfully. However, urinary tract infection may occur when catheterization technique is poor. In addition, noncompliance with self-catheterization may lead to partial obstruction and subsequent graft dysfunction.

In some studies, graft outcome in children with urologic problems is inferior to that of children with normal lower urinary tracts. In addition, in recipients with an abnormal bladder, there is an increased incidence of posttransplantation urologic complication and urinary tract infection. Nevertheless, in centers with skilled pediatric urologists, children with ESRD as a consequence of urologic malformations can be very successfully transplanted.

Renal Osteodystrophy

Aggressive diagnosis and treatment of hyperparathyroidism, osteomalacia, and adynamic bone disease are important in the pretransplant period. Control of hyperparathyroidism with vitamin D analogues, or even parathyroidectomy, may be required.

Failure to do so may predispose to posttransplant hypercalcemia and limit the growth potential of a successful transplant recipient.

Children Receiving Peritoneal Dialysis

It has been generally accepted that children being treated with peritoneal dialysis have graft and patient survival rates that are similar to those of children receiving hemodialysis. A retrospective study by the NAPRTCS, however, suggested that children treated with peritoneal dialysis are at significantly higher risk of graft thrombosis than children treated with hemodialysis, or those who received preemptive transplants independent of the age of the transplant recipient. The etiology of this observation is not clear. Peritoneal dialysis may, in fact, facilitate transplant surgery, especially in very young and small infants. Repeated peritoneal fluid cycling expands the abdomen, and creates adequate space for extraperitoneal placement of the relatively large adult kidney. Extraperitoneal placement of the graft is desirable because it may allow for continued peritoneal dialysis after transplantation in the event of DGF, and patients can tolerate oral feeds and medications sooner because of minimal bowel manipulation. However, intraperitoneal graft placement is not an absolute contraindication to posttransplant peritoneal dialysis, should it become necessary.

A recent episode of peritonitis or exit-site infection in a child awaiting a transplant does not preclude transplantation. Potential transplant recipients should be appropriately treated for 10 to 14 days and have a negative peritoneal fluid culture off antibiotic treatment before contemplating transplantation. In addition, the preoperative peritoneal cell count should not suggest peritonitis. If a chronic exit-site infection is present at the time of surgery, the catheter should be removed and appropriate parenteral antibiotics administered. An overt tunnel infection should be treated before transplantation. The incidence of posttransplant peritoneal dialysis-related infections is low. However, peritonitis and exit-site infection should be considered in the differential diagnosis in any child with unexplained fever after transplant, and early sampling of the peritoneal fluid should be pursued. Such infections typically respond to appropriate antibiotic therapy, although catheter removal may be necessary for recurrent infections. In the absence of infections, the peritoneal catheter may be left in place until good graft function has been established for 2 to 3 weeks.

Nephrotic Syndrome

In children with glomerular diseases, proteinuria usually diminishes as kidney function deteriorates and ESRD ensues. Occasionally, florid nephrotic syndrome may persist, particularly in children with FSGS. Persistence of heavy proteinuria causes a hypercoagulable state and increases the risk of graft thrombosis and thromboembolic complications at the time of surgery, and makes fluid management very difficult because of leakage of fluids into the extravascular space, which may lead to delayed graft function and adversely affect graft outcome. Control of heavy proteinuria prior to transplantation is important and can sometimes be achieved with prostaglandin inhibitors, although renal embolization or bilateral laparoscopic nephrectomy may be required.

In the child with CNSF, unilateral or bilateral nephrectomy is usually performed early in the course of the disease to allow for better skeletal growth while on dialysis, and to prevent infectious and thromboembolic complications. Congenital nephrotic syndrome caused by DMS usually requires early bilateral nephrectomy as part of the treatment of Wilms tumor or of its precursor, Denys-Drash syndrome, which is commonly present at the time of diagnosis.

Pretransplant Nephrectomy

Nephrectomy should be avoided if possible because leaving the kidneys *in situ* may facilitate fluid management during dialysis, an important consideration for small children in whom fluid balance may be tenuous. Nephrectomy may be indicated for severely hypertensive patients in whom blood pressure control is suboptimal despite optimal fluid removal, and use of a multiple antihypertensive agents. Intractable urinary tract infection, in the presence of hydronephrosis or severe reflux, may also require nephrectomy before transplantation. Occasionally, nephrectomy is required to create adequate space for placement of the adult graft in a small infant. This is frequently the case in autosomal recessive polycystic kidney disease, where the enlarged kidneys occupy the abdominal cavity, and may impair diaphragmatic movement, causing respiratory difficulty.

Portal Hypertension

Portal hypertension may occur in certain forms of ESRD common in children, such as congenital hepatic fibrosis, which may accompany autosomal recessive polycystic kidney disease, and nephronophthisis. The manifestations of congenital hepatic fibrosis must be controlled; esophageal varices require sclerotherapy or portosystemic shunting. If neutropenia and thrombocytopenia are present as a result of hypersplenism, partial splenectomy or splenic embolization may occasionally be required.

Prior Malignancy

Wilms tumor is the most common renal malignancy in children, and as such, it is the principal malignancy producing ESRD in children. Posttransplant recurrence of Wilms tumor has been described in up to 6% of patients. Patients with recurrent Wilms tumor tend to be younger and have a shorter interval from tumor recognition to transplantation. A disease-free period of 2 years from the time of remission should be observed before transplantation. Premature transplantation has been associated with overwhelming sepsis, which may be related to recent chemotherapy. The presence of a primary nonrenal malignancy is not an absolute contraindication to transplantation, although an appropriate waiting time must be observed between tumor extirpation and transplantation (see Chapter 6).

Preemptive Transplantation

Nearly 25% of all pediatric transplantations are now performed without the institution of dialysis. The percentage is even higher for recipients of living donors and is much higher than that achieved in adults. The incidence of preemptive transplantation is nearly double in white children (30%) as compared to African American and Hispanic children. In children and in adults, there is a significant improvement in graft survival for patients who have not received pretransplant dialysis (see Chapter 6).

Nutrition

Poor feeding is a prominent feature of uremia in children. Aggressive nutritional support is essential. Early gastrostomy or nasogastric tube feeding is often employed to improve caloric intake and promote growth, especially in children started on dialysis therapy at a young age. Because of technical difficulty and a resultant possibility of graft loss, a weight of 8 to 10 kg is used as a target weight for transplantation at most centers. This weight may not be reached until 2 years of age, even with the most aggressive nutritional regimens. Transplantation in children weighing less than 5 to 8 kg has been successfully performed at some centers.

PERIOPERATIVE MANAGEMENT OF THE PEDIATRIC RENAL TRANSPLANT RECIPIENT

Preparation for Transplantation

For living donor transplants some programs commence immunosuppression in the week prior to the transplant date. A final crossmatch is performed within 1 week of transplantation, and the patient is evaluated clinically to ensure medical stability. Laboratory tests obtained at admission permit detection of metabolic abnormalities that require correction by dialysis. Aggressive fluid removal is discouraged in the immediate preoperative period to reduce the risk for delayed graft function (see Chapter 8). Preoperative immunosuppression is discussed below.

Intraoperative Management

Methylprednisolone sodium succinate (Solu-Medrol), 10 mg/kg, is given intravenously at the beginning of the operation. Close attention is paid to blood pressure and hydration status in an attempt to reduce the incidence of DGF. Typically, a central venous catheter is inserted to monitor the central venous pressure (CVP) throughout the operation. To achieve adequate renal perfusion, a CVP of 12 to 15 cm H_2O should be achieved before removal of the vascular clamps; a higher CVP may be desirable in the case of a small infant receiving an adult-sized kidney. Dopamine is usually started in the operating room at 2 to 3 μg/kg per minute and increased as required and is continued for 24 to 48 hours postoperatively. It is used to facilitate diuresis and perhaps to effect renal vasodilatation. The mean arterial blood pressure is kept above 65 to 70 mm Hg by adequate hydration with a crystalloid solution or 5% albumin and, if necessary, the use of dopamine at higher doses. Blood transfusion with packed red blood cells may be required in very small recipients because the hemoglobin may drop as a result of sequestration of about 150 to 250 mL of blood in the transplanted kidney. Mannitol and furosemide may be given before removal of the vascular clamps to facilitate diuresis. Urine volume is replaced immediately with 0.5% normal saline. Occasionally, an intraarterial vasodilator, such as verapamil, is used to overcome vasospasm that may impair renal perfusion.

Postoperative Management

Because of the small size of young children, fluid management must be fastidious. Urine output should be replaced on a cc for cc basis with 0.45% or 0.9% normal saline continued for 24 to 48 hours. Insensible water losses are replaced with a dextrose-containing crystalloid. Potassium replacement may be required. Dextrose is not added to the replacement solution and is only used as part of the insensible water loss replacement solution. Withholding dextrose in the urine replacement solutions helps to prevent posttransplant hyperglycemia and osmotic diuresis. The lack of concentrating ability of the newly transplanted kidney accounts for an obligatory high urine output that may be observed in the first few posttransplantation days. As the kidney function improves and the serum creatinine levels fall close to normal values, urinary concentrating ability recovers, and urine output decreases from several liters per day to amounts that begin to match daily fluid intake. At this time, urine output replacement can be stopped, and daily fluid intake is usually set to provide about 150% to 200% of the normal daily maintenance needs, preferably administered orally.

Hypertension is commonly observed. Pain is an important cause of hypertension in the immediate postoperative period, and adequate analgesia may be all that is required to control blood pressure. Hypertension is rarely aggressively corrected in the immediate postoperative period to avoid sudden swings in blood pressure that may impair renal perfusion. Electrolyte disorders encountered early in the postoperative course are discussed

Table 15.2.   Cytomegalovirus (CMV) prophylaxis protocol at the Mattel Children's Hospital at UCLA pediatric renal transplant program using donor and recipient CMVIgG status

Donor Status	Recipient Status	Ganciclovir[a]	CMV Hyperimmune Globulin (Cytogam)[b]
Positive	Positive	Yes	No
Positive	Negative	Yes	Yes
Negative	Positive	Yes	No
Negative	Negative	No	No

[a] Ganciclovir is given intravenously initially (2.5 mg/kg daily) until oral intake is tolerated; oral ganciclovir dose = 20–30 mg/kg/dose orally t.i.d. for 10–12 weeks.
[b] Cytogam dose = 100 mg/kg/dose IV. The first dose is given immediately postoperatively; doses are then given every 2 weeks thereafter for a total of five doses.

elsewhere. Prophylaxis against CMV infection is outlined in Table 15.2 and in Chapter 10.

PEDIATRIC IMMUNOSUPPRESSIVE PROTOCOLS

Readers are referred to Chapter 4 for a full discussion of transplant immunosuppressive agents and protocols. The construction of the immunosuppressive protocol for pediatric transplantation is similar to that for adults. Most pediatric renal transplant centers employ combination drug therapy consisting of a calcineurin inhibitor and corticosteroids with an adjunctive agent, usually MMF (Tables 15.3 and 15.4). The NAPRTCS reported that in 2003, approximately 80% of transplanted patients were receiving a three-drug regimen at 6 months after transplantation. Induction therapy with a biologic agent is employed in approximately 60% of transplant recipients. Thymoglobulin can be used to provide adequate initial immunosuppression and allow delayed introduction of the calcineurin inhibitor in cases of DGF, or to provide intensified immunosuppression in the highly sensitized transplant recipient. When transplantation is contemplated in a child with prior malignancy, a two-drug regimen, or even monotherapy, may be considered to minimize the effect immunosuppressive drugs may have on immune surveillance. In this situation, the use of antibody induction is generally avoided, and living donation is encouraged to provide the best HLA match. Corticosteroids continue to be used in more than 95% of transplant recipients 1 year after transplantation. However, there has been a steady increase in the percentage of patients treated with steroid minimization protocols, especially alternate-day steroid regimens.

Corticosteroids

Corticosteroids remain an integral part of most pediatric immunosuppressive protocols despite their toxicity, although lower daily doses are now routinely used. In children, retarded skeletal growth is the most important side effect. Concerns remain about familiar side effects, such as hypertension, obesity, diabetes mellitus, hyperlipidemia, osteopenia, and aseptic necrosis. Cosmetic side effects, such as Cushingoid facies and acne, may tempt children and adolescents into stop taking their immunosuppressive drugs.

Corticosteroid Withdrawal/Avoidance

There are currently no reliable immunologic or clinical indicators to predict in which pediatric transplant recipients steroids can be safely withdrawn. Several investigators have reported single-center experience on the successful withdrawal of steroids using tacrolimus-based regimens. Long-term data and multicenter controlled studies are still lacking. In general, steroid withdrawal has led to improvement in blood pressure, lipid profiles, and statural growth. The benefits of steroid withdrawal have been overshadowed, however, by high rates of acute rejection that have been reported in from 25% to 70% of children.

Complete steroid avoidance is emerging as a strategy to prevent the steroid-associated morbidities, especially growth retardation in children. Complete steroid avoidance has been described using

Table 15.3. Immunosuppressive protocol for pediatric kidney transplantation at the Mattel Children's Hospital at UCLA

Pretransplant (1 wk in living donor recipients only)

- Prednisone: 0.5 mg/kg daily (minimum dose = 20 mg/d)
- MMF: 600 mg/m^2/dose b.i.d.
   + Famotidine: 1 mg/kg/dose b.i.d. (maximum = 40 mg b.i.d.: other H$_2$ blockers, except cimetidine, or H$^+$ pump blockers may be used)

Pretransplant (6–24 hr)

- Daclizumab: 1 mg/kg in 50 mL of normal saline IV over 30 min
- MMF: 600 mg/m^2 PO within 6 hr

Intraoperatively

- Solumedrol: 10 mg/kg IV at the beginning of surgery (maximum dose of 1 g)

Immediate postoperative period

- Solumedrol: 0.5 mg/kg/d IV (minimum dose = 20 mg/day)[a]
- MMF: 600 mg/m^2/dose IV q 12 hr[a]
- Cyclosporine: 10–15 mg/kg/d PO divided b.i.d. For children who weigh less than 10 kg or are younger than 6 yr of age, give 400–500 mg/m^2/d divided t.i.d.[b] The dose is adjusted to achieve trough levels of 250–350 ng/mL and/or C2 levels of 1200–1500 ng/mL.
   OR
   Tacrolimus 0.15–0.2 mg/kg/day PO divided b.i.d. to achieve levels of 8–12 ng/ml.[b]
   + Famotidine or H$_2$ blocker

Maintenance therapy

- Daclizumab: 1 mg/kg at 2, 4, 6, and 8 wk after transplantation
- Prednisone: Dose tapering is started 2 wk after transplantation and continued to reach a maintenance dose 0.07–0.1 mg/kg/d by 3–4 months.
- MMF: 600 mg/kg/dose PO b.i.d. with cyclosporine, 300–400 mg/kg/dose PO b.i.d. with tacrolimus[c]
- Cyclosporine/tacrolimus: Dose is adjusted to achieve the desired trough levels (see Chapter 4, Part I and Table 4.10).

H$_2$, histamine-2; MMF, mycophenolate mofetil.
[a] The drug is given orally when the patient tolerates oral intake.
[b] Cyclosporine/tacrolimus is started once urine output has been established and the serum creatinine level is below 2.5–3 mg/dL or less than 50% of its baseline value before transplantation.
[c] The dose can be spread to a three-times-daily schedule if gastrointestinal symptoms develop early.

Table 15.4. Guidelines for drug dose tapering in pediatric renal transplant recipients

1. Cyclosporine/Tacrolimus

Minimal or no change in the first 4 weeks to allow for faster tapering of prednisone.

Dose reduction should not exceed 10%–20%.

Cyclosporine/Tacrolimus and prednisone doses should not be lowered on the same day (risk of precipitating an acute rejection).

Serum creatinine and cyclosporine/tacrolimus levels should be checked 2–3 days after each change and before the next change is made.

(The same guidelines are applied to patients treated with tacrolimus.)

2. Prednisone

Start tapering the dose 2–3 weeks after transplantation if stable and cyclosporine/tacrolimus level is within the desired range.

Initial dose tapering is by 2.5 mg each time, about 10% (may reduce by 5 mg if total dose is >2 mg/kg). Once a 10-mg dose is reached, dose reduction is by 1 mg each time.

Longer periods of time should elapse before further tapering at the lower dose range.

Cyclosporine/Tacrolimus and prednisone doses should not be lowered on the same day.

Serum creatinine and cyclosporine/tacrolimus levels should be checked 2–3 days after each change and before the next change is made.

3. Mycophenolate mofetil

Dose reduction is only indicated if hematologic or gastrointestinal side effects develop.

Dose reduction is done in 30%–50% increments.

It can be safely withheld for a few days up to 2–3 weeks for severe side effects.

---

a regimen of tacrolimus with MMF, and an extended course of daclizumab, with frequent protocol biopsies. Rejection rates with this protocol are low and growth and renal function are significantly improved. Similar results have been described using Thymoglobulin induction followed by maintenance therapy with cyclosporine and MMF.

Calcineurin Inhibitors

There are some important differences in the use of cyclosporine and tacrolimus between adults and children. Children, particularly those younger than age 2 years, may require higher doses than adults when calculated on a milligram per kilogram of body weight basis. The higher dose requirement is believed to be the result of a higher rate of metabolism by the hepatic cytochrome P450, resulting in faster clearance. Dosing based on surface area, or thrice-daily dosing, appears to provide better therapeutic levels in smaller children and in children in whom metabolism is accelerated (e.g., patients receiving certain anticonvulsant medications). The use of peak-level monitoring of cyclosporine (C2 levels, see Chapter 4, Part I) that has been recommended for adults has not been independently validated in children. The recommended drug levels of cyclosporine and tacrolimus for children are similar to those recommended for adults (see Chapter 4, Table 4.10). Studies comparing the efficacy of cyclosporine and tacrolimus in children have tended to favor tacrolimus both in terms of the incidence of acute rejection and graft loss. In the NAPRTCS database, however, there was very little difference between the two drugs when used in combination with MMF. Concern, generated from data collected in the late 1980s, regarding a much higher incidence of PTLD in children receiving tacrolimus, has largely mitigated.

The side-effect profile of the calcineurin inhibitors in children is similar to that seen in adults (see Chapter 4, Part I). Hirsutism, gingival hyperplasia, and coarsening facial features may be troublesome in children receiving cyclosporine, particularly Hispanic and African American children. In the adolescent population, especially girls, these side effects may be devastating, causing severe emotional distress and possibly leading to dangerous noncompliance. Switching to tacrolimus may be helpful, although hair loss may follow. Seizures are observed more commonly in children treated with calcineurin inhibitors than in adults. Neurologic symptoms tend to be more severe with tacrolimus. Children, like adults, are more likely to develop hypercholesterolemia and hypertriglyceridemia with cyclosporine, and may be candidates for lipid-lowering agents. Glucose intolerance is less common than in adults, and occurs in less than 5% of children; it is more common with tacrolimus. Overt diabetes mellitus may occasionally occur. There has been a steady trend toward using tacrolimus rather than cyclosporine for children. As of 2002, NAPRTCS reported that slightly more than half of pediatric recipients were receiving tacrolimus-based therapy.

Mycophenolate Mofetil

MMF is used in approximately two-thirds of U.S. pediatric renal transplant recipients and has largely replaced azathioprine. The capacity of MMF to reduce the incidence of acute rejection episodes relative to azathioprine is similar in children to that described in adults (see Chapter 4, Part I and Fig. 4.8). In children, as in adults, gastrointestinal and hematologic side effects can be troublesome and may respond to dose reduction. Therapeutic drug monitoring of MMF has been proposed for children but has not achieved widespread use. MMF has been used successfully in children for the treatment of steroid-resistant acute rejection.

Sirolimus

Although early experience with sirolimus in pediatric renal transplantation is encouraging, long-term data are still lacking. Reported efficacy and side-effect profiles mimic the adult experience. The combination of rapamycin with low-dose tacrolimus is especially attractive in children in whom steroid withdrawal is contemplated to enhance skeletal growth. NAPRTCS-sponsored clinical trials are in progress to evaluate the use of sirolimus for chronic allograft nephropathy and as a primary agent in combination with low-dose tacrolimus in *de novo* pediatric renal transplant recipients. Metabolism of sirolimus may be more rapid in children than in adults and more frequent dosing may be advisable.

Biologic Immunosuppressive Agents

The indications for the use of antibody-induction are discussed in Chapter 4 and do not differ between adults and children. More than 60% of children are treated with antibody induction, most frequently with nondepleting agents. The side-effect profiles of these agents are also similar. In pediatric deceased donor transplantation, there is close to a 10% advantage in the 5-year graft survival rate when antibody induction is used. Acute rejection episodes are approximately 30% less frequent and tend to occur later.

The non–lymphocyte-depleting anti-CD25 monoclonal antibodies (daclizumab and basiliximab) may be of particular benefit in children because of their effectiveness, ease of administration, and absence of side effects. In an open-label multicenter pediatric study with daclizumab used in addition to a triple-drug regimen with either cyclosporine or tacrolimus together with MMF and prednisone, the rate of acute rejection was found to be only 7% at 6 months and 16% at 1 year after transplantation. All rejections were mild and steroid responsive. No first-dose or cytokine-release effect or anaphylactic reactions were observed. Rates of opportunistic infections were not increased.

ACUTE REJECTION IN PEDIATRIC TRANSPLANTATION

Acute rejection episodes in pediatric renal transplantation account for about 15% of graft failures. With standard immunosuppressive therapy, an acute rejection episode is experienced in approximately 26% of recipients of living donor transplants and 30% of deceased donor transplant recipients. The first rejection episode occurs within the first 3 months after transplantation in about half of patients, with higher frequency and earlier recurrence in recipients of deceased donor transplants. Black race, DGF, and poor HLA matching may predispose to rejection episodes. In children, as in adults, acute rejection is the single most important predictor of chronic rejection. It precedes graft failure from chronic rejection in more than 90% of cases. Chronic rejection is the most common cause of graft loss in children.

Diagnosis of acute rejection in the very young transplant recipient is not always straightforward and requires a high index of suspicion. Because most small children are transplanted with adult-sized kidneys, the elevation in serum creatinine may be a late sign of rejection as a result of the large renal reserve compared with the body mass. Significant allograft dysfunction may be present with little or no increase in the serum creatinine level. One of the earliest and most sensitive signs of rejection is the development of hypertension along with low-grade fever. In children, any increase in serum creatinine, especially if accompanied by hypertension, should be considered a result of acute rejection until proved otherwise. Late diagnosis and treatment of rejection are associated with higher incidence of resistant rejections and graft loss.

The differential diagnosis of acute allograft dysfunction in children is similar to that in adults (see Chapter 8). Renal biopsy is the gold standard for diagnosis. Urinalysis and culture, viral cultures, and ultrasound and radionuclide imaging studies (see Chapter 14) are used to diagnose other causes of graft dysfunction and should be performed without delay before allograft biopsy.

Treatment of Acute Rejection

The techniques used to treat acute rejection are similar in children to those used in adults (see Chapter 4, Part IV). Complete reversal of acute rejection, as judged by a return of the serum creatinine level to baseline, is achieved in about half of children; 40% to 45% achieve partial reversal, and graft loss occurs in the remainder. Complete reversal from acute rejection is even less likely with subsequent rejection episodes. Younger transplant recipients are at higher risk for graft loss from acute rejection.

Corticosteroids

In children, as in adults, high-dose corticosteroid pulses are the first line of treatment of acute rejection, and approximately 75% of episodes are responsive to treatment. After the diagnosis is made, intravenous methylprednisolone is given in doses that range from 5 to 10 mg/kg per day for 3 to 5 days. After completing therapy, the maintenance corticosteroid is resumed at the prerejection level, or is increased and then tapered to baseline levels over a few days. The serum creatinine level may rise slightly during therapy and may not go back to baseline until 3 to 5 days after therapy is completed.

OKT3

OKT3 reverses up to 90% of the acute rejection episodes that do not respond to steroids. The pediatric protocol for OKT3 administration is similar to that used in adults (see Chapter 4, Table 4.4). For children who weigh less than 30 kg, the standard dose is reduced from 5 mg to 2.5 mg; a lower first dose is sometimes given. For children, as in adults, OKT3 can be administered on an outpatient basis after the first few doses. Children may regenerate the CD3–T-cell receptor complex more rapidly than adults, and twice-daily dosing of OKT3 is occasionally necessary to effect successful rejection reversal. Before completion of the OKT3 course, the calcineurin inhibitor dose should be increased so that at completion of the course, blood levels are somewhat higher than they were before treatment; this may reduce the incidence of rebound rejections. When rebound rejections do occur, they may be amenable to high-dose steroid treatment.

The side effects of OKT3 are similar in children and adults. Children must be euvolemic before administration of the first dose to prevent pulmonary edema. Fever is nearly universal, and diarrhea and vomiting occur in nearly half of children treated. Severe headache is common and may represent a mild form of aseptic meningitis. Occasional fatalities have been associated with OKT3-mediated cerebral edema.

Refractory Rejection

Refractory rejection usually refers to those episodes of acute rejection that do not respond to, or reoccur after, treatment with steroid and OKT3. Approximately 75% of cases can be reversed by switching to tacrolimus or adding MMF, if this drug had not been part of the immunosuppressive protocol. Relatively high doses and trough levels are required. Sirolimus is a potential treatment option, although experience is limited. Whenever such aggressive immunosuppressive therapy is employed, the risk for opportunistic infections and posttransplant lymphoma increases. Viral prophylaxis and infection surveillance are critical.

NONCOMPLIANCE IN PEDIATRIC TRANSPLANTATION

At least half of pediatric deceased donor transplant recipients demonstrate significant noncompliance. In adolescents, this figure exceeds 60%. Noncompliance is the principal cause of graft loss in up to 15% of all pediatric kidney transplant recipients; for retransplanted patients, this figure may exceed 25%. Reversible and irreversible episodes of graft dysfunction related to noncompliance occur in up to 40% of adolescents and are somewhat less frequent in younger children. Patterns of noncompliance vary from partial compliance to complete noncompliance. Partial compliance ranges from the occasional missed dose to an occasional extra dose. It is most commonly the result of forgetfulness, misunderstanding of a dose change or modification, or the presence of events that lead to the belief that medications are not helping. In children, complete noncompliance is often the result of underlying emotional or psychosocial stress.

Measuring Compliance

Methods to measure compliance are crude and provide only a general estimate at best. The easiest method is asking patients directly about their compliance; patients, however, tend to tell physicians what they want to hear. Assessments made by patients of failure to take medications are often accurate, whereas denials of noncompliance are not. Serum drug-level monitoring is only helpful when the drug level is either inexplicably low or high. Other methods to measure noncompliance include pill counts and assessment of prescription refill rates. A continuous microelectronic device, usually attached to the cap of the medication bottle, records each opening of the bottle as a presumptive dose and records the time and frequency of taking the medication. Recorded data can then be retrieved and an assessment of compliance made.

Predicting Compliance

Pretransplantation prediction of posttransplantation noncompliance is difficult. Risk factors include a disorganized family structure, female sex, adolescence, and a history of previous graft loss as a consequence of noncompliance. Personality problems related to low self-esteem and poor social adjustment are found with higher frequency in noncompliant patients. Studies indicate that compliance has no correlation with intelligence, memory, education, or the number of drugs that a patient takes, although the daily frequency of taking medications may affect compliance greatly. A linear decline in compliance rates has been demonstrated with increasing number of doses per day. Frequent clinic visits may improve compliance. Noncompliance in children must be suspected when there is unexplained diminution in cushingoid features, sudden weight loss, or unexplained swings in graft function or trough blood levels of the calcineurin inhibitors.

Strategies to Improve Compliance

Education, planning dose regimens, clinic scheduling, communication, and getting patients involved in the medical management are the main strategies. The child should know that the physician is their advocate and is interested in how they take their medications. Providing patients with specific reminders or cues to which the medication can be tied can be of great help. These cues should be simple and preferably part of the patient's daily activities, such as meal times, daily rituals, specific clock times, a certain television program, tooth brushing, shaving, and so forth. Contracting with pediatric patients and rewarding them is another strategy to enhance compliance. Finally, asking the same questions about compliance each visit and explaining the consequences of noncompliance repeatedly reinforces the compliance message and physician interest.

Psychological Intervention

Behavior modification programs and other means of psychological intervention may be beneficial in some patients. In the pretransplant period, an ongoing program of counseling should be undertaken in high-risk patients. Clearly defined therapeutic goals should be set while the patient is receiving dialysis, and family problems that are recognized in the pretransplantation period should be addressed before activation on the transplant list. The presence of at least one highly motivated caretaker is a helpful factor in long-term graft success.

Adolescence brings with it rapid behavioral and bodily changes. The adolescent's strong desire to be normal conflicts with the continued reminder of chronic disease that the taking of medication engenders; this tendency is particularly true when medications are taken many times a day and alter the physical appearance. Ambivalence between the desire for parental protection and autonomy, combined with a magical belief in his or her invulnerability, sets the stage for experimentation with noncompliance. Adolescents with psychological or developmental problems may use impulsive noncompliance during self-destructive episodes. The transplantation teams must be aware of these developmental issues so that they can initiate appropriate psychological intervention before the onset of significant noncompliant behavior.

GROWTH

Retarded skeletal growth is a constant feature in children with chronic renal failure and ESRD. The severity of growth retardation is directly related to the age of onset of renal failure; the earlier the onset, the more severe. Renal osteodystrophy, metabolic acidosis, electrolyte disturbances, anemia, protein and calorie malnutrition, delayed sexual maturation, and accumulation of uremic toxins have all been implicated in the development of growth retardation.

Growth retardation is typically assessed by the *standard deviation score* (SDS) or height deficit score (also known as the *Z score*). These measure the patient's height compared with that of unaffected children of similar age.

Determinants of Posttransplant Growth

Growth improves after transplantation; however, full catch-up growth is not realized in most patients. The following factors have a major influence on posttransplantation growth.

Age

Children younger than 6 years of age have the lowest standard deviation scores before transplantation, and these exhibit the best improvement in their SDS after transplantation. Two years after transplantation, infants younger than 1 year of age have an improvement in their SDS by 1 full standard deviation (SD), compared with an improvement of only 0.5 SD for those between 2 and 5 years of age, and 0.1 SD in those between the ages of 6 and 12 years. Children older than 12 years of age tend to have minimal or no growth after transplantation. Older children occasionally continue to grow into puberty; however, the growth spurt experienced by most growing children at this age may be blunted or lost.

The fact that youngest children benefit the most in statural growth from early transplantation provides a strong argument for expedited transplantation in an attempt to optimize and perhaps normalize stature. In addition, earlier transplantation allows less time for growth failure while receiving dialysis and therefore a lesser requirement for catch-up growth.

Corticosteroid Dose

The precise mechanism by which steroids impair skeletal growth is unknown. They may reduce the release of growth hormone, reduce insulin-like growth factor (IGF) activity, directly impair growth cartilage, decrease calcium absorption, or increase renal phosphate wasting. Strategies to improve growth include the use of lower daily doses of steroids, the use of alternate-day dosing, or dose tapering to complete withdrawal. Conversion to alternate-day dosing should be considered in selected, stable patients in whom compliance can be assured.

Ideally, steroids are withdrawn completely. In tacrolimus-based immunosuppressive regimens, withdrawal of steroids within the first 6 months has been successfully performed in more than 70% of patients. The effect of this approach on growth has been remarkable, with improvement in the SDS at 2 years after transplantation in children younger than 13 years of 3.6 SD in the withdrawn group, as compared with 1.5 SD in the nonwithdrawn group. The rates of acute rejection in the withdrawn group, however, were high, which could adversely affect growth by virtue of a decline in graft function and the need for high-dose steroids to treat rejection. In adults in whom steroids were withdrawn, a decline in long-term graft function has been observed (see Chapter 4, Part IV), and long-term followup of steroid-withdrawn children is required before this regimen can be adopted on a widespread basis.

Growth Hormone

The use of recombinant human growth hormone (rhGH) in pediatric renal transplant recipients significantly improves growth velocity and SDS. The NAPRTCS reports that growth velocity almost tripled 1 year after starting rhGH therapy, with a slight slowing after 2 and 3 years of therapy. There is some evidence to suggest that rhGH increases allogeneic immune responsiveness, leading to acute rejection and graft loss in addition to direct adverse effects on graft function. These adverse effects were not observed in the NAPRTCS data. Growth hormone therapy is generally started in prepubertal children at least 1 year after transplantation and continued until catch-up growth is achieved or until puberty ensues. Cyclosporine levels may fall after initiation of rhGH therapy, and the dose should be increased by 10% to 15%.

Allograft Function

A GFR of less than 60 mL per minute per 1.73 m^2 is associated with poor growth and low IGF levels; optimal growth occurs with a GFR greater than 90 mL per minute per 1.73 m^2. Graft function is the most important factor after high corticosteroid dosage in the genesis of posttransplantation growth failure. The immunosuppressive properties of corticosteroids needed to control rejection and preserve kidney function must be balanced against the need to minimize steroids to maximize growth. Thus, an excessive steroid dose leads to impairment of growth and an inadequate dose to impairment of graft function. Administration of high-dose recombinant human growth hormone may induce acceleration of growth even in the presence of chronic graft dysfunction.

Posttransplant Sexual Maturation

Restoration of kidney function by transplantation improves pubertal development. This most likely occurs as a result of normalization of gonadotrophin physiology. Elevated gonadotrophin levels and reduced gonadotrophin pulsatility are observed in chronic renal failure, whereas children with successful kidney transplants demonstrate a higher nocturnal rise and increased amplitude of gonadotrophin pulsatility.

Female patients who are pubertal before transplantation typically become amenorrheic during the course of chronic renal failure. Menses with ovulatory cycles usually return within 6 months to 1 year after transplantation and potentially sexually active adolescents should be given appropriate contraceptive information. Adolescent female transplant recipients have successfully borne children; the only consistently reported neonatal abnormality has been an increased incidence of prematurity. Adolescent males should be made aware that they can successfully father children. No consistent pattern of abnormalities has been reported in their offspring.

Posttransplant Infections

The reader is referred to Chapter 10 for a full discussion of posttransplant infections. The spectrum of infections and their presentation may differ somewhat between children and adults and the following section focuses on these differences. Infection in the immunocompromised child remains the major cause of morbidity and mortality after transplantation, and is the most frequent reason for posttransplant hospitalization.

Bacterial Infections

Pneumonia and urinary tract infections are the most common posttransplantation bacterial infections. Urinary tract infection can progress rapidly to urosepsis and may be confused with episodes of acute rejection. Opportunistic infections with unusual organisms usually do not occur until after the first posttransplant month.

Viral Infections

The herpesviruses (CMV, herpesvirus, varicella-zoster virus, and EBV) pose a special problem in view of their common occurrence in children. Many young children have not yet been exposed to these viruses, and because they lack protective immunity, their predisposition to serious primary infection is high. The incidence of these infections is higher in children who receive antibody induction therapy and after treatment of acute rejection, and prophylactic therapy is advisable.

CYTOMEGALOVIRUS

The incidence of CMV seropositivity is approximately 30% in children older than 5 years of age and rises to about 60% in teenagers. The younger the child, the greater the potential for serious infection when a CMV-positive donor kidney is transplanted. CMV infection may have the same effect on the course of pediatric transplantation as on adult transplantation, and various strategies have been proposed to minimize its impact. It has been suggested that seronegative children receive only kidneys from seronegative donors; however, given the frequency of seropositivity in the adult population, this restriction would penalize seronegative children with a prolonged wait for a transplant at a critical growing period. CMV hyperimmune globulin, high-dose standard immune globulin, high-dose oral acyclovir, and oral ganciclovir are all potentially valuable therapeutic options. Ganciclovir is effective therapy for proven CMV infection in children. Volganciclovir is under study in pediatric transplantation.

VARICELLA-ZOSTER VIRUS

The most commonly seen manifestation of varicella-zoster virus infection in older pediatric transplant recipients is localized disease along a dermatomal distribution. In younger children, however, primary varicella infection (chickenpox) can result in a rapidly progressive and overwhelming infection with encephalitis, pneumonitis, hepatic failure, pancreatitis, and disseminated intravascular coagulation. It is important to know a child's varicella-zoster antibody status because seronegative children require prophylactic varicella-zoster immune globulin (VZIG) within 72 hours of accidental exposure. VZIG is effective in favorably modifying the disease in 75% of cases. With the development of a new varicella vaccine, it is likely that all seronegative children with ESRD will be appropriately vaccinated.

A child with a kidney transplant who develops chickenpox should begin receiving parenteral acyclovir without delay; with zoster infection, there is less of a threat for dissemination, although acyclovir should also be used. In both situations, it is wise to discontinue azathioprine or MMF until 2 days after the last new crop of vesicles has dried. The dose of other immunosuppressive agents will depend on the clinical situation and response to therapy.

EPSTEIN-BARR VIRUS

About half of children are seronegative for EBV, and infection will occur in about 75% of these patients. Most EBV infections are clinically silent. PTLD in children, as in adults, may be related to EBV infection in the presence of vigorous immunosuppression (see Chapter 9).

POLYOMAVIRUS

Polyomavirus nephropathy is emerging as an important cause of allograft dysfunction and is discussed in Chapters 8, 10, and 13. The virus has been detected in the urine of up to 26% of transplanted children; however, allograft dysfunction as a result of infection appears to be uncommon.

Posttransplant Antibiotic Prophylaxis

Protocols for posttransplant antibiotic prophylaxis in children vary from center to center. Most centers use an intravenous cephalosporin for the first 48 hours to reduce infection from graft contamination and the transplant incision. The use of nightly trimethoprim-sulfamethoxazole for the first 3 to 6 months serves as prophylaxis against *Pneumocystis carinii* pneumonia and urinary tract infections. Prophylactic oral miconazole (nystatin) minimizes oral and gastrointestinal fungal infections. CMV prophylaxis has been discussed. Children who have undergone splenectomy should be immunized with pneumococcal vaccine and should receive postoperative prophylaxis for both gram-positive and gram-negative organisms, both of which may cause overwhelming sepsis.

Posttransplant Hypertension and Cardiovascular Disease

Persistent posttransplant hypertension is a serious problem in children, as it is in adults. More than two-thirds of transplanted children treated with cyclosporine are hypertensive, and many require multiple medications for blood pressure control. The differential diagnosis is the same as that for adults. It should be emphasized, however, that late-onset hypertension, especially when accompanied by low-grade fever, is commonly the first sign of acute rejection and may be present before any change in the serum creatinine level. Calcium-channel blockers are generally well tolerated in children and are the agents of choice for blood pressure management.

Concern regarding long-term cardiovascular morbidity and mortality has generally been directed toward the older adult posttransplant population. Young adults who developed chronic renal disease in childhood must also be considered to be at high risk for cardiovascular morbidity. Risk factors should be addressed in children who will hopefully grow to adulthood with their transplants. Serum cholesterol levels are frequently higher than the

185 mg/dL "at-risk" level for children with transplants. Dietary measures are appropriate to reduce hyperlipidemia and vascular calcification. There are currently insufficient data to make firm recommendations for the use of pharmacologic measures in children, but the HMG-CoA reductase inhibitors are generally effective and safe.

REHABILITATION OF TRANSPLANTED CHILDREN

Successful reentry into school after transplantation requires coordinated preparation of the child, family or caregivers, classmates, and school personnel. Treatment side effects, social and emotional difficulties, academic difficulties, school resources, and caregiver attitudes all play a role and should be addressed.

Within a year of successful transplantation, the social and emotional functioning of the child and the child's family appears to return to preillness levels. Pretransplantation personality disorders, however, continue to manifest themselves. Within 1 year after transplantation, more than 90% of children attend school, and less than 10% are not involved in any vocational or education programs. Three-year followup shows that nearly 90% of children are in appropriate school or job placement. Surveys of 10-year survivors of pediatric kidney transplants report that most patients consider their health to be good; engage in appropriate social, educational, and sexual activities; and experience a very good or excellent quality of life.

Children carry with them many of the medical consequences of chronic kidney disease into their adult life. Nearly half of adult pediatric transplant recipients are severely short and more than 25% are obese. Rates of hypertension, orthopedic problems, and cataracts are high. Despite these health problems, the great majority of these adult "survivors" report a good quality of life and successful rehabilitation.

SELECTED READINGS

Abbott K, Sawyers ES, Oliver JD 3rd, et al. Graft loss due to recurrent focal segmental glomerulosclerosis in renal transplant recipients in the United States. *Am J Kidney Dis* 2001;37:366–373.

Al-Uzri A, Stablein D, Cohn R. Posttransplant diabetes mellitus in pediatric renal transplant recipients: a report of the North American Pediatric Renal Transplant Cooperative Study (NAPRTCS). *Transplantation* 2001;72:1020.

Bartosh S, Leverson G, Robillard D, et al. Long-term outcomes in pediatric renal transplant recipients who survive into adulthood. *Transplantation* 2003;76:1195–1200.

Bertelli R, Ginevri F, Caridi G. Recurrence of focal segmental glomerulosclerosis after renal transplantation in patients with mutations of podocin. *Am J Kidney Dis* 2003;41:1314–1319.

Dharnidharka V, Stablein D, Harmon W. Post-transplant infections now exceed acute rejection as cause for hospitalization: a report of the NAPRTCS. *Am J Transplant* 2004;4:384–389.

Dharnidharka V, Sullivan K, Stablein D. Risk factors for posttransplant lymphoproliferative disorder (PTLD) in pediatric kidney transplantation: a report of the North American Pediatric Renal Transplant Cooperative Study (NAPRTCS). *Transplantation* 2001; 71:1065–1070.

Englund M, Berg U, Tyden G. A longitudinal study of children who received renal transplants 10–20 years ago. *Transplantation* 2003;76:311–316.

Ettenger R. The practical problems of prednisone. *Transplant Proc* 2001;33:989–991.

Fivush BA, Neu AM. Immunization guidelines for pediatric renal disease. *Semin Nephrol* 1998;18:256–266.

Gjertson D, Cecka M. Determinants of long-term survival of pediatric kidney grafts reported to the United Network for Organ Sharing kidney transplant registry. *Pediatr Transplant* 2001;5:5–15.

Jungraithmayr T, Staskewitz A, Kirste G. Pediatric renal transplantation with mycophenolate mofetil-based immunosuppression without induction: results after three years. *Transplantation* 2003;75:454–461.

Kaskel F. Chronic renal disease: a growing problem. *Kidney Int* 2003;64:1141–1146.

Lilien MR, Stroes ES, Op't Roodt J, et al. Vascular function in children after renal transplantation. *Am J Kidney Dis* 2003;41:684–691.

Matteucci M, Ugo G, Calzolari U, et al. Total peripheral vascular resistance in pediatric renal transplant patients. *Kidney Int* 2002; 62:1870–1877.

Mitznefes M, Kimball T, Border W. Abnormal cardiac function in children after renal transplantation. *Am J Kidney Dis* 2004;43:721–726.

Neu A, Ho P, Fine R, et al. Tacrolimus vs. cyclosporine A as primary immunosuppression in pediatric renal transplantation: a NAPRTCS study. *Pediatr Transplant* 2003;7:217–224.

Oh J, Wunsch R, Turzer M, et al. Advanced coronary and carotid arteriopathy in young adults with childhood-onset chronic renal failure. *Circulation* 2002;106:100–105.

Ohta T, Kawaguchi H, Hatorri M. Effect of pre- and postoperative plasmapheresis on posttransplant recurrence of focal segmental glomerulosclerosis in children. *Transplantation* 2001;71:628.

Rianthavorn P, Ettenger R, Malekzadeh M, et al. Noncompliance with immunosuppressive medications in pediatric and adolescent patient receiving solid-organ transplants. *Transplantation* 2004;77:778–781.

Salvatierra O. Felix Rapaport memorial lecture: moving toward a perfect transplant for pediatric kidney recipients. *Transplant Proc* 2002;34:2763–2766.

Sarwal M, Vidhun J, Alexander S, et al. Continued superior outcomes with modification and lengthened follow-up of a steroid avoidance pilot with extended daclizumab induction in pediatric renal transplantation. *Transplantation* 2003;76:1331–1336.

Sindhi R. Sirolimus in pediatric transplant recipients. *Transplant Proc* 2003;35[Suppl 3A]:113.

Yorgin P, Belson A, Sanchez J. Unexpectedly high prevalence of posttransplant anemia in pediatric and young adult renal transplant recipients. *Am J Kidney Dis* 2002;40:1306–1311.

Psychiatric Aspects of Kidney Transplantation

Kirk J. Murphy

Patients who are candidates for renal and/or pancreatic transplantation present numerous challenging and clinically relevant psychiatric issues. Within academic medicine, the mental health needs of transplant recipients and donors lie within the scope of transplant psychiatry—a subsection of consultation–liaison psychiatry, which is, in turn, a subspecialty within psychiatry. In the face of such quaternary subspecialization, clinicians seeking to meet the mental health needs of transplant patients may mistakenly conclude that they require arcane and esoteric knowledge in order to care for these patients. Fortunately, the task is a manageable one. The focus of this discussion is to identify the conceptual, diagnostic, and clinical issues most likely to confront psychiatrists, physicians, and other health professionals with responsibility for the mental health needs of renal transplant patients.

GENERAL CONSIDERATIONS

Whereas the formal roles assumed in the transplant process by psychiatrists, psychologists, and social workers may vary from center to center, the clinical needs of transplant patients are similar. Although many of the clinical details involved in the provision of psychiatric care for transplant patients are unique, the so-called biopsychosocial model provides a robust framework on which to organize clinical impressions and plans. This model encourages the integration of diverse symptomatology and presentation within a heterogeneous group along three primary axes: the biological, psychological, and social characteristics of individual patients. The following general discussion explores the model in the context of clinical issues arising in the psychiatric care of transplant patients.

With respect to biology, the most obvious delineation is that between donors and recipients. For this reason, the special issues pertinent to donors are covered separately. Among recipients as a group, the most salient biologic issue common to the group is that of immunologic rejection of the transplanted organ. With the exception of recipients receiving allografts from identical twins, all transplant recipients will require immunosuppressive medications as long as they have a functioning transplant. Because optimal graft function is currently associated with the use of corticosteroids, transplant recipients will invariably be at risk for their psychiatric side effects. Moreover, because the majority of other immunosuppressants is associated with central (and often peripheral) neurotoxicity, patients are at significantly elevated risk for a variety of psychiatric symptoms.

Yet another important biologic consideration is the etiology of the condition that led to end-stage renal disease (ESRD). From a psychiatric perspective, the most significant etiologic distinction is between conditions known to be causally associated with central nervous system (CNS) disease or dysfunction and those that are not. Among the former group, diabetes mellitus, hypertension, and systemic lupus erythematosus are the most significant, although Alport syndrome (and any other diagnoses associated with impairment of visual or auditory acuity) may be of potential significance.

The psychological issues facing transplant patients are divisible along multiple planes. The most fundamental distinction is that between donor and recipient. Within the latter group, the psychiatric issues confronting patients prior to transplantation differ in many ways from those that might arise after transplantation. Among transplant recipients, the issues of acute medication side effects, surgical complications, and questions of acute rejection and/or delayed graft function are most relevant in the immediate posttransplant period, whereas issues such as quality of life, medication compliance, the risk of chronic rejection, and long-term sequelae of immunosuppression become more relevant as the posttransplant time interval lengthens. Moreover, the psychiatric issues confronting patients with a history of multiple complications or severe rejection after transplantation differ from those confronting patients whose treatment course has been relatively uneventful.

The extent to which a patient became accustomed to medical treatment prior to the onset of ESRD is an important variable affecting their psychological response to transplantation. The helplessness and loss of control that transplantation may incur can be far more intrusive for patients with no experience of dependence upon medical care prior to ESRD than for patients who have become familiar with medical care as a result of their own chronic illness or that of their relatives. The nature of these previous experiences is an additional variable, which may positively or negatively impact on their expectations of transplantation and the physicians and other providers caring for them. Finally, the extent to which a patient does or does not tolerate dialysis treatments (or insulin maintenance therapy for potential pancreas transplant recipients) may have a substantial impact on their reaction to the prospect of transplant failure.

Social issues have substantial implications for assessment and management of psychiatric issues in transplant patients. The most obvious social variable is the extent to which illness may have affected the patient's available social and emotional support system. The unanticipated onset of ESRD may pose a significant challenge to the emotional capacities and defense mechanisms of the patient, spouse, other individuals, or the larger social unit. Conversely, some individuals may have suffered the vicissitudes of chronic disease in childhood and early adult life. The result of the early onset of chronic disease may significantly impact developmental milestones of young adulthood such as differentiation from the family of origin and the establishment of outside support networks. In this context, health professionals must be mindful of the prospect that such alternatives to putative "norms" of psychosocial development are, in fact, creative adaptations by family systems. Another potential consequence of early onset ESRD is that the cosmetic and social consequences of posttransplant immunosuppression may lead some young recipients to forego adherence to medication regimens in order to facilitate acceptance by their peers. This specific example serves to illustrate that psychiatrists and other health professionals who maintain curiosity about the social and emotional matrices of their patients' lives are more likely to succeed in communicating with them regarding potentially deleterious behaviors.

The fortuitous fact that within the United States all individuals with ESRD become eligible for health insurance by Medicare serves to maximize the demographic diversity of the patient pool with potential access to renal transplantation. The association of increased risk for both hypertension and diabetes with various specific ethnic groups also plays a role in determining the extent to which patients of varying ethnicity will comprise the total pool of candidates for renal transplantation at various centers. Particularly among first-generation immigrants, ethnicity may be a covariant with cultural values, linguistic fluency, and economic status. Psychiatrists and other healthcare professionals must be cognizant of the role these variables play in the patient's capacity to navigate the complexities of the tertiary healthcare setting.

Regardless of national origin, the availability or absence of economic resources for a given patient can also be of critical importance to health professionals working with the emotional needs of transplant recipients. In the vast majority of healthcare systems, economic resources are one—and often the primary—factor in determining access to transportation, lodging (at healthcare centers distant from patients' residences), child and/or elder care permitting clinic attendance, and long-term access to immunosuppressant medications. Stressors arising directly or indirectly (from their very tangible implications for graft survival) from these issues have substantial psychological impact upon transplant recipients. The presence or absence of financial resources can also determine whether or not a transplant recipient experiences substantial economic burdens resulting from ESRD, and may impact on their expectation and emotions regarding the consequences of success or failure of the transplant.

Educational experience is another relevant demographic variable. It is of particular importance to the success or failure of attempts to adequately inform patients about immunosuppressant regimens and the potential risks and benefits of the transplant procedure. Mental health professionals can have a direct role in optimizing long-term transplant function by ensuring successful communication between transplant team members and transplant patients of all educational backgrounds.

PRETRANSPLANT ASSESSMENT

In broad terms, the purpose of the pretransplant psychosocial assessment of both transplant recipients and their potential donors is to afford both parties an opportunity to acquire sufficient information to maximize the probability of a successful outcome. For donors, this information must include a thorough and comprehensible discussion of the nature of the risks of renal donation and of the precise extent and limits of potential benefits to both the recipient and donor. For the recipients, the information must include a clear and accessible discussion of the potential risks arising from immunosuppression and the transplant surgery itself, as well as the extent and limits of potential benefits arising from transplantation.

The conduct of the evaluation must afford the opportunity to obtain a longitudinal history of psychiatric symptomatology (including psychoactive substance use). It should assess the patient's capacity to comprehend and thus give informed consent and adhere to the immunosuppressive regimen. It should also provide a cross-sectional evaluation of the presence or absence of symptomatology consistent with active psychiatric diagnoses of relevance to transplantation.

Although corticosteroids and other immunosuppressants may induce neuropsychiatric symptoms in individuals with no prior psychiatric history, such symptoms are most commonly observed in patients with a preexisting history of thought disorder, mood disorder, anxiety disorders, and cognitive disorder. Although schizophrenia and other thought disorders are relatively uncommon (estimated lifetime prevalence between one and two percent), the disorders tend to be chronic, and hence are more likely to be active during a single clinical visit. In contrast, the episodic nature of many mood and anxiety disorders may minimize the likelihood of symptoms being present at the time of examination. Moreover, the symptoms associated with anxiety and mood disorders are generally less obvious to general clinical observers than are the presentations associated with chronic thought disorders. The more subtle presentation of anxiety and mood disorders has perhaps served to obscure the fact that such diagnoses are relatively common. Estimates of lifetime prevalence rates of mood and anxiety disorders in the general population vary between 12% and 20%; in the population of individuals with diabetes mellitus, the lifetime prevalence rates are closer to 30% to 40%.

The symptoms of thought, anxiety, and mood disorders are clearly the manifestations of biologic perturbations in the central nervous system. Available evidence strongly suggests that as the number of episodes of mood or severe anxiety disorder increases over an individual's lifetime, so, too, does the likely severity and frequency of future episodes. Additional evidence also suggests associations between the presence of symptomatic mood and anxiety disorders, on the one hand, and increased probability and severity of chronic medical illnesses (including diabetes, coronary artery disease, and possibly hypertension), and morbidity and mortality from major surgical procedures. The obvious pertinence of such findings for the reduction of transplant morbidity mandates careful assessment of the longitudinal history of psychiatric symptoms in transplant candidates. The fact that such a history is necessary for the expeditious diagnosis and management of acute psychiatric symptoms (especially those associated with corticosteroids) in the immediate posttransplant period further underscores the importance of such information for the transplant team as a whole.

The fundamental importance of this clinical information for the management of conditions that may contribute to posttransplant morbidity and mortality mandates the use of thorough and valid techniques to elicit the presence or absence of psychiatric symptomatology. The use of structured clinical interviews employing diagnostic instruments of demonstrated validity allows the clinician conducting the pretransplant psychosocial assessment the maximal opportunity to accurately detect the presence of psychiatric diagnoses relevant to transplantation. The use of casual, unstructured questioning which places upon the patient the responsibility of defining and recognizing medical diagnoses ("Do you have depression? Do you have any psychiatric disorders?") is inadequate and may lead to the failure to recognize episodic conditions (particularly mood or anxiety disorders) which are relevant to the post-transplant management of psychiatric symptomatology. Although a detailed discussion of diagnostic instruments used in psychiatric assessment falls outside the scope of this chapter, the ADIS-R (Anxiety Disorders Interview Scale–Revised) is a convenient method to facilitate rapid and thorough evaluation of transplant candidates. The ADIS-R focuses upon anxiety and, to a lesser extent, mood disorders. For reasons discussed above, accurate diagnosis of anxiety and mood disorders is of cardinal importance in anticipating the impact of high-dose corticosteroid therapy associated with immunosuppression.

Assessment of the history of psychiatric symptoms is best prefaced with an explanation of the reason for seeking such information. The psychiatrist should explain that the brain, like many other organs in the body, is susceptible to disruption by immunosuppressants and other transplant-related events. The patient should appreciate that information obtained from the psychiatric history will allow for appropriate pretransplant prophylactic measures to optimize posttransplant comfort and function. Patients who are reluctant to discuss their psychiatric history should be reassured that the mere presence of such a history is not, in and of itself, a reason to deny access to transplantation, and that very few psychiatric diagnoses are absolute barriers to transplant. In the United States, the *Americans with Disabilities Act* forbids any attempt to restrict access to transplantation or other medical services merely because of the presence of psychiatric symptoms or history.

Evaluation of Transplant Donors

Living kidney donation is an act of profound human generosity and when appropriate consideration is given to all its medical and psychosocial aspects, it can be a source of much gratification for all the parties involved. The psychosocial assessment of potential transplant donors must focus wholly on the needs and issues relevant to the donor's well being. Given the highly asymmetric nature of the physical benefits arising from renal donation, few, if any, circumstances in medical or psychiatric practice demand a more rigorous application of the ancient principle of *primum non nocere* (first, do no harm) than does the evaluation of potential organ donors.

The increasing shortage of deceased donors has been a stimulus to broaden the traditional range of individuals who are being considered as living donors (see Chapter 5). Whereas living donors were typically first-degree relatives for whom the nature of the relationship with the recipient and the motivation for donation was typically clear-cut, donors are increasingly individuals who are not biologically related. The psychosocial evaluation of unrelated or "emotionally related" living donors requires particular attention to ensure that their psychiatric well-being is protected.

Most individuals undergoing assessment for renal donation have made a free, informed, and autonomous decision to participate in the process. The evaluating psychiatrist, however, can never take this fact for granted. For this reason, it must be stressed that the purpose of the interview is to elicit and implement the donor's desires regarding transplantation. Potential donors should be explicitly informed of the option to elect not to proceed. They should be able to trust that they can exercise this option without fear that the motives for their decision will become known to the prospective recipient or any other parties, without their approval. Some potential donors actually do not wish to serve as donors, yet find themselves unable or unwilling to communicate their wishes to the prospective recipient or other emotionally relevant parties. Others, when informed of the existence of deceased donor donation as an alternative, elect not to proceed as a donor. Donors may have been led to understand that the recipient's life may be at stake, a situation that is rare. The fact that donor nephrectomy is not wholly devoid of risk is sufficient to cause some to reconsider their participation. A more subtle, and hence more difficult to evaluate, situation is that of donors who do not directly report a desire to forego participation in transplant, but who provide information suggestive of strong ambivalence or emotional conflict regarding their participation.

The psychiatrist, therefore, is obliged to ensure that the prospective donor is acting in the absence of coercion and in the presence of accurate information regarding the consequences of the donor's decision for the health of the recipient. In this context, the psychiatrist's sole ethical and clinical obligation is to the prospective donor. The psychiatrist (or other mental health professional) conducting the psychosocial evaluation of the donor must have no previous clinical relationship with the potential recipient. Only by maintaining rigorous boundaries can psychiatrists be experienced and perceived as pursuing the interests of their patient—the potential donor.

For donors to enjoy a truly free choice regarding their participation, the transplant team must respect the donor's ethical and legal right to reach an independent decision within the context of strict medical confidentiality. A corollary to the requirement for adamant delineation of boundaries surrounding psychosocial assessment of the donor is that absolute confidentiality must be maintained during and after the donor's evaluation. Rigorous protection of the donor's privacy requires that information arising from this clinical encounter must be obtained and maintained in a fashion that prevents all possibility of disclosure to potential recipients, the recipients' family members and associates, and any healthcare providers extrinsic to the donor's transplant evaluation. For this reason, the physicians and other healthcare providers with direct responsibility for providing care for the potential recipient should not participate in the evaluation of prospective donors for the recipient. For the same reason, the donor and psychiatrist must meet in the absence of family members, significant others, friends, or anyone else (with the exception of a professional translator, if required).

Another consequence of the statutory and ethical imperative to protect donors' confidentiality is that when translators are required, the translator must be unknown to the donor or recipient. The use of professional healthcare translators free of any relationship to donor or recipient is most feasible in large medical care centers in areas with substantial linguistic diversity; even in these settings, however, arranging such translation services for healthcare may require some effort. In circumstances or localities in which the appropriate professional medical translators are unavailable, arranging donor psychosocial evaluations at other centers where such services are available is a potential option. The use of remote (e.g., telephonic) professional translators at other medical centers, when appropriate, provides an alternative to physical travel by the donor to such locations. Because of the specialized vocabulary and information required for medical translation, any of the foregoing arrangements is infinitely preferable to the use of general purpose translation services provided (in the United States) by commercial long-distance telephone services.

Although creation of such rigorous privacy standards is irrelevant to many donors and thus may potentially be regarded as excessive, the unwilling donors who arrive for pretransplant psychosocial evaluation after multiple encounters with other components of the transplant service offer convincing refutation of the hypothesis that such stringent confidentiality measures are unnecessary.

Evaluation of prospective donors must include consideration of the possibility of direct financial incentive to the donor in the form of payment or other remuneration by the recipient or third parties acting on the recipient's behalf. Financial inducements for solid organ donation are a violation of federal law in the United States (see Chapter 17). Any suggestion on the part of donors (or other involved parties) of such arrangements must be the focus of intense scrutiny. The presence of financial arrangements as an incentive for renal donation is incompatible with the donor's participation in transplantation.

Evaluation of Transplant Candidates

There has been a steady reduction in the psychiatric diagnoses or findings regarded as absolute contraindications to transplantation. Psychiatric and general medical evaluation of candidates (see Chapter 5) have in common the purpose of considering those issues that are of predictive value for the survival of the allograft itself and for the overall health of the transplant recipient.

Adherence/Compliance

The most critical psychiatric issue influencing graft survival is whether or not the patient has the capacity to comply with the various components of a complex immunosuppressive protocol and to the associated regimen of intense medical surveillance. ("Compliance" is the term most commonly used for this capacity, although many prefer the term "adherence," which implies greater autonomy on the patient's part.) There are surprisingly few variables with predictive value for compliance. Adolescence is robustly associated with noncompliance, although a history of florid noncompliance with immunosuppression as a teenager is often not predictive of noncompliance as an adult. Patients who, irrespective of age, display a relatively stable pattern of conflict with medical care recommendations despite deleterious consequences are at great risk of noncompliance with posttransplant immunosuppression. Patients with severe thought disorders, extremely severe personality disorders (especially borderline personality), severe mood disorders (especially bipolar disorder), or psychoactive substance disorders (excluding tobacco) are at extremely high risk of noncompliance unless their primary psychiatric disorders can be successfully mitigated by treatment or other interventions prior to transplantation (such as the creation of a conservatorship or other such external locus of responsibility).

Regardless of circumstance or etiology, the presence of substantial medication noncompliance in transplant candidates at the time of evaluation does correlate with increased risks of posttransplant noncompliance. In these candidates, it may be wise to require a period of some months of documented adherence to a medication regimen and/or dialysis schedule in order to assess whether the candidate currently possesses the capacity to tolerate the highly structured medication and clinical regimen which follows transplantation. Some candidates who display an incapacity to tolerate such a structured regimen can subsequently be assisted in gaining that ability through cognitive and/or interpersonal psychotherapies.

Cognitive Disorders

For patients with cognitive disorders or other psychiatric conditions unrelieved by or unamenable to treatment, transplant candidacy can only be meaningfully assessed in the context of the patient's external environment. The extent to which the caregivers in that environment can reliably compensate for aspects of the patient's condition that serve as barriers to compliance needs to be individually assessed. It should be emphasized that even individuals with severe cognitive impairment can comply with the posttransplant regimen if the patient's family and caregivers are committed to the success of transplantation.

From a psychiatric perspective, the detrimental effects of transplantation upon the overall function of recipients arise chiefly from either cognitive impairment or the provocation or exacerbation of psychiatric symptoms. For transplant recipients whose social life and emotional support is derived solely from their dialysis center, the result of successful renal transplantation may be to exacerbate isolation and loneliness—both of which can exacerbate or even engender cognitive and psychiatric dysfunction.

In the selection of transplant candidates, the presence of cognitive dysfunction raises at least two questions for evaluating psychiatrists: (a) Can transplantation be expected to ameliorate or exacerbate the cognitive dysfunction? (b) Will any probable or possible exacerbation of cognitive impairment result in functional restrictions for the recipient? As a rule, answering the former question requires a putative or differential diagnosis of the cognitive impairment. Such a diagnosis inevitably requires the longitudinal history of psychiatric symptoms discussed above, and almost always requires neurocognitive testing to assess the precise deficit that may underlie the observed cognitive impairment. In general, cognitive impairments associated with impaired attention which arises from mood disorders, anxiety disorders, endocrine abnormalities, or perturbations of sleep or metabolic disorders associated with ESRD may be expected to improve posttransplant. In contrast, cognitive impairments associated with irreversible neuronal loss arising from severe hypoglycemia, poorly controlled hypertension, cerebral infarct, or primary dementias such as Alzheimer disease are unlikely to demonstrate significant improvement. For these patients, the crucial question of whether neurotoxicity arising from immunosuppressant agents will lead to further functional impairments can be only be answered—if at all—on an individual basis.

Substance Abuse

Depending on the practices and values of an individual transplant center, the question of optimizing allograft and recipient survival may or may not extend to consideration of individual behaviors regarding dietary choices, exercise, or tobacco dependence. Psychiatrists who are cognizant of the risks, benefits, and efficacy of various forms of medical and nonmedical management of obesity and nicotine dependence are best able to serve the needs of both transplant candidates and the transplant teams.

The presence of active substance abuse or dependence is generally regarded as a contraindication to renal transplantation. In contrast, a past history of substance abuse that was followed by successful abstinence for 6 months or greater is seldom, if ever, a valid contraindication. Among transplant candidates who present with active substance abuse or dependence, the most appropriate course is generally to defer acceptance for transplantation pending successful completion of substance abuse treatment and a specified period of abstinence verified through random serum qualitative checks for substances of abuse. The possibility of false positives or other factors that diminish the validity of qualitative testing for patients with ESRD must be considered. For this reason, transplant teams should obtain confirmation of qualitative "drug screen" results via assays of the highest possible accuracy and specificity prior to making clinical assessments or decisions.

Among transplant candidates with current or previous substance abuse or dependence, the probability of comorbid psychiatric diagnoses is significantly greater than among candidates without such diagnoses. For this reason, careful assessment of psychiatric history and symptomatology is of particular importance in candidates with substance abuse diagnoses.

Psychiatric History

The extent to which the posttransplant medication regimen may itself lead to psychiatric symptomatology that decreases overall function is largely determined by the patient's previous psychiatric history. For the purposes of candidate selection, those patients with a history of moderate to severe symptoms of thought, mood, and/or anxiety disorders that have proven refractory to adequate medication trials are at greatest risk of compromised function arising from uncontrolled symptoms after transplant. This group of candidates, as well as those candidates with a history of thought disorder, recurrent mood disorder, or long-standing anxiety disorder who are unwilling to accept maintenance treatment, pose a difficult challenge. Fortunately, of all transplant candidates with a history of significant psychiatric symptoms, the proportion of those with either symptoms refractory to adequate treatment or a refractory refusal to allow treatment is extremely small. Far more common is the patient with a history of moderate to severe psychiatric symptoms that have gone undiagnosed or have received inadequate treatment. If these patients are willing and able to receive effective psychiatric treatment prior to transplantation, their history of symptoms should not be regarded as a contraindication to transplantation.

Treatment of Posttransplant Psychiatric Symptoms

Medication Withdrawal

With the possible exception of hallucinogens, almost any psychotropic agent administered or used on a chronic or frequent basis can lead to withdrawal symptoms mediated through the central nervous system. A common and easily avoided psychiatric condition arising in the immediate posttransplant period is the result of inadvertent discontinuation of psychoactive medications on admission to the hospital for transplantation. Psychoactive substance withdrawal in the posttransplant period is complicated because most immunosuppressants can act to increase neuronal excitability and thereby decrease seizure threshold.

This condition is most likely to occur when a patient has been using benzodiazepines (especially short-acting agents such as alprazolam or triazolam) or other sedative-hypnotics for the management of insomnia, anxiety disorders, or other conditions prior to transplant. In these patients, the clinical picture usually progresses along a continuum of hyperarousal ranging from nervousness and anxiety to disinhibition, delirium, and withdrawal seizures. Prompt treatment of the symptoms of benzodiazepine withdrawal is mandatory. For moderate withdrawal symptoms, a starting dose of 0.5 to 1.0 mg of intravenous lorazepam can be carefully titrated upwards with an endpoint of reversing significant tachycardia and systolic hypertension arising from the withdrawal. Significant reductions in respiratory rate or falling oxygen saturation are suggestive of respiratory depression arising from benzodiazepine administration. In the event of incorrect identification of benzodiazepine withdrawal, or overly enthusiastic management of a correctly identified episode of withdrawal, the benzodiazepine receptor antagonist, flumazenil, and the equipment and capacity for emergent intubation must be available. Avoiding abrupt or rapid discontinuation of benzodiazepines and other sedative-hypnotics is the safest way to prevent this potentially lethal complication from arising during transplantation.

Symptomatic withdrawal syndromes that include mental status changes are associated with the discontinuation of a variety of psychotropic medications. The most frequent are

1. Diphenhydramine (which many dialysis patients receive in high oral or parenteral dosages).
2. Selective serotonin reuptake inhibitors or SSRIs (the withdrawal symptoms may be delayed by up to 36 hours).
3. Postsynaptic serotonin receptor agonists (nefazodone and trazodone).
4. Dopamine receptor antagonists (commonly used to treat dysregulation of gastrointestinal motility in dialysis patients).

Resumption of the discontinued medication is the most effective short-term intervention to control withdrawal symptoms as long as potential drug interactions with immunosuppressants are considered. In the event of withdrawal, symptoms arising from the discontinuation of nonpharmaceutical substances such as ethanol or nicotine, provision of an agent with cross-tolerance properties (benzodiazepines for ethanol) or via an alternative route of administration (transdermal nicotine) may also be useful.

Delirium

The central nervous system makes exacting demands of the body in order to maintain functional homeostasis. Delirium is an acute manifestation of failure to maintain such homeostasis. Delirium is a clinical diagnosis characterized by (a) a disturbance in consciousness manifest in reduced capacity to focus, sustain, or shift attention; (b) a change in cognition or development of perceptual disturbance; and (c) the development and fluctuation of symptoms over a course of hours to days. Delirium is relatively familiar in acute care hospitals in general, and in posttransplant patients in particular, and its development is always a cause for concern. Delirium is robustly associated with increased risk of morbidity and mortality. Medication withdrawal, narcotic analgesia, infection, immunosuppressant neurotoxicity, and protracted sleep disturbance can cause delirium. Given the diversity of causal factors associated with delirium, effective management even in the absence of certainty regarding etiology is essential for clinicians responsible for the care of transplant recipients.

Oral or parenteral haloperidol is commonly used in the management of delirium, although more rapid control of both behavioral disinhibition and agitation may be attained with parenteral droperidol. Droperidol offers the dual advantage of more rapid onset and a lesser chance of akathisia (a subjective sense of restlessness arising from extrapyramidal dopamine receptor blockade), thus minimizing the possibility of a positive feedback loop in which greater amounts of dopamine receptor antagonist are administered in order to manage apparent restlessness. Droperidol should be administered initially in test doses of 0.625 to 1.25 mg every 5 minutes, with monitoring for the extremely rare, reported side effects of hypotension and bradycardia; if neither condition becomes manifest, the dosage may be titrated upward to 2.5 to 5.0 mg over 10 to 15 minutes until control of acute agitation is attained. In patients with clinically significant hypotension or bradycardia arising from cardiac dysfunction, parenteral haloperidol may be used as a substitute for droperidol. Given that the duration of onset of haloperidol in this context is generally 20 to 30 minutes, the frequency of repeat dose administrations must be reduced accordingly. As with any delirium, the use of "low-potency" agents (of which chlorpromazine may be regarded as a prototypical example) is contraindicated secondary to anticholinergic side effects which exacerbate cognitive impairment.

Insomnia

Insomnia is the most common subjective neuropsychiatric symptom in the posttransplant period. While acute or intensive care hospital settings are intrinsically capable of engendering insomnia, corticosteroids are the most powerful and most common cause of insomnia in the first days and weeks after transplantation. Management of insomnia arising can generally be attained via the use of temazepam, with a dose of 15 to 30 mg sufficing for most patients. The use of the hypnotic triazolam (Halcion) or other short-acting triazolobenzodiazepines, such as alprazolam (Xanax) and midazolam (Versed), is inappropriate. In the posttransplant period, short-acting benzodiazepines are associated with an increased risk of both rebound insomnia and cognitive and or perceptual disturbances that can progress to frank delirium, profound affective lability, or overt hallucinations.

Anxiety

In the acute posttransplant period, as many as 20% of all patients will complain of the affective state of anxiety or the subjective experience of restlessness. These symptoms are most typically associated with corticosteroids, but may also occur with nonsteroidal immunosuppressants. Patients with a preexisting history of anxiety disorders (panic disorder, agoraphobia and other phobias, obsessive-compulsive disorder, and posttraumatic stress disorder) are at highest risk for this complication. Initial management of anxiety should include careful attention to the possibility of inadvertent medication withdrawal as well as the possibility of akathisia arising from the use of dopamine receptor antagonists used most frequently to treat nausea. In these cases, relief of anxiety is best attained by resumption of the discontinued psychotropic agent or discontinuing the dopamine receptor antagonists. In the majority of transplant recipients who manifest anxiety, neither of the aforementioned etiologies are present and of anxiety can be treated with clonazepam 0.25 to 0.5 mg p.r.n. every 8 to 12 hours, with titration of dosage and frequency of administration upwards as required for symptomatic relief. For patients who require parenteral administration, or who develop sad mood or overt depression in the context of clonazepam administration, anxiety may be managed with lorazepam 0.25 to 0.5 mg orally or intravenously every 4 to 6 hours. As in the management of insomnia, alprazolam (Xanax) and other short-acting benzodiazepines should be avoided. Barbiturates, because of their low therapeutic index and immunosuppressant drug interactions, have no place in the management of posttransplant anxiety.

Mood Disorders

Broadly speaking, mood disorders are manifest as insufficient cerebral activation (depression) or excessive cerebral activation (mania). Transplant recipients may also develop a mixed state characterized by affective lability, pressured speech, and/or behavioral disinhibition in the presence of intact sensorium and maintenance of orientation. Patients exhibiting behavioral disinhibition should be acutely stabilized with parenteral droperidol, in doses equal to or greater than those discussed above in the management of delirium, while awaiting psychiatric consultation.

Depression is characterized by a persistent (greater than 2 weeks) state of sad mood, and/or anhedonia, together with changes in thought content (hopeless or suicidal ideation), thought process (rumination), attention (decreased concentration), social relatedness (withdrawal), and somatic function (diminished energy and perturbations in sleep or appetite). The diagnosis of a first episode of depression in the posttransplant period is complicated by the fact that corticosteroids and other immunosuppressants may produce diminished concentration as a function of disruption in attention. Corticosteroids also commonly increase appetite and cause insomnia. For these reasons, the onset of persistent sad mood and/or anhedonia, hopeless or negative ideation, and suicidal ideation are the most reliable indicators of depressive episodes in the posttransplant period.

Patients with a previous history of major depression or other affective disorder are at greatest risk for depression in the posttransplant period. Pretransplant identification of a history of recurrent (two or more episodes) major depression should trigger prophylactic therapy. SSRIs of moderate half-life such as sertraline (Zoloft) or paroxetine (Paxil) are generally the best choices. The capacity of paroxetine to enhance sleep quality is an added advantage for patients troubled by sleep disturbance associated with ESRD. In patients experiencing a first episode of depression, or in patients in whom the diagnosis of recurrent major depression was missed prior to transplantation, either sertraline (50 to 150 mg q.a.m.) or paroxetine (10 to 40 mg q.h.s.) will generally ameliorate the symptoms within several days to a few weeks. Use of temazepam for insomnia or a low dose of clonazepam (0.25 mg every 8 to 12 hours) for anxiety engendered by depressive ideation or related symptomatology, can be of great relief to patients awaiting the onset of antidepressants.

Mania is characterized by persistently elevated mood, which may be of an ego-syntonic (euphoric) or ego-dystonic (irritable) nature. It occurs together with alterations in concentration (diminished attention), thought process (flight of ideas or loosening of associations), speech process (rapid or pressured speech), somatic function (insomnia, restlessness, and/or hypersexuality), judgment (diminished impulse control and/or grandiosity), and/or behavioral disinhibition. Mania may range from mildly intrusive to catastrophically disruptive. Incorrectly managed mania can cause allograft loss (because of noncompliance with immunosuppression or followup appointments), severe disruption of clinical or domestic settings, and behavioral disinhibition, which can engender lethal events for the recipient or others. Psychiatric consultation for suspected mania is imperative. While awaiting psychiatric consultation, acute disinhibition requires environmental (constant observation), and pharmacologic management (parenteral droperidol as used in delirium, with the addition of parenteral lorazepam for more rapid onset of sedation if needed). Less-severe symptoms of mania may be managed by clonazepam (0.5 to 2.0 mg every 4 to 6 hours, with careful titration to avoid excessive sedation progressing to respiratory depression in patients without tolerance to benzodiazepines). Gabapentin in an initial dosage of 100 to 200 mg t.i.d. with titration up to 400 to 600 mg q.i.d. is also effective in the management of mania associated with transplantation. Exacerbation of preexistent bipolar affective (manic-depressive) disorder by high-dose corticosteroids is the rule, rather than the exception, and transplant patients should receive mood stabilizers (valproic acid or gabapentin) prior to transplant. As in the case of recurrent major depression, the safest and most effective way of managing mania after transplantation is for candidates with a preexisting history to be started on prophylactic medications prior to transplantation.

Hallucinations and Delusions

In the majority of patients, the presence of hallucinations (perturbations of perception) and delusions (perturbations of cognition) in the posttransplant period are manifestations of delirium. Appropriate management includes palliative treatment of the distressing symptoms and efforts to identify and treat correctable causes.

Occasionally, hallucinations and delusions may arise without disturbance or fluctuation in consciousness. This picture is most likely to arise in patients with auditory or visual impairment prior to transplantation, but may also occur without sensory impairment. In recipients with no other psychiatric symptoms who are unconcerned by occasional visual hallucinations in the form of small dots or streaks of light, pharmacologic intervention may be unnecessary. When pharmacologic intervention is desired either because of patient preference or because of more overt symptoms, low doses of risperidone (Risperdal) (0.25 to 0.5 mg q.h.s. or b.i.d.) are generally sufficient.

IMMUNOSUPPRESSANT/PSYCHOTROPIC DRUG INTERACTIONS

Careful choice of psychotropic medications for transplant candidates and recipients can minimize the risk of deleterious interactions with immunosuppressants and hence minimize the risk of avoidable allograft dysfunction or rejection. Ideally, the choice of psychotropic agents in transplant patients is informed by knowledge of the relevant metabolic pathways for psychotropic medications, immunosuppressants, and the adjunctive medications commonly used in transplantation. Although a detailed discussion of these matters exceeds the scope of this chapter, awareness of general principles promotes informed application of specific recommendations.

The majority of significant drug interactions with psychotropic medications arise from alterations in the rate of oxidative metabolism carried out by the cytochrome P450 hepatic enzyme system, which is particularly important for the metabolism of the calcineurin inhibitors and sirolimus (see Chapter 4). Psychotropics that perturb the baseline activity of the IID6 and IIIA3/4 isoenzymes have the greatest propensity for deleterious changes in immunosuppressant levels.

Specific Recommendations

1. Among "serotonergic" antidepressants, the capacity to raise calcineurin-inhibitor levels is in order of: fluvoxamine > nefazodon > fluoxetine > trazodone > paroxetine > sertraline > citalopram. (Sertraline doses that equal or exceed 200 mg per day result in increased isoenzyme inhibition and thus disproportionately increased serum levels.)

2. Among anxiolytics and hypnotics, serum levels and half-lives of the triazolobenzodiazepines (alprazolam, midazolam, and triazolam), propofol, buspirone, and zolpidem are potentially increased by azole antifungals, macrolide antibiotics, and cimetidine.

3. Among anticonvulsants used in mood stabilization, carbamazepine may lead to decreases in immunosuppressant levels as a result of isoenzyme induction. Valproate is chiefly metabolized by phase II (conjugative) pathways, and thus poses far less risk of untoward interactions. Gabapentin, which is excreted unchanged, appears to carry no risk of altered immunosuppressant levels arising from altered metabolism.

4. Among atypical antipsychotics, sertindole and olanzapine levels are increased by interaction with posttransplantation medications to a greater extent than are levels of risperidone. With appropriate dosage modifications, all may be used successfully in transplant recipients.

5. Among typical antipsychotics, low-potency agents such as chlorpromazine are subject to alterations in serum levels resulting from changes in hepatic enzyme activity. High-potency agents, such as haloperidol and droperidol, appear to be less liable to such changes. For this reason, and because anticholinergic properties can exacerbate cognitive dysfunction, low-potency agents are a suboptimal choice for most transplant recipients.

6. St. John's wort, a popular over-the-counter herbal remedy for depression, is associated with graft loss as a result of isoenzyme induction and accelerated metabolism of immunosuppressants. Its use is contraindicated in transplant patients.

7. Fluvoxamine and nefazodone can cause increases in cisapride levels resulting in lethal cardiac arrhythmias.

SELECTED READINGS

Abbott KC, Agodoa LY, O'Malley PG. Hospitalized psychosis after renal transplantation in the United States: incidence, risk factors, and prognosis. *J Am Soc Nephrol* 2003;14:1628–1635.

Benedetti E, Asolati M, Dunn T, et al. Kidney transplantation in recipients with mental retardation. *Am J Kidney Dis* 1998;31:509–512.

Schlitt HJ, Brunkhorst R, Schmidt HH, et al. Attitudes of patients before and after transplantation towards various allografts. *Transplantation* 1999;68:510–514.

Ethical and Legal Issues Surrounding Kidney Transplantation

Robyn S. Shapiro

Since the late 1960s, when kidney transplants became a standard therapy for treating kidney failure, the disparity between organ supply and organ demand has intensified (see Chapter 1), and pressure has grown to find new sources of organs and new paradigms for allocation of those that are available. Proposals that have been put forward in response to this pressure raise a number of challenging ethical and legal issues.

DECEASED DONOR TRANSPLANTATION

Current Situation

Most transplanted kidneys are taken from brain-dead[1] individuals whose respiration and circulation are artificially maintained so that the organs remain fully oxygenated until they are removed from the donor's body for transplantation (see Chapter 5). While the total pool of potential organ donors following brain death is estimated to be at a maximum close to 14,000 per year, only approximately 4,500 deceased donor organs are actually recovered each year.

Under existing federal law, all hospitals wishing to retain eligibility for Medicare and Medicaid reimbursement must adopt written procedures to "assure that families of potential organ donors are made aware of the option of organ or tissue donation and their option to decline." Unfortunately, however, these "required request" procedures are not always followed; and even when prospective donor families are approached, permission to remove organs is denied almost half of the time. Hospital policy typically requires family permission in order for organs to be recovered even for the deaths involving individuals who have filled out an organ donor card or otherwise indicated before death their desire to donate their organs.

Changing the Current Situation—Alternative Approaches

Presumed Consent

Under a presumed consent system, consent for deceased donor organ donation would be presumed, and the organs of the deceased would be removed unless an objection had been registered in advance by the donor or by the family. Some presumed consent

---

[1]The Uniform Determination of Death Act, which has been adopted in most states, provides that an individual is dead if there is irreversible cessation of circulatory and respiratory function, or if there is irreversible cessation of all brain functions of the entire brain, including the brain stem. Uniform Definition of Death Act §1, 12 U.L.A. 386 (1980).

proposals would require that reasonable efforts be made to contact the deceased's family to ensure the absence of an objection to removal of the organs, but a "pure" presumed consent system would allow organ removal without these efforts, in the absence of preexisting evidence of an objection.

Presumed consent advocates argue that this approach spares families from having to consider organ donation at a traumatic time, and that it would produce greater numbers of organs for transplantation. However, public opinion polls indicate ambivalence among the American public regarding presumed consent. Some families have mounted successful legal challenges to the validity of presumed consent laws, which exist in a number of states, for cornea donation. In light of this ambivalence, there is a risk that if presumed consent were adopted, the public would be generally less supportive of organ donation.

Mandated Choice

A mandated choice system is favored by some who contend that the main reason for family refusal to authorize organ donation from a loved one is that the deceased did not previously express his or her own views on the subject. Under a mandated choice system, individuals would be required to make a choice either for or against deceased donor organ donation in order to receive or renew a driver's license or to file tax returns, and a central registry of these responses would be maintained and consulted when an organ donation situation arose. If the preferences of the deceased in favor of organ donation were clear, it is contended, the deceased's family would be more likely to consent at the time of death. Disadvantages to this approach include the significant costs and logistics of operating such a system. Moreover, requiring individuals to make a donation decision would not, in itself, provide motivation for, or assure, affirmative responses.

Protocols for Donation After Cardiac Death

The term "donation after cardiac death" (DACD) is preferred to the more familiar but more confusing term "non–heart-beating donor." DACD protocols are discussed in some detail in Chapter 5. They rely on the use of "irreversible cessation of circulatory and respiratory functions," as opposed to "irreversible cessation of brain function," which is the principle criterion for donation after brain death. There are several problems with this approach. First, it appears to violate the rationale behind the Uniform Determination of Death Act (UDDA). The UDDA added brain death to the traditional definition of death in recognition of the fact that but for technology's ability to indefinitely maintain heartbeat and respiration, cessation of breathing and heartbeat is really a proxy for death of the brain, which coordinates the processes that sustain human life. Under the DACD protocols, however, the organs are removed *before* the brain is dead.

A second problem with DACD protocols arises on account of the fact that the removal of vital organs obviously cuts off any possibility for an "apparent death" (i.e., an *impermanent* cessation of cardiopulmonary functions) to reverse spontaneously. The

Pittsburgh Protocol for DACD requires that a 2-minute period follow cessation of mechanical respiration before organ recovery commences. It has been contended that the Pittsburgh Protocol was adopted without adequate data concerning the potential for spontaneous autoresuscitation *after* the 2-minute stoppage called for in the Protocol and, therefore, the validity of this approach for declaring death has been questioned. To address these concerns, it was recommended at an international workshop in Maastricht in 1995 that the period between cessation of mechanical respiration and organ recovery be set at 10 minutes.

Financial Incentives for Deceased Donor Donation

Some advocate for change of the prohibition of organ sales in current law[2] on the theory that people may be more willing to provide organs if they receive compensation. They argue that as a general matter, producers supply a good only when the price they will receive provides an adequate incentive for its production. Even when scarce natural or life-saving resources are involved (such as the provision of expensive medical treatment), some note, the government generally permits the market to determine the distribution of resources and to assure an adequate supply.

On the other hand, many characterize the notion of an open market for deceased donor organs, in which those needing transplants would buy organs directly from the families of deceased donors, with the price determined by the law of supply and demand, as inefficient, inequitable, and immoral. More specifically, opponents worry that an open-market approach would undermine altruism in society, be coercive to the poor, jeopardize the quality of the organ supply, and dehumanize society by treating individuals and their parts as mere commodities. There is good reason to believe that in many parts of the world exploitation of paid kidney donors is commonplace.

Arguably, these concerns about an unregulated organ market would apply, to some extent, to any kind of financial incentive to donate. Yet, the objections to an open organ market do not apply equally to other forms of financial incentives; and as bioethicist James Childress wrote in 1989, "... it may be possible to accommodate some types of transfer of some kinds of tissues for valuable consideration without major ethical costs. Future contracts for cadaver organs may be one approach using financial

[2]The National Organ Transplantation Act, 42 U.S.C. §274(e) (2002), enacted in 1984, prohibits the buying and selling of human tissue and organs for "valuable consideration" for use in human transplantation if the transfer affects interstate commerce. As defined, the term "valuable consideration" does *not* include "the reasonable payments associated with the removal, transportation, implantation, processing, preservation, quality control, and storage of a human organ or the expenses of travel, housing and lost wages incurred by the donor of a human organ in connection with the donation of the organ." Individuals violating this law are subject to a fine of up to $50,000, imprisonment for up to 5 years, or both. In addition, 1987 amendments to the Uniform Anatomical Gift Act, 8A U.L.A. 2, which has been adopted by a number of states, prohibits the sale of organs "if removal of the parts is intended to occur after the death of the decedent" (8A U.L.A. 58).

incentives for cadaver organ donation that involves fewer ethical concerns. Under this approach, an individual could agree to donate his or her organs after death, in return for financial remuneration of moderate value from the state to his or her family, estate, or designated beneficiary at the time of the donation. The amount and form of the financial remuneration could vary (i.e., the compensation offered could take the form of an income tax credit, funeral expense reimbursement or a direct monetary payment); and the organs would be allocated under the current system.

Arguments in favor of a future contracts system include that it could enhance donor autonomy, avoid the need for posing requests for organ donation to grieving families at the bedside, and increase organ donations. In addition, some note that this approach would remedy the injustice in the current system, which provides a benefit to all parties involved in a transplantation procedure *except* for the donor. Also, in contrast to presumed consent, compensation for organ donation appears to have more widespread support among the public in the United States.

LIVING DONOR TRANSPLANTATION

Living donors play a large role in supplying kidneys for transplantation. Between 1994 and 1998, there was a 38% increase in the number of transplants from living donors in the United States. In 2002, 6,233 of the 11,863 kidney donors in this country were living donors. Living donation has been controversial because of the basic "do no harm" tenet in medicine. Removal of a kidney, which is of no physical benefit to the donor, entails a finite degree of risk (see Chapter 5, Part I) and at least 20 people are thought to have died as a direct consequence of donating a kidney. In addition, some worry that living donors may experience depression and/or resentment if the donated kidney is rejected. On the other hand, living kidney donations offer a number of advantages. For example, living-related donors often provide a better tissue match with the recipient, which means a reduced risk of rejection and higher rate of graft survival. In addition, living-related kidney donors often enjoy substantial psychological benefits, because of the opportunity to make such a big difference in the life of a loved one. Studies report that most donors feel better about themselves for having donated and assess their donation to be a high point of their lives.

Approaches for increasing living kidney donations include unrelated donations and financial incentives, which are discussed below.

Unrelated Donations

Living organ donors were initially biologically related on the assumption that the risk of immune rejection would be minimized; the pool of potential donors now extends to biologically unrelated donors. Most nonrelated donations have been from the patient's spouse or other emotionally related individuals, such as in-laws and close friends. Some donors have been coworkers, business associates, or acquaintances of the recipient; and, most recently, some programs have instituted "nondirected donation" programs, in which altruistic strangers donate kidneys for transplant.

One concern in nondirected living donation is the level of risk that strangers, as opposed to relatives, should be allowed to accept, in light of the fact that related donors have more to gain from the donation. In other words, it is argued, facilitating continued life or improved health of a loved one is a far greater benefit than the psychological benefit that may accrue to an individual who performs an altruistic act for a stranger. On the other hand, others contend that both types of donors realize substantial benefit, and given the subjective nature of such benefit, it cannot be said that any one donor's benefit is of greater value.

In all cases, it is important for the donor to fully understand material information about the procedure, including risks, expected recovery time and predonation evaluation procedures. In addition, it is advisable for prospective donors to undergo a psychosocial evaluation to rule out underlying psychiatric disorders and to confirm their capacity to make an informed decision about the donation.

Another concern with nondirected donation relates to allocation of the donated organs. In the absence of a national system for allocating organs from altruistic living donors, centers that offer nondirected living donation have been left to devise their own allocation systems. To assure equity, and to maximize the benefits of such donations, some centers limit the pool of potential recipients to patients on their waiting list who are candidates for a first or second transplant and who have no history of noncompliance with a medical regimen, and then simply rank these potential recipients according to the same point system used to allocate cadaveric kidneys (i.e. taking into account the extent of human leukocyte antigen matching between donor and recipient and the length of time the recipient has been on the waiting list).

Donor–recipient contact issues also arise with nondirected living donations. Nondisclosure of the recipient's identity prior to the procedure, and routing communication between donor and recipient following the procedure through the transplant center, help to assure the donor's altruistic motives. In addition, if the prospective donor wishes to remain anonymous even after the transplant, that should be imposed as a condition of the recipient's receipt of the donated organ.

Financial Incentives for Living Donation

The strongest argument in favor of legalizing organ sales by living donors is that it would generate an increased supply of a scarce and lifesaving resource. In addition, some contend that people should be able to dispose of their body parts in whatever way they wish, and that just as firefighters and deep sea divers are paid for their dangerous (and sometimes painful) work, those who undertake risk to contribute their organs for the well-being of others should be compensated. Bolstering this argument is the inequity that arises from the fact that while hospitals, doctors, laboratories, and pharmaceutical companies charge patients for transplantation-related products and services, donors are not compensated. A third argument in support of legalizing payment for living donation is that it occurs, despite being illegal, and it would be better to legalize the practice so that it could be regulated appropriately.

On the other hand, there are several potent objections to permitting sales by living kidney donors. One is that it could result in unfair disadvantages for would-be recipients who are unable to pay. One response to this problem would be for the government, or a private organization under government contract, to purchase the organs and distribute them equitably, with no directed donations allowed. Another objection to living organ sales is that it could well undermine voluntary organ donation, just as blood sales resulted in a decrease in voluntary donations. Some respond that this consequence is not inevitable, noting, for example, that professional social work and charitable social work coexist.

A further objection is that payment for organs would represent an additional cost that would be passed on to recipients, thereby increasing total transplant costs. However, supporters of payment for organs note that the shortage of transplantable organs inflates the economic returns currently generated by organ transplant programs and that increased organ supply brought on by financial incentives for donation would decrease overall costs of transplant procedures.

Tissue Engineering

As an alternative to expanding the organ supply through encouraged donation, researchers are increasingly interested in tissue engineering to produce organs. Some scientists are working with human adult cells in attempts to create muscle cells and small intestines. Others are working with embryonic stem cells, aiming to be able to program such cells to create replacement tissues and organs for transplantation without rejection. Some object to such research because embryos must be destroyed in order to extract stem cells. Others argue that the very early embryo from which the stem cells are derived is not a human "person," and that many early embryos used for such research are left over after being cryopreserved for infertility treatment purposes and would be discarded if not so used; and that there are significant benefits to be gained from the research.

XENOTRANSPLANTATION

A number of factors have increased interest in xenotransplantation to meet the growing organ demand, including improved understanding of both human and animal immune systems; insight into histocompatibility; new agents to control graft versus host disease; animal breeding programs for the production of transgenic animals; and perfection of surgical techniques. Yet, xenotransplantation raises a number of ethical and legal issues.

First, some believe that transferring organs from animals to humans is "unnatural" and wrong (a charge that has been levied against a number of other medical innovations, including assisted conception). However, it is difficult to separate that which is "natural" from that which is "unnatural." One could say that everything that humans do is unnatural because it constitutes an interference with the nonhuman natural order, or one could say that nothing that humans do is unnatural because humans themselves are a part of nature. Moreover, even if one could distinguish that which is natural from that which is not, it is not clear why interference with nature should be regarded as being wrong—especially when one considers that by interfering with nature, we have protected human lives from destructive effects of such natural phenomena as droughts, hurricanes, and infectious agents.

A second ethical issue surrounding xenotransplantation relates to the morality of sacrificing animals for purposes that can only benefit human recipients. Some respond by noting that humans occupy a higher niche in creation and enjoy a relative moral superiority over nonhuman animals, and that just as animals may be sacrificed for use in the food chain, they may be sacrificed to preserve human life through xenotransplantation, provided that guidelines for xenotransplantation assure that it is performed responsibly.

A third ethical and legal issue concerns informed consent. There are risks that infectious agents could be transmitted from animals to human transplant recipients, and then to the recipient's family and even the public at large. In light of this infectious disease risk, Public Health Service guidelines on xenotransplantation state that patients should be informed of the potential for infection from a zoonotic agent, told that they must undergo lifelong surveillance, and be asked to inform their current and future contacts of the risk of transmission of infectious agents to them. Some contend that this is inadequate, and that consent of the recipient's intimate contacts and the community at large should be secured prior to the performance of any xenotransplant procedure. Currently, however, there is no legal requirement for obtaining consent of third parties prior to the performance of a medical procedure, and a number of practical obstacles would preclude obtaining "community" consent.

A fourth ethical issue relates to the possible impact of xenotransplantation on public support for allotransplantation donations. The worry is that aversion to xenotransplantation may undermine the symbolism of organ donation as the ultimate human gift and result in an even greater organ shortage.

SELECTED READINGS

Abecassis M, Adams M, Adams P, et al. Consensus statement on the live organ donor. *JAMA* 2000;284:2919–2926.

American Society of Transplantation. The AST statement on ethics in organ transplantation. 1999. http://www.a-s-t.org/about/generalethics.htm

Anderson MF. The future of organ transplantation: from where will the new donors come, to whom will their organs go? *Health Matrix* 1995;5:249.

Brook NR, Waller JR, Nicholson ML. Nonheart-beating kidney donation: current practice and future developments. *Kidney Int* 2003;63:1516–1529.

Childress JF. Ethical criteria for procuring and distributing organs for transplantation. *Journal of Health Politics, Policy and Law* 1989; 14(1):87–113.

Cronin DC, Siegler M. Ethical issues in living donor transplantation. *Transplant Proc* 2003;35:904–905.

Delmonico FL, Arnold R, Scheper-Hughes N, et al. Ethical incentives—not payment—for organ donation. *N Engl J Med* 2002; 346:2002–2005.

Grazi R, Wolowelsky JB. Nonaltruistic kidney donations in contemporary Jewish law and ethics. *Transplantation* 2003:75:250–252.

Kahn JP, Delmonico F. The consequences of public policy to buy and sell organs for transplantation. *Am J Transplant* 2004;4:178–180.

Matas AJ, Garvey CA, Jacobs CL, et al. Nondirected donation of kidneys from living donors. *N Engl J Med* 2000;343:433–436.

Matas AJ, Schnitzler M. Payment for living donor (vendor) kidneys: a cost effectiveness analysis. *Am J Transplant* 2004;4:216–221.

Schreiber HL. Present and future legal aspects of living donor transplantation. *Transplant Proc* 2003;35:903.

Sheehy E, Conrad SL, Brigham LE. Estimating the number of potential organ donors in the United States. *N Engl J Med* 2003;349:667–674.

Nutrition in the Kidney Transplant Recipient

Susan Weil Guichard

The nutritional management of the renal transplant recipient is an important determinant of outcome in terms of both morbidity and mortality. Diet can be used to prevent and ameliorate many transplant-related complications, although the precise nutrient requirements of kidney transplant recipients continue to be incompletely defined. The following recommendations provide a guide to nutrition care management in the pretransplant, acute posttransplant, and long-term posttransplant periods.

PRETRANSPLANT NUTRITION MANAGEMENT

Major Concerns

In the pretransplant period, a multidisciplinary approach should incorporate diet and lifestyle changes to help correct or improve malnutrition, dyslipidemia, obesity, renal osteodystrophy, and hypertension. To varying degrees, the presence of these comorbidities in the pretransplant recipient is a predictor of related complications in the posttransplant period. Although the etiology of these problems is multifactorial, it is reasonable to assume that aggressive nutritional management in the pretransplant period may help minimize posttransplant morbid events.

Malnutrition

The primary nutritional focus of the pretransplant period is the prevention and treatment of malnutrition, some element of which has been identified in up to 70% of the dialysis population, in whom a low serum albumin level is a powerful predictor of mortality risk and morbidity. In data from the Centers for Medicare and Medicaid Services (CMS) 2002 Clinical Performance Measures Project, only 36% of hemodialysis and 19% of peritoneal dialysis recipients in the U.S. had albumin levels equal to or greater than 4.0 g/dL. Inadequate dialysis can compound the effect of malnutrition. In addition, chronic inflammation may cause low albumin, malnutrition and progressive atherosclerotic cardiovascular disease in dialysis recipients. The causes of inflammation are multifactorial but proinflammatory cytokines such as interleukin (IL)-6 and tumor necrosis factor (TNF)-α may play a central role. Markers of inflammation, such as C-reactive protein, are elevated in both peritoneal and hemodialysis patients, and inflammation appears to be a cause of hypoalbuminemia via increased albumin catabolism.

It is not entirely clear how these findings before transplantation may affect transplant outcome. Low serum albumin levels and other evidence of poor protein status are predictors of surgical risk and risk of infection. Aggressive treatment of malnutrition with oral supplements, tube feeding, or parenteral nutrition (PN), as well as careful attention to dialysis adequacy and intervening causes of poor intake, may not only ultimately improve transplant outcome, but allow transplantation to be an option for recipients who may otherwise have been excluded.

Obesity, Dyslipidemia, and Cardiovascular Disease

The incidence of postoperative wound complications, and in some studies, delayed graft function, and recipient and graft survival, may be increased in recipients with pretransplant obesity, defined as a body mass index (BMI) of more than 30 kg/m^2 or more than 130% of ideal body weight. Meier-Kriesche and his group, in a retrospective analysis of the U.S. Renal Data Systems transplant registry found that extremes in BMI (less than 18 and greater than 36 kg/m^2) were associated with significantly worse recipient and graft survival independent of other known risk factors for recipient and graft survival. Conflicting findings from Johnson's group suggest that obese recipients experience an increase in wound complications, such as perioperative infections and wound dehiscence, but not patient or graft survival, when those with preexisting cardiac disease were excluded from transplantation (see "Selected Readings," below). Posttransplant hyperlipidemia, hypertension, and glucose intolerance have been observed in obese recipients and play a role in the development of cardiovascular disease. It has been suggested that obese recipients with a cardiac history should not undergo transplantation until weight loss to a BMI of less than 30 kg/m^2 has been achieved. Chronic kidney disease (CKD) stage V is associated with dyslipidemia, as evidenced by moderate hypertriglyceridemia with a normal total cholesterol; normal or increased triglyceride-rich low-density lipoprotein (LDL); decreased high-density lipoprotein (HDL); increased cholesterol-rich very-low-density lipoprotein (VLDL); and increased susceptibility of LDL to oxidation. Decreased levels of apoprotein A-I, and increased apoprotein B, apoprotein C-III, and lipoprotein (a) have also been described, and contribute to the increased incidence of cardiovascular disease in this population. In addition, abnormalities of mineral metabolism (elevated phosphorus and calcium–phosphorus product), as well as secondary hyperparathyroidism, have been implicated in the etiology of nonatherogenic cardiovascular disease in the CKD population. Attention to dialysis adequacy, treatment of anemia, dyslipidemia, secondary hyperparathyroidism, hypertension, diabetes, and weight management in the transplant candidate can potentially improve certain outcomes once they become transplant recipients.

Nutritional Assessment of the Transplant Candidate

Nutritional assessment of the transplant candidate should include the following:

- History—medical and dialysis history including comorbidities; current intake; gastrointestinal/appetite symptoms; use of medications including vitamins and herbal preparations; physical activity and limitations; psychosocial and financial impediments to adherence to diet therapy, allergies or food intolerances

- Physical/anthropometric assessment—evidence of muscle wasting and depletion of subcutaneous fat stores determined by subjective global assessment or other measurements, although triceps skinfold, arm muscle circumference, and mid-arm circumference may be less reliable as a consequence of variations in fluid status; height; weight; weight changes; physical evidence of vitamin deficiencies
- Laboratory data—serum albumin; lipid profile; anemia profile including hemoglobin, ferritin, transferrin saturation; bone disease profile including parathyroid hormone, phosphorus and calcium; Kt/V; glycosylated hemoglobin (HGA_{1C}) in diabetics

ACUTE POSTTRANSPLANT NUTRITION MANAGEMENT

Major Concerns

Protein Catabolism

The acute posttransplant period generally refers to the 4- to 6-week period after surgery when the stress of surgery combined with the use of high-dose corticosteroids can lead to severe protein catabolism, particularly in recipients with underlying malnutrition. The primary goal is to provide adequate protein and calories to counteract protein catabolism, promote wound healing, and decrease susceptibility to infection associated with protein malnutrition.

Fluid and Electrolyte Balance

During the postoperative period, fluid and electrolyte requirements vary depending on the level of renal function, volume status, and drug–nutrient interactions. Needs are reassessed daily to balance between adequate hydration and volume overload. Specific guidelines are discussed in the section "Acute Posttransplant Nutrient Requirements," below.

Drug–Nutrient Interactions

Drug–nutrient interactions, important in the long-term management of the transplant recipient, should also be considered in the acute period. Table 18.1 lists both short- and long-term side effects, including nutrient interactions, of immunosuppressive agents. A special concern is the interaction between grapefruit and cyclosporine. Grapefruit or grapefruit juice inhibits the metabolic activities of cytochrome P450 (CYP)3A4 isoenzyme, the most abundant P450 enzyme, which is found primarily in liver and intestinal epithelial tissues. Grapefruit is thought to inhibit gut wall CYPA34 and thereby increase absorption when taken concomitantly with cyclosporine. This interaction is thought to also be pertinent to tacrolimus and sirolimus.

Acute Posttransplant Nutrient Requirements

In the following sections, the recommendations listed as "per kilogram of body weight" should be based on actual body weight in the underweight/appropriate weight patient, or body weight adjusted for obesity in the obese patient.

Table 18.1.   Side effects of immunosuppressive agents

Immunosuppressive Agent	Side Effect
Corticosteroids	Polyphagia, glucose intolerance, hyperlipidemia, osteoporosis, gastritis and peptic ulcer disease, fluid retention, hypertension, protein catabolism, altered mood
Cyclosporine	Nephrotoxicity, neurotoxicity, hypertension, glucose intolerance, hyperlipidemia, hyperkalemia, hypomagnesemia, hyperuricemia, gingival hypertrophy
Azathioprine	Leukopenia, thrombocytopenia, megaloblastic anemia, nausea and vomiting, hepatic dysfunction
Atgam and Thymoglobulin	Chills, fever, leukopenia, thrombocytopenia, hyperglycemia (rare), diarrhea, nausea, vomiting
OKT3	Chills, fever, arthralgias, hypertension, pulmonary edema, nephrotoxicity, headache, encephalopathy, nausea, vomiting, diarrhea
Tacrolimus	Anemia, leukocytosis, hypertension, hyperglycemia, hyperkalemia or hypokalemia, hyperuricemia, hypomagnesemia, nausea, abdominal pain, gas, vomiting, anorexia, constipation, diarrhea, leukopenia
Mycophenolate mofetil (MMF)	Anorexia, nausea, epigastric pain, gas, diarrhea, abdominal pain
Sirolimus	Hypertriglyceridemia, hypercholesterolemia, thrombocytopenia, leukopenia, hypokalemia, delayed wound healing (at high doses)
Basiliximab and daclizumab	None identified

Protein

In the acute postoperative period, protein requirements are generally accepted to be 1.3 to 2.0 g/kg body weight. These levels are compatible with neutral or positive nitrogen balance, provided caloric intake is adequate. For recipients who continue to require dialysis, these levels of protein intake do not result in an increased dialysis requirement and therefore are used in patients with a functioning or nonfunctioning graft. With evidence of protein depletion, protein is provided at the upper end of the recommended range.

Calories

For the uncomplicated recipient, caloric requirements are 30 to 35 kcal/kg or 1.3 to 1.5 × basal energy expenditure (BEE) as determined by the Harris-Benedict equation, although this equation has not been systematically studied in kidney transplant recipients. This calorie level appears to be compatible with maintaining or achieving neutral or positive nitrogen balance.

Carbohydrates

Recommendations are 50% to 70% of calories should be from carbohydrate sources with diabetic diet modifications as needed in the presence of hyperglycemia. Several small, early studies demonstrated that limitation of carbohydrates in combination with a high-protein diet minimized cushingoid facies in renal transplant recipients; however, these studies have not been repeated in a larger population or on a long-term basis.

Fat

Diet modification for hyperlipidemia, a key issue in the long-term management of the transplant recipients, can be introduced in the early postoperative period, assuming calorie requirements are easily met. Up to 35% of calories from fat can be provided, in keeping with the National Heart, Lung, and Blood Institute Adult Treatment Panel III Guidelines (Table 18.2).

Sodium

Hypertension and volume overload are common in the posttransplant period. Cyclosporine-related hypertension is, in part, salt dependent (see Chapter 9). In these circumstances, control of sodium intake to 2 g per day is appropriate. Normotensive recipients who are edema-free do not require strict sodium restriction.

Potassium

Hyperkalemia, often seen in the posttransplant period in the presence of cyclosporine/tacrolimus toxicity or impaired graft function, may be exaggerated with the use of β-adrenergic

---

Table 18.2. Adult Treatment Panel III (ATP III) guidelines[a]

Therapeutic Lifestyle Changes (TLC) in Low-Density Lipoprotein (LDL)-Lowering Therapy

Major features
- TLC diet
  - Reduced intake of cholesterol-raising nutrients (same as previous step II diet)
    - Saturated fats <7% of total calories
    - Dietary cholesterol <200 mg/day
  - LDL-lowering therapeutic options
    - Plant stanols/sterols (2 g/day)
    - Viscous (soluble) fiber (10–25 g/day)
- Weight reduction
- Increased physical activity

---

[a]The ATP III guidelines were developed by The National Heart, Lung, and Blood Institute of the National Institutes of Health and the U.S. Department of Health and Human Resources.

blocking agents, angiotensin-converting enzyme inhibitors, acidosis, and potassium-containing phosphorus supplements. Treatment of hyperkalemia may require dietary potassium restriction or more aggressive measures. If potassium restriction is warranted, approximately 1 mEq of potassium should be allowed per gram of protein in the diet, so as not to interfere with adequate protein intake.

Phosphorus

Hypophosphatemia is a common finding after transplantation, primarily as a result of increased urinary excretion of phosphate both mediated by and independent of residual secondary hyperparathyroidism. In addition, glucocorticoid-induced gluconeogenesis in the renal proximal tubule contributes to phosphaturia. Increased intake of high-phosphorus foods may not be sufficient for repletion, and oral replacement is often necessary.

In the presence of delayed graft function, the use of phosphate-binding antacids may be temporarily warranted to control hyperphosphatemia. A drug interaction has been identified between sevelamer hydrochloride and mycophenolic acid that results in lowered mycophenolic acid levels. Peak levels and the area under the curve (AUC) were reduced by a mean of 25% of the AUC as a result of a 30% mean decrease in maximal drug concentration (C_{max}) after coadministration with sevelamer hydrochloride, so caution should be used when both medications are prescribed.

Magnesium

Hypomagnesemia, which may exacerbate cyclosporine-induced nervous system toxicity, is a common postoperative finding secondary to cyclosporine- and tacrolimus-induced hypermagnesuria. Dietary replacement of magnesium is likely to be inadequate, necessitating the use of magnesium supplements.

Fluid Intake

Early posttransplant fluid management is discussed in Chapter 8. For a normovolemic recipient with a well-functioning graft, a reasonable minimum fluid intake is 2,000 mL per day. For an oliguric recipient, a volume of fluid should be provided to equal urine output plus a minimum of 500 to 750 mL to cover insensible losses. Variations should be determined by volume status and blood pressure, typically erring on the positive side, as urine output increases.

Vitamins

Replacement of water-soluble vitamins containing B complex and up to 100 mg of vitamin C should be continued as long as posttransplant dialysis is required. See "Nutrient Recommendations for the Stable Transplant Recipient," below.

Trace Minerals
IRON

Iron deficiency, defined as a transferrin saturation (iron/total iron-binding capacity) of less than 20% or a serum ferritin level of less than 100 ng/mL, is a common finding in CKD recipients receiving erythropoietin, particularly those not treated with hemodialysis, where intravenous iron is typically provided. A preoperative evaluation of iron status and correction of deficiency is indicated to optimize treatment of anemia.

OTHER TRACE MINERALS

Posttransplant trace mineral requirements have not been well investigated. Zincuria is associated with steroid therapy, although its clinical significance is not well substantiated. Routine supplementation of trace minerals is not indicated in recipients on an oral diet.

NUTRITIONAL SUPPORT IN THE POSTTRANSPLANT PERIOD

In nutritionally high-risk recipients, early nutritional support is indicated. Use of aggressive nutritional support in recipients with CKD and septic complications, including posttransplant recipients, reduces mortality rates.

In the typical posttransplant course, progression to oral intake and solid foods occurs within 2 to 3 postoperative days. The length of hospitalization may be less than 1 week, and aggressive nutritional support is rarely necessary. The following guidelines, however, can be used for recipients of combined pancreas–kidney transplants, who may not be able to tolerate oral nutrition for prolonged periods (see Chapter 14).

Indications for Aggressive Nutritional Intervention

Delayed Oral Intake

Nutritional support in the form of PN may be warranted if postoperative oral intake is delayed for more than 5 days because of complications such as protracted ileus, intractable nausea and vomiting, or graft pancreatitis. The decision to begin PN should be made only after failed attempts at oral intake and tube feeding, or if either route is contraindicated.

Inadequate Intake

Any recipient unable to sustain adequate intake to meet protein and calorie needs after the fifth postoperative day is considered a potential candidate for some type of nutritional intervention. The decision to intervene will depend on the nutritional status of the recipient, degree of catabolism (either measured by urea generation rate or estimated by type and degree of surgical or medical complication), and the amount of intake deficit.

Choice of Feeding Modality

Oral Supplements

Supplements are considered 4 to 5 days after surgery in any recipient in whom protein and calorie needs are not being met on a standard diet. Correctable reasons for inadequate oral intake should be assessed, such as overly restrictive diet, unnecessarily slow progression to a full diet, and interference with meals by dialysis, scheduled tests, and procedures.

Tube Feeding

Tube feeding, rarely required after kidney transplant, is considered in the postoperative period in any recipient with a functional gastrointestinal tract who, by postoperative day 5, is unable to maintain adequate protein and calorie nutrition with the use of diet or oral supplements. Small bowel access and use of continuous feeding are preferred when tube feeding is indicated. Tube feeding is preferred over parenteral nutrition because of a decreased risk for infection related to central line use, and because with tube feeding, production of secretory immunoglobulins help to prevent adverse bacterial growth in the intestinal mucosal lining, as well as maintain normal intestinal function and integrity.

A wide variety of high nitrogen oral and enteral products are commercially available to meet the needs of the transplant recipient.

Total Parenteral Nutrition

A mixture of both essential and nonessential amino acids, fat, and dextrose should provide a daily intake of at least 1.5 g protein/kg and 30 to 35 kcal/kg. Preferably, calorie requirements are assessed by indirect calorimetry.

Dietary Considerations During Acute Rejection Episodes

During acute rejection episodes, provision of optimal protein and calorie intake is the primary nutritional concern. High-dose steroids produce a dose-related increase in protein catabolic rate, leading to severe catabolism. Protein intake providing at least 1.5 g/kg is appropriate.

Special Considerations for the Simultaneous Pancreas–Kidney Recipient

For the well-functioning combined pancreas–kidney transplant, nutritional guidelines are essentially the same as for solitary kidney transplants, except with regard to fluid and electrolyte intake. In the bladder-drained pancreas transplant, persistent exocrine pancreatic drainage into the bladder results in sizable urinary losses of sodium chloride and sodium bicarbonate (see Chapter 14). Extracellular fluid volume contraction and metabolic acidosis may ensue, necessitating sodium and bicarbonate replacement. Enteric drainage of the exocrine pancreas secretions and resultant reabsorption of pancreatic secretions is now commonly used and avoids these metabolic complications, although diarrhea may be present until the bowel adapts.

LONG-TERM NUTRITION MANAGEMENT

For many recipients, a successful kidney transplant represents a long-awaited opportunity to be liberated from the certain diet restrictions required while on dialysis. When providing diet instruction, this need for "liberation" should be recognized and directed in a manner that will permit the recipient a well-deserved sense of dietary freedom without potentially morbid dietary indiscretion. For some recipients, it is hard to "loosen up" from years of compulsive dietary control, but instruction by a skilled renal dietitian helps to facilitate this transition. In the presence of varying degrees of chronic allograft nephropathy, nutrition guidelines should be implemented in accordance with National Kidney Foundation Disease Outcome Quality Initiative recommendations for CKD stages I to IV, with adjustments as appropriate considering the use of immunosuppressive agents and other comorbidities.

Major Concerns

Hyperlipidemia

Cardiovascular disease remains the main cause of long-term mortality in the transplant population. Risk factors for atherosclerotic disease commonly found in the transplant population include hyperlipidemia, diabetes, obesity, and hypertension, and are directly affected by immunosuppressive agents. Posttransplant hyperlipidemia occurs in up to 82% of transplant recipients and is associated with use of glucocorticoids, cyclosporine, and sirolimus and potentially aggravated by obesity. In addition to the development of cardiovascular disease, chronic allograft nephropathy may be enhanced by the presence of hyperlipidemia.

Transplant recipients treated with cyclosporine typically present with elevated VLDL cholesterol and LDL levels thought to be a direct effect of cyclosporine on cell membrane cholesterol concentration and regulatory pools, resulting in both increased synthesis of cholesterol and decreased clearance of LDL. HDL levels are typically normal or elevated in the absence of obesity; however, the cardioprotective HDL^2 fraction may remain low. Cyclosporine has also been associated with an increase in lipoprotein (a). The hyperlipidemic effect of corticosteroids is well established and is thought to result from increased hepatic VLDL synthesis and a resultant increase in cholesterol and triglycerides. Sirolimus appears to increase hepatic synthesis of triglyceride, secretion of VLDL, and hypertriglyceridemia as a result of alteration in insulin signaling pathways and, thereby, increased adipose tissue lipase activity, decreased lipoprotein lipase activity, or a combination of both. Diet therapy and exercise may be at least partially effective in lipid reduction after transplantation, although the "statin" drugs are often required.

Homocysteine

Homocysteine is a sulfur-containing amino acid produced in all cells; it is formed from the essential amino acid methionine through methylation. Hyperhomocysteinemia has been identified as a risk factor for the development of cardiovascular disease in the general population. Several B complex vitamins play a role in the metabolic pathway of methionine. Pyridoxine (vitamin B_6) is a cofactor for cystathionine-beta-synthase, by which homocysteine is transformed to cystathionine—the initial step in the transsulfuration pathway and renal excretion of sulfur. Roughly half of the homocysteine formed from a normal diet is remethylated to methionine by a pathway requiring folic acid and vitamin B_{12}. Low levels of these B vitamins, serum albumin levels, age, renal impairment, and a genetic mutation in methylenetetrahydrofolate reductase, which limits the conversion of homocysteine to methionine, correlate with homocysteine levels. A high prevalence of hyperhomocysteinemia has also been identified in the renal transplantation population, and an inverse relationship has been identified between renal function and high homocysteine levels. Renal transplant recipients do not respond to the usual B-vitamin doses used to correct hyperhomocysteinemia in the general population, and behave much like the early stage CKD population in terms of etiology and treatment response. Supraphysiologic doses of B vitamins do seem to lower homocysteine in this population, and they are more responsive than the CKD dialysis-dependent population. Studies in the CKD population also suggest a link between risk for cardiovascular disease and hyperhomocysteinemia. Marcucci's group demonstrated that supplementation (5 mg folic acid, 50 mg vitamin B_6, and 400 μg vitamin B_{12}) over a 6-month period not only lowered homocysteine levels in renal transplant recipients, but resulted in a decrease in carotid-intima thickness, an early sign of atherosclerosis. An ongoing, randomized clinical trial involving 4,000 renal transplant recipients is attempting to determine whether lowering homocysteine with high-dose B complex supplementation will reduce cardiovascular disease outcomes over a 5 year period. The daily doses used in this study were 5 mg folic acid, 50 mg vitamin B_6, and 1 mg vitamin B_{12}.

Obesity and Weight Gain

Hyperphagia associated with steroid therapy, together with a sense of liberation from the dietary constraints of dialysis and an increased sense of well-being, contribute to the propensity for weight gain after transplantation. Obesity can contribute to the development or exacerbation of hypertension, hyperlipidemia, cardiovascular disease, and diabetes mellitus.

The reported prevalence of posttransplant obesity varies, although approximately 50% of recipients experience weight gain after transplantation. Demographic factors such as female gender, young age (18 to 29 years), and African American race are associated with the most weight gain in the first 2 years posttransplant. Pretransplant obesity, cumulative corticosteroid dose, donor source, posttransplant renal function, time on dialysis before transplantation, and rejection history do not appear to correlate with weight gain.

MANAGEMENT OF OBESITY

In addition to limitation of caloric intake, management of posttransplant obesity includes behavior modification, an exercise program, and early intensive nutritional counseling. Frequent followup by members of the healthcare team, including a physician, dietitian, and nurse, along with group support techniques, may optimize adherence to weight management programs. Lopes' group demonstrated that diet intervention resulted in weight loss and body fat reduction as measured by bioelectrical impedance, and improvement in hyperlipidemia using the American Heart Association step I diet. Medications used to treat obesity in the general population have not been well studied in the renal transplant population. Potential side effects of increased blood pressure with sibutramine and interference with cyclosporine absorption with orlistat, a nonsystemic gastrointestinal lipase inhibitor, mandate careful usage and monitoring.

A final consideration is that of immunosuppression. In a retrospective comparison of recipients on and off 5-mg maintenance steroid therapy, Van Den Ham determined that in the first year posttransplant, weight gain was not associated with maintenance or cumulative steroid dose, age, gender, rejection, or renal function, but rather with pretransplant BMI and dialysis treatment modality. Higher weight gains in year 1 were seen in recipients with low BMI (less than 20 kg/m^2) and those treated with hemodialysis. After the first year posttransplant, the cumulative steroid dose alone correlated positively and significantly with weight gain (see "Selected Readings," below).

Bone Disease

Diet plays both a palliative and a preventive role in certain posttransplant bone abnormalities. Osteoporosis has been associated with long-term glucocorticoid use as a result of decreased intestinal absorption of calcium, decreased osteocalcin, decreased gonadal hormone synthesis, decreased production of skeletal growth factors, and increased urinary calcium excretion, as well as inhibition of preosteoblast transformation to osteoblasts. Lumbar bone loss is associated with glucocorticoid use and a history of alcohol intake. Although *in vitro* and *in vivo* experiments show conflicting results of cyclosporine on bone, most studies do not demonstrate a toxic effect on bone or any effect to be minor. No bone loss has been demonstrated with other immunosuppressive agents. Hyperparathyroidism may persist long after transplantation in as many as 30% of transplant recipients with normal renal function and vitamin D metabolism, and influences the severity of bone loss. Montalban's group looked at long-term transplant recipients with normal renal function and found a frequent occurrence of slight increases in parathyroid hormone. No effect on bone histology was identified, although a delay in mineralization was common (see "Selected Readings," below). Most of the bone loss occurs in the first 6 months posttransplant. Provision of adequate calcium, phosphorus, and vitamin D may attenuate these problems. The efficacy of using calcitriol versus 25-hydroxy vitamin D in this setting has not been fully elucidated. Given the newly appreciated presence of poor vitamin D nutrition in recipients with CKD, and the advice imparted on transplant recipients regarding limiting sun exposure (a major source of vitamin D), assessing vitamin D nutrition in the transplant recipient and supplementing accordingly may be prudent. Weight-bearing exercise is also beneficial. Additional manifestations of transplant-related bone disease are reviewed in Chapter 9.

Hypertension

The prevalence of hypertension in transplant recipients is reported in most series to be at least 50% of patients. Hypertension is an important risk factor for cardiovascular disease, as well as for graft survival. Although posttransplant hypertension is multifactorial in origin, cyclosporine is known to enhance sympathetic nervous system activity, renal vasoconstriction, and sodium/water retention (see Chapter 4, Part I). Recipients who are hypertensive and treated with cyclosporine should be on a sodium-controlled diet. Recent data from multicenter trials suggest that renal transplant recipients under tacrolimus-based therapy showed less arterial hypertension than did cyclosporine-treated recipients. New immunosuppressive drugs, including mycophenolate mofetil and rapamycin, are not nephrotoxic and they do not have a hypertensive effect. A study by Moeller and his group (see "Selected Readings," below) suggested no relationship between salt intake and the prevalence of hypertension in posttransplant recipients. Routine sodium restriction of all transplant recipients is not justified and sodium recommendations should be individualized. Weight loss in the obese hypertensive recipient may also play an important role in its treatment. Exercise provides a beneficial adjuvant. The beneficial effect of other nonpharmacologic influences, such as calcium, potassium, and magnesium intake, and avoidance of alcohol use have not been well defined.

Posttransplant Diabetes Mellitus

Transplant recipients who develop diabetes are at greater risk of graft-related complications, including graft rejection, graft loss, and infection. In addition, hyperglycemia, if chronic, poses a long-term risk of vascular complications. The cumulative incidence of new-onset posttransplant diabetes mellitus (PTDM), as determined in a retrospective analysis, was 9.1%, 16%, and 24% at 3 months, 12 months, and 36 months, respectively. Risk factors for development of PTDM include age older than 40 years, family history of diabetes, obesity, hepatitis C viral infection, and African American or Hispanic ethnicity. Both prednisone and calcineurin-inhibitors provide additional risk factors, with tacrolimus conveying an increased risk, as compared to cyclosporine. Corticosteroids have been shown to produce peripheral insulin resistance and to cause an alteration in pancreatic beta-cell insulin secretion. Cyclosporine and tacrolimus also appear to alter peripheral insulin sensitivity and to diminish islet cell function. Other possible risk factors include glucose intolerance or gestational diabetes prior to transplantation, the presence of metabolic syndrome, and deceased donor source.

A referral to a dietitian for diet and weight loss counseling, if appropriate, and exercise, along with decreased dosing of corticosteroids, provide the basis for initial management. Oral hypoglycemic agents or insulin may be warranted (see "Selected Readings," below).

Progression of Renal Disease in Kidney Transplants

The role of diet in the progression of renal disease in the transplanted kidney requires further study. Although there is a lack of data in transplant recipients with normal renal function, several studies indicate that protein restriction may be helpful in the presence of chronic allograft nephropathy and may help to decrease the associated proteinuria. This finding has been identified in recipients with diabetes and with kidney diseases of various etiologies. Protein status must be closely monitored to avoid exacerbation of hypoalbuminemia, a predictor of mortality in the transplant recipient. The optimal dose of protein remains to be determined, although 0.6 to 0.8 g protein/kg has been shown to be efficacious. Evidence of continued protein wasting has been described even with low doses of corticosteroids, necessitating ongoing assessment of nutritional status for recipients on low-protein diets. Metabolic predictors of early graft failure include elevated serum triglycerides (more than 300 mg/dL) and elevated cholesterol (more than 250 mg/dL) and diabetes. Normal levels of cholesterol, triglycerides, and glucose both before and after transplantation predicted prolonged graft survival. Chronic allograft nephropathy risk factors, independent of acute rejection and proteinuria and not attributable to immune mechanisms, include low serum albumin levels (less than 3.5 g/dL) and high triglyceride levels (more than 200 mg/dL) and the development of PTDM. Various donor-specific risk factors and nonmetabolic risk factors also play a role in both acute and chronic graft survival (see Chapter 9).

Hypoalbuminemia

In addition to its possible role as a risk factor for decreased renal graft survival, a retrospective analysis of 232 simultaneous pancreas–kidney transplant recipients by Becker and coworkers (see "Selected Readings," below) indicated that hypoalbuminemia was associated with increased risk for cytomegalovirus infection, graft loss, and decreased survival rate. Low albumin levels have also been described as a strong independent risk factor for all causes of mortality after renal transplantation.

Foodborne Infectious Complications

Even the nonnutritionally compromised transplant recipient may be susceptible to an increased incidence of infection (see Chapter 10). Infectious complications in the renal transplant recipient have been reported to occur at a level 10 times higher than anticipated in the presence of malnutrition, defined as a serum albumin of less than 2.8 g/dL. Attention to potentially pathogenic organisms commonly found in food may provide a relatively simple, preventive measure to avoid certain infections. Providing education on safe and sensible food habits may help to minimize the morbidity associated with certain posttransplant infectious disease complications.

Food vehicles for *Listeria monocytogenes* include raw milk, soft cheeses, and hot dogs. *Nocardia asteroides,* although ubiquitous in the environment and not uncommonly nosocomially acquired, can be present in decaying vegetables. *Salmonella* species infections are associated with undercooked, contaminated meat, poultry, and eggs, as well as raw milk. The potential for *Legionella* species infection exists in areas with a contaminated or unsafe water supply. *Salmonella Kottbus, Salmonella enteritidis,* and *Escherichia coli* are associated with ingestion of raw sprouts, while *Salmonella serotype Poona* infections have resulted from imported cantaloupe. *Anisakiasis,* caused by human infection *Anisakis larvae,* and *Vibrio cholerae O1 and O139* are linked to eating raw or undercooked fish. Prevention includes proper food selection, handling, preparation, storage, and pasteurization, and careful selection when eating out.

Foodborne Noninfectious Complications

Transplant recipients with impaired renal function should be advised to avoid ingestion of star fruit (*Averrhoa carambola*). Although formerly a rare fruit typical to some Asian cuisines, it is now commonly available in grocery stores. Intake of star fruit in people with impaired renal function is associated with severe neurologic symptoms and death.

Use of Herbal Supplements

The use of herbal medicines and inclusion of herbal medicines in food items, such as juices, is increasingly common. In the United States, herbal medicines are regulated as food products and dietary supplements and are not tested for safety or efficacy by the Food and Drug Administration. These products pose a special potential risk for transplant recipients for several reasons. One concern is the lack of information about drug–nutrient interactions and whether these substances increase or decrease the effectiveness of immunosuppressants or other prescribed medications. A well-described example is the interaction between St. John's wort and cyclosporine. St. John's wort, a potent inducer of CYP3A4, enhances plasma clearance of a number of drugs, such as cyclosporine. Coadministration of cyclosporine and St. John's wort results in a rapid and significant reduction of plasma cyclosporine concentrations and alterations in cyclosporine metabolite kinetics that may affect the toxicity profile of the drug. Red yeast rice (*Monascus purpureus*) an herbal preparation used to lower cholesterol, has induced rhabdomyolysis in a stable renal transplant recipient. Rice fermented with red yeast contains mevinic acids, including monacolin K, which is the same as lovastatin, an beta-hydroxy-β-methylglutaryl-coenzyme A reductase inhibitor with known potential at higher doses for rhabdomyolysis, when taken with cyclosporine.

A second related concern is that certain herbs and food products, such as Echinacea, Astragalus, and Noni juice, appear to contain immune-enhancing properties. *In vitro* lymphocyte proliferation tests using phytohemagglutinin, mixed lymphocyte culture (MLC) assay, and IL-2 and IL-10 production from MLC, demonstrated that dong quai, ginseng, and milk thistle had nonspecific immunostimulatory effects on lymphocyte proliferation. Ginger and green tea had immunosuppressive effects. Dong quai and milk thistle increased alloresponsiveness in MLC, whereas ginger and green tea decreased these responses. The immunostimulatory effects of dong quai and milk thistle were consistently seen in both cell-mediated immune response and nonspecific lymphoproliferation. The immunosuppressive effect of green tea and ginger were mediated through a decrease in IL-2 production, but the immunostimulatory effects of dong quai and milk thistle were not. Green tea, dong quai, ginseng, milk thistle, and ginger have varying effects on *in vitro* immune assays that may be relevant in transplant recipients and should be avoided or used with caution.

Some herbal preparations have been found to contain heavy metals and toxic botanicals. Because there are no sanitation standards for herbal medicines, the potential for microbial contamination poses a particular risk for the immune-suppressed recipient. Until and unless adequate research and appropriate regulations exist, herbal product use should be discouraged in transplant recipients.

Nutrient Recommendations for the Stable Transplant Recipient

Protein and Calories

Posttransplant protein requirements for stable transplant recipients are not well defined, with muscle wasting identified even at corticosteroid doses of 0.20 mg/kg per day. A daily protein intake of 1.0 g/kg has been recommended for stable posttransplant recipients with good renal function. Negative nitrogen balance has been reported in short-term studies of protein intake levels of 0.6 g/kg per day unless calorie intake is maintained above 25 kcal/kg per day. A daily protein intake approaching 1 g/kg, combined with an adequate calorie intake, appears to be compatible with neutral or positive nitrogen balance. Lower levels may be appropriate for recipients with chronic allograft nephropathy as discussed previously.

For stable transplant recipients who require weight reduction, a daily calorie intake of 25 kcal/kg ideal body weight is a reasonable starting point. Caloric restriction should be combined with exercise, behavior modification techniques, and regular team followup.

Fat and Carbohydrate

Given the incidence of posttransplant hypercholesterolemia, the propensity toward weight gain, and the potential contribution of lipids to decreased graft survival, a reduced fat and reduced cholesterol diet is appropriate for most long-term recipients.

The recommendations of the Third Report of the National Cholesterol Education Program's Adult Treatment Panel (ATP III) (see "Selected Readings," below) incorporate a Therapeutic Lifestyle Change (TLC) program that includes diet. These diet recommendations have supplanted what formerly was referred to as the American Heart Association's (AHA) steps I and II diets, which are no longer promoted by the AHA for people with cardiac risk factors. The National Kidney Foundation Disease Outcome Quality Initiative Guidelines for management of dyslipidemias considers all CKD recipients to be in the high-risk category and advocates use of the TLC guidelines. The diet component of the TLC guidelines incorporates the benefits of keeping *trans*-fatty acid intake low, and the addition of viscous fiber and plant stanol/sterol esters to reduce low-density lipoprotein cholesterol beyond that seen with the step II diet. It also deemphasizes total fat and focuses more specifically on the kinds of fat ingested. Other health-promoting aspects of the diet include use of fish and omega-3 fatty acids.

For recipients who ultimately require pharmacologic management for control of hypercholesterolemia, diet guidelines should continue to be encouraged as adjunctive therapy. Table 18.3 lists the TLC diet guidelines for fat and carbohydrate. For transplant recipients with PTDM or diabetes mellitus, which predates transplantation, complex carbohydrates should be emphasized with limitation of simple sugars as needed to control glucose levels. A high fiber intake (25 to 30 g per day) can assist with blood glucose and blood cholesterol control.

Fish Oil

Further studies are needed to clarify and evaluate the effect of n-3 fatty acids, in the form of fish oil in the posttransplant recipient. Treatment with fish oil during the first 3 months posttransplant does not appear to benefit acute rejection rate, renal function, or graft survival as had been reported earlier. Fish oil may be of

Table 18.3.   Adult Treatment Panel III (ATP III) guidelines—nutrient composition of the Therapeutic Lifestyle Changes diet[a]

Nutrient	Recommended Intake
Saturated fat	Less than 7% of total calories
Polyunsaturated fat	Up to 10% of total calories
Monounsaturated fat	Up to 20% of total calories
Total fat	25%–35% of total calories
Carbohydrate	50%–60% of total calories
Fiber	20–30 g/day
Protein	Approximately 15% of total calories
Cholesterol	Less than 200 mg/day
Total calories (energy)	Balance energy intake and expenditure to maintain desirable body weight and to prevent weight gain

[a]The ATP III guidelines were developed by The National Heart, Lung, and Blood Institute of the National Institutes of Health and the U.S. Department of Health and Human Resources.

benefit in control of posttransplant hyperlipidemia and for recipients with immunoglobulin A nephropathy. The precise role of fish oil in this setting remains controversial.

Sodium
Sodium restriction to 2 to 3 g per day is warranted in cyclosporine-treated recipients with hypertension. In normotensive, nonedematous recipients, strict sodium restriction is not warranted.

Potassium
Hyperkalemia, associated with the use of cyclosporine and tacrolimus, may continue to be observed in otherwise stable transplant recipients. Guidelines, as discussed in the section on nutritional support in the posttransplant period, continue to apply in this setting. Potassium levels up to 5.5 mEq/L are common and are rarely a source of concern in stable recipients.

Calcium, Phosphorus, and Vitamin D
Calcium should be provided at the level of 1,000 to 1,500 mg per day by a combination of diet and supplements. Vitamin D, either in the 25-hydroxyvitamin D_2 (400 IU) and/or 1,25-dihydroxyvitamin D_3 (0.25 μg) form should be supplemented based on vitamin D and vitamin D metabolite status with 1,25-dihydroxyvitamin D_3 generally instituted in recipients with a glomerular filtration rate (GFR) of less than 30 mL per minute. Whether routine use of calcidiol should be used as opposed to calcitriol at higher GFRs is under debate. Hypophosphatemia may persist into this period, necessitating phosphate supplementation. Hypercalcemia may persist in as many as one-third of recipients in the first year, and subsequently in as many as 10% after 1 year, as a result of secondary hyperparathyroidism. In chronic

allograft nephropathy, hyperphosphatemia should be treated using guidelines for CKD.

Magnesium

Hypomagnesemia may persist into the long-term posttransplant period, and magnesium supplements are often prescribed. Magnesium supplementation may favorably influence the blood lipid profile, primarily by increasing HDL cholesterol levels. The role of magnesium in controlling blood pressure in this population remains equivocal.

Vitamins

To ensure adequate intake, water-soluble vitamin supplementation is warranted for recipients on diets restricting protein (to less than 60 g per day), potassium, or calories (to less than 1,200 kcal per day). The efficacy of routine supplementation of certain water-soluble vitamins, specifically pyridoxine, B_{12}, and folic acid, is under investigation regarding their role in treating hyperhomocysteinemia and decreasing the risk of cardiovascular events in this population (see discussion of "Homocysteine," above). Early studies suggested that elevated vitamin A levels, associated with CKD stage V, persist after transplantation. Studies to further evaluate this issue and to determine whether supplementation is contraindicated have not been performed. In the cardiac transplant recipient, Fang's group demonstrated that supplementation with antioxidant vitamins C (500 mg) and E (400 IU) retards the early progression of transplant-associated coronary arteriosclerosis as measured by intimal index (plaque area divided by vessel area) (see "Selected Readings," below). The application to renal transplant recipients has not been examined, although the potential value in reducing oxidative stress will need to be balanced with the potential for secondary oxalosis in those recipients with impaired renal function.

The role of vitamin E supplementation in focal segmental glomerulosclerosis and for reducing oxidative stress in the transplant recipients is yet undefined, as is the efficacy of routine vitamin E supplementation for kidney transplant recipients. Of concern is an interaction between cyclosporine and water-soluble vitamin E (D-α-tocopherol-polyethlene-glycol-1000-succinate) resulting in increased bioavailability of cyclosporine. The mechanism appears to be water-soluble vitamin E-induced inhibition of p-glycoprotein, an adenosine triphosphate-dependent efflux pump found primarily in the gastrointestinal tract, which limits the transport of "foreign" compounds. Tacrolimus, sirolimus, and cyclosporine are all p-glycoprotein substrates. Although this interaction has only been seen with water-soluble vitamin E, and it is unclear whether the vitamin or the other ingredients in this particular formulation are the responsible components, caution should be used in concomitant intake of vitamin E and these immunosuppressive agents.

Alcohol

Excessive alcohol intake interferes with the metabolism and therefore increases the potential toxicity of cyclosporine, although moderate amounts may be tolerated without a marked effect. An interaction has been identified specifically between cyclosporine and red wine, similar to that of grapefruit juice. Red wine inactivated CYP3A4 at a rate approximately 16% that of grapefruit juice.

Heavy alcohol use is also associated with increased risk for avascular necrosis and bone loss, as well as hypertension. Other medications prescribed to transplant recipients should be screened for drug and alcohol interactions.

Exercise

Physical training is a vital part of the management of the transplant recipient. It attenuates some of the side effects of immunosuppressive therapy, such as protein catabolism and muscle wasting, hyperlipidemia, hypertension, osteoporosis, and obesity. A randomized trial of exercise training after transplantation by Painter's group demonstrated higher measured and self-reported physical functioning, although it did not by itself affect body composition (see "Selected Readings," below). Glucose control in diabetic recipients can also be improved with a regular exercise program. Quality of life may also improve as a result of a regular exercise program. Although the optimal exercise program is not defined in the transplantation population, recommendations for the general population, which include cardiovascular conditioning and muscle strengthening, are appropriate for most recipients.

Nutrient Recommendations for the Pregnant Transplant Recipient

The protein needs of stable pregnant transplant recipients are 0.8 g/kg pregravida ideal or adjusted body weight plus 10 g per day. Caloric requirements can be calculated using basal energy expenditure times an activity factor of 1.2 to 1.4; an additional 300 kcal per day should be consumed in the second and third trimesters. Other nutrient requirements are the same as for nontransplanted pregnant women, although close monitoring is appropriate in terms of weight gain and glucose control because of the risk for glucose intolerance. Residual secondary hyperparathyroidism may also require adjustments in phosphorus, calcium, and vitamin D intake.

SELECTED READINGS

Baum CL, Thielke K, Westin E, et al. Predictors of weight gain and cardiovascular risk in a cohort of racially diverse kidney transplant recipients. *Nutrition* 2002;18(2):139–146.

Becker BN, Becker YT, Heisey DM, et al. The impact of hypoalbuminemia in kidney-pancreas transplant recipients. *Transplantation* 1999;68:72–75.

Bernardi A, Biasia F, Pati T, et al. Long-term protein intake control in kidney transplant recipients: effect in kidney graft function and in nutritional status. *Am J Kidney Dis* 2003;41[3 Suppl 1]):S146–S152.

Brookhyser J, Wiggins K. Medical nutrition therapy in pregnancy and kidney disease. *Adv Ren Replace Ther* 1998;5(1):53–63.

Chan LN. Drug-nutrient interactions in transplant recipients. *J Parenter Enteral Nutr* 2001;25(3):132–141.

Davidson J, Wilkinson A, Dantal J, et al. New-onset diabetes after transplantation. *Transplantation* 2003;75(10):SS3–SS24.

De Sevaux RG, Hoitsma AJ, Corstens FH, et al. Treatment with vitamin D and calcium reduces bone loss after renal transplantation: a randomized study. *J Am Soc Nephrol* 2002;13(6):1608–1614.

Fang JC, Kinlay S, Beltrame J, et al. Effect of vitamins C and E on progression of transplant-associated arteriosclerosis: a randomized trial. *Lancet* 2002;359(9312):1108–1113.

Friedman AN, Rosenberg IH, Selhub J, et al. Hyperhomocysteinemia in renal transplant recipients. *Am J Transplant* 2002;2(4):308–313.

Hansen HP, Tauber-Lassen E, Jensen BR, Parving HH. Effect of dietary protein restriction on prognosis in recipients with diabetic nephropathy. *Kidney Int* 2002;62(1):220–228.

Hasse JM. Nutrition assessment and support of organ transplant recipients. *J Parenter Enteral Nutr* 2001;25(3):120–131.

Hasse JM, Blue LS, eds. *Comprehensive guide to transplant nutrition,* 1st ed. Chicago: American Dietetic Association, 2002.

Heaf JG. Bone disease after renal transplantation. *Transplantation* 2003;75(3):315–325.

Hernandez D, Guerra R, Milena A, et al. Dietary fish oil does not influence acute rejection rate and graft survival after renal transplantation: a randomized placebo-controlled study. *Nephrol Dial Transplant* 2002;17(5):897–904.

Johnson DW, Isbel NM, Brown AM, et al. The effect of obesity on renal transplant outcomes. *Transplantation* 2002;74(5):675–681.

Lopes IM, Martin M, Errasti P, et al. Benefits of a dietary intervention on weight loss, body composition, and lipid profile after renal transplantation. *Nutrition* 1999;15:7–10.

Marcucci R, Zanazzi M, Bertoni E, et al. Vitamin supplementation reduces the progression of atherosclerosis in hyperhomocysteinemic renal transplant recipients. *Transplantation* 2003;75(9):1551–1555.

Meier-Kriesche HU, Arndorfer JA, Kaplan B. The impact of body mass index on renal transplant outcomes: a significant independent risk factor for graft failure and recipient death. *Transplantation* 2002;73(1):70–74.

Mikuls TR, Julian BA, Bartolucci A, et al. Bone mineral density changes within six months of renal transplantation. *Transplantation* 2003;75(1):49–54.

Moeller T, Buhl M, Schorr U, et al. Salt intake and hypertension in renal transplant recipients. *Clin Nephrol* 2000;53(3):159–163.

Montalban C, De Francisco AL, Marinoso ML, et al. Bone disease in long-term adult kidney transplant recipients with normal renal function. *Kidney Int Suppl* 2003;85:S129–S132.

National Kidney Foundation. K/DOQI clinical practice guidelines for managing dyslipidemias in chronic kidney disease. *Am J Kidney Dis* 2003;41(3):S1–S92.

Neto MM, Da Costa JA, Garcia-Cairasco N, et al. Intoxication by star fruit (*Averrhoa carambola*) in 32 uraemic patients: treatment and outcome. *Nephrol Dial Transplant* 2003;18(1):120–125.

Painter PL, Hector L, Ray K, et al. A randomized trial of exercise training after renal transplantation. *Transplantation* 2002;74(1):42–48.

Patel MG. The effect of dietary intervention on weight gains after renal transplantation. *J Ren Nutr* 1998;8:137–141.

Ponticelli C, Villa M. Role of anaemia in cardiovascular mortality and morbidity in transplant recipients. *Nephrol Dial Transplant* 2002;17[Suppl 1]:41–46.

Suliman ME, Stenvinkel P, Barany P, et al. Hyperhomocysteinemia and its relationship to cardiovascular disease in ESRD: influence of hypoalbuminemia, malnutrition, inflammation, and diabetes mellitus. *Am J Kidney Dis* 2003;41[3 Suppl 1]:S89–S95.

Third Report of the National Cholesterol Education Program (NCEP) Expert Panel on Detection, Evaluation, and Treatment of High Blood Cholesterol in Adults (Adult Treatment Panel III) final report. Circulation 2002;106(25):3143–3421.

2002 Annual Report ESRD Clinical Performance Measures Report, Department of Health and Human Services, Centers for Medicare and Medicaid Services.

Van Den Ham EC, Kooman JP, Christiaans MH, et al. Weight changes after renal transplantation: a comparison between recipients on 5-mg maintenance steroid therapy and those on steroid-free immunosuppressive therapy. *Transpl Int* 2003;16(5):300–306.

Wilasrusmee C, Siddiqui J, Bruch D, et al. *In vitro* immunomodulatory effects of herbal products. *Am Surg* 2002;68(10):860–864.

Psychosocial and Financial Aspects of Transplantation

Robert S. Gaston and Marci H Gitlin

The diagnosis of advancing kidney disease is life changing, not only for the patient, but also for family members. Many questions and concerns may arise that can be addressed by the social worker who is highly invested in patient care and treatment, including the following:

- What treatment choice is best for me?
- How will my life change because of my illness?
- How will my illness affect my family?
- How will I pay for my treatments?
- Will I be able to continue working and return to my daily activities?

The nephrology or transplant social worker can help patients understand and cope with their feelings, and adjust to a new lifestyle with dialysis or a transplant. They can assist patients with their concerns about employment, insurance, changing roles in marriage and family life, problems with sex and intimacy, and concerns about death and dying.

The social work team member is an expert on community resources and can refer patients and family members to the appropriate programs that they need, such as vocational rehabilitation, social security disability, home health care services, medical equipment, support groups, and financial assistance. They also complete a comprehensive psychosocial assessment on every patient being considered for transplant candidacy. When a patient begins their assessment for transplant candidacy, it is recommended that a comprehensive psychosocial assessment be completed by the transplant team's social worker. It is during this process that compliance, family system dynamics, financial resources, and mental health are examined. Table 19.1 identifies the areas that should be covered in a social work assessment.

This chapter discusses the psychosocial benefits and potential risks of transplantation, concerns with patient nonadherence, information regarding social security disability, vocational rehabilitation, financial concerns, psychosocial assessment, and the availability of community resources.

PSYCHOSOCIAL BENEFITS OF TRANSPLANTATION

The quality of life for transplant patients is generally better than the quality of life for dialysis patients. Approximately 80% of transplant recipients function psychosocially at nearly normal levels, as compared to approximately 50% of dialysis patients. Dialysis patients show more morbidity on the General Health Questionnaire (which evaluates loss of emotional control and

Table 19.1. Major Areas Covered in Psychosocial Assessment

Illness assessment
1. Illness history and impact on patient's functioning, understanding, reaction, and adjustment
2. Patient's knowledge of transplantation, process of being referred to transplant center, understanding of the assessment process for candidacy, feelings about transplantation.

Patient assessment
1. Personal
   Age, lifecycle stage
   Physical functioning
   Intellectual functioning
   Emotional functioning
   Sexual functioning
   Major stressful events
   Coping style and approaches
   Religious beliefs and faith
   History of substance abuse
   Ability to comply with medical regime
2. Educational
   Level of education attained
3. Vocational
   Type of occupation
   Length of employment
   Stability of present/recent job
4. Financial
   Sources of income and other resources, their adequacy for current lifestyle, and their adequacy for transplantation and for future medical needs

Support system assessment
1. Family
   Composition—spouse and children; age, education, occupation; needs, availability
   Role structure—effect of illness on roles
   Interactions—patterns and quality of communication
   Functioning—quality of family life
   Problem-solving approach and skills
2. Social
   Extended family—quality of contacts
   Friends, neighbors, colleagues—quality of relationships
   Others—religious, cultural, and social affiliations
3. Environmental
   Housing and transportation
   Need for relocation
   Need for travel alternatives

depression) than do transplant patients and healthy controls. It is important to note, however, that these studies do not address the effects of transplant failure, which may result in a significant decrease in quality of life.

The obvious benefit of kidney transplantation is freedom from the constraints of dialysis. Successful transplantation permits much more personal time and independence for an individual who is freed of the necessity of being connected to a machine several times a day, or at night, or going to an outside facility two to three times a week for several hours each visit. On average, patients spend anywhere from 40 to 50 hours a month on hemodialysis, 60 to 70 hours on continuous ambulatory peritoneal dialysis (CAPD), or 280 hours on continuous cycling peritoneal dialysis (CCPD).

There is significant psychosocial stress associated with dialysis. Patients are faced with the conflict of maintaining independence despite being forced to depend upon a machine, with difficulties in remaining financially solvent, with reduced activity in the family household, and with loss of spontaneity.

Transplantation permits greater flexibility and more convenience when traveling. Patients need not worry about having to make arrangements ahead of time, or having to travel only to those cities that have dialysis centers. For many patients who have been on dialysis, transplant offers the freedom to actually plan a vacation (more than a weekend getaway). Many patients report they have not taken an extended trip since commencing dialysis because of the inconvenience and because of their concerns about being either too far away from their dialysis centers or going to an unfamiliar dialysis unit.

There also is greater dietary flexibility (see Chapter 18). Specifically, the fluid restrictions are often difficult to adhere to in warmer climates, or during the summer season. Many patients complain of having a difficult time finding enough protein in their diet without having to eat foods that were previously considered "unhealthy" (red meat, starchy carbohydrates, etc.).

Transplant patients generally have more energy and stamina and can spend more time dealing with issues outside of their own health problems. The time alone saved in being off dialysis is approximately 50 hours a month, or 600 hours a year. This results in an increased earning potential and increased family and personal time. The long-term complications of dialysis may be avoided by transplantation (see Chapter 1) and many patients view a transplant as a symbol of freedom and restored health.

Ideally, after receiving a kidney transplant, patients are able to return to normal functioning by going back to work or school, and working toward getting themselves off disability. Patients are encouraged to engage in vocational rehabilitation while they are on dialysis, because the waiting time for deceased donor transplant may be years, during which time they may complete training courses or school programs. Social Security offers vocational training for patients while they are receiving disability benefits, and assists with job placement to help individuals get back into the work force when they are medically able to do so.

Financial Benefits of Transplantation

Successful kidney transplantation is more cost-effective than hemodialysis and provides a relative net saving after a period of approximately 3 years. Although data may vary from center to center, transplantation costs to Medicare average $107,000 by the end of the first year, with cumulative costs decreasing each successive year, as a consequence of avoidance of dialysis and reduction in dosage of immunosuppressive drugs. The reduction continues so that cumulative cost is approximately $117,000 by the end of the second year and $126,000 by the end of the third year. These figures do not reflect the costs associated with rehospitalization (beyond the first year). The cost of providing dialysis is approximately $54,000 per year. Therefore, kidney transplantation is a more cost-effective alternative than dialysis if the graft remains viable for more than 2 to 3 years. Depending on donor source 80% to 90% of transplanted kidneys remain viable long enough to recoup this dividend.

PSYCHOSOCIAL RISKS OF TRANSPLANTATION

The social worker can offer support for the patient, family, and friends with issues that can have a negative impact on transplant results, such as the hesitancy to leave the dependent sick role, concerns about reentering the workforce, importance of being needed rather than needing, maintenance of hope during periods of rejection, and the need to escape feelings of distinctiveness, both in terms of psychological and physical symptoms.

Although patients are educated about medication side effects, until they are faced with them, it is uncertain how they will cope. Patients who have a prior psychiatric history of anxiety or depression are particularly susceptible to an exacerbation of their symptoms once immunosuppressive therapy begins, although patients with no prior history are also at risk (see Chapter 16). Family members should be comforted by the assurance that such symptoms are generally temporary and treatable. The physical side effects of transplant medications, such as hirsutism, gum overgrowth, and weight gain, may impact on body image in a manner that is not always easy to detect and sensitive probing may be required. Side effects are almost inevitable posttransplant and they can cause patients to stop or skip doses of their medication. Patients should be systematically questioned about their attitude toward their side effects.

Multiple lifestyle changes occur for the transplant patient. Their place may change within their family system and work environment. Their capacity to reenter the workforce after many years may be changed. There may be a risk of losing financial support, such as disability income and health insurance. Personal relationships may be at risk and posttransplant stress may lead to divorce and separation. Sexual functioning may change posttransplant (see Chapter 9) and engender new hopes and fears. The newly found posttransplant freedom may be a threat to patients whose identity has been associated with their "sick role" as a dialysis patient. The shift to health may be difficult and an identity crisis may occur. Counseling and support groups can aid in this transition.

Employment is a topic that weighs heavily on many patients who have been receiving disability payment from various sources and is often tied into their health insurance coverage. There can be fear of losing Medicare or Medicaid benefits and not being able to obtain health insurance from a new employer. Government legislation (The Ticket to Work and Work Incentives Act of 1999, known as "the ticket" and the Health Insurance Portability and Accountability Act) offers some protection for transplant recipients who face this hurdle.

Many patients live in fear of suffering rejection episodes and losing their transplants, or suffering from other catastrophic complications. These fears are not irrational, although they may be exaggerated; they can be best addressed by an open and factual discussion of the extent of the risk at all phases of treatment. Patients may also suffer feelings of guilt at having received a kidney at someone else's expense. Patients should be assured that these are common feelings and reminded that they are deserving beneficiaries of the wishes of the donor and the donor's loved ones.

NONCOMPLIANCE

Graft survival is dependent on providing adequate long-term pharmacologic immunosuppression. As a consequence, transplant recipients who do not adhere to often complex medical regimens are at substantial risk of graft loss. The term "noncompliance" is used to indicate failure of transplant recipients to ingest medications as prescribed, for whatever reason. Few patients consciously decide to discontinue immunosuppression. For most, noncompliant behavior evolves gradually as a consequence of many interacting variables.

Noncompliance with medical therapies affects treatment outcomes in many chronic diseases, and it is estimated that only a half of the 1.6 billion prescriptions written in the United States each year are taken properly. To quote former surgeon general Dr. C. Everett Koop, "Drugs don't work in patients who don't take them!" A series of variables have been linked to medication noncompliance (Table 19.2) and each is evident in transplant immunosuppressant regimens. In renal transplantation, clinically

Table 19.2.   Attributes of pharmacologic therapies that enhance the risk of noncompliance

Multiple medications
Prolonged duration of therapy
Short dosing intervals
Palatability of medication
Definable adverse effects
Financial expense
Beliefs about severity of illness
Failure to understand treatment regimen
Increasing intervals between contacts with providers

Adapted from Cramer JA. Practical issues in medication compliance. *Transplant Proc* 1999; 31:[Suppl 4A]:7S–9S.

important noncompliance occurs in approximately 20% of recipients, substantially increasing risk of adverse immunologic events and even death. Occasional noncompliance and "forgetfulness" is widespread, although its clinical significance is difficult to assess. Both multiple and late episodes of acute rejection predict subsequent graft loss to chronic rejection (see Chapter 9), and medication noncompliance significantly enhances the risk for both. Noncompliance increases the risk of graft loss by up to sevenfold. It has been estimated that noncompliance contributes up to 36% of cases of graft loss.

Several demographic variables appear to affect the likelihood of noncompliance. Diabetic patients, accustomed to the demands of living with chronic illness, are less likely to have problems with compliance after transplantation. Younger patients, particularly adolescents, and those with a limited educational background are more likely to be noncompliant. Psychiatric illness and a history of substance abuse also increase risk. At least some noncompliant behavior is attributable to either financial hardship or the relative inability to procure appropriate medication when no funds are available. Low socioeconomic status is a strong predictor of noncompliance and poorer long-term outcomes in renal transplantation. Knowledge of these demographic risk factors, however, is of only limited benefit in dealing with individual patients. It does little to facilitate identification of noncompliant behavior early enough to allow remedy, nor does it provide insight into what that remedy should be.

The interventions required to alter noncompliant behavior vary from patient to patient. At the very least, transplant recipients must have access to immunosuppressants, the annual cost of which may exceed that of housing for many patients (Table 19.3). For patients with private insurance or Medicaid coverage,

Table 19.3. Financial costs of commonly used immunosuppressive regimens in the United States

Immunosuppressive Regimen	Cost per Annum[a]
Tacrolimus, MMF, prednisone	$ 17,500
Neoral, MMF, prednisone	$ 14,700
Neoral, sirolimus, prednisone	$ 14,700
Generic CyA, MMF, prednisone	$ 14,000
Tacrolimus, azathioprine, prednisone	$ 9,500
Neoral, prednisone	$ 6,600
Generic CyA, azathioprine, prednisone	$ 6,000

CyA, cyclosporine; MMF, mycophenolate mofetil.
[a]Annual charges (for an average patient weighing 70 kg, at a retail pharmacy in Birmingham, AL, 2003) assuming the following medication doses: cyclosporine (Neoral or generic) 4 mg/kg/day; mycophenolate mofetil (MMF) 2,000 mg/day; tacrolimus 0.1 mg/kg/day; Sirolimus 3 mg/day. It must be recognized that dose reduction in various protocols will impact retail costs. For example, MMF dosing (1–1.5 g/day) that is now common with tacrolimus will decrease overall costs by 15%–25%.

finances may not pose a significant problem. Medicare policy now provides immunosuppressant coverage for the life of the allograft, but only for those beneficiaries who retain Medicare eligibility beyond the 3 years allowed for end-stage renal disease (ESRD) patients after transplantation. Others patients must navigate (usually with the assistance of social workers) a complex network of indigent care programs and state kidney networks. There is a significant risk of late rejection and graft loss for patients who discontinue immunosuppressant medications because of financial hardship; when patients are provided with drugs, outcomes improved dramatically. In the 1990s, extension of Medicare coverage for immunosuppressants from 1 to 3 years was shown to attenuate income-related differences in long-term graft survival.

In addition to ensuring financial access to proper medications, other interventions might improve patient compliance. Electronic monitoring of drug dosing can allow earlier detection of noncompliance, although such devices have not become widely accepted. Drug regimens should be simplified, with perhaps optimal compliance as a more compelling goal than optimal pharmacokinetics. Patients should be helped to develop daily routines that foster compliance. The facilitation of adherence of transplant recipients to their medical regimen requires both recognition of its importance in ensuring long-term graft survival and ongoing trust between patient and provider.

DISABILITY INSURANCE FOR TRANSPLANT PATIENTS

State Disability Insurance

In California, state disability insurance (SDI) is available for those patients who are employed and are paying state income taxes. Patients are also eligible to apply if they are unable to work because of disabilities that are not work-related (e.g., while they are receiving medical treatments, recovering from illness or surgery, or non–work-related accidents). SDI eligibility begins 1 week after the patient stops work because of any of the above reasons, and continues for a maximum of 1 year, or until the patient is able to return to work, or until their SDI funds run out (usually up to 6 months). Patients who continue to be disabled after 1 year need to apply for long-term disability. The maximum financial benefit is approximately $336.00 a week, based on the individual's highest quarter wage. It is often supplemented by employer disability plans to approximate the original salary.

For transplant recipients, the estimated amount of time off work is 2 to 3 months, although some patients may return to work sooner. Because transplant recipients require close medical followup in the first 1 to 2 months, it is generally recommended that they do not return to work prior to 2 months posttransplant. Some patients are unable to cope financially on SDI for more than a month, and request to return to work sooner. A decision needs to be made as to whether or not the patient is medically stable and can be cleared to return to work.

Social Security Disability Income

Social Security disability income (SSDI) is long-term disability program for those patients who are considered "permanently" disabled for at least 1 year. Patients who run out of temporary disability and yet are still unable to return to work will often apply for SSDI, even prior to 1 year of being disabled, because the eligibility process can take several months.

Social Security payments are monthly, and are based on a patient's individual earnings in the highest quarter. Patients with ESRD who are on dialysis or who have had a transplant are eligible for Social Security disability if they have paid FICA (Federal Insurance Contributions Act) taxes. Patients are encouraged to continue working even after starting on dialysis, because they may be able to have flexible work hours or reduce their work schedule to part-time. Patients may choose CAPD or CCPD, so as not to interrupt their work schedules by having to go to a hemodialysis center several times a week. Patients receiving SSDI may return to work on a limited basis without having their Social Security benefits stopped. They can still collect SSDI as long as they do not earn more than $500 per month for more than 8 months.

Patients should be encouraged to return to work after a transplant because many of them will lose their benefits and insurance. Some patients continue on SSDI, particularly if they have disabling conditions in addition to ESRD (e.g., diabetes, retinopathy, blindness, or other physical disabilities).

Consolidated Budget Reconciliation Act of 1985

The Consolidated Budget Reconciliation Act (COBRA) of 1985 provides additional help to employees and their dependents who would normally lose their health insurance coverage because of job loss, divorce, or the death or retirement of a spouse. This is a federal law that requires companies with 20 or more employees to extend their insurance coverage to employees and their dependents for 18 months (up to 36 months) when benefits would otherwise end. Although a person may receive extended coverage through COBRA, they are still fully responsible for premium payments to the group health plan.

An employee covered by a group health plan may continue coverage for up to 18 months if the employee left work voluntarily or involuntarily (for reasons other than misconduct), or the working hours are reduced beyond the minimum amount to qualify for health benefits. Patients considered disabled under Social Security guidelines at the time work is discontinued can choose to continue their health coverage for up to 29 months, after which time they become eligible for Medicare. They must show that they are insurable in order to continue coverage. If a person leaves work because of disability, they may be able to keep their life insurance policy if there is a disability waiver. The insurer must be notified and proof of disability provided.

Family Medical Leave Act

The Family Medical Leave Act (FMLA) requires employers to provide up to 12 weeks of unpaid job-protected leave to "eligible" employees for certain family and medical reasons that make the employees unable to perform their work. Employees are eligible if they have worked for an employer for at least 1 year (minimum of 1,250 hours over the previous 12 months).

The employee may be required to provide advance leave notice and medical certification. Leave may be denied if requirements are not met. The employee ordinarily must provide 30 days advance notice when leave is "foreseeable." An employer may require a medical certificate (and may require a second opinion at the employer's expense) to support a request for leave because of a serious health condition.

For the duration of FMLA leave, the employer must maintain the employee's health coverage under any "group health plan." Upon return from FMLA leave, most employees must be restored to their original or equivalent positions with equivalent pay, benefits, and other employment terms.

The use of FMLA leave cannot result in the loss of any employment benefit that accrued prior to the start of an employee's leave. The U.S. Department of Labor is authorized to investigate and resolve complaints of violations. An eligible employee may bring a civil action against an employer for violations.

Vocational Rehabilitation

Many transplant patients are not working at the time of the transplant for various health reasons. They may be eligible for vocational rehabilitation, as are patients who are unable to return to their prior employment because their job responsibilities are in conflict with transplant-related restrictions.

Vocational rehabilitation is a service that provides people with disabilities the tools they need to be able to return to work, enter a new line of work, maintain work, or start work for the first time. Following a transplant, it is important that the patient enter a rehabilitation program as soon as the patient is well enough to protect their disability coverage.

The Social Security Administration (SSA) can help people with disabilities get the vocational rehabilitation services they need. Patients need to inquire at their local SSA office about these services; they may also contact their state rehabilitation agency. Vocational rehabilitation providers furnish a variety of services designed to provide the training or other services that are needed to help patients acquire gainful employment.

Once a person is able to successfully return to work, special rules, called "work incentives," help them retain their current cash benefits (SSD, SSI) and health insurance coverage (Medicare, Medicaid) during a trial work period. There are different work incentives for people who receive SSD and SSI benefits. These incentives help people with disabilities to work by allowing them to test their ability to work for a specified period of time without losing any benefits.

SELECTED READINGS

Butkus DE, Dottes AL, Meydrech EF, et al. Effect of poverty and other socioeconomic variables on renal allograft survival. *Transplantation* 2001;72:261–266.

Butler JA, Roderick P, Muller M, et al. Frequency and impact of nonadherence to immunosuppressants after renal transplantation: a systematic review. *Transplantation* 2004;77:769–789.

Chapman JR. Compliance: the patient, the doctor, and the medication. *Transplantation* 2004;77:782–785.

Field MJ, Lawrence RL, Zwanziger L, eds. *Extending Medicare coverage for preventive and other services*. Washington, DC: National Academy Press, 2000.

Gaston RS, Hudson SL, Ward M, et al. Late allograft loss: noncompliance masquerading as chronic rejection. *Transplant Proc* 1999; 31[Suppl 4A]:21S–23S.

Greenstein S, Siegal B. Evaluation of a multivariate model predicting noncompliance with medication regimens among renal transplant patients. *Transplantation* 2000;69:2226–2228.

Kalil RS, Heim-Duthoy KL, Kasiske BL. Patients with a low income have a reduced allograft survival. *Am J Kidney Dis* 1992;20: 63–69.

Markell MS, DiBenedetto A, Maursky V, et al. Unemployment in inner-city renal transplant recipients: predictive and sociodemographic factors. *Am J Kidney Dis* 1997;29:881–887.

Nevins TE, Kruse L, Skeans MA, et al. The natural history of azathioprine compliance after renal transplantation. *Kidney Int* 2001; 60:1565–1570.

Prieto LR, Miller DS, Gayowski T, et al. Multicultural issues in organ transplantation: the influence of patients' cultural perspectives on compliance with treatment. *Clin Transpl* 1997;11:529–535.

Rudman, L, Gonzales, MH, Borgida, E. Mishandling the gift of life: noncompliance in renal transplant patients. *J Appl Soc Psych* 1999; 29:4–9.

Sanders CE, Julian BA, Gaston RS, et al. Benefits of continued cyclosporine through an indigent drug program. *Am J Kidney Dis* 1996;28:572–577.

Thamer M, Henderson SC, Fox Ray N, et al. Unequal access to cadaveric transplantation in California based on insurance status. *Health Serv Res* 1999;34:879–884.

Woodward RS, Schnitzler MA, Lowell JA, et al. Effect of extended coverage of immunosuppressive medications by Medicare on the survival of cadaveric renal transplants. *Am J Transplant* 2001;1: 69–73.

Websites

**SELECTED U.S. KIDNEY TRANSPLANT-RELATED
RESOURCES, WEBSITES AND THEIR ACRONYMS**

American Association of Kidney Patients (AAKP)
  http://www.aakp.org

American Society for Histocompatibility & Immunogenetics
(ASHI)
  http://www.ashi-hla.org

American Society of Nephrology (ASN)
  http://www.asn-online.org/

American Society of Transplantation (AST)
  http://www.a-s-t.org/

American Society of Transplant Surgeons (ASTS)
  http://www.asts.org/

Association of Organ Procurement Organization (AOPO)
  http://www.aopo.org

Centerspan
  http://www.centerspan.org/

Centers for Medicare and Medicaid Services (CMS)
  http://www.hcfa.gov

Coalition on Donation
  http://www.shareyourlife.org

Division of Transplantation, U.S. Dept. of Health and Human
Services (HRSA)
  http://www.hrsa.gov/osp/dot

Health Resources and Services Administration (HRSA)
  http://hrsa.dhhs.gov

Israel Penn International Transplant Tumor Registry (IPITTR)
  http://www.ipittr.uc.edu

National Kidney Foundation (NKF)
  http://www.kidney.org

National Transplantation Pregnancy Registry
  http://www.tju.edu/ntpr

North American Pediatric Renal Transplant Cooperative Study
(NAPRTCS)
  www.spitfire.emmes.com/studt/ped

Scientific Registry of Transplant Recipients (SRTR)
  http://www.ustransplant.org

The Transplantation Society
  http://www.transplantation-soc.org/

Transplant Recipients International Organization (TRIO)
  http://www.trioweb.org

TransWeb: All About Transplantation and Donation
http://www.transweb.org/

United Network for Organ Sharing (UNOS)
http://www.unos.org/

United States Renal Data System (USRDS)
http://www.usrds.org

University Renal Research and Education Association (URREA)
http://www.urrea.org

Subject Index

Page numbers followed by f denotes figure; those followed by t denote tables.